Pheromone
Biochemistry

Pheromone Biochemistry

Edited by

Glenn D. Prestwich

Department of Chemistry
State University of New York at Stony Brook
Stony Brook, New York

Gary J. Blomquist

Department of Biochemistry
University of Nevada
Reno, Nevada

1987

ACADEMIC PRESS, INC.

Harcourt Brace Jovanovich, Publishers

Orlando   San Diego   New York   Austin
Boston   London   Sydney   Tokyo   Toronto

ACADEMIC PRESS, INC.
Orlando, Florida 32887

United Kingdom Edition published by
ACADEMIC PRESS INC. (LONDON) LTD.
24–28 Oval Road, London NW1 7DX

Library of Congress Cataloging in Publication Data

Pheromone biochemistry.

  Includes index.
    1. Insect hormones.   2. Pheromones.   I. Prestwich,
Glenn D.   II. Blomquist, Gary J.   [DNLM: 1. Biochemistry.
2. Insects.   3. Pheromones.   QP 190 P5422]
QL495.P48   1987   595.7'0142   86-30224
ISBN 0–12–564485–X (alk. paper)

To our families
Barbara, Steven, and Jocelyn
and
Cheri, Carianne, A.J., and Scotty
for their love and understanding

Contents

3.   Pheromone Biosynthesis in Lepidopterans: Desaturation and Chain Shortening

L. B. Bjostad, W. A. Wolf, and W. L. Roelofs

4.   Pheromone Biosynthesis: Enzymatic Studies in Lepidoptera

David Morse and Edward Meighen

7. Biosynthesis and Endocrine Regulation of Sex Pheromone Production in Diptera

Gary J. Blomquist, Jack W. Dillwith, and T. S. Adams

8. Alkaloid-Derived Pheromones and Sexual Selection in Lepidoptera

Thomas Eisner and Jerrold Meinwald

9. Neuroendocrine Regulation of Sex Pheromone–Mediated
    Behavior in Ixodid Ticks
    Daniel E. Sonenshine

10. Cantharidin Biosynthesis and Function in Meloid Beetles
    John P. McCormick and James E. Carrel

II. RECEPTION AND CATABOLISM OF PHEROMONES

11. Functional Morphology of Pheromone-Sensitive Sensilla
Rudolf Alexander Steinbrecht

12. The Molecular Basis of Pheromone Reception: Its Influence on Behavior
Richard G. Vogt

13. The Neurobiology of Pheromone Reception

Jacobus Jan De Kramer and Jürgen Hemberger

14. Chemical Studies of Pheromone Reception and Catabolism

Glenn D. Prestwich

15. Molecular Mechanisms of Vertebrate Olfaction: Implications for Pheromone Biochemistry

U. Pace and D. Lancet

Index

Preface

In the last three decades, chemists and biologists have developed sophisticated techniques for determining the chemical structures of pheromones, for making pure stereoisomers on a kilogram scale, for dissecting the behavioral sequences elicited by pheromones, for visualizing the ultrastructural details of receptive sensillae, and for using pheromones for mating disruption and for monitoring in integrated pest-management schemes. Several recent books have appeared highlighting these successes, yet we still find ourselves a long way from a thorough understanding of the practical use of insect sex pheromones. Until very recently there has been a paucity of biochemical studies on pheromone-relevant macromolecules which would provide a connection between small molecules and whole organisms. Specifically, we feel that much more intensive effort is required now in the basic areas of pheromone biochemistry and neurobiology to solve problems of biosynthesis, perception, transduction, and metabolism.

Current awareness of this new direction in pheromone research has resulted in at least five symposia in the last two years: two within the American Chemical Society, two in the Entomological Society of America, and one at an AAAS meeting. The latter elicited an editorial comment in *Science* [**226,** 1343 (1985)] by Philip Abelson, in which he voiced support for focusing attention on the biochemical details of how pheromones and their associated macromolecules work on a molecular level. Although "early enthusiasm about the use of pheromones to control insect populations has dwindled," there is a consensus that basic research in pheromone biosynthesis, binding, and degradation may reinvigorate optimism for the utility of pheromone analogs in pest management.

This book is designed as a sourcebook for the next decade of research, and we hope it fulfills this expectation. We have assembled contributed chapters from experts who are at the frontiers of pheromone chemistry, glandular and antennal morphology, neurobiology, and biochemistry. Although there is considerable emphasis on the Lepidoptera, this is balanced by chapters on ticks, flies, beetles, and even vertebrate olfactory biochemistry. We hope that researchers in the areas of chemistry, biochemistry, entomology, neurobiology, molecular biology, enzymology, morphology, behavior, and ecology will be able to use this volume as an entry into the literature of pheromone biochemistry.

The book is divided into two major sections. The first deals with pheromone production and its regulation in female insects, while the second covers reception, perception, and degradation of pheromones by male insects. Each author has included a review of the literature, examples of detailed practical methodology, very current and often unpublished data from their own laboratories, and a healthy amount of interpretation and speculation on how their particular subdiscipline will grow interdependently with others.

The chemicals used as sex pheromones exhibit considerable diversity, reflecting a variety of unique biochemical processes that occur in pheromone-producing tissues. The biosynthetic pathways for the pheromones from a number of species have been determined, and work is progressing toward description of the enzymes involved. From the results of studies to date, it appears that these specific and unique chemicals are produced by the addition of one or two ancillary enzymes to alter the products of ''normal'' metabolism, rather than the elaboration of an entire set of unique enzymes in the pheromone glands. Pheromone production in many species must be under endocrine regulation to optimize mating strategies. Products of the corpora allata, brain, and ovary have been implicated as agents which regulate pheromone production. The studies of the biosynthesis and regulation of pheromone production are still embryonic, and we hope that this book will stimulate further research in this area.

In many ways, insects are ideal models for determining the details of olfactory reception and transduction. They are easy to obtain in large numbers, and the collection of biosynthetic and olfactory tissues is mechanically straightforward. Most insects show strong male–female dichotomy in the production of and response to pheromone blends. The blends are simple, and single-receptor sensory cells can be located for many pheromone components. Insects grow rapidly, and the appearance of new mRNA and new proteins for pheromone biosynthesis, reception, and catabolism can be timed accurately. The olfactory organs are exterior to the organism and are readily accessible for chemical, electrical, and mechanical manipulation in experimental protocols. Olfactory mutants and a genetically diverse population of olfactory responses and olfactant proteins are readily identified and provide materials for uncovering the molecular biology of pheromone-mediated behavior. The odorants are simple lipids, often a few closely related components, rather than highly complex ''gestalt'' mixtures. Thus, highly specific, high-affinity receptor proteins are expected in contrast to the less specific, lower affinity olfactory receptors in many vertebrates. Finally, many of the target insects for olfactory studies are pests of serious agricultural or medical importance. We believe that the intellectual exercise of unraveling the olfactory mechanism is in reality a necessity for the development of the behavior-modifying agrochemicals of the future.

May 1987   Glenn D. Prestwich
                                                     Gary J. Blomquist

Acknowledgments

We owe a tremendous debt to our colleagues and co-workers for their advice and encouragement, unpublished results, and moral support during the preparation of this book. Special thanks are due to Ms. Marie Dippolito (Stony Brook) for her tireless assistance in preparing the index and coordinating the contributions of the various authors. We are grateful to the authors of the individual chapters for preparing scientifically exciting and visually stimulating contributions. Most important, we thank our mentors, postdocs, and students for making this work fun and rewarding. Financial support to us and our laboratories by the National Science Foundation, the National Institutes of Health, the United States Department of Agriculture, the Herman Frasch Foundation, the Nevada Agricultural Experiment Station (GJB), the Alfred P. Sloan Foundation (GDP), the Camille and Henry Dreyfus Foundation (GDP), Rohm and Haas Co. (GDP), and Stuart Pharmaceuticals (GDP) made the research possible and the book preparation a reality.

I

Pheromone Biosynthesis and Its Regulation

1

Relationship of Structure and Function to Biochemistry in Insect Pheromone Systems

J. H. TUMLINSON
P. E. A. TEAL
Insect Attractants, Behavior, and Basic Biology Research Laboratory
Agricultural Research Service
U.S. Department of Agriculture
Gainesville, Florida 32604

I. INTRODUCTION

Chemical cues are major sources of information used by most insects to interpret environmental stimuli. This reliance on chemical stimuli undoubtedly stems from the development of chemosensory organs and cells early in evolutionary history, perhaps even before the development of light-sensitive organs (Snodgrass, 1926). Broadly speaking, these chemical stimuli are categorized as semiochemicals. They function as pheromones when used for intraspecific communication. When used at the interspecific level, they are termed kairomones when the species responding to the chemical message benefits and allomones when the species emitting the signal gains some advantage over the receiving organism. There is considerable overlap between these classes, and often the same compounds serve both intra- and interspecific functions. Therefore, in order to elucidate the roles of individual semiochemicals it is necessary to study all aspects of the communication system from biosynthesis of the compounds to the perception and integration of the compounds by all of the organisms responding.

3

Pheromone Biochemistry

Of the three classes of semiochemicals mentioned above, pheromones are the most extensively studied. Although all insect orders use pheromones in communication, the highly social Hymenoptera and Isoptera have developed the most complex and sophisticated pheromone systems. In fact, Blum (1974) suggests a strong evolutionary relationship between the development of insect societies and diversification of pheromone communication. Among subsocial insects, pheromones have been shown to play major roles in (1) the initiation of gregarious behavior during group oviposition among certain mosquitoes (Hudson and Mclintock, 1967) and the desert locust *Schistocerca gregaria* (Forsk.) (Norris, 1963); (2) the formation of aggregations at food sites, particularly among scolytid beetles (Birch, 1984) and *Drosophila* species (Bartelt *et al.*, 1985); (3) dispersal behavior among generally gregarious species during predator attack (Nault and Phelan, 1984); (4) the synchronization of gamete maturity among species exhibiting aggregative behaviors (Blum, 1974); and (5) mate attraction among species that maintain a solitary life style.

According to Inscoe (1977), conspecific attractancy among lepidopteran species has been known since 1690, when John Ray reported several male *Biston betularia* (L.) flying around a caged female. This knowledge of the attractive capacity of female Lepidoptera also was used by such great naturalists as Fabré for collection of rare specimens; the procedure used was essentially the same as that of Ray (Kettlewell, 1946; Inscoe, 1977). The use of live females for population monitoring of the gypsy moth, *Lymantria dispar* (L.), began in 1914, but by 1920 the females had been replaced by crude abdominal tip extracts that remained active for longer periods than females (Collins and Potts, 1932). Attempts to isolate the chemical components of lepidopteran sex attractants also began in the 1920s. Unfortunately, the methods then available for chemical analysis were not adequate, requiring large sample quantities and necessitating continuous rearing of large numbers of insects. As a consequence, little headway was made. The first sex pheromone identified was that of *Bombyx mori* (L.), the silkworm moth, by Butenandt *et al.* (1959). The elucidation of bombykol [(E,Z)-10,12-hexadecadien-1-ol] required 20 years and 500,000 female abdomens.

Subsequent to the identification of "bombykol," considerable emphasis was placed on the identification of pheromone components of pest Lepidoptera, and, in 1966, (Z)-7-dodecenyl acetate was identified as the sex pheromone of the cabbage looper moth (Berger, 1966). Following this, single components of the pheromones of a number of noctuid and tortricid moths were identified. This led to the "magic bullet" theory of pheromone communication, which hypothesized that every insect species used a single compound for pheromone communication and that each species was isolated from closely related species by differences in the functionality or number and geometry of double bonds within the pheromone molecule. This hypothesis was generally accepted by many researchers working on Lepidoptera until about 1970. However, early work on bark beetles by Silverstein *et al.* (1966) in which three terpenes, (*S*)-(−)-ipsenol (**I**), (*S*)-(+)-ipsdienol (**II**), and (*S*)-(+)-*cis*-verbenol (**III**), were identified as a synergistic pheromone blend for *Ips paraconfusus* Lanier, indicated that multicomponent pheromones were used by Coleoptera. This has since been shown to be true for most insects, and now single-component pheromones are the exception rather than the rule.

I   II   III

Our knowledge of the chemistry, behavior, physiology, and biochemistry of insect communication systems has increased dramatically over the past 25 years. Early studies were aimed at two different goals. The first was development of a basic knowledge about the biological aspects of pheromone communication, as is indicated by the early work of Shorey and co-workers (e.g., Shorey, 1964; Shorey and Gaston, 1965). The second area was the identification and synthesis of pheromones based on simple bioassays. The bioassays used for these studies tended to rely on single behaviors, such as flight or clasper extension, of groups of insects and failed to monitor observations of the whole range of reproductive behaviors exhibited by individual males. Additionally, the chromatographic and spectroscopic instrumentation available in the 1960s was incapable of resolving complex isomeric mixtures or of detecting minor components present in only nanogram amounts. Thus, usually only the components present in greatest quantity were identified. This is illustrated by the identification of (Z)-7-dodecenyl acetate as the sex pheromone of the cabbage looper moth (Berger, 1966). While this compound is an effective attractant for males for this species, the insects do not exhibit the entire range of behaviors performed in response to females. It was not until 1984 that Bjostad *et al.* (1984) and Linn *et al.* (1984) accurately defined the complete pheromone blend of this insect. The additional components identified by Bjostad *et al.* (1984) are present in very small amounts and were not found until studies on biosynthesis identified the precursors of the additional components. This demonstrates the need for studies on all aspects of semiochemical-mediated biology.

The next step in the evolution of studies on pheromone communication came with the development and common use of electrophysiological techniques including the electroantennogram and single cell recording. These studies aided the identification process greatly and, in conjunction with electron microscopic studies, also formed the foundations on which our theories of pheromone perception are based. These advances coupled with tremendous improvements in analytical instrumentation (Heath and Tumlinson, 1984) and the use of flight tunnel studies (see Fig. 1, Section III) to sequentially analyze the responses of individual insects have led us to the realization that insects use complex chemical systems, rather than single unrelated signals, for communication. Frequently there is considerable overlap in signals, particularly among closely related species.

While present methods of study have been highly effective in defining the actual pheromone blends released and the behavioral roles of the chemical components, as exemplified by the work of Baker and Cardé (1979) on the oriental fruit moth, Linn *et al.* (1984) on the cabbage looper, and Teal *et al.* (1986) on the tobacco budworm moth, we have not been able as yet to completely unveil the total communication system from biosynthesis to perception and neural integration. Although initial studies on biosynthesis of pheromones were begun in the 1970s when Kasang *et al.* (1974) induced female gypsy moths to synthesize tritiated disparlure and Jones and Berger (1978) succeeded in inducing female cabbage loopers to produce ^{14}C-labeled (Z)-7-dodecenyl acetate by injecting [1-^{14}C]acetate, only limited work on pheromone anabolism and catabolism had been conducted until recently. This type of research is needed to provide the insight into the regulation of pheromone production and perception that will allow us to exploit the inherent weaknesses in the communication systems for development of more effective control strategies. The chapters that follow will present stimulating new results of molecular studies in pheromone biosynthesis, perception, and catabolism.

II. CHEMICAL STRUCTURE OF INSECT PHEROMONE SYSTEMS

A wide range of compounds have been identified as insect pheromone components. While carbon, hydrogen, and oxygen are the usual atoms incorporated into these molecules, nitrogenated and chlorinated compounds have been identified also (see Tamaki, 1985). Usually, small molecules are used for communication when rapid dispersal of the signal is needed, while larger, less volatile compounds tend to function in attraction and stimulation when prolonged exposure is necessary. The former case is exemplified by 4-methyl-3-heptanone (**IV**), used by numerous species of myrmicine ants as an alarm pheromone (Moser *et al.*, 1968; Riley *et al.*, 1974). The latter is illustrated by numerous lepidopteran sex pheromone components which are generally between 10 and 24 carbons in length [for example, the lesser peachtree borer, *Synanthedon pictipes* (Grote and Robinson), pheromone, (*E,Z*)-3,13-octadecadien-1-ol acetate (**V**)] and are much less volatile than the alarm pheromone mentioned above.

IV   **V**

In addition to the different molecular sizes, which reflect behavioral functions, pheromone structures vary greatly between different orders of insects, and even within orders tremendous diversity in molecular structure exists. Coleopteran species provide an excellent example of this, with structures varying from the terpenes used by bark beetles (Silverstein *et al.*, 1966) and the boll weevil (Tumlinson *et al.*, 1969) to the 8-methyl-2-decanol propanoates used by *Diabrotica* species (Guss *et al.*, 1982) and the lactone, (*Z*)-5-(1-decenyl)dihydro-2(3*H*)-furanone (**VI**), of the Japanese beetle (Tumlinson *et al.*, 1977). Nonetheless, generic themes of structural type exist within groups as is evidenced by the use of the same or structurally related compounds by many species of the same genus. These themes are the result of the development of common biosynthetic pathways with differences in blend ratios and components being the result of minor permutations in the enzymatic steps involved.

VI

The activity of a semiochemical is imparted by many factors including size, shape, chirality, degree of unsaturation, and the functional group of the molecule. Among many insects the position, number, and geometry of double bonds are critical for activity. Even so, structurally similar molecules may be active although at greatly reduced levels, and positional isomers often have electrophysiological activity (Priesner, 1968). For example, ''hexalure'' [(*Z*)-7-hexadecenyl acetate] is attractive to pink bollworm males but is considerably less active than the 1:1 blend of (*Z,Z*)- and (*Z,E*)-7,11-hexadecadienyl acetates, which comprise the pheromone blend (Hummel *et al.*, 1973).

Similarly, the functional group may be changed in some instances with the resulting compounds eliciting behavioral responses similar to those triggered by the actual pheromone components. Formates, for example, have been substituted for the aldehydic pheromone components of some noctuid moths (Beevor *et al.*, 1977; Mitchell *et al.*, 1975, 1978) with apparently little effect on the resulting attraction of males. In these cases, there is some specificity, however, and not all formate analogs mimic the corresponding aldehydes. Thus, (Z)-9-tetradecenyl formate (**VII**) substitutes for (Z)-11-hexadecenal (**VIII**) in *Heliothis zea* (Boddie) and *H. virescens* (F.) blends. However, when (Z)-7-dodecenyl formate was substituted for (Z)-9-tetradecenal in the *H. virescens* pheromone blend, *H. virescens* males were not attracted (Mitchell *et al.*, 1978).

Finally, some molecules differing in both the number of olefinic bonds and the functional moiety can substitute for actual pheromone components. This is demonstrated by the diolefinic hydrocarbon analog, (Z)-1,12-heptadecadiene (**IX**), of the major aldehyde component (**VIII**) of the corn earworm (Carlson and McLaughlin, 1982), which is active behaviorally even though it lacks the aldehyde functionality. However, **IX** had no effect on *H. virescens* behavior despite the fact that **VIII** is the major component of both *H. virescens* and *H. zea* pheromone blends. Similarly, Silk *et al.* (1985) showed that (E)- and (Z)-1,12-pentadecadiene, analogs of both (E)- and (Z)-11-tetradecenal, the pheromone of the spruce budworm moth, were active in behavioral experiments.

In all of the above cases the analogs have chemical structures quite similar to the pheromone components. These features show that insect communication systems are not as rigid as once thought, and it has been suggested that this fluidity might be exploited by developing active pheromone analogs that are more economical to synthesize and/or more stable, and that would therefore be of more practical value in pest management (Carlson and McLaughlin, 1982).

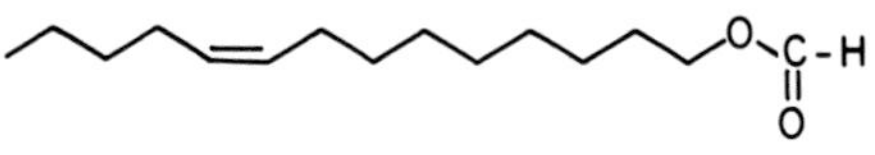

VII

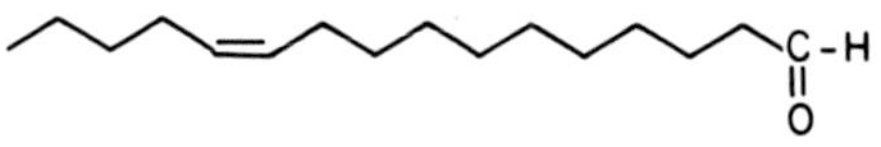

VIII

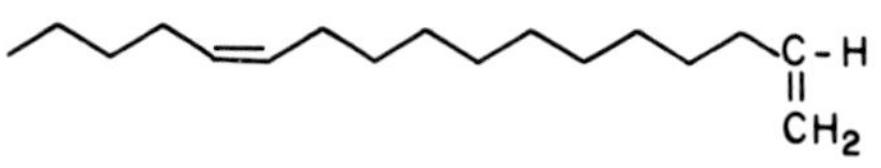

IX

While there is a degree of structural flexibility in the molecules that can be perceived by some species, particularly when the molecules are fatty acid-like, the existence of chirality in a pheromone usually imparts a much higher degree of rigidity to the system. Chirality plays a very important role in the specificity of many pheromone molecules, and often one enantiomer gives a positive biological response while the other enantiomer inhibits the behavior. For example, as little as 1% of the S-(+) enantiomer of **VI** significantly reduces the response of male Japanese beetles to their pheromone, (R)-($-$)-**VI**. The greatest number of chiral pheromones have been discovered in coleopteran species, and examples within this order serve to exemplify a number of the nine possible categories of behavioral response to enantiomers or diastereomers hypothesized by Silverstein (1979). The western corn rootworm provides an example of two of the response categories. The naturally produced pheromone of this species is (R,R)-8-methyl-2-decyl propanoate (**X**), and males are neither inhibited nor attracted to the $2R,8S$ or $2S,8S$ isomers. However, the $2S,8R$ isomer is attractive, although at a much lower level than the natural $2R,8R$ (Guss et al., 1984). A closely related species, the northern corn rootworm, is strongly inhibited by the $2S,8R$ stereoisomer but uses the $2R,8R$ for communication (Guss et al., 1985; Dobson and Teal, 1987). Thus, when an enantiomer or a single stereoisomer is used for communication, the other enantiomer or stereoisomers may elicit positive or inhibitory responses or may not elicit any response.

X

Often the communication systems and the role of chirality in these systems can be even more complicated. The pheromone systems of the various strains of *Ips pini* (Say) serve as a good example. Initially, the pheromone of *I. pini* in California was identified as (R)-($-$)-ipsdienol [the R-($-$) enantiomer of **II**]. As little as 3% of the S-(+) enantiomer, a component of the pheromone of the competitive *I. paraconfusus*, completely interrupted the *I. pini* response to the R-($-$) (Birch et al., 1980a). However, *I. pini* in New York produces a 65:35 ratio of (+):($-$) ipsdienol and responds more strongly in the field to synthetic racemic ipsdienol (Lanier et al., 1980). A survey of the literature on *Ips* pheromones indicates that the species in this genus use varying combinations of components and chiralities to achieve the necessary pheromone specificity. The stereospecificity of pheromone biosynthesis in this beetle is summarized by Vanderwel and Oehlschlager (Chapter 6, this volume).

Blends and the regulation of blends also are critical factors in determining pheromone specificity and are, therefore, two of the most important aspects of pheromone biosynthesis. As indicated earlier, the first multicomponent pheromone identified was that used by *Ips paraconfusus*, composed of (S)-($-$)-

ipsenol (**I**), (*S*)-(+)-ipsdienol (**II**), and (*S*)-(−)-*cis*-verbenol (**III**) (Silverstein *et al.*, 1966). These compounds were found to be synergistic in that little or no attraction occurred when the individual components were tested, but the combination of the three was highly attractive. Similar cases have been documented for many species, particularly among the Lepidoptera. For example, both (Z)-9-tetradecenal and (Z)-11-hexadecenal act in concert to induce upwind flight by males of *H. virescens,* but neither component shows significant activity when released alone (Vetter and Baker, 1983). Another interesting feature of pheromone blends is that in many instances the individual components function in concert to maximize each sequential step in the behavioral sequence. Thus, rather than each component being responsible for the elicitation of a single behavior, the essence of the whole blend is required for maximizing the behavioral sequence. This is exemplified by studies conducted by Baker and Cardé (1979) on the oriental fruit moth, Linn *et al.,* (1984) on the cabbage looper, and Teal *et al.* (1986) on the tobacco budworm moth.

Within closely related taxa variations in blends, or ratios of components in blends, play critical roles in affecting species specificity. Interestingly, differences in these blends reflect very minor differences in the basic biosynthetic processes that produce the components but have major ramifications with regard to the behaviors elicited by the species involved. Mechanisms by which multicomponent pheromones can increase reproductive isolation are many and include (1) the release of a component having no effect on conspecifics but an inhibitory effect on males of another species, (2) the addition of components necessary for reproductive behaviors among conspecific males and which are inhibitory to males of other species, and (3) differences in the component ratios among species using the same chemicals.

Although cases are few in which a component is produced solely for the purpose of decreasing the reproductive responses of males of other species, such a case is indicated between the gypsy moth, *Lymantria dispar,* and the nun moth, *L. monacha* (L.). The sex pheromone of the gypsy moth was identified as (Z)-7,8-epoxy-2-methyloctadecane (disparlure, **XI**) by Bierl *et al.* (1970). Studies using the (+) and (−) enantiomers and the racemic mixture have indicated that males respond only to the (+) enantiomer and are inhibited by very small amounts of (−)-disparlure (Cardé *et al.,* 1977b; Miller *et al.,* 1977; Miller and Roelofs, 1978). Male gypsy moths have two antennal neurons that respond to the pheromone. However, one neuron responds solely to the (+) enantiomer, while the other cell responds only to (−)-disparlure (Hansen, 1984). The nun moth also is attracted to (+)-disparlure, but studies have indicated that the (−) enantiomer has no effect on the attraction of this moth (Klimetzek *et al.,* 1976; Vite *et al.,* 1976). However, Hansen (1984) reported that extracts of nun moth pheromone glands elicited responses from both receptor cells in gypsy moth male antenna and produced evidence to indicate that the nun moth females produce a 90 : 10

blend of (−)- and (+)-disparlure. Therefore, reproductive isolation between gypsy moth males and nun moth females appears to result from the release by the latter species of a compound that is not perceived by conspecific males.

7S, 8R (−)   7R, 8S (+)

XI

The addition of a compound or compounds required for upwind anemotaxis and/or courtship by conspecific males, and which are inhibitory to males of other species, is particularly evident among the tortricids. For example, the two closely related, co-occurring species, *Argyrotaenia velutinana* (Walker) and *Choristoneura rosaceana* (Harris), both use a 9:1 ratio of (Z)- to (E)-11-tetradecenyl acetate in their pheromone blends, but in addition to these *A. velutinana* also produces dodecyl acetate (Cardé *et al.*, 1977a). The addition of the dodecyl acetate increases conspecific male atraction and effectively inhibits the response of male *C. rosaceana* (Roelofs and Cardé, 1974). Similarly, in the communications systems of *I. pini* and *I. paraconfusus*, which are competing species, the pheromone of each functions as an allomone for the other by interrupting response to conspecific semiochemicals (Birch *et al.*, 1977, 1980a,b; Light and Birch, 1979).

The function of differences in pheromone blend ratios in reproductive isolation is also evident among the Tortricidae. Cardé *et al.* (1977a) have shown it to effect the isolation of two species, *Archips argyrospilus* (Walker) and *A. mortuanus* Kearfott, which share four components. Unfortunately, little work has been done on the roles of such ratios, on individual components therein, or on the behavioral steps leading to mating, so that it is unknown if each component performs the same role in each species.

As we have indicated, there is much interspecific communication with pheromones, particularly among closely related species. There is another type of interspecific communication in which a pheromone may function in another capacity. For example, components of the sex pheromone of *H. zea* also act as kairomones that increase searching efficiency of the egg parasite *Trichogramma pretiosum* (Riley) (Lewis *et al.*, 1982). Similarly, parasites, for example, *Tomicobia tibialis* Ashmead (Rice, 1969), and predators, including *Temnochila chlorodia* (Mannerheim) (Bedard *et al.*, 1969, 1980), both respond to pheromones released by their beetle hosts, *I. paraconfusus* and *Dendroctonus brevicomis* LeConte, respectively.

Another complicating factor, largely unexplored, is the interaction between

pheromones and host-produced kairomones in chemical communication systems. For example, the aggregation pheromone of the bark beetle, *D. brevicomis,* consists of frontalin produced by males and *exo*-brevicomin released by females. These two components, however, are synergized by myrcene released by the tree under attack (Birch, 1984). Another synergistic kairomone–pheromone system has been documented for aggregations of Japanese beetles (Klein *et al.,* 1973, 1980). In this case, the sex pheromone produced by females is synergized by eugenol and phenylethyl propionate, which are found in several host plants of the Japanese beetles. Both males and females are attracted to the combined lure in much greater numbers than to either the pheromone or the plant attractant alone. These cases exemplify complexities inherent to semiochemical communication systems and serve to illustrate the major importance of chemical stimuli for the insect.

III. BEHAVIORAL AND PHYSIOLOGICAL RESPONSES OF INSECTS TO PHEROMONES

The bioassay is critical in determining the identity of compounds involved in semiochemical communication. More often than not, the design of the bioassay effectively determines the compounds that will be identified as pheromone components. For example, the use of activation bioassays like that described by Gaston and Shorey (1964) has often led to the identification of only the major components in a pheromone blend, which may have only limited or no activity in the field.

The many difficulties encountered in the development of effective bioassays all relate to the basic semiochemical-mediated behavior of the species in question. Therefore, it is crucial that the whole behavioral sequence involved in communication between the insects be critically evaluated prior to analysis of the behavioral effects of the semiochemicals alone. This behavioral analysis is extremely complicated and is often hampered by variation in environmental parameters such as temperature and humidity. Thus, analysis of semiochemically mediated behavior is often best accomplished in laboratory flight tunnel studies (Fig. 1) (Baker and Linn, 1984). Such assays allow for variations in single parameters such as blend ratios, concentrations, and wind speed while maintaining other factors constant. Thus, single effects can be analyzed, and pheromone components and the roles played by the components in chemically mediated behavior can be identified. The final test, however, is observation under field conditions because of the complex environmental factors that must interact with and modify the effect of the blend in the natural environment (Cardé and Elkington, 1984).

Electrophysiological studies are of considerable value in determining the abil-

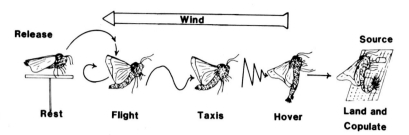

Fig. 1. Typical responses of male noctuid moths to the sex pheromone released by female moths.

ity of an insect to perceive semiochemicals. The electroantennogram (EAG) is widely used in isolation and identification studies because of the ease of operation and because a large number of candidate compounds can be screened with this method (Roelofs, 1984). This technique has even been interfaced to capillary gas chromatographs for use as a highly sensitive detector (Struble and Arn, 1984). The EAG indicates only that a compound stimulates receptor cells, however, and does not give information regarding the behavioral response to the compound. Therefore, compounds such as (Z)-11-hexadecen-1-ol, which was identified in pheromone gland extracts of the corn earworm, give significant EAG recordings, but the compound is a potent inhibitor to male behavior when used in pheromone traps (Teal *et al.*, 1984). Furthermore, behaviorally inactive compounds like positional or geometrical isomers often give significant EAG responses (Roelofs, 1984).

Single-cell electrophysiological recordings are much more selective in their responses. These studies involve monitoring responses of single receptor cells within the antennae and, more recently, the responses of neurons within the antennal lobe of the brain. A number of studies have suggested that the sensillar cells that respond to pheromone components, the so-called specialists, have binding macromolecules specific for pheromone molecules (Kaissling, 1979; Priesner, 1979; Mustaparta, 1979; Mayer and Mankin, 1985). Evidence presented by Mayer and Mankin (1985) on the cabbage looper moth suggests that an across-fiber response pattern of the different types of receptor cells within the antenna which respond to pheromone molecules sets up the coding necessary to elicit a behavioral response. Studies also have demonstrated that the responses to two components of a pheromone can be synergistic when the compounds are mixed together (O'Connell, 1972, O'Connell *et al.*, 1986). Therefore, it appears that the first step in pheromonal discrimination occurs in the peripheral nervous system. Studies like that reported by the Matsumoto and Hildebrand (1981) on the tobacco hornworm, *Manduca sexta* (L.), in which pheromone-responsive neurons in the brain cells were stained, have shown that pheromone-specific

neurons are present only in the brains of the responding sex. Therefore, although the behavioral response by females to an oviposition site and males to a sexually receptive female may be identical (Schneiderman et al., 1986), only males respond to the sex pheromone because of the presence of sex-specific receptors in the antenna and neurons in the brain. Studies of these types are critical for developing an understanding of the mechanisms of perception and central nervous system processing of pheromone-mediated events.

Recently, several groups have developed novel methods for probing the mechanisms involved in physiological and behavioral response to pheromones. Schneiderman et al. (1982) successfully grafted the antennal imaginal discs of fifth-instar male tobacco hornworm moths into female larvae and showed that a macroglomerular complex normally found only in the antennal lobes in the brain of an adult male developed in these gynandromorphic females during metamorphic adult development. Furthermore, neurons in these macroglomerular complexes responded when pheromone-sensitive neurons in the transplanted antenna were stimulated with the female sex pheromone. Subsequent studies have indicated that the gynandromorphic females responded to the female-produced sex pheromone in a flight tunnel with the same behavioral pattern shown by normal males (Schneiderman et al., 1986). Studies of this nature have demonstrated sex-specific pathways in the central nervous system which are important in understanding the male responses of insects to pheromones.

Another technique used to probe the mechanism of response to pheromones is the analysis of an insect's behavior after it is treated with sublethal amounts of neurotoxins. Studies with male oriental fruit moths have established that topical application of sublethal amounts of a number of neuroactive compounds results in changes in specific behaviors associated with male response to pheromones and that a dose–response curve can be established for each neuroactive compound (Linn and Roelofs, 1984). For example, exposure to permethrin caused a significant reduction in the number of males that entered taxis, while chlordimeform affected all of the response categories with hairpencil display being reduced to the greatest extent. Linn and Roelofs (1984) also studied the effect of dual treatment with antagonistic compounds like octopamine and yohimbine and found that normal response was restored in these cases. These studies have demonstrated that the neurotoxins do not affect peripheral reception but rather seem to affect perception by the central nervous system and the motor responses regulated by the central nervous system.

Studies in one of our laboratories (P. E. A. Teal, unpublished) support the idea that the ability to respond to pheromone is not hindered by exposure to some neurotoxins. In our experiments, we loaded rubber septum lures with both 2 mg of (±)-disparlure, the pheromone of the gypsy moth, and up to 20 mg of either fluvalinate or dichlorvos. Both field trapping and flight tunnel studies indicated

no differences in taxis or landing of male gypsy moths between pheromone–pesticide lures and the pheromone lures alone, although all males tested in the flight tunnel died within 24 hr after contacting the pesticide lure (Teal, 1986). If the effect of these pesticides were to cause dysfunction of the receptor neurons immediately on contact, then even small numbers of pesticide molecules encountered by the antennae in the pheromone plume would have disrupted behavior and certainly would have caused differences after males contacted the lure. However, the number of moths reorienting to the lures and subsequently landing a second time was no different for lures containing pesticide plus pheromone or pheromone alone. While the results of our flight tunnel study are preliminary they do support the hypothesis expressed by Linn and Roelofs (1984) that neuroactive substances function on the central rather than peripheral nervous systems.

Still other studies are being conducted using inhibitors for sensory disruption. Compounds that are structural analogs of pheromone molecules can be used to block pheromone receptors (Prestwich, Chapter 14, this volume). For example, the acyl fluoride mimic of (Z)-9-tetradecenal has been shown to change dramatically the response of tobacco budworm moths to their pheromone. These studies will facilitate the development of an understanding of the role of macromolecular pheromone receptors in semiochemical-medicated communication.

IV. BIOCHEMISTRY OF PHEROMONE SYSTEMS

While research in the areas of pheromone isolation and identification and the behavioral aspects of pheromone communication has been extensive over the past 25 years, studies on pheromone biosynthesis and the biochemistry associated with pheromone perception are relatively new. The biochemical investigations build on and complement work in the areas of pheromone identification and behavioral analysis, and they are thus important in accurately defining pheromone communication systems.

Pheromone biosynthesis determines the compounds that will be produced and emitted as pheromones and also establishes the ratio of components in the blend that is released. This is demonstrated by the pheromone blends used for communication by members of the *Spodoptera* genus of noctuid moths. The southern armyworm, *S. eridania* (Cramer), uses a series of four mono- and diunsaturated 14-carbon acetates and a monounsaturated 16-carbon acetate for communication (Teal *et al.*, 1985). Beet armyworm moths, *S. exigua* (Hübner), do not respond to this blend of acetates in the field (Teal *et al.*, 1985) but are attracted when (Z)-9-tetradecenol, a major component of its pheromone (Tumlinson *et al.*, 1981), is included in the blend. Interestingly, this alcohol is present in pheromone gland extracts of the southern armyworm but is not released, suggesting a close biosynthetic relationship between alcohols and acetates among members of this genus.

Gene expression is ultimately responsible for establishing pheromone communication systems. While the majority of species produce and respond to a reasonably constant blend of pheromone components, there are examples where isolated subgroups of a species have modified the biosynthetic pathways and produce altered blends. Miller and Roelofs (1980) have demonstrated that a laboratory strain of the redbanded leafroller moth has a significantly lower proportion of (E)-11-tetradecenyl acetate than does the feral population in New York. While this situation is artificial and may reflect selective pressures due to laboratory rearing, cases have been documented in which feral populations produce and respond to different blends. For example, two pheromone races of the European corn borer, *Ostrinia nubilalis* (Hübner), exist in North America, having been imported from different areas of Europe. The pheromone used by this species is a blend of (E)- and (Z)-11-tetradecenyl acetates, but apparently during a period of geographic isolation two pheromonally distinct races of moths evolved. One strain uses a $96:4$ $E:Z$ blend while the other responds to a $3:97$ $E:Z$ ratio of the acetates (Klun *et al.*, 1973; Kochansky *et al.*, 1975). In areas of North America where the two races exist in sympatry, evidence indicates that males respond preferentially to the pheromone of their own race and that the races are not interbreeding freely (Cardé *et al.*, 1978). Studies by Klun and Maini (1979) on hybrid and backcross individuals of the two strains have indicated that both pheromone blend production and perception are controlled by the simple autosomal inheritance of a single pair of alleles. However, the F_1 hybrids of both parental crosses contained a $65:35$ $E:Z$ ratio of the acetates rather than the expected $1:1$ blend. Klun and Maini (1979) explain the disparate ratio in terms of incomplete dominance by the allele governing the E isomer of the acetate.

A similar case has been documented for eastern and western strains of *I. pini*. In this case, the western population produces and responds preferentially to $(-)$-ipsdienol while the eastern race uses a $65:35$ blend of both enantiomers (Lanier *et al.*, 1980). Both races preferentially respond to their own pheromone (Lanier *et al.*, 1972), and hybrids of the two populations respond maximally to the hybrid pheromone blend (Lanier *et al.*, 1980). As in the case of the European corn borer, the genetics of both pheromone production and attraction are governed by autosomal genes.

Studies on pheromone biosynthesis are useful in defining the pheromone blends produced by insects and in establishing the biosynthetic mechanisms responsible for maintaining pheromonally regulated reproductive isolation. Furthermore, by comparing the biosynthetic pathways used by males and females for pheromone production we can obtain valuable information regarding the molecular genetics of pheromone production. Recent studies conducted in our laboratory on the terminal steps in pheromone biosynthesis in both males and females of a number of species of *Heliothis* moths serve to illustrate these features. Females of *H. virescens* release a volatile sex pheromone blend composed of tetradecanal, (Z)-9-tetradecenal, hexadecanal, and (Z)-7-, (Z)-9-, and (Z)-11-hexadecenals (Pope *et al.*, 1982; Teal *et al.*, 1986), but the corresponding alcohols are also present in the pheromone gland in approximately the same ratio as the aldehydes (Teal *et al.*, 1986). The major alcohol component, (Z)-11-hexadecen-1-ol, has no apparent effect on males of this species (Vetter and Baker, 1983), and while it is present in the pheromone glands of two other species, *H. subflexa* (Teal *et al.*, 1981; Klun *et al.*, 1982) and *H. zea* (Teal *et al.*, 1984), inclusion of it in pheromone lures of these species results in decreased capture of males.

In vivo application of hexadecan-1-ol and other primary alcohols to the surface of the pheromone gland of *H. virescens* indicated that the alcohols were rapidly converted to the corresponding aldehydes (Fig. 2). Secondary alcohols were not converted to the corresponding ketones. Conversion of the alcohols to aldehydes was inhibited when preparations were treated with the primary alcohol substrates under nitrogen. However, the conversion proceeded when air was substituted for N_2 after 15 min (Teal and Tumlinson, 1986). These results demonstrated that the enzyme responsible for the alcohol to aldehyde conversion was an alcohol oxidase specific for primary alcohols. Further, the production of a $1:3.5$ ratio of (Z)-9-tetradecenal : hexadecanal when a $1:3$ ratio of the corresponding alcohols were applied, coupled with the similar ratios of alcohol precursors and aldehyde pheromone components found in gland extracts (Teal *et al.*, 1986), demonstrated that substrate-level competition for the enzyme by the alcohol precursors regulates the blend of aldehydes produced as pheromone components. A similar biosynthetic system which utilizes an alcohol oxidase has been identified for the spruce budworm moth (Morse and Meighen, 1984, 1986 and Chapter 4, this volume), and suggests that oxidases may be common among Lepidoptera species that produce aldehyde pheromone components.

Subsequent studies (Teal and Tumlinson, 1987) established that the conversion of the alcohols to aldehydes occurred within and on the surface of the cuticle overlying the sex pheromone gland while the alcohols were present in the gland cells alone. This is the first instance in which the insect cuticle has been demonstrated to contain enzymes involved in pheromone biosynthesis and supports Percy-Cunningham's hypothesis that the cuticle is an integral part of the sex pheromone gland (see Percy-Cunningham and MacDonald, Chapter 2, this volume). Studies on both *H. zea* and *H. subflexa* have shown that a similar enzymatic conversion occurs in aldehyde production by these species (Teal and Tumlinson, 1986, 1987). In fact, in the laboratory we have overcome pheromone-mediated reproductive isolation between *H. zea* and *H. virescens* by

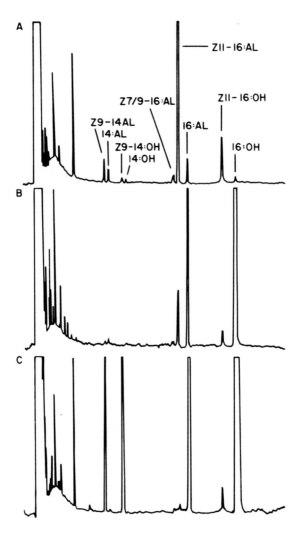

Fig. 2. Chromatograms of gland extracts of *Heliothis virescens* on a 30 m × 0.25 mm fused silica capillary column coated with methyl silicone. (A) Extract of untreated gland. (B) Extract of gland treated with 1 μg of 16:OH in DMSO. (C) Extract of gland treated with a 3:1 ratio of 16:OH and Z9-14:OH.

inducing *H. zea* females to produce the same blend used by *H. virescens*. Appropriate amounts of the two 14-carbon alcohols that correspond to the aldehydes lacking from the *H. zea* blend were applied to the pheromone gland of *H. zea* females (Teal and Tumlinson, 1986). Female *H. zea* treated in this manner were attractive to *H. virescens* males, and repeated interspecific copulation attempts were recorded in laboratory flight tunnel studies.

The sex pheromone used by *H. subflexa* differs from the above species in that, in addition to the alcohols and aldehydes, the sex pheromone gland also contains the corresponding acetates in a ratio that approximates that of the aldehydes (Teal *et al.*, 1981; Klun *et al.*, 1982). The acetates are important for maximizing the behavioral response of males to pheromone lures, and as such we anticipated that the alcohols were precursors of both the acetate and aldehyde components. However, *in vivo* application studies showed that the acetate was, in fact, the precursor of the alcohol that was then rapidly converted to the aldehyde. Our present hypothesis is that the major portion of the acetate is converted to the analogous alcohol within the pheromone gland cells and that both the acetate and the alcohol are secreted into the cuticle. Thus, the pheromone released from the surface is composed of acetates and aldehydes. Strangely, the pheromone gland of *H. virescens* females also contains enzymes capable of converting acetates to the corresponding alcohols (Ding and Prestwich, 1986; Teal and Tumlinson, 1987) even though no acetates are present in the gland of this species. The presence of this enzyme in the *H. virescens* pheromone gland shows the close phylogenetic relationship between *H. subflexa* and *H. virescens*.

The similarities in pheromone biosynthesis between *H. virescens* and *H. sub-flexa* become clearer when considering the pheromone blend produced by the hairpencil glands of males of *H. virescens* and the biosynthesis of these components. Recently we undertook a detailed study on the chemistry and biology of the pheromone components produced by the male hairpencil glands. Gas chromatographic (GC) and GC–mass spectral analysis of extracts of the whole gland complex or the hairpencil scales alone obtained from individual males indicated that the compounds present in greatest amount were hexadecyl acetate (212.4 ng/♂), hexadecen-1-ol (27.3 ng/♂), and hexadecenoic acid (22.2 ng/♂). In addition, each male equivalent of these samples contained an average of 14.2 ng of octadecyl acetate and 7.5 and 6.3 ng of the corresponding alcohol and acid, respectively. Gas chromatographic analysis of these extracts on both polar and apolar capillary columns also revealed the presence of a number of other compounds as indicated in Table I. However, adequate mass spectra have not been obtained to confirm the identities of these compounds (Teal and Tumlinson, 1987).

Assuming that our assignments for all of these components are correct, then, in addition to the 18-carbon compounds, acetates corresponding to all of the aldehydic pheromone components released by females of *H. virescens* are present in the hairpencil pheromone produced by males. However, as indicated in Table I, the acetates were always present in much greater amounts than either the corresponding acids or alcohols, and the saturated compounds were present in much greater concentration than the monounsaturates of equal chain length. The latter feature suggests that although both sexes of *H. virescens* possess enzymes involved in desaturation (see Bjostad and Roelofs, 1983), the activities of these enzymes are regulated differently by each sex. Topical application studies indi-

TABLE I

**Compounds Present in Hairpencil Gland Extracts of
Males of *H. virescens* based on Gas Chromatographic
Analysis ($n = 20$)**

Compound	Mean amount (ng)	SD	Mean percentage
14 : OH	0.35	0.22	0.118
14 : Ac	1.2	0.92	0.405
Z9-14 : Ac	0.19	0.09	0.064
14 : Acid	2.7	2.1	0.91
16 : OH	27.3	15.6	9.2
Z11-16 : OH	0.27	0.25	0.09
16 : Ac	212.4	78.4	71.665
Z7-16 : Ac	0.52	0.40	0.175
Z9-16 : Ac	0.18	0.15	0.061
Z11-16 : Ac	3.5	1.0	1.181
16 : Acid	22.2	7.3	7.490
18 : OH	7.5	3.6	2.531
18 : Ac	14.2	2.2	4.791
18 : Acid	6.3	1.15	2.126

cated that the acetates are the immediate precursors of the alcohol components. Esterases capable of the same conversion of acetates to alcohols play an integral role in pheromone biosynthesis by females of *H. subflexa* (Teal and Tumlinson, 1987) and, as indicated above, are also present in the pheromone gland of females of *H. virescens*. The presence of the corresponding acids as volatile components is somewhat of an enigma. However, conversion of the alcohol to the aldehyde with immediate and complete conversion to the acid (Ding and Prestwich, 1986) might explain both the presence of the acids and absence of the aldehydes.

Thus, within the members of the genus *Heliothis* we see a common biosynthetic theme of pheromone production. Variations on the theme that result in the production of specific blends can be attributed to the evolution of genes responsible for the production of specific enzymes and to genetically controlled specific enzyme activities.

As indicated earlier, a complete understanding of semiochemically mediated communication systems should lead to development of more effective methods of pest management using pheromones. Continued studies on the actual blends of components released by calling insects will allow the development of lures that are fully competitive with females, thereby increasing the effectiveness of mating disruption programs. Similarly, studies on the use of inhibitors may lead to control techniques based on inhibiting responses to pheromones. Finally, knowledge of the biochemistry and enzyme systems involved in pheromone biosynthesis may lead to the development of control programs based on enzyme or hormone inhibition or may allow for the development of control programs based on genetically altered insects. Thus, while studies on the biosynthesis and catabolism of pheromones are just beginning, the field promises to be one of the most exciting areas of study for the future from both the purely scientific and practical standpoints.

Knowledge of the biochemistry of putative pheromone receptor proteins and the associated neurophysiological responses is limited, and it is important that we increase our knowledge in this area. This will lead to the elucidation of the mechanisms of perception and central nervous system processing that could lead ultimately to the development of new methods of insect control. These subjects are covered in detail by Prestwich (Chapter 14, this volume) and by Vogt (Chapter 12). It would not be surprising to find that a close link between pheromone biosynthesis and catabolism exists.

REFERENCES

Baker, T. C., and Cardé, R. T. (1979). Analysis of pheromone-mediated behavior in male *Grapholitha molesta,* the oriental fruit moth (Lepidoptera: Tortricidae). *Environ. Entomol.* **8,** 956–968.

Baker, T. C., and Linn, C. E. (1984). Wind tunnels in pheromone research. *In* "Techniques in Pheromone Research" (H. E. Hummel and T. A. Miller, eds.), pp. 75–110. Springer-Verlag, New York.

Bartelt, R. J., Jackson, L. L., and Schaner, A. M. (1985). Ester components of aggregation pheromone of *Drosophila virilis* (Diptera: Drosophilidae). *J. Chem. Ecol.* **11,** 1197–1208.

Bedard, W. D., Tilden, P. E., Wood, D. L., Silverstein, R. M., Brownlee, R. G., and Rodin, J. O. (1969). Western pine beetle: Field response to its sex pheromone and synergistic host terpene myrcene. *Science* **164,** 1284–1285.

Bedard, W. D., Wood, D. L., Tilden, P. E., Lindahl, K. O., Jr., Silverstein, R. M., and Rodin, J. O. (1980). Field responses of the western pine beetle and one of its predators to host- and beetle-produced compounds. *J. Chem. Ecol.* **6,** 625–641.

Beevor, P. S., Hall, D. R., Nesbitt, B. F., Dyck, V. A., Arida, G., Lippold, P. C., and Oloumi-Sadeghi, H. (1977). Field trials of synthetic sex pheromones of the striped rice borer, *Chilo suppressalis* (Walker) (Lepidoptera: Pyralidae), and of related compounds. *Bull. Entomol. Res.* **67,** 439.

Berger, R. S. (1966). Isolation, identification and synthesis of sex attractant of the cabbage looper, *Trichoplusia ni. Ann. Entomol. Soc. Am.* **59,** 767–771.

Bierl, B. A., Beroza, M., and Collier, C. W. (1970). Potent sex attractant of the gypsy moth: Its isolation, identification and synthesis. *Science* **170,** 87–89.

Birch, M. S. (1984). Aggregation in bark beetles. *In* "Chemical Ecology of Insects" (W. J. Bell and R. T. Cardé, eds.), pp. 331–343. Sinauer Associates, Sunderland, Massachusetts.

Birch, M. C., Light, D. M., and Mori, K. (1977). Selective inhibition of response of *Ips pini* to its pheromone by the (*S*)-(−)-enantiomer of ipsenol. *Nature (London)* **270,** 738–739.

Birch, M. C., Light, D. M., Wood, D. L., Browne, L. E., Silverstein, R. M., Bergot, B. J., Onloff,

G., West, J. R., and Young, J. C. (1980a). Pheromonal attraction and allomonal interruption of *Ips pini* in California by the two enantiomers of ipsdienol. *J. Chem. Ecol.* **6**, 703–717.

Birch, M. C., Suihra, P., Paine, T. D., and Miller, J. C. (1980b). Influence of chemically mediated behavior on host tree colonization by four cohabitating species of bark beetles. *J. Chem. Ecol.* **6**, 395–414.

Bjostad, L. B., and Roelofs, W. L. (1983). Sex pheromone biosynthesis in *Trichoplusia ni:* key steps involve Δ^{11} desaturation and chain shortening. *Science* **220**, 1387–1389.

Bjostad, L. B., Linn, C. E., Du, J. W., and Roelofs, W. L. (1984). Identification of new sex pheromone components in *Trichoplusia ni* predicted from biosynthetic precursors. *J. Chem. Ecol.* **10**, 1309–1323.

Blum, M. S. (1974). Pheromonal sociality in the Hymenoptera. In "Pheromones" (M. C. Birch, ed.), pp. 224–229. North Holland Biomedical Press, Amsterdam.

Butenandt, A., Beckmann, R., Stamm, D., and Hecker, E. (1959). Über den Sexual-Lockstoff des Seidenspinners *Bombyx mori*. Reindarstellung und Konstitution. *Z. Naturforsch.* **14**, 283–284.

Cardé, R. T., and Elkington, J. S. (1984). Field trapping with attractants: methods and interpretation. In "Techniques in Pheromone Research" (H. E. Hummel and T. A. Miller, eds.), pp. 111–129. Springer-Verlag, New York.

Cardé, R. T., Cardé, A. M., Hill, A. S., and Roelofs, W. L. (1977a). Sex pheromone specificity as a reproductive isolating mechanism among the sibling species *Archips argyrospilus* and *A. mortuanus* and other sympatric tortricine moths (Lepidoptera: Tortricidae). *J. Chem. Ecol.* **3**, 71–84.

Cardé, R. T., Doane, C. C., Baker, T. C., Iwaki, S., and Murumo, S. (1977b). Attraction of optically active pheromone for male gypsy moths. *Environ. Entomol.* **6**, 768–772.

Cardé, R. T., Roelofs, W. L., Harrison, R. G., Vawter, A. T., Brussard, P. E., Mutuura, A., and Monroe, E. (1978). European corn borer: Pheromone polymorphism or sibling species. *Science* **199**, 555–556.

Carlson, D. A., and McLaughlin, J. R. (1982). Diolefin analog of a sex pheromone component of *Heliothis zea* active in disrupting mating communication. *Experientia* **38**, 309–310.

Collins, C. W., and Potts, S. F. (1932). Attractants for flying gypsy moths as an aid in locating new infestations. *U.S. Dept. Agric. Tech. Bull.* **336**, 1–43.

Ding, Y. S., and Prestwich, G. D. (1986). Metabolic transformations of tritium-labeled pheromone by tissues of *Heliothis virescens* moths. *J. Chem. Ecol.* **12**, 411–429.

Dobson, I. D., and Teal, P. E. A. (1987). Analysis of the long range reproductive behavior of male *Diabrotica virgifera virgifera* LeConte and *D. barberi* Smith and Lawrence to stereoisomers of 8-methyl-2-decyl propanoate under laboratory conditions. *J. Chem. Ecol.* **13**, 1331–1341.

Gaston, L. K., and Shorey, H. H. (1964). Sex pheromones of noctuid moths: IV. An apparatus for bioassaying the pheromones of six species. *Ann. Entomol. Soc. Am.* **67**, 779–780.

Guss, P. L., Tumlinson, J. H., Sonnet, P. E., and Proveaux, A. T. (1982). Identification of a female-produced sex pheromone of the western corn rootworm. *J. Chem. Ecol.* **8**, 545–556.

Guss, P. L., Sonnet, P. E., Carney, R. L., Branson, T. F., and Tumlinson, J. H. (1984). Response of *Diabrotica virgifera virgifera, D. v. zea,* and *D. porracea* to stereoisomers of 8-methyl-2-decyl propanoate. *J. Chem. Ecol.* **10**, 1123–1121.

Guss, P. L., Sonnet, P. E., Carney, R. L., Tumlinson, J. H., and Wilkin, P. J. (1985). Response of northern corn rootworm, *Diabrotica barberi* Smith and Lawrence, to stereoisomers of 8-methyl-2-decyl propanoate. *J. Chem. Ecol.* **11**, 21–26.

Hansen, K. (1984). Discrimination and production of disparlure enantiomers by the gypsy moth and nun moth. *Physiol. Entomol.* **9**, 9–18.

Heath, R. R., and Tumlinson, J. H. (1984). Techniques for purifying, analyzing and identifying pheromones. In "Techniques in Pheromone Research" (H. E. Hummel and T. A. Miller, eds.), pp. 287–332. Springer-Verlag, New York.

Hudson, A., and Mclintock, J. (1967). A chemical factor that stimulates oviposition by *Culex tarsalis* Coquillet (Diptera: Culicidae). *An. Behav.* **15**, 336–343.

Hummel, H. E., Gaston, L. K., Shorey, H. H., Kaae, R. S., Byrne, K. J., and Silverstein, R. M. (1973). Clarification of the chemical status of the pink bollworm sex pheromone. *Science* **181**, 873–875.

Inscoe, M. (1977). Chemical communication in insects. *J. Wash. Acad.* **67**, 16–33.

Jones, I. F., and Berger, R. S. (1978). Incorporation of [1-^{14}C]acetate into *cis*-7-dodecen-1-ol acetate, a sex pheromone in the cabbage looper (*Trichoplusia ni*). *Environ. Entomol.* **7**, 666–669.

Kaissling, K. E. (1979). Recognition of pheromones by moths, especially in Saturniids and *Bombyx mori*. *In* "Chemical Ecology: Odor Communication in Animals" (F. J. Ritter, ed.), pp. 43–56. Elsevier/North Holland, Amsterdam.

Kasang, G., Knauer, B., and Beroza, M. (1974). Uptake of the sex attractant [^{3}H]disparlure by male gypsy moth antennae (*Lymantria dispar*) (=*Porthetria dispar*). *Experientia* **30**, 147–148.

Kettlewell, H. B. D. (1946). Female assembling scents with reference to an important paper on the subject. *Entomologist* **79**, 8–14.

Klein, M. G., Ladd, T. L., and Lawrence, K. O. (1973). Simultaneous exposure of phenethyl propionate–eugenol (7 : 3) and virgin female Japanese beetles as a lure. *J. Econ. Entomol.* **66**, 373–374.

Klein, M. G., Tumlinson, J. H., Ladd, T. L., Jr., and Doolittle, R. E. (1980). Japanese beetle (Coleoptera: Scarabaeidae): Response to synthetic sex attractant plus phenethyl propionate : eugenol. *J. Chem. Ecol.* **7**, 1–7.

Klimetzek, D., Loskant, G., Vite, J. P., and Mori, K. (1976). Disparlure. Differences in pheromone perception between gypsy moth and nun moth. *Naturwissenschaften* **63**, 581.

Klun, J. A., and Maini, S. (1979). Genetic bases of an insect chemical communication system: The European corn borer. *Environ. Entomol.* **8**, 423–426.

Klun, J. A., Chapman, O. L., Mattes, K. C., Wojtkowski, P. W., Beroza, M., and Sonnet, P. E. (1973). Insect sex pheromones: Minor amount of opposite geometrical isomer critical to attraction. *Science* **181**, 661–663.

Klun, J. A., Leonhardt, B. A., Lopez, J. D., Jr., and LeChance, L. E. (1982). Female *Heliothis subflexa* (Lepidoptera: Noctuidae) sex pheromone: Chemistry and congeneric comparisons. *Environ. Entomol.* **11**, 1084–1090.

Kochansky, J., Cardé, R. T., Liebherr, J., and Roelofs, W. L. (1975). Sex pheromone of the European corn borer, *Ostrinia nubilalis* (Lepidoptera: Pyralidae) in New York. *J. Chem. Ecol.* **1**, 225–231.

Lanier, G. N., Birch, M. C., Schmitz, R. F., and Furniss, M. M. (1972). Pheromones of *Ips pini* (Coleoptera: Scolytidae): Variation in response among three populations. *Can. Entomol.* **104**, 1917–1923.

Lanier, G. N., Classen, A., Stewart, T., Piston, J. J., and Silverstein, R. M. (1980). *Ips pini*: The basis for interpopulational differences in pheromone biology. *J. Chem. Ecol.* **6**, 677–687.

Lewis, W. J., Nordlund, D. A., Gueldner, R. C., Teal, P. E. A., and Tumlinson, J. H. (1982). Kairomones and their use for management of entomophagous insects. XIII. Kiromonal activity for *Trichogramma* spp. of abdomen tips, excretion and a synthetic sex pheromone blend of *Heliothis zea* (Boddie) moths. *J. Chem. Ecol.* **8**, 1043–1055.

Light, D. M., and Birch, M. C. (1979). Inhibition of the attractive pheromone response in *Ips paraconfusus* by (*R*)-(−)-ipsdienol. *Naturwissenschaften* **66**, 159–160.

Linn, C. E., and Roelofs, W. L. (1984). Sublethal effects of neuroactive compounds on pheromone response thresholds in male Oriental fruit moths. *Arch. Insect Biochem. Physiol.* **1**, 331–334.

Linn, C. E., Bjostad, L. B., Du, J. W., and Roelofs, W. L. (1984). Redundancy in a chemical signal: Behavioral responses of male *Trichoplusia ni* to a 6-component sex pheromone blend. *J. Chem. Ecol.* **10**, 1635–1658.

Matsumoto, S. G., and Hildebrand, J. G. (1981). Olfactory mechanisms in the moth *Manduca sexta:* Response characteristics and morphology of central neurons in the antennal lobes. *Proc. R. Soc. London* **B213**, 249–277.

Mayer, M. S., and Mankin, R. W. (1985). Neurobiology of pheromone production. *In* "Comprehensive Insect Physiology, Biochemistry and Pharmacology" (G. A. Kerkut and L. I. Gilbert, eds.), pp. 95–144. Pergamon, New York.

Miller, J. R., and Roelofs, W. L. (1978). Gypsy moth responses to pheromone enantiomers as evaluated in a sustained-flight tunnel. *Environ. Entomol.* **7**, 42–44.

Miller, J. R., and Roelofs, W. L. (1980). Individual variation in sex pheromone component ratios in two populations of the redbanded leafroller moth, *Argyrotaenia velutinana*. *Environ. Entomol.* **9**, 359–363.

Miller, J. R., Mori, K., and Roelofs, W. L. (1977). Gypsy moth field trapping and electroantennogram studies with pheromone enantiomers. *J. Insect Physiol.* **23**, 1447–1453.

Mitchell, E. R., Jacobson, M., and Baumhover, A. H. (1975). *Heliothis* spp.: Disruption of pheromonal communications with (Z)-9-tetradecen-1-ol formate. *Environ. Entomol.* **4**, 577–579.

Mitchell, E. R., Tumlinson, J. H., and Baumhover, A. H. (1978). *Heliothis virescens:* Attraction of male to blends of (Z)-9-tetradecen-1-ol formate and (Z)-9-tetradecenal. *J. Chem. Ecol.* **4**, 709–716.

Morse, D., and Meighen, E. (1984). Detection of pheromone biosynthetic and degradative enzymes *in vitro*. *J. Biol. Chem.* **259**, 475–480.

Morse, D., and Meighen, E. (1986). Pheromone biosynthesis and the role of functional groups in pheromone specificity. *J. Chem. Ecol.* **12**, 335–351.

Moser, J. C., Brownlee, R. G., and Silverstein, R. M. (1968). Alarm pheromones of the ant *Atta texana*. *J. Insect Physiol.* **14**, 529–535.

Mustaparta, H. (1979). Chemoreception in bark beetles of the genus *Ips:* Synergism, inhibition and discrimination of enantiomers, *In* "Chemical Ecology: Odor Communication in Animals" (F. J. Ritter, ed.), pp. 147–158. Elsevier/North Holland, Amsterdam.

Nault, L. R., and Phelan, P. L. (1984). Alarm pheromones and sociality in pre-social insects. *In* "Chemical ecology of insects," (W. J. Bell and R. T. Cardé, eds.), pp. 237–256. Sinauer Associates, Sunderland, Massachusetts.

Norris, M. J. (1963). Laboratory experiments on gregarious behavior in ovipositing females of the desert locust [*Schistocerca gregaria* (Forsk.)]. *Entomol. Exp. Appl.* **6**, 279–303.

O'Connell, R. J. (1972). Responses of olfactory receptors to the sex attractant, its synergist and inhibitor in the redbanded leafroller. *In* "Olfaction and Taste" (D. Schneider, ed.), Vol. 4, pp. 180–186. Wissenschaftliche, Stuttgart.

O'Connell, R. J., Beauchamp, J. T., and Grant, A. J. (1986). Insect olfactory receptor responses to components of pheromone blends. *J. Chem. Ecol.* **12**, 469–482.

Pope, M. M., Gaston, L. K., and Baker, T. C. (1982). Composition, quantification, and periodicity of sex pheromone gland volatiles from individual *Heliothis virescens* females. *J. Chem. Ecol.* **8**, 1043–1055.

Priesner, E. (1968). Die interspezifischen Wirkungen der sexuallockstaffe der Saturniidae (Lepidoptera). *Z. Vergl. Physiol.* **61**, 263–297.

Priesner, E. (1979). Specificity studies on pheromone receptors of noctuid and tortricid lepidoptera. *In* "Chemical Ecology: Odor Communication in Animals" (F. J. Ritter, ed.), pp. 57–71. Elsevier/North Holland, Amsterdam.

Rice, R. E. (1969). Response of some predators and parasites of *Ips confusus* (LeC.) (Coleoptera: Scolytidae) to olfactory attractants. *Cont. Boyce Thompson Inst. Plant Res.* **24**, 189–194.

Riley, R. G., Silverstein, R. M., and Moser, J. C. (1974). Biological responses of *Atta texana* to its alarm pheromone and the enantiomer of the pheromone. *Science* **183**, 760–762.

Roelofs, W. L. (1984). Electroantennogram assays: Rapid and convenient screening procedures for pheromones. *In* "Techniques in Pheromone Research" (H. E. Hummel and T. A. Miller, eds.), pp. 131–159. Springer-Verlag, New York.

Roelofs, W. L., and Cardé, R. T. (1974). Sex pheromones in the reproductive isolation of lepidopterous species. *In* "Pheromones" (M. C. Birch, ed.), pp. 96–114. Elsevier/North Holland, Amsterdam.

Schneiderman, A. M., Matsumoto, S. G., and Hildebrand, J. G. (1982). Trans-sexually grafted antennae influence development of sexually dimorphic neurons in moth brain. *Nature (London)* **298**, 844–846.

Schneiderman, A. M., Hildebrand, J. G., Brennan, M. M., and Tumlinson, J. H. (1986). Trans-sexually grafted antennae alter pheromone-directed behavior in a moth. *Nature (London)* **323**, 801–803.

Shorey, H. H. (1964). Sex pheromones of noctuid moths. II. Mating behavior of *Trichoplusia ni* (Lepidoptera: Noctuidae): The role of the sex pheromone. *Ann. Entomol. Soc. Am.* **57**, 371–377.

Shorey, H. H., and Gaston, L. K. (1965). Sex pheromones of noctuid moths. V. Circadian rhythm of pheromone responsiveness in males in *Autographa californica, Heliothis virescens, Spodoptera exigua* and *Trichoplusia ni* (Lepidoptera: Noctuidae). *Ann. Entomol. Soc. Am.* **58**, 604–608.

Silk, P. J., Juenen, L. P. S., and Lonergan, G. C. (1985). A biologically active analogue of the primary sex-pheromone components of spruce budworm, *Choristoneura fumiferana* (Lepidoptera: Noctuidae). *Can. Entomol.* **117**, 257–260.

Silverstein, R. M. (1979). Enantiomeric composition and bioactivity of chiral semiochemicals in insects. *In* "Chemical Ecology: Odor Communication in Animals" (F. J. Ritter, ed.), pp. 113–146. Elsevier, Amsterdam.

Silverstein, R. M., Rodin, J. O., and Wood, D. L. (1966). Sex attractants in frass produced by male *Ips confusus* in ponderosa pine. *Science* **154**, 509–510.

Snodgrass, R. E. (1926). The morphology of insect sense organs and the sensory nervous system. *Smithsonian Misc. Coll.* **77**, 1–88.

Struble, D. L., and Arn, H. (1984). Combined gas chromatography and electroantennogram recording of insect olfactory responses. *In* "Techniques in Pheromone Research" (H. H. Hummel and T. A. Miller, eds.), pp. 161–178. Springer-Verlag, New York.

Tamaki, Y. (1985). Sex pheromones. *In* "Comprehensive Insect Physiology, Biochemistry and Pharmacology" (G. A. Kerkut and L. I. Gilbert, eds.), Vol. 9, pp. 145–191. Pergamon, New York.

Teal, P. E. A. (1986). Control of the gypsy moth using sex pheromone lures containing pesticide. [Renewable Resources Research Seminar (Abstract).] *Ont. Min. Nat. Res.*, 9.

Teal, P. E. A., and Tumlinson, J. H. (1986). Terminal steps in pheromone biosynthesis by *Heliothis virescens* and *H. zea. J. Chem. Ecol.* **12**, 353–366.

Teal, P. E. A., and Tumlinson, J. H. (1987). Induced changes in pheromone biosynthesis of *Heliothis* moths (Lepidoptera: Noctuidae). *In* "Molecular Entomology," (J. H. Law, ed.). Allan R. Liss, New York (in press).

Teal, P. E. A., Heath, R. R., Tumlinson, J. H., and McLaughlin, J. R. (1981). Identification of a sex pheromone of *Heliothis subflexa* (Gn.) (Lepidoptera: Noctuidae) and field trapping using different blends of components. *J. Chem. Ecol.* **7**, 1011–1022.

Teal, P. E. A., Tumlinson, J. H., McLaughlin, J. R., Heath, R. R., and Rush, R. A. (1984). (Z)-11-Hexadecenol: A behavioral modifying chemical present the pheromone gland of female *Heliothis zea* (Lepidoptera: Noctuidae). *Can. Entomol.* **116**, 777–779.

Teal, P. E. A., Mitchell, E. R., Tumlinson, J. H., Heath, R. R., and Sugie, H. (1985). Identification of volatile sex pheromone components released by the southern armyworm, *Spodoptera eridania* (Cramer). *J. Chem. Ecol.* **11**, 717–725.

Teal, P. E. A., Tumlinson, J. H., and Heath, R. R. (1986). Chemical and behavioral analyses of volatile sex pheromone components released by calling *Heliothis virescens* (F.) females (Lepidoptera: Noctuidae). *J. Chem. Ecol.* **12**, 107–126.

Tumlinson, J. H., Hardee, D. D., Gueldner, R. C., Thompson, A. C., Hedin, P. A., and Minyard, J. P. (1969). Sex pheromones produced by male boll weevil: Isolation, identification and synthesis. *Science* **166**, 1010–1012.

Tumlinson, J. H., Klein, M. G., Doolittle, R. E., Ladd, T. L., and Proveaux, A. T. (1977). Identification of the female Japanese beetle sex pheromone: Inhibition of male response by an enantiomer. *Science* **197**, 789–792.

Tumlinson, J. H., Mitchell, E. R., and Sonnet, P. S. (1981). Sex pheromone components of the beet armyworm, *Spodoptera exigua*. *J. Environ. Science Health* **A16**, 189–200.

Vetter, R. S., and Baker, T. C. (1983). Behavioral responses of *Heliothis virescens* in a sustained-flight tunnel to combinations of the 7 compounds identified from the female sex pheromone gland. *J. Chem. Ecol.* **9**, 747–759.

Vite, J. P., Klimetzek, D., Loskant, G., Hedden, R., and Mori, K. (1976). Chirality of insect pheromones: Response interruption by inactive antipodes. *Naturwissenschaften* **63**, 582–583.

2

Biology and Ultrastructure of Sex Pheromone–Producing Glands

JEAN E. PERCY-CUNNINGHAM
Austin, Texas 78748

J. A. MacDONALD
Forest Pest Management Institute
Sault Sainte Marie, Ontario, Canada P6A 5M7

I. INTRODUCTION

Among insects, pheromone-producing glands exhibit as many differences in location and gross morphology as functions assigned to them. Their complexity may be as simple as individual unicellular glands distributed throughout the integument or as elaborate as an internal cellular aggregate distinct from, but connected to, a reservoir. Regardless of its complexity, a gland is usually composed of epidermal cells, ultrastructurally modified after they have secreted the overlying cuticle. The cellular modifications, in general, reflect a change in function. Organelles related to differentiation or cuticle biosynthesis and secretion are replaced with organelles involved in lipid biosynthesis and secretion, but, for most gland cells, the specific involvement of the organelles in the biosynthesis and secretion of the sex pheromones has not been determined.

This chapter will encompass recent contributions to the literature concerning the structure and function of pheromone glands. Material published prior to 1974 has been covered in an earlier review (Percy and Weatherston, 1974) and will be used here only when needed for comparison. Furthermore, this chapter will

27

emphasize pheromone glands producing airborne sex pheromones, particularly those of female Lepidoptera.

II. ELUCIDATION OF STRUCTURAL DETAILS

Ideally, an elucidation of the structure and function of pheromone gland cells should include all of the following investigative areas (Sections II,A to II,D, below). Often, however, certain events preclude the completion of the ideal regime of study using a particular insect. For example, if the insects are field collected rather than lab reared, and if behavioral and/or chemical studies have not been completed, then ages appropriate for ultrastructural study cannot be accurately determined. If examination of pupae reveals no useful character for determining age and onset of differentiation of the gland cells, then determining the relationship of organelle structure to function can be extremely difficult.

A. Whole Insects

A pheromone-producing gland is often located initially during observations of the insect's precopulatory behavior. The gland may appear as a bulbous eversion as in, for example, many female Lepidoptera, the female praying mantis, and the male scorpion fly. If there is no obvious eversion, the site may be pinpointed by the rhythmical pumping of certain parts of the body or by the insect's tendency to rub legs or wings against other parts of the body. Another method of locating the gland is through observation of the response of the recipient and recording of the part of the emitter's body to which the recipient pays particular attention. Since release of the pheromone is both age and diel specific, these observations are also very important for ultrastructural studies, and they suggest the appropriate times for preparing material for detailed observation.

The results are usually recorded by macrophotography. Single lens reflex cameras with a system of bellows or tube extensions and lenses of about 100 mm focal length, used in conjunction with electronic flash equipment, are invaluable for recording insect calling behavior and evidence of gland eversion. Infrared-sensitive emulsions with suitable illumination and filters are sometimes necessary for recording the behavior of nocturnal insects. The advent of video camera equipment, now widely used by sex pheromone scientists, has further enhanced the ability to record and analyze precopulatory behavior.

B. Whole Mounts

Isolated and properly prepared whole mounts are extremely useful in determining not only the differentiation of glandular tissue during the development of the adults but also the relationship of the gland to the surrounding tissue. Material to be used as whole mounts does not need to be fixed with complicated fixing techniques. A solution of 70% ethanol is adequate for certain stains. We have found that a modification of Grenacher's borax carmine (Humasson, 1967; Percy and George, 1979) works very well for glands from female Lepidoptera. This method has a short preparation time in comparison to other techniques, e.g., the Feulgen technique, which has also been used in the preparation of whole mounts (Bronskill, 1970; Lalanne-Cassou *et al.*, 1977; Percy, 1978a). Other techniques used include fixation in Bouin's fluid and staining with a 1% methylene blue solution or examination of the whole mounts using interference microscopy and without staining (Menon, 1981).

C. Surface Studies

It is particularly important to study the surface of the gland in order to determine the disseminating mechanisms related to pheromone emission. The primary instrument involved in surface studies is the scanning electron microscope (SEM). However, there are very few published studies despite the widespread availability of the SEM, the facility with which it can be used, and the relative ease with which insect material can be prepared. Maintenance of the turgidity of the cuticle in the vacuum can be difficult, but proper preparation can be accomplished.

One technique involves virtually no fixation, as exemplified by the examination of the sex pheromone gland of the spruce budworm, *Choristoneura fumiferana* (Weatherston and Percy, 1970). The gland was extruded by a dental matrix retainer with pressure being applied dorsoventrally to abdominal segments six and seven of living insects; the abdominal tip was excised and immediately affixed to a copper specimen holder using conductive silver paint. The specimens were allowed to air dry before being examined in the SEM. An example of the result obtained is shown in Fig. 1a.

Other studies have involved complex fixation and preparation procedures. For example, the gland from the tobacco budworm, *Heliothis virescens,* shown in Fig. 1b was fixed in 4% osmic acid before dehydration through an ethanol series to ethanol–Freon and critical-point dried from Freon (Teal *et al.,* 1983). Other methods used have included vacuum immobilizing the specimen (*Trogoderma glabrum,* a dermestid beetle), followed by mounting it on a metal specimen holder with silver paint and subsequently gold coating (Hammack *et al.,* 1973). Excellent SEM results were also obtained after the specimen, a braconid wasp, *Apanteles melanoscelus,* was freeze dried and sputter coated with gold (Weseloh, 1980). Yet another method utilized oven drying of specimens and subsequent gold coating (Quennedey, 1978; Sreng, 1984).

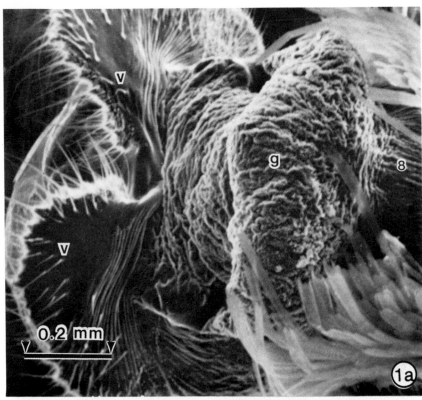

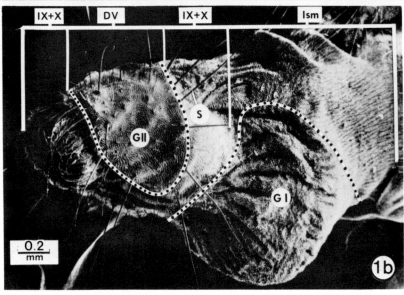

D. Sectioned Material

Both structural and functional information can be obtained from glandular tissue which has been fixed and prepared for microscopic examination. The function of structural modifications within cells can be inferred by comparison with tissues from other orders (or even classes). A more convincing structural–functional relationship can be derived by using histochemical techniques. The interpretation of results from these techniques requires knowledge of the glands and their secretion, and, since it is not always possible to have such a complete interdisciplinary study, comparative studies have become very important.

Some studies have used, for light microscopy, the thick sections of material prepared for the transmission electron microscope. The tissue generally exhibits very good fixation and reveals many details about the cells. For example, with an appropriate stain, the sections will reveal immediately whether globular deposits are lipid and whether there are deposits of lipid within the cuticle. Such a stain is toluidine blue (a 1% solution in pH 11 borate buffer) where osmicated lipid appears green (de Martino *et al.,* 1968; Percy, 1979). This test requires many repetitions to identify lipid deposits in the cuticle since, during fixing and embedding, lipid is prone to extraction.

The preparative procedure routinely used is the double fixation method using aldehydes and osmium tetroxide, as described in standard texts (Glauert, 1975; Hayat, 1970, 1972). Modifications are often dictated by special characteristics of the tissue and the scope of the study. Some tissues are more vulnerable to extraction than others during primary fixation, thus the length of fixation may be shortened. A considerable degree of flexibility in applying standard techniques and an empirical approach, when dealing with pheromone gland ultrastructure, is conducive to success.

We have also found that during preparation special attention must be paid to peculiarities of gland morphology and associated structures which may prevent adequate fixation and infiltration of stains and embedding media. For example, the pheromone gland of the female tussock moth, *Orgyia leucostigma* (Percy, 1975), is underlain by a dense web of tracheoles which must be removed or fixation and subsequent processing will be unsuccessful. In addition, the glands of very small insects tend to form a cul-de-sac which prevents proper infiltration

---

Fig. 1. Topography of sex pheromone glands. (a) *Choristoneura fumiferana.* The sex pheromone gland (g) is a modification of the dorsal part of the intersegmental membrane between the eighth (8) and ninth abdominal segments. [The ninth segment is integrated into the dorsal part of the valves (v)]. ×120. From Weatherston and Percy (1970). (b) *Heliothis virescens.* The gland complex consists of two regions: the ventrolateral part (GI) of the intersegmental membrane (Ism) between the eighth abdominal segment and the ninth/tenth abdominal segments (IX + X) and the dorsal valves (GII/DV). There are two types of gland cells in the valves, columnar and modified trichogen cells, and the latter underlie long setae (S). ×40. From Teal *et al.* (1983).

as, for example, that of the grapevine moth, *Lobesia botrana* (LaLanne-Cassou *et al.*, 1977). Careful dissection, adapted to the characteristics of the gland is a prerequisite for successful ultrastructural study.

If histochemical techniques are contemplated during the study of a pheromone gland, it may be necessary to alter the routine fixing procedures. The length of fixation should be as short as possible, and certain aldehydes and buffers should be avoided in order to maintain optimal enzyme activity (Glauert, 1975). In practice, the altered techniques must provide an acceptable compromise between adequate penetration and preservation, and a useful level of enzyme activity. Few histochemical techniques have been used to date, primarily because of the lack of complete studies on individual glands. One histochemical study used a technique designed to identify the enzyme catalase in other tissues (Locke and MacMahon, 1971; Novikoff *et al.*, 1972, 1980; Percy, 1978a). Other histochemical techniques in which organic solvents are employed have been unsuccessful in identifying parts of the cuticle involved in the release and possible production of the pheromone (Percy, 1978a).

III. DISTRIBUTION OF GLANDS

A. Topography

Examination of the surfaces of glands have revealed different methods of disseminating the pheromone. Gland cuticle is seldom without projections which, in an eversible gland, probably function to retain the pheromone on the surface of the inverted gland and to retard immediate evaporation of all the pheromone from the surface of the everted gland. In a noneversible gland, the projections could prevent collapse of glands and provide excess cuticle, if elastic reexpansion of glands is necessary. Such a hypothesis has been proposed for the noneversible glands of the arctiid moth, *Utetheisa ornatrix* (Conner *et al.*, 1980).

Cuticular projections in the form of ''spikes'' (Weatherston and Percy, 1970), ''spines'' (Conner *et al.*, 1980), or ''microspines'' (Aubrey *et al.*, 1983) are most frequently encountered. The cuticular surface of the gland in the cucumber beetle, *Diabrotica virgifera*, was found to have polygonal structures with tubercules on their posterior margins (Lew and Ball, 1978). Polygonal structures, which are probably not related to pheromone dissemination, are also found on the house cricket cuticle (Hendricks and Hadley, 1983). However, similar structures are also found over pheromone glands in the cockroach subfamily Oxyhaloinae (Sreng, 1984) where they likely serve this function. More elaborate projections have been observed in the Eri-silkmoth, *Samia cynthia ricini*, where the glandular surface is composed of irregular mammiform protuberances each with a spinescent process at the apex (Kawakami and Tanaka, 1978).

Modified scales are also utilized by many insects, primarily male Lepidoptera. These can be very elaborate and consist of many different types. Hairpencil scales of the oriental fruit moth, *Grapholitha molesta* (George and Mullins, 1980), and the Mediterranean flour moth, *Anagasta kuehniella* (Corbet and Lai-Fook, 1977), are hollow shafts with honeycombed walls. In females of the noctuid moth, *Noctua fimbria,* certain body scales have been modified to form a tuft of hair which serves as a scent brush (Urbahn, 1913).

Large pores are easily seen in surface studies as, for example, those of the glands in roaches where they are 1.5–6 μm in diameter (Sreng, 1984). Smaller pores of the order of 150–200 Å are not easily observed although there are several reports of such pores being seen in sectioned material (Steinbrecht, 1964a; Percy, 1974; Quennedey, 1978) (Fig. 2a). Perhaps it would be necessary to devise a technique such as that used for the unmodified cuticle in the house cricket, *Acheta domesticus* (Hendricks and Hadley, 1983).

B. Histological Characteristics

In many pheromone glands the epidermal cells are hypertrophied, and the resulting glandular cells are in direct contact with the overlying surface cuticle which is produced by the cells themselves. The pheromone is produced within the cells, transported through the cuticle, and disseminated from the surface of the cuticle. Cells may be cuboidal, columnar, modified columnar, or goblet shaped. The histological features characteristic of these cells include a large nucleus, many vacuoles, and sometimes an apical "brush border"; some cells, however, differ very little, histologically, from unmodified cells. Ultrastructural studies reveal that they contain smooth endoplasmic reticulum (often tubular), lipid spheres, microvilli, or apical folds (Percy and Weatherston, 1974; Bode, 1978; Quennedey, 1978; Ismail and Zachary, 1984). The cuticle overlying these gland cells is usually untanned. There are no large pores in the cuticle.

An interesting modification of this type of gland has been reported for males of the subterranean beetle, *Speonomus hydrophilus,* where the glands are internal but are tubular invaginations of the eighth/ninth sternal intersegmental membrane. Cuboidal glandular cells surround the tubules and presumably have secreted the cuticular lining. However, this cuticle is extremely modified, contains many unusual layers of mesocuticle, and also appears to lack epicuticle. In addition, the tubule does not open through the cuticle, but rather through a porous plate (Cazals and Juperthie-Jupeau, 1983).

In other pheromone glands which have secretory units instead of hypertrophied cells, several different glandular cells may participate in pheromone production, and not all are necessarily in direct contact with the surface cuticle. The chemicals produced by one gland cell may be combined with those of modified or unmodified cells and transported to the cuticle surface. Modified

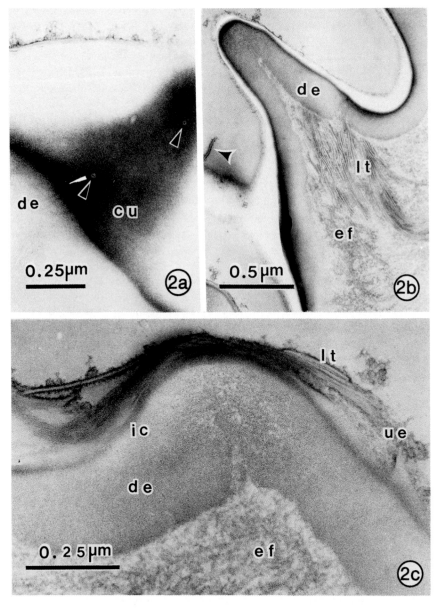

Fig. 2. External layers of gland cuticle in *Trichoplusia ni*. (a) Glancing section through pores (arrows) in the cuticulin (cu) overlying the dense epicuticle (de). ×66,900. (b) Lipid tubules within (lt) and outside (arrow) the cuticle over adult gland cells. The epicuticular filaments (ef) underlying the dense epicuticle (de) are not as distinct as the lipid tubules. ×40,000. (c) Lipid tubules (lt) on the outer surface of the cuticle intermingle with the outer, uneven layer (ue). Also shown are epicuticular filments (ef), inner cuticulin (ic), and dense epicuticle (de). ×100,350. From Percy (1979).

cells may be hypertrophied columnar cells or may be associated with a cuticle-lined duct or modified scale. There are often other cells in the unit which do not participate in the production or release of the pheromone. These may be unmodified cuticle-secreting duct or epidermal cells or nerve cells.

Secretory units with modified epidermal oenocytes as primary glandular cells and unmodified cells as secondary cells are found in the gland of the sand fly, *Culicoides nubeculosus* (Ismail and Zachary, 1984). Secretory units also with modified oenocytes as primary glandular cells but with hypertrophied epidermal cells as secondary cells are found in the sternal glands of several termites (Quennedey, 1978).

In secretory units where the pheromone is transported to the surface by a duct and emitted through its pore, there are at least two cells associated with each duct. The duct itself is formed by one or more duct cells which envelop it from its origin within the inverted apical membrane of the secretory cell to its merging with the body cuticle. The histological characteristics of these cells are the same as other cuticle-secreting cells, i.e., they have small nuclei and cytoplasm composed mainly of rough endoplasmic reticulum. The secretory cell has as a primary identifying feature an "end apparatus" composed of fibrillar or filamentous material partially enclosed in the thin cuticular termination of the duct cell cuticle. In addition, there may be unmodified epidermal cells between the secretory units and the body cuticle. These types of cells are found in the pheromone glands of males of the lacewing, *Chrysopa perla* (Wattebled *et al.*, 1978); the thoracic gland of males of three species of ant lions, *Myrmeleon formicarius, Grocus bare,* and *Euroleon nostras* (Eloffson and Lofqvist, 1974); and the male scorpion fly, *Harpobittacus australis* (Crossley and Waterhouse, 1969). The glandular cells may not be organized into a discrete unit as is the case in the pentatomid bug, *Nezara viridula,* where ducted unicellular glands are scattered throughout the abdominal integument. These are found only in males, and it has been suggested that they produce a sex attractant (Carayon, 1981). The ultrastructural characteristics of these secretory cells are very similar to those of the hypertrophied individual glandular cells. The cuticle overlying these cells varies since often the part surrounding the pore does not belong to the gland.

In secretory units where the pheromone-disseminating mechanism is a modified scale (hair), the glandular cells are modified trichogen cells which do not degenerate after the scent hair has been secreted. The modified scales are usually enlarged and circular in cross section, hence the term hair. Gland cells appear as enlarged goblet cells at the base of each hair, with the inverted apical membrane exhibiting many microvilli and surrounding an extension of fibrous endocuticle from the hair. Cells have very large, lobed nuclei often surrounded by active Golgi complexes, numerous mitochondria, and both rough and smooth endoplasmic reticulum. The base and periphery of the cells have noticeably deeper involutions of the plasma membrane than in the female pheromone glands.

Deposits of glycogen are often observed toward the base of the cell; lipid droplets and electron-dense spheres of unknown secretion are frequently observed at the apex. A tormogen cell participates in the formation of the hair shaft and remains as part of the secretory unit. The lepidopteran species examined to date include *Grapholitha molesta* (George and Mullins, 1980), *Phragmatobia fuliginosa* (Nielson, 1979), *Anagasta kuehniella* (Corbet and Lai-Fook, 1977), and *Trichoplusia ni* (J. E. Percy and J. A. MacDonald, unpublished observations). A similar sort of gland has recently been identified in females of the pyralid moth, *Eldana saccharina,* where there are scent scales with enlarged trichogen cells at the posterior margin of the seventh tergite (Atkinson, 1982).

This type of secretory unit may be further complicated by having a separate disseminating mechanism which may be found on almost any part of the insect's body. This separation of function requires a behavioral adaptation on the part of the insect in order to enable the secretory part to contact the disseminating part. In several thyridid moths, *Stringlia* spp., the scent brush is located in the hind wing and is inserted into a pouch or groove in the abdomen where the pheromone is presumably secreted (Whalley, 1974). Male tortricid moths in the genus *Archips* possess costal folds on the fore wings which have hairpencil scales whose tips lie in contact with small glandular pocket scales whose cells produce the mating pheromone (Grant, 1978).

A pheromone system which has been studied in some detail is that of some noctuid moths. The system has two parts: an internal structure known as Stobbe's gland and eversible scent brushes. The scent brushes are composed of numerous modified scales which, when the insect is at rest, are located within a large, ventrolateral abdominal pocket. The cells of Stobbe's gland produce the precursor to the pheromone and secrete it into the pocket where it is enzymatically converted to the pheromone. Scales of the gland show little surface folding, whereas scales of the scent brushes, the disseminating organs, have a large, complex evaporative surface (Birch, 1970; Clearwater, 1975a,b). In the noctuid moth, *Mamestra configurata,* the pheromone has been identified and is phenethyl alcohol, the immediate precursor is phenethyl-β-glucoside, and a biosynthetic pathway has been proposed from *in vivo* and *in vitro* experiments (Clearwater, 1975c; Weatherston and Percy, 1976). The ultrastructural details of this type of gland have not been reported although the information accumulated concerning the biosynthesis of the pheromone of *M. configurata* is extensive enough to provide a good basis for an in-depth ultracytochemical analysis.

There have been two attempts at producing a classification scheme to encompass the various types of epidermal glands. The first scheme defines three classes of gland cells based on whether the surface cuticle is secreted by the gland cell and on the mode of egress of the secretion (Noirot and Quennedey, 1974). Class 1 cells include the individual glandular cells which are in direct contact with the overlying cuticle and which secrete the cuticle themselves. A special group within this class are the secretory units with a modified scale as a disseminating mechanism. Class 2 cells are those gland cells where the pheromone crosses the cuticle only after transfer into more or less modified epidermal cells (the latter may be similar to Class 1 gland cells). Class 3 cells are those secretory units where the pheromone is transported to the surface by a duct and where the gland cells do not secrete the surface cuticle. This scheme does not attempt to correlate any developmental homologies which may be present.

An attempt has been made at a classification scheme which would allow for possible homologies for the pheromone glands. In this scheme there are two groups based on the spindle axis of the primary mitotic division of the imaginal epidermal cells. The first group, the individual glandular cells, originates from mitotic divisions occurring along a horizontal axis. The second group, the organules or secretory units, originates from mitotic divisions which occur along the vertical or oblique axis. The two types of secretory units involving ducts or modified scales are merely different modifications of cells arising from vertical or oblique mitotic divisions (Corbet and Lai-Fook, 1977). This scheme appears to make no allowances for those glands in which the primary glandular cell is a modification of an epidermal oenocyte, although oenocytes could also be considered to arise from a vertical to oblique mitotic division in which one cell loses contact with the cuticle.

C. Location of Glands

1. Antennae

Antennal modifications presumably related to the production of sex pheromones are found in the genera *Batrisus* and *Batrisodes,* beetles in the family Pselaphidae (De Marzo and Vit, 1983), and in several species of Trichoptera (Roemhild, 1980). In the male beetles, morphological and histological studies of the apical antennal segments showed them to be glandular whereas in male microcaddisflies similar studies identified the basal segments as glandular as well as occipital areas of the head. The gland cells of the microcaddisflies are trichogen cells with modified scales as dispensing mechanisms.

2. Thorax

Internal metathoracic glands producing sex pheromones have been found in two orthopteran and three neuropteran species. In females of the grasshopper, *Poecilocerus pictus,* the gland is a bilobed sac located mid-dorsally with a duct opening at a transverse slit in the intersegmental membrane between the metathorax and first abdominal segment. The gland appears to originate as an invagination of the intersegmental membrane (Gupta, 1978). Females of the grasshopper, *Taeniopoda eques,* emit the perhomone through the metathoracic spiracle and produce it in tracheal glands surrounding the spiracular trunks (Whitman, 1982). The illustration in the paper suggests that the gland is composed of hyperdeveloped tracheal cells, although this is not definitely stated.

Male ant lions produce a presumed pheromone in ducted gland cells of elongated internal thoracic glands which open behind and below the metathoracic spiracle. The glands are present in the females but are very poorly developed. Distribution of the pheromone is aided by a club-shaped organ, Eltringham's organ, which projects from the posterior margin of the hind wing and fits into a pit near the opening of the gland when the insect is at rest. The functions of the glands and distributing organ are postulated since neither calling male ant lions nor copulating pairs have been observed (Elofsson and Lofqvist, 1974).

The thorax has been identified as the source of the pheromone in two species of bagworm moths. An anterior site of pheromone production would be advantageous to the bagworm moth. Bagworm moth larvae pupate in the "head-down" position, and upon eclosion female adults normally expose only the head and thorax through the opening of the pupal case ("bag") (Bosman and Brand, 1971; Leonhardt et al., 1983).

3. Legs

The sex pheromone glands of many male moths are found on the legs and were described in many earlier reports (references in Percy and Weatherston, 1974). In a study of the geometriid, *Semiothisis eleonora,* the pheromone-producing glands have been found as brush organs at the ventral junction of the femur and tibia of the hind leg. The brushes fan out ventrally on stretching the hind leg at right angles to the long axis of the body (DasGupta, 1979).

4. Abdomen—General

Tergal glands associated with the intertergal membrane have been identified in representatives of several orders. Eversible modifications of intertergal membranes are present in the scorpion fly, *Harpobittacus australis* (Mecoptera) (Crossley and Waterhouse, 1969); the praying mantis, *Acanthops falcata* (Orthoptera) (Robinson and Robinson, 1979); the crane fly; *Emodotipula* (Diptera) (Tjeder, 1979); as well as females of many species of Lepidoptera (see Section IV). Glands are located in intertergal membranes between tergites six and seven and seven and eight for *Harpobittacus;* between six and seven for *Acanthops;* and between nine and ten (sometimes eight and nine as well) for *Emodotipula.* Between eight and nine is the usual modification in Lepidoptera. Only male *Harpobittacus* and the female Lepidoptera have been studied histologically. Cells with ducts are found in *Harpobittacus* whereas hypertrophied cells are characteristic of the Lepidoptera.

Noneversible intertergal glands which have been implicated in the production of sex pheromones have been found in Hemiptera, specifically, the pentatomid,

Podisus modestus. The glands are present in both males and females but are much larger in males (Aldrich *et al.,* 1978). Gland cells are ducted and resemble the cells of anterior glands in larvae of the pentatomid, *Apateticus bracteatus* (Percy *et al.,* 1980; J. A. MacDonald, unpublished observations). Noneversible tergal glands opening through the intertergal membrane have been located in the sawfly, *Neodiprion sertifer.* The glands are found in both sexes but are better developed in the males. Glands are paired and are located laterally within tergite two, opening via a duct between tergites two and three. Although the function has not been conclusively proved, the suggestion has been made that this is the gland which produces the sex pheromone. The secretory cells are associated with ducts and ductile cells. The cells have one or more microvilli-lined cavities, and within the cavities the usual fibrillar material is found. Golgi complexes are numerous, rough endoplasmic reticulum predominates, but there is no mention of smooth endoplasmic reticulum (Hallberg and Lofqvist, 1981).

Sex pheromone glands are also found ventrally within the abdomen in representatives from several orders. In male Lepidoptera the scent brushes, or hairpencils, are often found ventrally or ventrolaterally and may have more than one glandular site. Additional sites are found on almost any part of the body. The suggestion has frequently been made that the different sites produce pheromones with different functions during the mating process. The arctiid moth, *Phragmatobia fuliginosa,* has an eversible bilobed gland with each lobe containing two glandular areas. The gland, located in the intersegmental membrane between segments six and seven, consists of scent brushes which are folded within the pouches while the insect is relaxed and everted during pheromone release. The individual scent hairs are supported by a very large goblet cell typical of hairpencil cells (Nielson, 1979). The evagination of the gland is controlled in part by evaginator muscles and in part by hemolymph and tracheal pressure (Nielson, 1982).

The gland in the pyralid moth, *Tryporyza incertulas,* is composed of several ventral groups of scent tufts. The anteriormost of these tufts is located on the posterior margin of the seventh abdominal segment, the mid tuft is found ventromedially on the anterior third of the eighth segment, and the posterior tuft is found on the distal margins of a small cuticular flap between the bases of the saccular processes. The gland cells of the anterior and mid groups disappear soon after eclosion while the posterior cells persist; they are typical of hairpencil cells (Ahmad *et al.,* 1977). In this respect they resemble the cells of the noctuids (Birch, 1970; as discussed in Percy and Weatherston, 1974). The gland in the pyralid moth, *Eldana saccharina,* is more complex and includes ventral scent brushes, wing glands, and also gland cells on the claspers. The scent brushes are found between the seventh and eighth segments. All gland cells are modified trichogen cells (Atkinson, 1982).

In a representative of Thysanoptera, *Thrips validus,* the glands are found in males and are located mid-ventrally in segments three to eight. Gland cells are hypertrophied and columnar and are not associated with ducts although there is a very distinct surface "pore plate" associated with each glandular area. On the basis of observations with a related species, *T. dianthi,* it is concluded that these glands produce both an attractant and aphrodisiac pheromone (Bode, 1978).

The pheromone gland complex of male roaches in the subfamily Oxyhaloinae (Dictyoptera) consists of both tergal and sternal glands, but only the sternal glands produce the sex pheromone which attracts females from a distance. The number of glands in each species is variable; there may be as few as three or as many as six. Externally, each gland is identified by large numbers of pores found on the concealed anterior and extreme posterior margins of the modified sternites. The glandular tissue is composed of ducted glandular cells separated laterally from each other by cells which are modified oenocytes (Sreng, 1984). The gland cells are separated from the overlying cuticle by a layer of squamous cells. The height of the entire epithelium varies with the age in *Nauphoeta cinerea;* the greatest height occurs at the time the males are most attractive to the females (Menon, 1981, 1986).

In many families of termites (Isoptera), tergal glands, when present, produce the sex pheromones. When these glands are not present, the sternal glands assume this role (Quennedey, 1978, and references therein). For example, in *Hodotermes mossambicus* it is the male which calls the female by flexing the abdomen dorsally to expose a large, well-developed sternal gland; in a resting insect this gland is covered by the preceding sternite (Leuthold and Bruinsma, 1977). The gland is also present in workers and adult females but is much smaller than it is in the males. In workers the gland produces a trail pheromone. Detailed studies have shown that the gland is composed of an anterior and a posterior zone; the anterior zone is more highly developed in adult males with the posterior zone being more highly developed in workers and females. The anterior zone is composed entirely of columnar cells while the posterior zone is composed of columnar cells and a nodule of modified cells reminiscent of epidermal oenocytes. The columnar cells of the anterior zone in males contains accumulated lipid spheres; the material is apparently stored there and is released during calling (Quennedey, 1978).

There is at least one termite species in which the sex pheromone is produced by both tergal and sternal glands. In *Trinervitermes bettonianus,* both glands are exposed when the female is calling the male. The sternal gland is also present in workers and dealate males where it produces the trail pheromone, although in these castes it is much smaller than it is in the females (Leuthold and Luscher, 1974). The difference in size of the gland is due solely to a difference in the height of the cells; morphologies of the cells and characteristic organelles are the same in all castes. The function of the secretion produced by sternal glands in workers and males is determined by its concentration since, in behavioral studies, when the concentration is increased, the pheromone attracts males and behaves as a sex pheromone (Quennedey and Leuthold, 1978).

Other species have pheromone glands both dorsally and ventrally in the abdomen. Females of the chrysomelid beetle, *Diabrotica virgifera,* have two groups of secretory cells, one of which is situated dorsally between the seventh and eighth tergites and a second situated ventrally between the seventh and eighth sternites. In both groups of cells there are both columnar and ducted cells. The ducts open through the cuticle, and the pores are readily observable with the SEM. Many sensilla and cuticular polygonal structures are associated with the pores (Lew and Ball, 1978). Many female Lepidoptera have glands both dorsally and ventrally within the terminal abdominal segments (Section IV).

Lateral sternal glands are part of the sex pheromone gland complex in male dung beetles, *Kheper nigroaenus* (Tribe, 1975). The glands are found on each side of the first abdominal sternite and produce a white flocculent secretion. It is thought that the pheromone is incorporated into this waxy carrier and is disseminated by the insect's simultaneously brushing the secretion with its metatarsal fringes of setae against rows of abdominal bristles. The histology of the gland has not been studied. Laterally situated scent glands (brushes) have been described from the olethreutid, *Grapholitha molesta* (George and Mullins, 1980).

5. Abdomen—Genital

Sex pheromone production and release is often associated with the genital region of the abdomen. The glands of this region may be associated with glands in another part of the body, as the scent brushes of male Lepidoptera. However, epidermal glands which appear to be the sole source of the pheromones have also been identified in several orders. Scorpion flies of the genus *Panorpa* have a ventral glandular patch on the genital bulb which projects anteriorly into the bulb but is eversible. The secretion from this gland attracts females, for the purpose of mating, from a distance of 8 m (25 ft). The gland is composed of columnar glandular cells which are adjacent to cuticular inpocketings. These cells are separated laterally by accessory cells, the apical surfaces of which do not reach the cuticle. Apparently unmodified epidermal cells, "matrix cells," separate the gland cells from the cuticle which has not been used to form inpocketings. A similar gland has been found in the genus *Brachypanorpa,* and a similar function has been postulated for it (Thornhill, 1973).

Many species of lacewings have two vesicles which are everted during courtship, and, although their exact function is not known, it is generally thought that the secretion influences the female during mating. The vesicles are paired and encircle a dorsomedial hooked-shaped pseudopenis. The gland cells of *Chrysopa perla* are ducted and are in close association with a sensory hair (Wattebled *et al.,* 1978).

In females of parasitic wasps in the genus *Apanteles* there are glandular fields which are found at the bases of the second valvifers and on the ninth tergite. Morphological studies, reinforced by behavioral studies, led Tagawa (1977, 1983) to conclude that the glandular fields associated with the second valvifers were the sites of production and release of the sex pheromone. The glands are composed of two types of glandular cells: modified trichogen cells with associated setae and ducted columnar cells. These results contradict those of Weseloh (1980), who stated that glands on the eighth tergite (equivalent to the ninth tergite) actually produced the pheromone. The contradiction by Tagawa (1983) was based on the observation that the tergal glands occur in both sexes and that, furthermore, the glandular cells are hyperdeveloped in both males and females. Confusing responses in the behavioral bioassays appear to stem from the fact that it is difficult to separate the ninth tergite from the valvifers when conducting the experiments.

6. Internal

There are at least two different types of internal abdominal glands associated with the production of sex pheromones: those whose sole function is pheromone production and those which are modified tissues devoted to other functions. Those whose sole function is the production of pheromones have been found in two families of beetles. Females of the tobacco beetle, *Lasioderma serricorne* (Anobiidae), have large glands which originate in the second abdominal segment and open at an orifice below the genital pore. The gland is a lobate structure clustered around a central duct, which is actually a modified apodeme. Behavioral bioassays and electroantennograms have identified this gland as the source of the pheromones (Levinson *et al.*, 1983). Males of *Speonomus hydrophilus* (Silphidae) have internal tubular glands opening via a porous plate toward the posterior margin medially in sternite eight. The glands vary in size and complexity from a small median sac to a large intricate network of tubules underlying sternites six through eight. The cells are enlarged and are cuboidal to goblet shaped (Juberthie-Jupeau and Cazals, 1984).

Other glands are modified parts of tissues obviously devoted to other functions. Within the Diptera, specifically, two species of tephritids (*Dacus tryoni* and *D. oleae*) and one drosophilid (*Drosophila grimshawi*), the glands are associated with the digestive tract. Lobes, consisting of modified tissue of the posterior part of the rectum, form the gland. The glands are eversible in *Dacus oleae* (Economopoulos *et al.*, 1971) and *Drosophila grimshawi* (Hodosh *et al.*, 1979) but not in *Dacus tryoni* (Fletcher, 1969). The glandular cells are hypertrophied columnar cells. In males of several species of bumblebees, *Pyrobombus lapidarius, P. hypnorum,* and *Megabombus hortorum,* the cephalic part of the labial glands produces a long-range sex pheromone (Agren *et al.*, 1979). Mandibular glands in the cincindelid beetle, *Cincindela sexpunctata,* have also been implicated in the production of sex pheromones (Singh and Gupta, 1982). A secretion from the poison gland is used by young females of the slave-making ants to attract the males for mating. Thus, males of *Harpagoxenus canadensis* and *H. sublaevis* respond to the secretion from females of both species but are prevented from mating by behavioral differences. Males of a third species, *H. americanus,* respond only to the conspecific pheromone (Buschinger and Alloway, 1979).

7. Other

Sex pheromone has been identified as a component of the nonpolar cuticular lipids in the screwworm fly, *Cochliomyia hominivorax* (Mackley and Broce, 1981); the housefly, *Musca domestica* (Blomquist *et al.,* Chapter 7, this volume); and the staphylinid beetle, *Aleochara cartula* (Peschke, 1978). By comparison, initial studies of the sand fly, *Culicoides nubeculosus,* also indicated that abdominal cuticular hydrocarbons contained the pheromone (Ismail and Kremer, 1983). Subsequently, the site of pheromone emission was more specifically determined to be four atrichial areas on each of the first eight sternites. Pheromone is produced by a pair of large cells located in the vicinity of, and lateral to, each of the atrichial areas. These large cells appear to be modified oenocytes and are found either in direct contact with the epidermis or within clumps of subepidermal adipose tissue. The evidence in favor of this hypothesis is the lack of enlarged cells in association with dorsal atrichial areas and the bioassay evidence that the pheromone is produced by the ventral cuticle (Ismail and Zachary, 1984).

IV. GLANDS OF FEMALE LEPIDOPTERA

A. Morphology of Glands

The glands of female Lepidoptera are more consistent in their location and histological composition than are glands of other orders. For this reason, studies to determine the comparative functional features of these glands are a little easier to design. Glands are most commonly found as modifications of the intersegmental membrane between the eighth and ninth abdominal segments. The cells are hypertrophied epidermal cells, and the cuticle is modified intersegmental membrane cuticle. The extent to which the membrane has become glandular is extremely variable. However, there has been enough consistency in the location within the membrane to enable the use of common descriptive phrases when comparing the glands of the different families. Thus, when the entire intersegmental membrane is modified as a pheromone-producing gland, it is termed a *ring gland.* This description is accurate when based on the gland's appearance in a calling insect, since the everted gland encircles the abdomen. However, histo-

as small and squamous to cuboidal. In contrast, another report concerning *Pectinophora gossypiella* states that the both the dorsal and ventral parts of the intersegmental membrane are modified to form the gland. The gland cells are columnar until the insect has mated, at which time the cells become cuboidal (El-Sawaf *et al.,* 1968).

3. Plutellidae

Two separate studies of the diamondback moth, *Plutella xylostella,* have yielded somewhat conflicting results. According to Su and Lee (1977), the pheromone is produced by a ventral gland, a suggestion based on morphological and topological studies of the intersegmental membrane. According to Chow *et al.* (1976), there are three distinct areas in the terminal abdominal segments with hyperdeveloped cells. These are (i) the epithelium of the ninth tergite, (ii) the epithelium at the opening of the ostium bursa and, (iii) the dorsal part of the intersegmental membrane. Extracts from all three sites give a positive response in bioassays.

4. Acrolepidae

Morphological and histological studies have identified a ring gland in the leek moth, *Acrolepia asectiella.* The cells are larger than those of an unmodified intersegmental membrane and are columnar (Thibout, 1972).

5. Tortricidae

a. Olethreutinae. Eleven species of Olethreutinae have been examined histologically, and in ten species the modified intersegmental membrane of a resting insect is invaginated to form a compact dorsal sac. The species include the grape vine moth, *Lobesia botrana* (LaLanne-Cassou *et al.,* 1977); the oriental fruit moth, *Grapholitha molesta* (George, 1965; Roelofs and Feng, 1968); the codling moth, *Cydia pomonella* (Barnes *et al.,* 1966; Roelofs and Feng, 1968); *Endopiza viteana; Hedya nubiferana* (Roelofs and Feng, 1968); the Nantucket pine tip moth, *Rhyacionia frustrana;* the pitch pine tip moth, *R. rigidana;* the pine tip moth, *R. subtropica* (Baer *et al.,* 1976); the European pine shoot moth, *R. buoliana;* and the Douglas fir cone moth, *Barbara colfaxiana* (J. E. Percy and J. A. MacDonald, unpublished observations). There is no apparent modification of the intersegmental membrane or hyperdevelopment of epidermal cells in the strawberry leaf roller, *Ancylis comptrana fragiariae* (Roelofs and Feng, 1968).

b. Tortricinae. Nine species have been examined histologically to determine the presence of a sex pheromone gland, and all have the intersegmental membrane modified to form a dorsal saddle in the resting insect. The glands are less compact than those of the olethreutines and many have deep longitudinal folds which disappear when the gland is everted (see Fig. 1a). The species examined include the spruce budworm, *Choristoneura fumiferana* (Weatherston and Percy, 1970; Percy and Weatherston, 1971; Percy, 1974); the jack pine budworm, *C. pinus* (Percy and Weatherston, 1971); the oblique banded leaf roller, *C. rosaceana;* the ugly nest caterpillar, *Archips cerasivoranus;* the fruit tree leaf roller, *A. argyrospilus; A. mortuanus* (Roelofs and Feng, 1968; Bronskill, 1970); the three-lined leaf roller, *Pandemis limitata* (Roelofs and Feng, 1968); the redbanded leaf roller, *Argyrotaenia velutinana* (Roelofs and Feng, 1968; Bronskill, 1970; Feng and Roelofs, 1977); and *A. quadrifasciana* (Roelofs and Feng, 1968; Bronskill, 1970).

6. Pyralidae

a. Pyraustinae. The sex pheromone gland in the European corn borer, *Ostrinia nubilalis,* is a ring gland with the cells located ventrally being much larger than the cells located dorsally (Hammad, 1961).

b. Ancylomiinae. The gland in the yellow rice stem borer, *Tryporyza incertulas,* is a modification of the anterodorsal part of the intersegmental membrane to form paired noneversible tubes which open to the outside by small slits. The cells are columnar and near the edge of the gland become squamous. The outer surface of the gland is covered with spines (Ahmed *et al.,* 1977).

c. Crambinae. In the webworm, *Crambus hammelus,* paired dorsolateral folds in the intersegmental membrane form the gland (Fig. 3b). Between the folds the cells and cuticle are modified for muscle insertion and not for lipid production. The gland in the sugar cane borer, *Diatraea saccharalis,* is also a dorsal bilobed sac, but the lobes are situated anteroposteriorly rather than laterally as in *C. hammelus* (White *et al.,* 1972). In *Chilo simplex* the gland is a ring gland with columnar cells although the cells are larger in the ventral part than in the dorsal part (Hammad, 1961).

d. Phycitinae. Six species of Phycitinae have been examined in this subfamily. The species include the bumblebee wax moth, *Vitula edmandsae* (Figs. 3a, 3c, and 3d) (Weatherston and Percy, 1968); *Dioryctria abietiella* (Fatzinger, 1972); the Mediterranean flour moth, *Anagasta kuehniella;* the tobacco moth, *Ephestia elutella;* and the almond moth, *E. cautella* (Dickens, 1936); all have been reported to have ring glands.

The Indian meal moth, *Plodia interpunctella.* has been the subject of several investigations, and not all authors agree on the extent to which the gland is developed. Two reports suggest that it is a ring-shaped gland (Dickens, 1936; Han *et al.,* 1979), with the latter report stating that it is more deeply invaginated

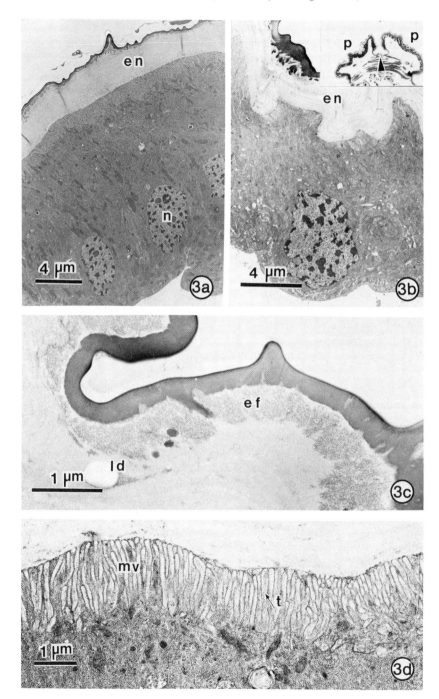

ventrally than dorsally and adding that it is interrupted laterally by the posterior apophyses. Four other reports maintain that it is a ventral gland (Barth, 1937; Smithwick and Brady, 1977a,b; Srinivasan *et al.*, 1979). The histological differentiation of the cells was traced from pupae through to the adult, and it was found that the cells increase in depth throughout pupation and reach their maximum height at eclosion. Microvilli appear at eclosion, they are consistent in width but vary in length, and they have a distinct central "fiber." Granular endoplasmic reticulum is common before eclosion but disappears afterward. On the other hand, smooth tubular endoplasmic reticulum is rare in pupae but is the main component of the cytoplasm in newly eclosed and 2-day adults. Some cisternal endoplasmic reticulum is present. Mitochondria increase in number throughout maturation. The basement membrane is finely granular and thin (Smithwick, 1970; Smithwick and Brady, 1977b).

7. Pterophoridae

There has been only one plume moth examined histologically. Hyperdeveloped cells, presumed to represent the gland of *Oidaematophorus hornodactylus*, are found in the dorsal part of the intersegmental membrane and its gross morphology is that of a median sac (J. A. MacDonald and J. E. Percy, unpublished observations).

8. Geometridae

a. Ennominae. Each of the species examined from this subfamily has glandular tissue in a different position. In the western hemlock looper, *Lambdina fiscellaria lugubrosa*, the gland is composed of eversible paired ventrolateral folds in an otherwise unmodified intersegmental membrane. Gland cells are goblet shaped (Ostaff *et al.*, 1974). We have examined the eastern hemlock looper, *L. fiscellaria fiscellaria*, on several occasions, at different ages, both field collected and lab reared, and throughout the terminal abdominal segments and have not identified any distinctly differentiated hyperdeveloped cells. In addition, *Petrophora subaequaria* and *Lomographa vestaliata* have also been examined; in the former hyperdeveloped cells are found in the dorsal part of the

---

Fig. 3. Pyralidae. (a) *Vitula edmandsae.* Columnar gland cells underlie the endocuticle (en) of the intersegmental membrane. The nucleus (n) is found near the base of each cell. ×2350. (b) *Crambus hammelus.* Cuboidal gland cells underlie the endocuticle (en) of two dorsolateral pouches in the intersegmental membrane. ×4200. *Insert:* The two pouches (p) are separated by a medial region modified for muscle insertion (arrow). ×67. (c) *Vitula edmandsae.* The epicuticular filaments (ef) form a dense mat underneath the epicuticle. Lipid deposits (ld) are also found within the endocuticle. ×19,325. (d) *Vitula edmandsae.* The apical microvilli (mv) of gland cells are very uniform in their dimensions. Each contains a tubule of smooth endoplasmic reticulum (t). ×11,625.

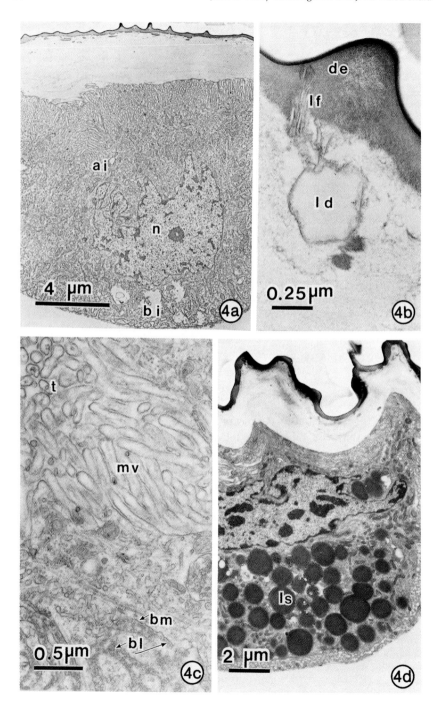

intersegmental membrane (Figs. 4a, 4b, and 4c), and in the latter the entire intersegmental membrane has glandular cells similar to *P. subaequaria*. In contrast, the sex pheromone gland of *Boarmia selenaria* is represented by two noneversible ventrolateral sacs which are partly on the ninth/tenth intersegmental membrane and open through them. The gland cells are cuboidal to columnar. The site was identified through electroantennograms and behavioral bioassays of extracted compounds (Wysoki *et al.*, 1985).

b. Larentiinae. Only one species of Larentiinae, the spear-marked black moth, *Rheumaptera hastata,* has been examined histologically for the presence of a sex pheromone gland. The gland is composed of two noneversible tubes which open at a single dorsal opening located dorsal to the anus and between the papillae anales. The paired glands were identified as the source of the pheromone by behavioral bioassays. During calling the female pulsates the abdomen, and this is probably the method whereby the pheromone is dispersed into the atmosphere (Werner, 1977).

9. Bombycidae

The sex pheromone gland in *Bombyx mori* is represented by a pair of eversible ventrolateral sacs in the intersegmental membrane. These sacs have been called the *sacculi laterales*. The gland cells are cuboidal, contain smooth tubular endoplasmic reticulum, and have apical folds (Steinbrecht, 1964a,b; Steinbrecht and Schneider, 1964; Waku and Sumimoto, 1969).

10. Lasiocampidae

Reexamination of the sex pheromone gland of the forest tent caterpillar, *Malacosoma disstria,* has shown that it is ring shaped only in the anterior part of the intersegmental membrane. The ring-shaped portion of the gland is more developed dorsally, as noted earlier (Percy and Weatherston, 1971; J. E. Percy and J. A. MacDonald, unpublished results). The posterior part of the membrane contains hyperdeveloped cells only between the posterior apophyses (Figs. 5a, 5b, and 5e).

Fig. 4. Geometridae. (a) *Petrophora subaequaria.* The hyperdeveloped cells of the dorsal part of the intersegmental membrane are somewhat goblet shaped in that they have a deep involution of the apical plasma membrane (ai). There are also many basal involutions (bi). Nuclei (n) are large and lobed. ×4600. (b) *Petrophora subaequaria.* Within the cuticle both lipid deposits (ld) and lipid filaments (lf) are observed close to the surface; the lipid filaments pass through the dense epicuticle (de). ×45,825. (c) *Petrophora subaequaria.* Involutions of the apical and basal plasma membranes almost appose each other when both penetrate deeply within the cells. Each apical microvillus (mv) contains a tubule of smooth endoplasmic reticulum (t). The basal lamina (bl) follows the contours of the involuted basal plasma membrane (bm). ×27,500. (d) *Lambdina fiscellaria fiscellaria.* Lipid spheres (ls) accumulate in all epidermal cells of this species. × 6050.

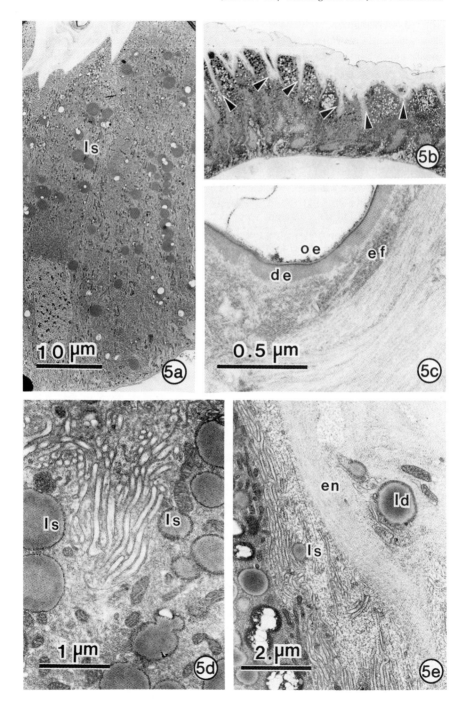

11. Saturniidae

a. Citheroniinae. *Citheronia laocoon* is the only species to have been studied. It has a ring gland with cuboidal cells modified in a manner similar to *Malacosoma disstria*. The cells contain lipid spheres (Barth, 1960).

b. Saturniinae. Sex pheromone glands have been identified in four species. Ring glands are found in *Caligula japonica* (Urbahn, 1913) and in the Eri-silkmoth, *Samia cynthia ricini* (Kawakami and Tanaka, 1978). The surfaces of glands in both species are covered with minute spikes. In the emperor moth, *Saturnia pavonia,* and the nailspot, *Aglia tau,* there are ventral glands. In the former there is a ventral sac while in the latter there is a ventral field (Urbahn, 1913). *Aglia tau* is rather unusual in that there is also a scent tuft on the eighth sternite which overlies the scent field. This scent tuft is everted during calling. There are no hyperdeveloped cells underlying the scent scales; the cells of the scent field are columnar and are particularly so in the region where the field comes into contact with the scent brush. Urbahn (1913) surmised that the scent tuft was used to disseminate the scent produced by the scent field.

12. Sphingidae

A histological examination of the terminal abdominal segments in the oleander hawk moth, *Daphnis nerii,* has revealed three distinct areas of hyperdeveloped cells. Two of the areas, a pair each of ventrolateral patches (Fig. 6a) and deep dorsolateral folds (Fig. 6b), are found on the intersegmental membrane. The third is comprised of epidermal cells of most of the valves (Fig. 6c).

13. Notodontidae

Eight species of Notodontidae have been examined for the presence of hyper-developed cells in the terminal abdominal segments. There is little consistency between species with regard to the location of hyperdeveloped cells. In the yellow-necked caterpillar, *Datana ministra,* modified cells are found posteriorly within the dorsal part of the intersegmental membrane (Fig. 7a). In the saddled prominent, *Heterocampa guttivitta,* they are found medially in the ninth tergite

---

Fig. 5. Lasiocampidae, *Malacosoma disstria.* (a) Lipid spheres (ls) in the modified columnar gland cells have the same appearance and distribution in both developing and mature gland cells. ×1825. (b) The modified columnar cells have an enlarged apical membrane produced by peripheral involutions of the apical membranes of apposing cells (arrows). ×425. (c) Epicuticular filaments (ef) form a dense mat underneath the dense epicuticle (de). Externally, the outer, uneven layer (oe) is very evident. ×49,500. (d) The lipid spheres (ls) have a peculiar surface deposit of reduced osmium. ×19,000. (e) Lipid spheres (ls) pass from the cell into the endocuticle (en) by eversion of the apical plasma membrane. They are stored as distinct lipid deposits (ld). ×9,300.

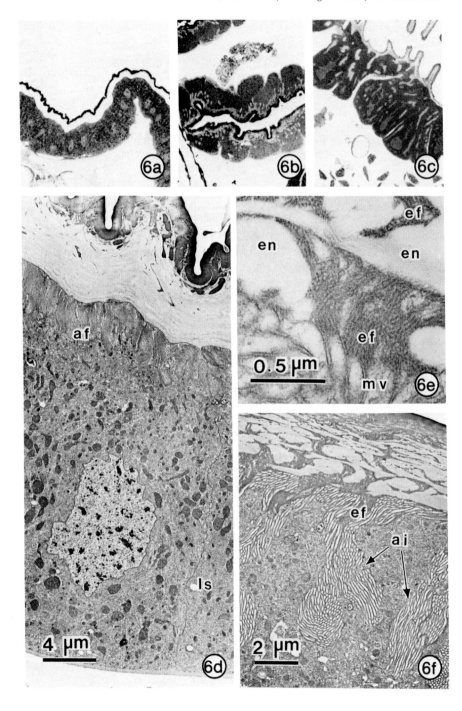

(Figs. 7b and 7c). In the unicorn caterpillar, *Schizura unicornis,* a single long, internal sac with a funnel-shaped orifice is found ventrally in the intersegmental membrane (Fig. 7d). In the red-humped caterpillar, *S. concinna,* modified cells are located in the dorsal part of the intersegmental membrane and in the valves (Fig. 7e). In the moonspot, *Phalera bucephala,* there is a dorsal scent field in the intersegmental membrane which is protruded during calling (Urbahn, 1913). Both *Clostera pigra* and *C. curtula* have ring glands formed from the distal half of the eighth/ninth intersegmental membrane; the gland is better developed ventrally, but the entire structure is everted during calling (Urbahn, 1913).

14. Arctiidae

Seven species of Arctiidae have been examined. There was no evidence of hyperdeveloped cells in the terminal abdominal segments of *Platarcha parthenos.* In the scarlet tiger moth, *Callimorpha dominula* (Urbahn, 1913); *Tyria jacobeae;* and *Utetheisa ornatrix* (Conner *et al.,* 1980) there are dorsally situated internal noneversible tubes. The tubes are forked and extend internally to the seventh segment, they open with a funnel-shaped opening in the eighth/ninth intersegmental membrane. The cells are modified columnar cells and are separated from each other near the bases. The surface of the cuticle is covered with a thick layer of spines. In *T. jacobeae* and *C. dominula* there are also two ventrolateral scent pits opening at two grooved depressions in the eighth/ninth intersegmental membrane (Urbahn, 1913). It has been shown that *Utetheisa ornatrix* pulse-releases its pheromone during calling as exemplified by the rhythmic extrusion of the terminal abdominal segments (Conner *et al.,* 1980).

In the fall webworm, *Hyphantria cunea,* the gland is not as large but is also composed of the dorsal part of the intersegmental membrane. It is invaginated deeply within the insect so as to make a W shape in cross section. Cells are columnar, and the cuticle is covered by a dense mat of spines (Lee *et al.,* 1983). In the saltmarsh caterpillar, *Estigmene acrea,* there are several areas of hyperdeveloped cells. They are found on the internal ventral surface of the dorsal part of the papillae anales, laterally on the ninth segment, and ventrally on the internal surface of the papillae anales. They are not found on the tergum of the

---

Fig. 6. Sphingidae, *Daphnis nerii.* (a) The ventrolateral patches contain cuboidal cells and are located anteriorly within the intersegmental membrane. ×240. (b) The deep dorsolateral folds contain modified goblet cells and are found posteriorly within the intersegmental membrane. ×250. (c) The epidermal cells of the valves are enlarged and goblet shaped. ×280. (d) The cuboidal cells of the ventrolateral patches have apical folds (af) and contain very few lipid spheres (ls). ×3700. (e) Within the cuticle overlying the cells of the dorsolateral folds the epicuticular filaments (ef) completely fill all pore canals of the endocuticle (en) and are especially noticeable near the microvilli (mv). ×40,700. (f) Each of the cells of the dorsolateral folds has several apical involutions (ai). The epicuticular filaments (ef) fill the invaginations formed by the apical involutions. ×6000.

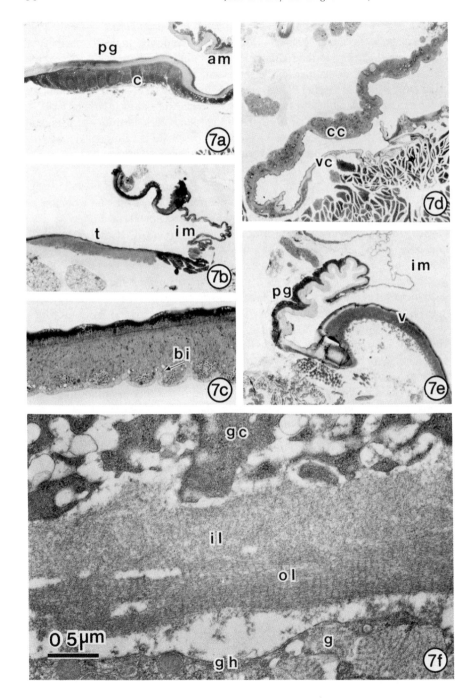

ninth segment or on the dorsal part of the eighth/ninth intersegmental membrane. The cells are cuboidal, and the cuticle is covered with a thick layer of spines. The ventral part of the intersegmental membrane has internal tubular structures, which can be everted only under extreme pressure. The cells of this gland are also cuboidal. Behavioral bioassays elicit sexual responses from all areas except the ventral internal tubular glands (MacFarlane and Earle, 1970).

15. Lymantriidae

The lymantriids are somewhat more consistent than other families in that, of the 12 species examined, all but two have the pheromone gland present as a dorsal modification of the intersegmental membrane. The species include the pine tussock moth, *Dasychira pinicola* (J. E. Percy and J. A. MacDonald, unpublished observations); the whitemarked tussock moth, *Orgyia leucostigma* (Percy *et al.*, 1971; Percy, 1975); *O. vetusta* (Percy, 1975); *Euproctis similis; Penthophora morio; O. gonostigma;* the rusty tussock moth, *O. antiqua; Dasychira selentica;* the pale tussock moth, *D. pudibunda;* and *D. fascelina* (Urbahn, 1913). The glands are crescent shaped and extend laterally to the point of the insertion of the posterior apophyses. The cells are goblet shaped, clustered around internal extensions of the endocuticle as illustrated for *D. pinicola* (Fig. 8).

The two exceptions to the above pattern are the nun moth, *Lymantria monacha*, where no hyperdeveloped cells were found (Urbahn, 1913), and the gypsy moth, *Lymantria dispar*, where both dorsal and ventral portions of the intersegmental membrane form the sex pheromone gland (Hollander *et al.*, 1982). The dorsal part is mainly composed of columnar cells although there are some cuboidal and goblet cells; the ventral part is composed of only cuboidal cells. Both parts produce positive responses in bioassays. All species disseminate pheromone through rhythmic protrusion and retraction of the terminal abdominal segments.

Fig. 7. Notodontidae. (a) *Datana ministra.* The presumed gland (pg) is found posteriorly and dorsally within the intersegmental membrane. The anterior part of the intersegmental membrane (am) is unmodified. The cells (c) are columnar. ×95. (b) *Heterocampa guttivitta.* The presumed gland is found medially within the ninth tergite (t). The intersegmental membrane (im) is unmodified. ×85. (c) *Heterocampa guttivitta.* The cells are columnar but are modified somewhat with deep peripheral involutions of the basal plasma membrane (bi). ×420. (d) *Schizura unicornis.* The presumed gland is a single, long internal sac found ventrally within the intersegmental membrane. The cells located dorsally within the sac are columnar (cc); the ventral cells are unmodified (vc). ×125. (e) *Schizura concinna.* The presumed gland (pg) is located dorsally within the intersegmental membrane (im) and the valves (v). The cells in both regions are columnar. ×45. (f) *Datana ministra.* A bilayered basal lamina underlies the presumed gland cells (gc). The inner layer (il) is amorphous while the outer layer (ol) is banded and appears to be formed from the contents of granules (g) within the underlying granular hemocytes (gh). ×30,200.

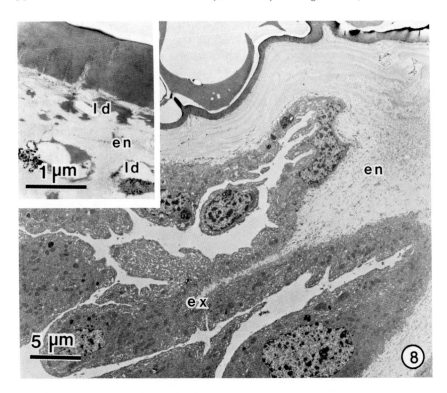

Fig. 8. Lymantriidae, *Dasychira pinicola*. The gland cells are goblet shaped and are clustered around inward extensions (ex) of endocuticle (en). ×2850. *Insert:* Lipid deposits (ld) are present within the endocuticle (en) even though lipid spheres do not accumulate in the cells. ×16,300.

16. Noctuidae

There have been more species examined in the Noctuidae than in other families. The species are representative of eight subfamilies.

a. *Plusiinae.*   The five species examined to date include the cabbage looper, *Trichoplusia ni* (Jefferson *et al.*, 1966; Miller *et al.*, 1967; Percy, 1978b, 1979); the alfalfa looper, *Autographa californica; Rachiplusia ou;* the soybean looper, *Pseudoplusia includens* (Jefferson *et al.*, 1968); and *Syngrapha circumflexa* (Hammad, 1961). In all species except the last, the gland is a dorsal modification of the intersegmental membrane. In *S. circumflexa* the gland is a ring gland. Gland cells are columnar and contain lipid spheres.

b. *Sarrothripinae.*   In *Erias insulana* the gland is a ring-shaped gland and is composed of columnar cells (Hammad, 1961).

During this time, (1) the microvilli change in appearance to those characteristic of adult cells; (2) smooth endoplasmic reticulum begins to appear to replace the large amounts of rough endoplasmic reticulum; (3) lipid deposits accumulate; (4) glycogen deposits accumulate; and (5) the shape of the cells changes. In short, the cells are changing from primarily protein-secreting cells to primarily lipid-secreting cells.

4. Mature Adult Gland Cells

The specific morphological features characteristic of mature adult gland cells are often distinctive for each species. However, there are certain similarities in the organelles which predominate in cells during the time when insects are most attractive to males. Generally, whether the female remains a virgin or mates, there is little visible difference in the ultrastructural appearance of gland cells during its adult life. This would lead one to speculate that the amount of pheromone manufactured by the insect is in excess of what is needed.

a. *Plasma Membrane.* The basal plasma membrane of gland cells has extensive basal involutions, the function of which is presumably to provide a larger surface area for the uptake of pheromone precursors (Percy, 1979). The extent to which the basal involutions may reach within the presumed gland cells is best exemplified by the geometriids where the basal plasma membrane nearly apposes the apical plasma membrane (see Fig. 4c). It is also interesting that in these particular glands the basal lamina follows the plasma membrane. This has not been observed in glands of other insects.

The apical membrane of all gland cells has an increased surface area produced by the presence of microvilli or apical folds. Tent caterpillar gland cells have a further modification with the apical membrane being enlarged and everted as well as containing microvilli (see Figs. 5b and 5e). This is the opposite of the inverted apical membrane of the tussock moths (Fig. 8); the geometriid, *Petrophora subaequaria* (Fig. 4a); and the sphingid, *Daphnis nerii* (Fig. 6d). Microvilli contain a tubule of smooth endoplasmic reticulum throughout their length (*Vitula edmandsae,* Fig. 3d). Penetration of microvilli with smooth endoplasmic reticulum has also been reported for cells of other epidermal glands (Percy *et al.,* 1980, 1983). It is noteworthy that these cells, in which the structure of the microvilli is basically similar, all secrete lipid-soluble substances. However, other sex pheromone glands have apical folds which have no internal organization, for example, *Bombyx mori* (Steinbrecht, 1964a), *Lobesia botrana* (Lalanne-Cassou *et al.,* 1977), and *Argyrotaenia velutinana* (Feng and Roelofs, 1977). The lack of internal organization is not characteristic of all lipid-producing epidermal glands with folds since certain of these types of glands have a complex interrelationship with the smooth endoplasmic reticulum (Percy and MacDonald, 1979; Waku and Foldi, 1984; Weatherston *et al.,* 1986). The dif-

certain that the presence of smooth endoplasmic reticulum is indicative of lipid synthesis in pheromone gland cells as is the case in other lipid-secreting cells.

There is some variability in the type of smooth endoplasmic reticulum encountered and the position it occupies within the cells. For example, in the spruce budworm it is tubular and mainly located between the nucleus and the apical membrane although there is some near the lipid spheres (Percy, 1974). In the tussock moth it is both cisternal and tubular and, when present, is located throughout the cell (Percy, 1975). In the cabbage looper it is mainly tubular and is located primarily near the lipid spheres (Percy, 1979). In *Lobesia botrana* it is tubular and is present throughout the cells (Lalanne-Cassou *et al.*, 1977). The presence of smooth cisternal endoplasmic reticulum in the tussock moths does not seem to be related to the lack of lipid spheres, since in several other species the presumed pheromone gland cells have neither cisternal endoplasmic reticulum nor lipid spheres. However, the ages of the latter group were unknown since they were field-collected insects.

Other organelles which appear to be universally characteristic of these pheromone gland cells are the microbodies. These organelles have been found in many cells but are especially prominent in cells engaged in the metabolism of cholesterol, steroids, and lipids (Tolbert and Essner, 1981). They have also been found in all 26 species in which we found hyperdeveloped cells in the terminal abdominal segments. In several species, they occur in large numbers during the time when females are most attractive to males and therefore during the time when most pheromone is being produced. In three species, it has also been shown that these organelles are in fact spherical to cylindrical enlargements of the smooth tubular endoplasmic reticulum and that they contain a granular material which consists, at least in part, of the enzyme catalase. In the insects where catalase has been demonstrated in the microbodies, the organelles are more correctly called microperoxisomes (Figs. 10a–10c).

The microbodies are often more numerous near lipid spheres, indicating that they may be involved in its production or processing. In fact, as a result of the elucidation of the biosynthetic pathway of the pheromone in the cabbage looper, it seems likely that the microperoxisomes are responsible for chain-shortening the immediate precursors to the pheromone (Bjostad and Roelofs, 1983; Bjostad *et al.*, Chapter 3, this volume). The microbodies do not appear to be involved in the release of lipid from the cell, at least in the cabbage looper, since they are not associated with the lipid spheres when they are in the vicinity of the apical membrane and are being released from the cell to the cuticle (Percy, 1979).

d.   Glycogen.   Several of the species examined, including the spruce budworm (Percy, 1974) have deposits of glycogen within the cells. It is not known what relationship the glycogen bears toward pheromone synthesis although it is

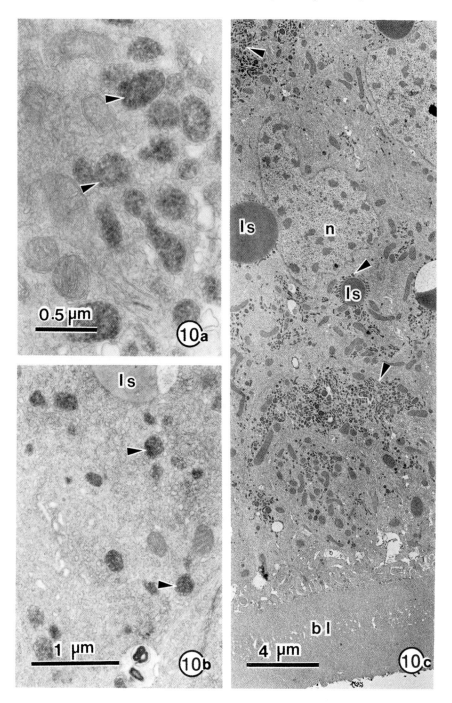

known that smooth endoplasmic reticulum participates in glycogenolysis (Fawcett, 1981).

e. *Gland Cuticle.* The structural characteristics of the cuticle overlying the gland cells differ only in two respects from those of cuticle overlying unmodified epidermal cells. First, the number of epicuticular filaments are frequently very much greater in the gland cuticle. The filaments may form a very dense mat under the epicuticle as in *Vitula edmandsae* (see Fig. 3c) or the tent caterpillar (Fig. 5c); they may be particularly noticeable near the apical membrane where they are found between the apical folds (Lalanne-Cassou *et al.,* 1977) or within the inversions of the apical membrane where they may penetrate the cell for some distance as in cells of the dorsolateral fold of the sphingid, *Daphnis nerii* (Figs. 6e and 6f). These filaments thus seem to be related to the pheromone but are not a structural representation of free lipid in the cuticle, since they are structurally unaltered after extraction with hexane or methylene chloride. They do change, however, in both modified and unmodified cuticle, after extraction with chloroform/methanol (Percy, 1975, 1978a).

Gland cuticle also differs from unmodified cuticle in some species where its function in the storage and transport of lipid is easily determined from the presence of distinct deposits of lipid. The lipid passes from the gland cell into the cuticle by eversion of the apical plasma membrane and is stored there while still within the confines of the cell membrane (Fig. 5e). Near the outer layers of the cuticle a filamentous form of lipid appears and passes through pores to lie on the external surface of the cuticle (Figs. 2b and 2c) (Percy, 1978a, 1979). These relationships have been studied in some detail in the cabbage looper, but survey studies of gland cells in other species indicate a similar pattern when both lipid deposits and lipid filaments occur together, as illustrated for the geometriid, *Petrophora subaequaria* (Fig. 4b). The accumulation of lipid deposits does not occur in the gland cuticle of many species—these may or may not have lipid filaments in addition to the epicuticular filaments.

Assuming that the lipid stored within the cuticle represents (or includes) the pheromone, then several explanations may be given for its appearance in some species and not in others: (1) more pheromone may be produced by the cells in glands with lipid stored in the cuticle; (2) the insect may be more parsimonious in

Fig. 10. Positive reaction for catalase as exhibited by microbodies when incubated in alkaline DAB (diaminobenzidine) medium containing hydrogen peroxide. (a) *Orgyia leucostigma.* Both elongate and circular profiles of microperoxisomes (arrows) are observed within the cells. ×33,500. (b) *Choristoneura fumiferana.* Circular profiles of microperoxisomes (arrows) are observed near but not adjacent to a lipid sphere. ×24,240. (c) *Trichoplusia ni.* Low magnification to illustrate the immense number of microperoxisomes (arrows), particularly adjacent to the lipid spheres (ls). Basal lamina (bl) and nucleus (n) are also shown. ×5900.

its use of pheromone than other species; or (3) only in those species with stored lipid is the pheromone present in the cuticle as free lipid. In other insects, the pheromone may be present as lipoproteins or phospholipids possibly bound as structural components of the cuticle, e.g., epicuticular filaments which would require an enzymatic reaction to release them.

Some storage of pheromone occurs on the surface of the pheromone glands. This is exemplified in representative sections of many species by an outer, uneven layer (see Fig. 5c) and, occasionally, by outer lipid filaments similar to those observed within cuticle (Figs. 2b and 2c). After solvent extraction of glands, an outer ''uneven'' layer (which also contains the lipid filaments) disappears entirely (Percy, 1975, 1978a). The solvents used are the lipid solvents, hexane and methylene chloride, which are also used in the extraction of pheromones. This outer layer of insect cuticle, the so-called wax layer, is found on the surface of all insects (Neville, 1975). The uneven layer is extracted from the gland cuticle using lipid solvents; therefore, it is safe to assume that this layer represents the wax layer which in a pheromone gland cuticle consists, at least in part, of the sex pheromone.

V. CONCLUDING REMARKS

Over the past decade, considerable information has accumulated concerning the structure of the cells and cuticle comprising sex pheromone glands, but the studies are far from complete and the biochemical elucidation of the structural–functional interrelationships has barely begun. Of specific importance in the general study of lipid biosynthesis and transport is the role played by the modified microvilli. It would also be most beneficial to elucidate the pathway of biosynthesis in gland cells where lipid spheres do not accumulate during pheromone production.

Finally, much benefit would be derived from a biochemical elucidation of the function of the individual cell types in those glands composed of several different gland cells. These are but a few of the investigative areas which are available to challenge pheromone scientists interested in complementary interdisciplinary ventures in the exciting field of pheromone research.

ACKNOWLEDGMENTS

The results of research reported herein were obtained while the senior author (J. E. P.-C.) was employed at the Forest Pest Management Institute. Gratitude is extended to the Director, Dr. George Green, for assistance during preparation of the manuscript. We also thank Dr. J. Weatherston for his critical review of the manuscript and Mrs. Irene Cunningham for her assistance with the proofreading.

REFERENCES

Adessan, C., Tamhankar, A. J., and Rahalkar, G. W. (1969). Sex pheromone gland in the potato tuberworm moth, *Phthorimaea operculella*. *Ann. Entomol. Soc. Am.* **62,** 670–671.

Agren, L., Cederberg, B., and Swensson, B. G. (1979). Changes with age in ultrastructure and content of male labial glands in some bumblebee species (Hymenoptera, Apidae). *Zoon* **7,** 1–14.

Ahmed, I., Afzal, M., and Islam, M. Z. (1977). Studies on the pheromone glands of *Tryporyza incertulas* (Walker) (Lepidoptera: Pyralidoidea). *Philos. J. Sci.* **106,** 147–164.

Aldrich, J. R., Blum, M. S., Lloyd, H. A., and Fales, H. M. (1978). Pentatomid natural products. Chemistry and morphology of III–IV dorsal abdominal glands of adults. *J. Chem. Ecol.* **4,** 161–172.

Atkinson, P. R. (1982). Structure of the putative pheromone glands of *Eldana saccharina* Walker (Lepidoptera: Pyralidae). *J. Entomol. Soc. S. Africa* **45,** 93–104.

Aubrey, J. G., Boudreaux, H. B., Grodner, M. L., and Hammond, A. M. (1983). Sex pheromone producing cells and their associated cuticle in female *Heliothis zea* and *Heliothis virescens* (F.) (Lepidoptera: Noctuidae). *Ann. Entomol. Soc. Am.* **76,** 343–348.

Baer, R. G., Berisford, C. W., and Hermann, H. R. (1976). Bioassay, histology and morphology of the pheromone-producing glands of *Rhyacionia frustrana*, *R. rigidana* and *R. subtropica*. *Ann. Entomol. Soc. Am.* **69,** 307–310.

Barnes, M. M., Peterson, D. M., and O'Connor, J. J. (1966). Sex pheromone gland in the female codling moth, *Carpocapsa pomonella* (Lepidoptera: Olethreutidae). *Ann. Entomol. Soc. Am.* **59,** 732–734.

Barth, R. (1937). Herkunft, Wirkung und Eigenschaften des Weiblichen Sexualduftstoffes einiger Pyraliden. *Zool. Jahrbucher* **5,** 653–662.

Barth, R. (1960). Sobre a glandula abdominal da femea de *Citheronia laocoon* (Cr., 1777) (Lepidoptera: Adeocephalidae). *Inst. Oswaldo Cruz Mem.* **58,** 125–128.

Barth, R. (1961). Die Drusenorgane des weibchens von *Prodenia ornithogalli* Gn. (Lepidoptera: Noctuidae). *An. Acad. Brasil Ciencas* **33,** 429–433.

Birch, M. (1970). Structure and function of pheromone-producing brush organs in males of *Phlogophora meticulosa* (L.) (Lepidoptera: Noctuidae). *Trans. R. Entomol. Soc. London* **122,** 277–292.

Bjostad, L. B., and Roelofs, W. L. (1983). Sex pheromone biosynthesis in *Trichoplusia ni:* Key steps involve Δ^{11} desaturation and chain-shortening. *Science* **220,** 1387–1389.

Bode, W. (1978). Ultrastructure of the sternal glands in *Thrips validus* Uzel (Thysanoptera, Terebrantia). *Zoomorphology* **90,** 53–65.

Bosman, T., and Brand, J. M. (1971). Biological studies of the sex pheromone of *Kotochalia junodi* Heyl. (Lepidoptera: Psychidae) and its partial purification. *J. Entomol. Soc. S. Africa* **34,** 73–78.

Bronskill, J. (1970). Permanent whole mount preparation of lepidopterous genitalia for complete visibility of the female sex pheromone gland. *Ann. Entomol. Soc. Am.* **63,** 898–900.

Buschinger, A., and Alloway, T. A. (1979). Sexual behaviour in the slave-making ant, *Harpagoxenus canadensis* M. R. Smith, and sexual pheromone experiments with *H. canadensis*, *H. americanus* (Emery), and *H. sublaevis* (Nylander) (Hymenoptera: Formicidae). *Z. Tierpsychol.* **49,** 113–119.

Carayon, J. (1981). Dimorphisme sexuel des glandes tegumentaires et production de pheromone chez les Hemipteres Pentatomoidea. *C. R. Acad. Sci. III* **292,** 867.

Cazals, M., and Juberthie-Jupeau, L. (1983). Ultrastructure d'une glande sternale tubuleuse des males de *Speonomus hydrophilus* (Coleoptera: Bathysciinae). *Can. J. Zool.* **61,** 673–681.

Chow, Y. S., Chen, J., and Chow, S. L. (1976). Anatomy of the female sex pheromone gland of the diamondback moth, *Plutella xylostella*. (Lepidoptera: Plutellidae). *Int. J. Insect Morphol. Embryol.* **5**, 197–203.

Clearwater, J. R. (1975a). Structure, development and evolution of the male pheromone system in some Noctuidae (Lepidoptera). *J. Morphol.* **146**, 129–176.

Clearwater, J. R. (1975b). Synthesis of a pheromone precursor in the male noctuid moth, *Mamestra configurata. J. Insect Biochem.* **5**, 737–746.

Clearwater, J. R. (1975c). Pheromone metabolism in male *Pseudoletia separata* (Walk) and *Mamestra configurata* (Walk) (Lepidoptera: Noctuidae). *Comp. Biochem. Physiol. B* **50**, 77–82.

Conner, W. E., Eisner, T., Van der Meer, R. K., Guerrero, A., Ghiringelli, D., and Meinwald, J. (1980). Sex attractant of an arctiid moth *(Utetheisa ornatrix),* a pulsed chemical signal. *Behav. Ecol. Sociobiol.* **7**, 55–63.

Corbet, S. A., and Lai-Fook, J. (1977). The hairpencils of the flour moth, *Ephestia kuehniella. J. Zool. (London)* **181**, 377–394.

Crossley, A. C., and Waterhouse, D. F. (1969). The ultrastructure of a pheromone-secreting gland in the male scorpion-fly, *Harpobittacus australis* (Bittacidae: Mecoptera). *Tiss. Cell.* **1**, 273–294.

DasGupta, B. (1979). Brush organ of male *Seminothesis eleonora* (Lepidoptera: Geometridae). *Zool. Anz.* **203**, 182–188.

de Martino, C., Natali, P. G., Bruni, C. B., and Accini, L. (1968). Influence of plastic embedding media on staining and morphology of lipid bodies. *Histochemie* **16**, 350–360.

De Marzo, L., and Vit, S. (1983). Antennal male glands of *Batrisus* and *Batrisodes:* Morphology, histology and taxonomic implications. *Entomologia* **18**, 77–110.

Dickens, G. P. (1936). The scent glands of certain Phycitidae. *Trans. R. Entomol. Soc. London* **85**, 331–362.

Economopoulos, A. P., Giasnnakakis, A., Tzanakakis, M. E., and Voyadjoglou, A. V. (1971). Reproductive behaviour and physiology of the olive fruit fly. I. Anatomy of the adult rectum and odours emitted by adults. *Ann. Entomol. Soc. Am.* **64**, 1112–1116.

Elofsson, R., and Lofqvist, J. (1974). The Eltringham organ and a new thoracic gland: Ultrastructure and presumed pheromone function. (Insecta, Myrmeieontidae). *Zool. Scripta* **3**, 31–40.

El-Sawaf, B. M., Kashef, A. H., and Soliman, A. A. (1968). Development and histology of the scent gland in the cotton leafworm, *Prodenia litura* F. and the pink bollworm, *Pectinophora gossypiella* S. (Lepidoptera). *Zeit. Agnew. Entomol.* **61**, 229–239.

Fatzinger, C. W. (1972). Bioassay, morphology and histology of the female sex pheromone gland of *Dioryctria abietiella* [Lepidoptera: Pyralidae (Phycitinae)]. *Ann. Entomol. Soc. Am.* **65**, 1208–1214.

Fawcett, D. W. (1981). "The Cell," 2nd Ed. Saunders, Philadelphia.

Feng, K. C., and Roelofs, W. (1977). Sex pheromone gland development in redbanded leafroller moth, *Argyrotaenia velutinana*, pupae and adults. *Ann. Entomol. Soc. Am.* **70**, 721–732.

Fletcher, B. S. (1969). The structure and function of the sex pheromone glands in the male Queensland fruit fly. *J. Insect Physiol.* **15**, 1309–1322.

George, J. A. (1965). Sex pheromone of the oriental fruit moth, *Grapholitha molesta* (Busck) (Lepidoptera: Tortricidae). *Can. Entomol.* **97**, 1002–1007.

George, J. A., and Mullins, J. (1980). Hairpencils on males of the oriental fruit moth, *Grapholitha molesta* (Busck) (Lepidoptera: Tortricidae). *Proc. Entomol. Soc. Ont.* **111**, 21–31.

Glauert, A. M. (1975). Fixation, dehydration and embedding of biological specimens. *In* "Practical Methods in Electron Microscopy," (A. M. Glauert, ed.), Vol. 3, Part 1. North Holland, Amsterdam.

Grant, G. G. (1978). Morphology of the presumed pheromone glands on the forewings of tortricid and phycitid moths. *Ann. Entomol. Soc. Am.* **71**, 423–431.

Gupta, B. D. (1978). Sex pheromone of *Poecilocerus pictus* (Fabricus) (Acridoidea: Pyrogomorphidae): I. Experimental identification and external morphology of the female sex pheromone gland. *Biochem. Exp. Biol.* **14**, 143–148.

Hallberg, E., and Lofqvist, J. (1981). Morphology and ultrastructure of an intertergal pheromone gland in the abdomen of the pine sawfly *Neodiprion sertifer* (Insecta, Hymenoptera): A potential source of sex pheromones. *Can. J. Zool.* **59**, 47–53.

Hammack, L., Burkholder, W. E., and Ma, M. (1973). Sex pheromone localization in females of six *Trogoderma* species. *Ann. Entomol. Soc. Am.* **66**, 545–550.

Hammad, S. M. (1961). The morphology and histology of the sexual scent glands in certain female lepidopterous moths. *Bull. Soc. Ent. Egypt* **45**, 471–482.

Han, S. S., Nam, S. H., Kim, W. K., and Kim, C. W. (1979). A morphological study on the sex pheromone gland in the Indian meal moth, *Plodia interpunctella* Hubner. *Kor. J. Entomol.* **9**, 11–13.

Hayat, M. A. (1970). "Principles and Techniques of Electron Microscopy." Vol. 1. Van Nostrand-Reinhold, Toronto.

Hayat, M. A. (1972). "Basic Electron Microscopy Techniques." Van Nostrand-Reinhold, Toronto.

Hendricks, G. M., and Hadley, N. F. (1983). Structure of the cuticle of the common house cricket with location of lipids. *Tiss. Cell.* **15**, 761–779.

Hodosh, R. J., Keough, E. M., and Ringo, J. M. (1979). The morphology of the sex pheromone gland in *Drosophila grimshawi*. *J. Morphol.* **161**, 177–184.

Hollander, A. L., Yin, C. M., and Schwallse, C. P. (1982). Location, morphology and histology of sex pheromone glands of the female gypsy moth, *Lymantria dispar* (L.). *J. Insect Physiol.* **28**, 513–518.

Humasson, G. L. (1967). "Animal Tissue Techniques," 2nd Ed. Freeman, San Francisco, California.

Ismail, M. T., and Kremer, M. (1983). Determination of the site of pheromone emission in the virgin female *Culicoides nubeculosus* Mg. (Diptera, Ceratopogonidae). *J. Insect Physiol.* **29**, 221–224.

Ismail, M. T., and Zachary, D. (1984). Sex pheromones in *Culicoides nubeculosus* (Diptera: Ceratopogonidae): Possible sites of production and emission. *J. Chem. Ecol.* **10**, 1385–1398.

Jefferson, R. N., Shorey, H. H., and Gaston, L. K. (1966). Sex pheromones of noctuid moths. X. The morphology and histology of the female sex pheromone gland of *Trichoplusia ni* (Lepidoptera: Noctuidae). *Ann. Entomol. Soc. Am.* **59**, 1166–1169.

Jefferson, R. N., Shorey, H. H., and Rubin, R. E. (1968). Sex pheromones of noctuid moths. XVI. The morphology of the female sex pheromone glands of eight species. *Ann. Entomol. Soc. Am.* **61**, 861–865.

Jefferson, R. N., Sower, L. L., and Rubin, R. E. (1971). The female sex pheromone gland of the pink bollworm, *Pectinophora gossypiella* (Lepidoptera: Gelechiidae). *Ann. Entomol. Soc. Am.* **64**, 311–312.

Juberthie-Jupeau, L., and Cazals, M. (1984). Physiologie animale. Les differentes types de la glande sternale tubuleuse propre aux males de certains Coleopteres Bathysciinae souterraines. *C. R. Acad. Sci.* **298**, 14.

Kawakami, T., and Tanaka, T. (1978). Surface structure of the alluring gland in the Eri-silkmoth, *Philosamia cynthia ricini* D. (Lepidoptera: Saturniidae)—Opening of the sex pheromone secretory duct. *Appl. Entomol. Zool.* **13**, 12–17.

Lalanne-Cassou, B., Percy, J., and MacDonald, J. A. (1977). Ultrastructure of sex pheromone gland cells in *Lobesia botrana* Den & Schiff (Lepidoptera: Olethreutinae). *Can. J. Zool.* **55**, 672–680.

Lee, J. J., Lee, H. P., and Lee, K. R. (1983). Morphological studies on sex pheromone gland and chemoreceptor of the fall webworm, *Hyphantria cunea* Drury. *Kor. J. Entomol.* **13**, 61–66.

Leonhardt, B. A., Neal, J. W., Jr., Klun, J. A., Schwartz, M., and Plimmer, J. R. (1983). An unusual lepidopteran sex pheromone system in the bagworm moth. *Science* **219**, 314–316.

Leuthold, R. H., and Bruinsma, O. (1977). Pairing behaviour in *Hodotermes mossambicus* (Isoptera). *Psyche* **84**, 109–119.

Leuthold, R. H., and Luscher, M. (1974). An unusual caste polymorphism of the sternal gland and its trail pheromone production in the termite, *Trinervitermes bettonianus*. *Insectes Soc.* **21**, 335–342.

Levinson, H. Z., Levinson, A. R., Kahn, G. E., and Schafer, K. (1983). Occurrence of a pheromone producing gland in female tobacco beetles. *Experientia* **39**, 1095–1097.

Lew, A. C., and Ball, H. J. (1978). The structure of apparent pheromone-secreting cells in female *Diabrotica virgifera*. *Ann. Entomol. Soc. Am.* **71**, 685–688.

Locke, M. (1969). The structure of an epidermal cell during the development of the protein epicuticle and the uptake of moulting fluid in an insect. *J. Morphol.* **127**, 7–40.

Locke, M., and McMahon, J. T. (1971). The origin and fate of microbodies in the fat body of an insect. *J. Cell Biol.* **48**, 61–78.

MacFarlane, J. H., and Earle, N. W. (1970). Morphology and histology of the female sex pheromone gland of the salt-marsh caterpillar, *Estigmene acrea*. *Ann. Entomol. Soc. Am.* **63**, 1327–1331.

Mackley, J. W., and Broce, A. B. (1981). Evidence of a female sex recognition pheromone in the screwworm fly, *Cochliomyia hominivorax*. *Environ. Entomol.* **10**, 406–408.

Menon, M. (1981). Morphological evidence for probable secreting site for the pheromone "seducin" in males of *Nauphoeta cinerea*. 1. Light microscope studies. *J. Morphol.* **168**, 229–237.

Menon, M. (1986). Morphological evidence for a probable secretory site of the male sex pheromones of *Nauphoeta cinerea* (Blattaria, Blaberidae). 2. Electron microscope studies. *J. Morphol.* **187**, 69–79.

Miller, J. R., and Roelofs, W. L. (1970). Sex pheromone titer correlated with pheromone gland development and age in the redbanded leafroller moth, *Argyrotaenia velutinana*. *Ann. Entomol. Soc. Am.* **70**, 136–139.

Miller, T., Jefferson, R. N., and Thomson, W. W. (1967). Sex pheromones of noctuid moths. XI. The ultrastructure of the apical region of cells of the female sex pheromone gland of *Trichoplusia ni*. *Ann. Entomol. Soc. Am.* **60**, 707–708.

Neville, A. C. (1975). "Biology of the Arthropod Cuticle." Springer-Verlag, New York.

Nielson, M. (1979). Morphologie de la glande a pheromone sexuelle male de *Phragmatobia fuliginosa* (Arctiidae). *Arch. Biol. (Bruxelles)* **90**, 161–176.

Nielson, M. (1982). Glande aphrodisiac de *Phragmatobia fuliginosa* (Lepidoptera: Arctiidae). *An. Soc. R. Zool. Belg.* **112**, 61–67.

Noirot, C., and Quennedey, A. (1974). Fine structure of insect epidermal glands. *Ann. Rev. Entomol.* **19**, 61–80.

Novikoff, A. B., Novikoff, P. M., Davis, C., and Quintana, N. (1972). Studies on microperoxisomes. II. A cytochemical method for light and electron microscopy. *J. Histochem. Cytochem.* **20**, 1006–1023.

Novikoff, A. B., Novikoff, P. M., Rosen, O. M., and Rubin, C. S. (1980). Organelle relationships in cultured 3T3-L1 preadipocytes. *J. Cell Biol.* **87**, 180–196.

Ostaff, D. P., Shepherd, R. F., and Borden, J. H. (1974). Sex attraction and courtship behavior in *Lambdina fiscellaria lugubrosa* (Lepidoptera: Geometridae). *Can. Entomol.* **106**, 493–501.

Percy, J. E. (1974). Ultrastructure of sex pheromone gland cells and cuticle before and during release of pheromone in female eastern spruce budworm, *Choristoneura fumiferana* (Clem.) (Lepidoptera: Tortricidae). *Can. J. Zool.* **52**, 695–705.

Percy, J. E. (1975). Development and ultrastructure of cells of the sex pheromone gland in the whitemarked tussock moth, *Orgyia leucostigma* (Lepidoptera: Lymantriidae). *Int. J. Insect Morphol. Embryol.* **4,** 567–579.

Percy, J. E. (1978a). Structure and function of glands producing airborne semiochemicals in four species of Lepidoptera. Ph.D. thesis, University of Western Ontario, London, Ontario, Canada.

Percy, J. E. (1978b). Haemocytes associated with the basement membrane of the sex pheromone gland of *Trichoplusia ni* (Lepidoptera: Noctuidae). Ultrastructural observations. *Can. J. Zool.* **56,** 238–245.

Percy, J. E. (1979). Development and ultrastructure of sex pheromone gland cells of the cabbage looper moth, *Trichoplusia ni* (Hubner) (Lepidoptera: Noctuidae). *Can. J. Zool.* **57,** 220–236.

Percy, J. E., and George, J. A. (1979). Abdominal musculature in relation to sex pheromone gland eversion in three species of Lepidoptera. *Can. Entomol.* **111,** 817–825.

Percy, J. E., and MacDonald, J. A. (1979). Cells of the thoracic defensive gland of the red-humped caterpillar, *Schizura concinna* (J. E. Smith) (Lepidoptera: Notodontidae): Ultrastructural observations. *Can. J. Zool.* **57,** 80–94.

Percy, J. E., and Weatherston, J. (1971). Studies of physiologically active arthropod secretions. IX. Morphology and histology of the pheromone producing glands of some female Lepidoptera. *Can. Entomol.* **103,** 1733–1739.

Percy, J. E., and Weatherston, J. (1974). Gland structure and pheromone production in insects. *In* "Pheromones, Frontiers of Biology" (M. Birch, ed.), Vol. 32, pp. 12–34. North Holland, Amsterdam.

Percy, J. E., Gardiner, E. J., and Weatherston, J. (1971). Studies of physiologically active arthropod secretions. VI. Evidence for a sex pheromone in *Orgyia leucostigma* (Lepidoptera: Lymantriidae). *Can. Entomol.* **103,** 706–712.

Percy, J. E., MacDonald, J. A., and Weatherston, J. (1980). Ultrastructure of scent glands in larvae of *Apateticus bracteatus* (Hemiptera: Pentatomidae) and the chemical composition of the secretion. *Can. J. Zool.* **58,** 2015–2115.

Percy, J. E., Blomquist, G. J., and MacDonald, J. A. (1983). The wax-secreting glands of *Eriocampa ovata* L. (Hymenoptera: Tenthredinidae): Ultrastructural observations and chemical composition of the wax. *Can. J. Zool.* **61,** 1797–1804.

Peschke, K. (1978). The female sex pheromone gland of the staphylinid beetle *Aleochara cartula*. *J. Insect Physiol.* **24,** 197–200.

Quennedey, A. (1978). Les glandes exocrines des termites; ultrastructure comparee des glandes sternales et frontales. Ph.D. thesis, Universite de Dijon, Dijon, France.

Quennedey, A., and Leuthold, R. H. (1978). Fine structure and pheromonal properties of the polymorphic sternal gland in *Trinervitermes bettonianus* (Isoptera: Termitidae). *Insectes Soc.* **25,** 153–162.

Robinson, M. H., and Robinson, B. (1979). By dawn's early light: Matutinal mating and sex attractants in a neotropical mantid. *Science* **205,** 825–827.

Roelofs, W. L., and Feng, K. C. (1968). Sex pheromone specificity tests in the Tortricidae—an introductory report. *Ann. Entomol. Soc. Am.* **61,** 312–316.

Roemhild, G. (1980). Pheromone glands of microcaddisflies, (Trichoptera: Hydroptilidae). *J. Morphol.* **163,** 9–12.

Sedlak, B., and Gilbert, L. I. (1976). Epidermal cell development during the pupal–adult metamorphosis of *Hyalophora cecropia*. *Tiss. Cell.* **4,** 637–648.

Singh, T., and Gupta, S. (1982). Morphology and histology of the mandibular gland in *Cincindela sexpunctata* (Coleoptera: Cincindelidae). *Uxtar Pradish J. Zool.* **2,** 14–18.

Smithwick, E. E. B. (1970). Development of the sex pheromone gland and of the production of sex pheromone in female Indian meal moth. Doctoral dissertation, University of Georgia, Athens.

Smithwick, E. B., and Brady, U. E. (1977a). Histology of the sex pheromone gland in developing female Indian meal moths, *Plodia interpunctella*. *J. Georgia Entomol. Soc.* **12**, 13–29.

Smithwick, E. B., and Brady, U. E. (1977b). Site and production of sex pheromone in developing female meal moths, *Plodia interpunctella*. *J. Georgia Entomol. Soc.* **12**, 1–13.

Snodgrass, R. E. (1935). "Principles of Insect Morphology." McGraw-Hill, New York.

Sreng, J. (1984). Morphology of the sternal and tergal glands producing the sexual pheromones and the aphrodisiacs among cockroaches of the subfamily Oxyhaloinae. *J. Morphol.* **182**, 279–294.

Srinivasan, A., Coffelt, J. A., and Oberlander, H. (1979). *In vitro* maintenance of the sex pheromone gland of the female Indian meal moth, *Plodia interpunctella* (Hubner). *J. Chem. Ecol.* **5**, 653–662.

Steinbrecht, R. A. (1964a). Feinstruktur und Histochemie der Sexualduftdruse des Seidenspinners *Bombyx mori* L. *Zeit. Zellforsch.* **64**, 227–261.

Steinbrecht, R. A. (1964b). Die Abhangigheit der Lockwirkung des Sexualduftorgans weiblicher seidenspinner (*Bombyx mori*) von alter und kopulation. *Z. Vergleich. Physiol.* **48**, 341–346.

Steinbrecht, R. A., and Schneider, D. (1964). Die Faltung du ausseren Zellmembran in den Sexu-allockstoff–Drusenzellen des Seidenspinners. *Naturwissenschaften* **51**, 41.

Su, C. Y., and Lee, W. Y. (1977). Study of morphological and histological structure of the female sex pheromone gland of the diamondback moth, *Plutella xylostella* (Lepidoptera: Plutellidae). *Plant Protection Bull.* **19**, 149–156.

Tagawa, J. (1977). Localization and histology of the female sex pheromone-producing gland in the parasitic wasp, *Apanteles glomeratus*. *J. Insect Physiol.* **23**, 49–56.

Tagawa, J. (1983). Female sex pheromone gland in the parasitic wasps, genus *Apanteles*. *Appl. Entomol. Zool.* **18**, 416–427.

Teal, P. E. A., and Philogene, B. J. R. (1980). The structure and function of the epidermal glands in the ovipositor of *Euxoa* species (Lepidoptera: Noctuidae). *Rev. Can. Biol.* **39**, 233–240.

Teal, P. E. A., Carlyle, T. C., and Tumlinson, J. H. (1983). Epidermal glands in terminal abdominal segments of female *Heliothis virescens* (F.) (Lepidoptera: Noctuidae). *Ann. Entomol. Soc. Am.* **76**, 242-247.

Thibout, E. (1972). Glandes exocrines males et femelles intervenant dans le comportement de pariade d'*Acrolepia assectiella* (Lepidoptera: Plutellidae). *Ann. Soc. Entomol. Fr. (N.S.)* **8**, 475–480.

Thornhill, A. R. (1973). The morphology and histology of new sex pheromone glands in male scorpionflies, *Panorpa* and *Brachypanorpa* (Mecoptera: Panorpidae and Panorpididae). *Great Lakes Entomol.* **6**, 47–55.

Tjeder, B. (1979). Presence of abdominal sacculi laterales in female of the subgenus *Emodotipula* (Diptera: Tipulidae). *Entomol. Scand.* **10**, 241–243.

Tolbert, N. G., and Essner, E. (1981). Microbodies: Peroxisomes and glyoxysomes. *J. Cell Biol.* **91**, 2715–2835.

Tribe, G. D. (1975). Pheromone release by dung beetles (Coleoptera: Scarabeidae). *S. African J. Sci.* **71**, 277–278.

Turgeon, J. T., McNeil, J., and Roelofs, W. L. (1983). Responsiveness of *Pseudoletia unipuncta* males to the female sex pheromone. *Physiol. Entomol.* **8**, 339–344.

Urbahn, E. (1913). Abdominale Duiftorgans bei weiblichen Schmetterlingen. *Z. Naturwiss.* **50**, 277–355.

Waku, Y., and Foldi, I. (1984). The fine structure of insect glands secreting waxy substances. *In* "Insect Ultrastructure" (R. C. King and H. Akai, eds.) Vol. 2, pp. 303–322. Plenum, New York.

Waku, Y., and Sumimoto, K. (1969). Ultrastructure and secretory mechanism of the alluring gland cells in the silkworm, *Bombyx mori* L. (Lepidoptera: Bombycidae). *Appl. Entomol. Zool.* **4,** 135–146.

Wattebled, S., Bitsch, J., and Rosset, A. (1978). Ultrastructure of pheromone-producing vesicles in males of *Chrysopa perla* L. (Insecta, Neuroptera). *Cell Tiss. Res.* **184,** 481–496.

Weatherston, J., and Percy, J. E. (1968). Studies of physiologically active arthropod secretions. 1. Evidence for a sex pheromone in female *Vitula edmandsae* (Lepidoptera: Phycitidae). *Can. Entomol.* **100,** 1065–1070.

Weatherston, J., and Percy, J. E. (1970). Studies of physiologically active arthropod secretions. IV. Topography of the sex pheromone producing gland of the eastern spruce budworm, *Choristoneura fumiferana* (Clem.) (Lepidoptera: Tortricidae). *Can. J. Zool.* **48,** 569–571.

Weatherston, J., and Percy, J. E. (1976). The biosynthesis of phenethyl alcohol in the male bertha armyworm, *Mamestra configurata. Insect Biochem.* **6,** 413–417.

Weatherston, J., MacDonald, J. A., Miller, D., Riere, G., Percy-Cunningham, J. E., and Benn, M. H. (1986). The ultrastructure of the exocrine prothoracic gland of *Datana ministra* (Drury) (Lepidoptera: Notodontidae) and the nature of its secretion. *J. Chem. Ecol.* **12,** 2039–2050.

Werner, R. A. (1977). Morphology and histology of the sex pheromone gland of a geometrid, *Rheumaptera hastata. Ann. Entomol. Soc. Am.* **70,** 264–266.

Weseloh, R. M. (1980). Sec pheromone gland of the gypsy moth parasitoid, *Apanteles melanoscelus:* Reevaluation and ultrastructural survey. *Ann. Entomol. Soc. Am.* **73,** 576–580.

Whalley, P. E. S. (1974). Scent dispersal mechanisms in the genus *Striglia* Guenee with a description of a new species (Lepidoptera: Thyrididae). *J. Entomol. (B)* **43,** 121–128.

White, M. R., Amborski, R. L., Hammond, A. M., and Amborski, C. F. (1972). Organ culture of the terminal abdominal segments of an adult female lepidopteran. *In Vitro* **8,** 30–36.

Whitman, D. W. (1982). Grasshopper sexual pheromone: A component of the defensive secretion in *Taeniopoda eques. Physiol. Entomol.* **7,** 111–115.

Wysoki, M., Scheepens, M. H. M., Moore, I., Beckert, D., and Cyjon, R. (1985). Location of the sex pheromone glands of female *Boarmia selenaria* (Lepidoptera: Geometridae). *Ann. Entomol. Soc. Am.* **78,** 446–450.

3

Pheromone Biosynthesis in Lepidopterans: Desaturation and Chain Shortening

L. B. BJOSTAD
W. A. WOLF
W. L. ROELOFS
Department of Entomology
New York State Agriculture Experimental Station
Geneva, New York 14456

I. INTRODUCTION

The first chemical identification of a pheromone, that of the silkmoth *Bombyx mori,* was the result of a 20-year study (Butenandt *et al.,* 1959). This identification touched off an intense research effort into all areas of pheromone biology, a dramatic increase in interest due largely to the chemical simplicity of the silkmoth pheromone. With the identification of the pheromones of the wild pest species *Trichoplusia ni* (Berger, 1966) and *Argyrotaenia velutinana* (Roelofs *et al.,* 1975), it became apparent that most sex pheromones were likely to be equally simple. The simplicity of structure was important, because it meant that the compounds involved would be fairly easy to synthesize, and also fairly inexpensive. The demonstration by Shorey *et al.* (1967) that these compounds could be used to suppress insect pest populations by disrupting their sexual communication, a demonstration concurrent with an emerging interest in nontoxic methods of insect control (Carson, 1962), provided an impetus to understand

77

all aspects of chemical communication in moths, including the chemical nature of the sex pheromones produced by females, the specific components of this signal that direct the behavioral repertoire of males, the neurophysiological basis for male response to sex pheromones, and the biosynthetic pathways involved in sex pheromone production.

To date, the sex pheromones of more than 200 species of moths have been chemically identified (Tamaki, 1985). Several themes have emerged regarding the chemical features of sex pheromones. For most of these species, the sex pheromone consists of a precise blend of compounds, and female variability in the proportions of the blend is very low. The compounds that comprise the sex pheromone blends of Lepidopterans are usually characterized by the following elements:

1. Chain length: 10, 12, 14, 16, or 18 carbon atoms in a straight chain
2. Functional group: a primary alcohol, acetate, or aldehyde
3. Double bonds: one, two, or three double bonds, at a variety of positions and with *Z* or *E* configuration.

This three-element theme may have been observed most commonly in part because pest species of moths tend to fall into just a few families, such as the Noctuidae, Pyralidae, Tortricidae, and Olethreutidae. Rather different constructions are often found in other species. For example, the pheromones of some gelechiid moths, the tomato pinworm and the potato tuberworm, have straight chains with 13 carbon atoms, an odd number instead of the even number observed for most other species. The pheromone of the gypsy moth (disparlure) is a methyl branched compound instead of a straight chain compound, has an epoxide group instead of a double bond, and does not have a terminal functional group. The pheromones of many Arctiidae also lack terminal functional groups and often have odd numbers of carbon atoms (Tamaki, 1985).

All the pheromones identified seemed to be closely related to the fatty acids that are common in nature, but with some interesting differences. Most fatty acids in nature are 16, 18, or 20 carbon atoms long. Pheromone molecules similarly tend to have a chain with an even number of carbon atoms, but a great variety of chain lengths is common, including chains of 10, 12, 14, 16, or 18 carbon atoms. Pheromone molecules usually have a single functional group, but this is usually the more reduced alcohol or aldehyde moiety.

A standard shorthand notation has been developed for pheromone molecules of this type (see Roelofs *et al.*, 1975). For example, (*Z*)-11-tetradecen-1-yl acetate is abbreviated Z11-14 : Ac. The corresponding alcohol is abbreviated Z11-14 : OH, the corresponding aldehyde is abbreviated Z11-14 : Al, the fatty acyl analog is abbreviated Z11-14 : Acyl, and the methyl ester is abbreviated Z11-14 : Me.

Early studies on sex pheromone biosynthesis were concerned more with individual steps in the pathway than with the pathway as a whole, and usually with steps near the end of the pathway for which the probable precursors were more apparent. Inoue and Hamamura (1972) demonstrated that glands of *Bombyx mori* incubated with radiolabeled hexadecanoic acid were able to produce radiolabeled bombykol, but individual fatty acyl transformations and the possible role of glycerolipid intermediates were not evaluated. Kasang and Schneider (1974) demonstrated that gypsy moth females were able to produce radioactive disparlure, the epoxide pheromone, after injection with the tritium-labeled olefin that is structurally analogous. The nature of early precursors in biosynthetic pathways was first addressed by Jones and Berger (1978), who demonstrated that cabbage looper females were able to biosynthesize the pheromone component (Z)-7-dodecenyl acetate *de novo* from acetate. The radiolabel was distributed throughout the molecule, consistent with a pathway that involved fatty acid synthesis from the radiolabeled acetate precursor and reduction and acetylation to generate the pheromone component.

A list of questions began to accumulate about the biosynthetic routes leading to sex pheromones of moths:

1. Are fatty acids the precursors?

The even carbon atom number in most pheromone molecules seemed to argue that this was the case. Fatty acids are constructed by joining together acetate molecules, so that chain length increases in two-carbon increments (Volpe and Vagelos, 1976).

2. Even if fatty acids are the precursors, is it technically possible to demonstrate that this is the case?

Fatty acid synthase in eukaryotes is a multienzyme complex, where the association of the enzymes is so intimate that they are even translated contiguously as a single polypeptide chain. Working out the separate biosynthetic steps of fatty acid synthesis in eukaryotes proved to be extremely difficult because the product of one enzyme was immediately transferred to the next for further processing, so that a large pool of each biosynthetic intermediate had no opportunity to accumulate in the cell. From the biochemist's perspective, it appeared that acetate went into the reaction and hexadecanoic acid came out, with no intermediates experimentally discernible in between. The separate steps were worked out largely in prokaryotes, in which the enzymes occur as separate molecules and appreciable amounts of the intermediates accumulate (Volpe and Vagelos, 1976). It seemed a possibility that the enzymes in sex pheromone biosynthesis might similarly be intimately associated, and that we might be able to dissect the pathway only by postulating structures of various intermediates and then observing whether or not radiolabeled versions were incorporated into the end product pheromone components.

3. How do different chain lengths arise?

Fatty acid synthase in a particular tissue usually makes predominantly or entirely hexadecanoate (octadecanoate is often a major product as well in insects). Longer chain lengths are made by separate chain-lengthing enzymes. Shorter chain length components are made by several mechanisms, including a modified thioesterase that cleaves nascent fatty acids from fatty acid synthase before they reach 16 carbon atoms in length (Ryan et al., 1982).

4. What determines the double bond positions?

Most fatty acids in nature acquire double bonds from desaturases, which remove a pair of hydrogen atoms to construct the double bond. Most desaturases determine the double bond position by measuring with respect to the carboxylate functional group, but some are known to measure with respect to the methyl end of the molecule. In bacteria, the double bond is introduced after partial chain construction, and the remainder of the chain is then added (Wakil, 1970). Pheromone components usually have one, two, or three double bonds, but, unlike the common fatty acids in nature, the double bond positions occur at many different locations and rarely occur at the ninth, twelfth, or fifteenth chain positions.

5. How does the functional group arise?

The acetate, alcohol, and aldehyde functional groups that predominate in the sex pheromones of moths are reduced derivatives of fatty acids. A single reduction step would produce an aldehyde, two reduction steps would produce a fatty alcohol, and esterification of an alcohol by acetyl coenzyme A would produce an acetate derivative. Reductases that convert fatty acyl groups to fatty aldehydes and alcohols have been found in other organisms (Kolattukudy and Rogers, 1978; Rock et al., 1978). Enzyme systems that carry out ester synthesis in insects have been characterized by Blomquist and Ries (1979) and by Lambremont and Wykle (1979). The functional group transformations in Choristoneura fumiferana have been studied by Morse and Meighen (1984, 1986), and a discussion of the enzymatic transformations appears in the next chapter (Morse and Meighen, Chapter 4, this volume).

6. If fatty acids are involved in sex pheromone biosynthesis, in what form do they occur in the pheromone gland, given that fatty acids are rarely free in most animal tissues and usually occur as derivatives of glycerol?

Phospholipids, including choline phosphatides and ethanolamine phosphatides, are common constituents of membranes in animal cells. Neutral lipids including triacylglycerols, diacylglycerols, and monoacylglycerols often occur as discrete droplets in the cell (Bell and Coleman, 1980).

7. How are the precise pheromone blends regulated?

In the family Tortricidae, many species include the compounds Z11-14:Ac and E11-14:Ac as components of their pheromones, using them in different proportions (Roelofs and Brown, 1982). Regulation of these blends could involve control by a single enzyme, or might involve a suite of enzymes that shaped the blend at each of several steps.

8. What is the biosynthetic basis for the phylogenetic pattern observed in pheromone composition?

Although many different compounds appear in sex pheromone blends, they are not random combinations of functional group, chain length, and double bond position. For example, in the Noctuidae, chains with 10 carbon atoms usually have the double bond at the fifth carbon atom, chains with 12 carbon atoms usually have the double bond at the seventh carbon atom, chains with 14 carbon atoms usually have the double bond at the ninth carbon atom, and chains with 16 carbon atoms usually have the double bond at the eleventh carbon atom (Steck *et al.*, 1982). In each case, the double bond is five carbon atoms from the methyl end of the chain ($n - 5$). Other double bond positions are much less common. A different pattern is found in the Tortricidae, in which chains with 14 carbon atoms usually have a double bond at the eleventh carbon atom, and chains with 12 carbon atoms usually have a double bond at the ninth carbon atom ($n - 3$).

II. METHODOLOGY

A. Characterization of Biosynthetic Intermediates

1. Tissues

In most species of moths, the sex pheromone is produced by a specialized gland on the ovipositor of the female, and the female releases the sex pheromone according to a circadian rhythm, exhibiting pheromone release behavior during a discrete portion of the day or night (Tamaki, 1985). Some moths store appreciable amounts of the sex pheromone in the gland, although the amounts vary considerably among species. For example, the redbanded leafroller moth stores an average of 100 ng in the gland (Roelofs *et al.*, 1975), the cabbage looper moth stores nearly 1 μg of the pheromone (Berger, 1966), and the saltmarsh caterpillar stores almost 10 μg (Hill and Roelofs, 1981). Other moth species store practically no sex pheromone at all, biosynthesizing the pheromone only during the normal pheromone release period and immediately volatilizing it from the gland. This has been found particularly in species whose pheromones include an aldehyde component, such as *Choristoneura rosaceana* (Weatherston *et al.*, 1971) and *Heliothis zea* (Klun *et al.*, 1980).

a. *Gland Morphology.* Female sex pheromone glands of different species have radically different morphologies, and this affects the ease of doing biosynthetic investigations. The three main categories of sex pheromone glands are as follows:

1. Eversible sacs: In *Trichoplusia ni* (Percy, 1979), *Argyrotaenia velutinana* (Feng and Roelofs, 1977), and many other Tortricidae and Noctuidae, the female keeps the gland retracted within the ovipositor during inactive periods, but everts the gland fully during sex pheromone release.
2. Internal glands: In *Estigmene acrea* (Hill and Roelofs, 1981) and many other Arctiidae, the gland is a pair of long, permanent invaginations of the ovipositor.
3. Surface glands: In *Lymantria dispar* (Bierl *et al.*, 1970) and *Ostrinia nubilalis* (Klun and Brindley, 1970), the epithelium of the sex pheromone gland is arranged as a flattened sheet that may be restricted to a patch on the dorsal surface of the ovipositor or may be arranged as a nearly continuous ring around the ovipositor.

b. *Gland Dissection.* Considerable rigor in tissue dissection is desirable for the study of sex pheromone biosynthesis. Extraneous lipids from tissues other than the sex pheromone gland itself can obscure the roles of lipids that are involved in biosynthesis of the pheromone. Dissecting the glandular epithelium from the ovipositor is best accomplished with fine forceps (sometimes sold as "watchmaker's forceps" or as "electron microscopy forceps" for handling small grids).

The dissection is particularly easy for pheromone glands that are simple, eversible sacs. The live female is held with a pair of soft forceps (or with thumb and forefinger if the moth is larger), exerting pressure at the tip of the abdomen to force out the ovipositor and then the pheromone gland. A pair of fine forceps, the tips of which have been rinsed with 2 : 1 chloroform : methanol, is used to grip the anterior and posterior faces of the gland at its base and pluck it cleanly from the ovipositor. Only tiny fragments of the glandular epithelium remain attached to the ovipositor.

The long, internal glands of *Estigmene acrea* and many other arctiid species emerge at the dorsal surface of the ovipositor as a pair of small papillae. Each papilla is gripped with fine forceps, and a sudden tug with the forceps breaks the papilla cleanly from the adjacent cuticle on the ovipositor, allowing the long gland to be withdrawn from within the ovipositor.

A pheromone gland that lies as a sheet covering much or most of the surface of the ovipositor is the most difficult to dissect. The ovipositor is gripped tightly near the base with fine forceps, and a solvent-rinsed razor blade is used to shear through the ovipositor along the anterior face of the forceps. A second pair of fine forceps is used to grip the distal (posterior) end of the ovipositor, and the first pair of forceps is released. Eggs and hemolymph in the ovipositor are expelled from the cut anterior end when the forceps are released. The first pair of forceps is used to stroke the ovipositor gently along its length to expel additional material. The ovipositor can now be turned inside out, and residual tissue can be scraped from the ovipositor with the forceps.

c. *Gland Extracts.* Extraction can be conveniently accomplished with 2 : 1 chloroform : methanol, as this solvent mixture allows recovery of lipids with a wide range of polarities (Folch *et al.,* 1957). All solvents should be glass distilled.

Once a gland has been dissected, a capillary tube (50 μl) with a small amount of 2 : 1 chloroform : methanol held in the tip by capillarity can be used to scrape the gland from the fine forceps in one motion, transferring the gland to the solvent in the capillary. The capillary is then set into a 4-ml vial containing about 200 μl of 2 : 1 chloroform : methanol. When all glands have been dissected, a bulb is used to blow out solvent and glands from the tip of the capillary into the vial.

Macerating the glands is usually not necessary for efficient extraction. Glands should be allowed to stand overnight in 2 : 1 chloroform : methanol at 4°C in an explosion-proof refrigerator. If glands are allowed to stand at room temperature in 2 : 1 chloroform : methanol for several days, the lipids that are extracted from the gland can react with methanol to form small amounts of methyl esters that appear as artifacts in subseqent analyses.

2. Separation of Lipids

a. *Thin-Layer Chromatographic Separation of Glycerolipids.* It is desirable to work with a smaller solvent volume than that of the original extract. The 200-μl extract is transferred with a 10-μl syringe (Hamilton Co., Reno, NV 89510) to a small test tube with a pointed end, made from glass tubing (5 mm ID, 50 mm long) with a torch (Wale Apparatus, Hellertown, PA 18055). The test tube is cleaned with 2 : 1 chloroform : methanol, and a nitrogen stream is used to reduce the solvent volume by evaporation. Most pheromone components and glycerolipid biosynthetic intermediates are not appreciably volatile by comparison with the solvent, and the extract can usually be evaporated completely to apparent dryness with no loss of material.

Thin-layer chromatography (TLC) plates prepared in the lab almost never have adequate resolution for separating the lipid intermediates in pheromone biosynthesis. Large TLC plates (20 × 20 cm, Anasil O, Analabs Inc., North Haven, CT 06473) can be broken down with the aid of a diamond scribe into smaller plates (2 × 10 cm) that are suitable for lipid separations. The resolution of the lipids equals or exceeds that obtained with larger plates, and the development time is much shorter (10 instead of 30–40 min). Coplin staining jars with ground glass lids can be used as development tanks. The small TLC plates are marked with a pencil line 2 cm from the end to mark the origin where an extract will later be applied and are placed in a Coplin staining jar filled with distilled methanol to extract contaminants from the plate. After soaking for 1 hr, the plates are dried in an oven at 100°C for 1 hr. Plates that are not dried in the oven give poorer resolution.

A lipid extract is applied to the origin of a clean TLC plate with a 10-μl syringe. The plate is removed from the 100°C oven and allowed to cool for 10 min. The extract is applied to the pencil line at the origin of the plate, with the top of the syringe leaning gently against the jaws of a thermometer clamp attached to a ring stand. The TLC plate is heated at 40°C for 10 min to allow complete drying (an inverted Petri dish on top of a drying oven works well), and the plate is then developed. The development tank is filled with the appropriate solvent system to a depth of 1.5 cm, well below the origin of a TLC plate. A clean TLC plate is added to the tank to assure a solvent-saturated atmosphere.

The lipids in the sex pheromone gland can be separated effectively by successively developing the plate with solvent systems that decrease in polarity each time (Fig. 1). The best initial solvent system is 62 : 34 : 4 chloroform : methanol : water. This allows separation of very polar lipids, such as ethanolamine phosphatides and choline phosphatides, and less polar lipids travel near the solvent front (Mangold, 1969). For pheromone gland extracts of all moth species we have examined, it is only necessary to develop the 10-cm TLC plate 2 cm above the origin with 62 : 34 : 4 chloroform : methanol : water. No detectable lipids remain at the origin, and a clear separation of both phosphatide classes is obtained.

For most applications, all the lipid classes that travel as a mixture near the solvent front during the first development can be separated with 80 : 20 : 2 hexane : ether : acetic acid, a less polar second solvent system. Prior to this development, the plate is dried briefly in a hood and then heated for 10 min at 40°C to remove solvent completely. The ethanolamine phosphatides and choline phosphatides do not noticeably migrate in the second development, but diacylglycerols, triacylglycerols, and the pheromone components themselves separate cleanly.

A third solvent of intermediate polarity is useful in some applications where it may be advantageous to separate with special rigor compounds of intermediate polarity, such as cholesterol, the 1,2-diacylglycerols, and the 1,3-diacylglycerols. This solvent system consists of benzene : diethyl ether : ethanol (25 : 10 : 2). The TLC plate should be developed first with 62 : 34 : 4 chloroform : metha-

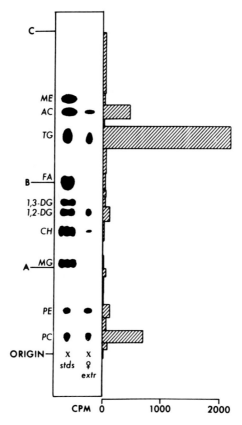

Fig. 1. Incorporation of sodium [1-^{14}C]acetate into lipid classes in sex pheromone glands of *Argyrotaenia velutinana*. The plate was developed to A with 62 : 34 : 4 chloroform : methanol : water, to B with 200 : 250 : 10 : 1 ether : benzene : ethanol : acetic acid, to C with 80 : 20 : 2 hexane : ether : acetic acid, and again to C with 93 : 5 hexane : ether. PC, Choline phosphatides; PE, ethanolamine phosphatides; MG, monoacylglycerols; CH, cholesterol; DG, diacylglycerols; FA, free fatty acids; TG, triacylglycerols; AC, acetates; ME, methyl esters. Lipid standards were chromatographed in the left lane, and a female extract was chromatographed in the right lane. Reproduced from Bjostad and Roelofs (1984a), by permission of Plenum Publishing Corp.

nol : water to 2 cm beyond the origin, then with benzene : diethyl ether : ethanol (25 : 10 : 2) to 4 cm beyond the origin, and finally to the top of the plate with 80 : 20 : 2 hexane : ether : acetic acid, drying the plate between developments as described above (Bjostad *et al.*, 1981; Bjostad and Roelofs, 1984a).

Because the compounds of interest are glycerolipids containing unsaturated fatty acids, staining with iodine is the most convenient means of visualization. The developed TLC plate is dried in a hood for 10 min and placed in a closed glass jar containing iodine crystals. If fractions are to be scraped from the TLC plate, spots are marked lightly with a probe, and the TLC plate is placed in a hood for 10 min to allow iodine to volatilize from the plate.

b. *Gas–Liquid Chromatographic Separation of Fatty Acyl Methyl Esters.* Fatty acyl methyl esters of interest can usually be resolved completely with a polar gas–liquid chromatography (GLC) column. The best separations are achieved with fused silica capillary columns, such as the Supelcowax 10 column (25 m × 0.25 mm ID); for analysis by flame-ionization detection (FID), use of such a column is the method of choice. Separation can also be achieved with packed GLC columns, but obtaining adequate separation of Z and E isomers, essential to the analysis of pheromone blends and their biosynthetic precursors, is often difficult. A glass column (3 m × 2 mm ID) filled with 10% XF-1150 (50% cyanoethyl methyl silicone) on 100–120 mesh Chromosorb W-AW-DMCS is appropriate. Alternatively, 15% OV-275 (dicyanoallyl silicone) on 100–120 Chromosorb P-AW-DMCS is suitable as a polar packing.

The main drawback of capillary columns in the past has been their limited capacity. Injection of more than a few micrograms of a mixture of compounds resulted in significant overloading and loss of resolution. This was a problem in biosynthetic studies. In short-term incubations with a radiolabeled precursor, only a tiny amount of radiolabel is incorporated into the compounds of interest. It is necessary to work with large numbers of pheromone glands in order to accumulate enough of a radiolabeled product to allow detection, but this means that large amounts of the unlabeled compounds are also present, making it difficult to avoid overloading a GLC column. The much larger capacity of packed GLC columns (which may allow injection of up to a milligram of a lipid mixture without overloading) has made them more useful for most biosynthetic work so far. Wide-bore capillary columns (0.75 mm ID) that are now becoming commercially available (Alltech Co. and Supelco Co.) have a larger capacity than was previously available, and may prove acceptable alternatives to packed columns.

For collection of radiolabeled compounds from a packed GLC column, a piece of Teflon tubing that connects the end of the column to the FID is disconnected from the FID and the end is passed out of the GLC oven through a stainless steel tube that lines a hole in the GLC oven wall (for Teflon connectors, the temperature must be below 250°C). A glass capillary tube (1.5 mm OD) is connected to the end of the Teflon tubing and inserted into the stainless steel tube until the end of the glass capillary tube barely protrudes beyond the oven wall. Glass capillary tubes are replaced at intervals to collect individual peaks.

3. Characterization of Glycerolipids

a. *Methanolysis and Gas/Liquid Chromatographic Analysis.* Methanolysis (Fig. 2) cleaves the fatty acyl groups of glycerolipids from the glycerol backbone and converts them to methyl esters that can be analyzed by gas–liquid chromatography (GLC). Methanolysis can be conducted under basic (Litchfield, 1972) or acidic (Nichols *et al.*, 1965) conditions. An important feature of base methanolysis is that fatty acyl groups of glycerolipids react to form methyl esters but free fatty acids do not form methyl esters. Acid methanolysis forms methyl esters from fatty acyl groups of glyderolipids and also from free fatty acids.

Acid methanolysis (Nichols *et al.*, 1965) is performed with a solution of methanol : benzene : sulfuric acid (30 : 15 : 1 v : v : v). The sample to be methanolyzed (typically less than 1 mg) is evaporated to apparent dryness with a nitrogen stream in a 4-ml screw-cap vial, and 1 ml of the acid methanolysis reagent is added. The vial is closed tightly with a Teflon-lined screw cap and heated at 100°C for 1 hr. The vial is cooled, and 1 ml of hexane and 1 ml of water are added. The vial is shaken vigorously, and the upper hexane extract layer is transferred to a second vial. The remaining methanol–water level is extracted a second time with 1 ml hexane, which is combined with the previous hexane extract. The hexane extract is washed twice with water, filtered through a small piece of cellulose tissue, and concentrated with a nitrogen stream for later GLC analysis. A disadvantage of acid methanolysis is that it destroys some fatty acyl groups. Bjostad and Roelofs (1984b) found that the sex pheromone of the silkmoth is completely destroyed by acid methanolysis, as is its fatty acyl precursor. Both the pheromone component and its fatty acyl precursor were stable under base methanolysis conditions.

It is important to preclean the vial for the reaction by heating the vial at 100°C for 1 hr with 2 ml of acid methanolysis reagent, which is then discarded. If a vial is merely cleaned with an organic solvent, acid methanolysis of the supposedly clean vial is found to generate small amounts of fatty acid methyl esters. A common problem with acid methanolysis is that the screw-cap vial used for the reaction may not seal adequately, allowing the solvent to boil away. Rubber-faced screw caps (with a Teflon liner added) provide a better seal than paper-faced caps.

Base methanolysis is conducted at room temperature (Litchfield, 1972). A solvent extract of the lipid to be methanolyzed is evaporated to apparent dryness with a nitrogen stream in a 4-ml vial, and 0.5 ml of base methanolysis reagent (0.5 M KOH in methanol) is added. The vial is allowed to stand 30 min at room temperature, and 1 ml of 1 M aqueous HCl is added. This is extracted twice with 1 ml of hexane, which is washed, filtered, and concentrated with a nitrogen stream for GLC analysis of the methyl esters as described above for acid methanolysis. It is advisable to test the remaining aqueous solution with pH test paper to be sure that enough aqueous HCl was added to make the solution acidic. An advantage of base methanolysis is that the solvent cannot boil away as with methanolysis.

Methanolysis converts pheromone components that are acetates to the corre-

4. Characterization of Fatty Acyl Methyl Esters

a. Gas–Liquid Chromatography. Analysis with two GLC columns, a polar column and a nonpolar column, is usually adequate for characterization according to GLC retention times. An appropriate choice for a polar column is a Supelcowax 10 column (25 m × 0.25 mm ID). An appropriate choice for a nonpolar column is a RSL 150 polydimethylsiloxane column (25 m × 0.25 mm ID).

b. Ozonolysis. Double bond positions of pheromone components and the methyl esters of their fatty acyl precursors are conveniently determined with ozonolysis (Beroza and Bierl, 1966). Ozonolysis cleaves the double bond to produce two aldehydes that can be analyzed by GLC. Ozonolysis of a compound whose double bond position is not known generates aldehydes whose GLC retention times can be compared with those of the ozonolysis products of a series of synthetic compounds with known double bond positions. Ozonolysis as described by Beroza and Bierl (1966) involves generating ozone within a solution of the unknown compound. Ozonolysis is not a high-yield reaction, and yields in the range 10–40% are typical. The possibility that excess ozone may cause lower yields has prompted alternative techniques. Bjostad and Roelofs (1983) generated a saturated solution of ozone in 50 μl of hexane in a small pointed test tube kept at −78°C in a bath of dry ice and acetone, and added a 10 μl hexane solution of the unsaturated compound to the ozone solution to effect ozonolysis. Excess ozone was dispelled immediately with a nitrogen stream, and a solution of triphenylphosphine was added to break the ozonide and generate the pair of aldehydes.

Another variation of ozonolysis has been developed by Dr. Thomas Bellas (CSIRO, personal communication), in which a glass capillary tube is used to collect an unsaturated compound from a GLC column and is then connected to a piece of Teflon tubing conveying an ozone supply for a few seconds. The collected compound on the inside wall of the capillary tube is ozonized *in situ* and is simultaneously cleaved to the aldehydes and recovered in solution by rinsing through the capillary tube with 50 μl of a hexane solution of triphenylphosphine. This technique minimizes handling losses of the compound of interest.

c. Mass Spectrometry. Mass spectra of pheromone components and the methyl esters of their fatty acyl precursors are most conveniently obtained with a mass spectrometer (MS) interfaced with a GLC (GLC–MS), so that mass spectra of all methanolysis products of a pheromone gland extract can be obtained with a single GLC run. Fatty acyl methyl esters can be analyzed by electron-ionization mass spectrometry or by chemical-ionization mass spectrometry. Electron-ionization mass spectrometry produces diagnostic peaks at M^+ (the mass of the methyl ester), and also at $(M - 31)^+$, $(M - 32)^+$, and $(M - 74)^+$ (Biemann, 1962). Chemical ionization with isobutane produces a prominent peak at $(M + 1)^+$, and other peaks are usually less than 10% the height of this base peak.

B. Radiolabeling Studies

1. Synthesis of Radiolabeled Fatty Acids

a. Carbon-14 Compounds. A simple, inexpensive way to label fatty acids is to use $K^{14}CN$ to add a single radioactive carbon atom. A sequence of four reactions (Bjostad and Roelofs, 1986) can be used to add carbon atoms sequentially, allowing the preparation of a fatty acid with a radioactive carbon at a defined position and with nonradioactive carbon atoms at other positions in the molecule. Each of the four reactions has a high yield and allows easy purification of the product from any unreacted precursors. In addition, all four reactions can be carried out in 4-ml screw-cap vials, so that all materials used for the radiosynthesis can be disposed of in a radioactive waste container and the possibility of radioactive contamination from reusing glassware is minimized.

As an example, the synthesis of $[3\text{-}^{14}C]$hexadecanoic acid can be carried out as follows. Bromotridecane (1 mg) is added to a solution of $K^{14}CN$ [4 mBq (millibecquerels)] in distilled dimethyl sulfoxide (0.5 ml) in a 4-ml vial with a Teflon-lined screw cap. After 1 hr at 25°C, water (2 ml) is added and the product $[1\text{-}^{14}C]$tetradecanonitrile is extracted twice with hexane (1 ml each time). The hexane extract is filtered through a small wad of Kimwipe in a Pasteur pipette to remove traces of water, and the extract is applied to a small chromatograph column Unreacted bromotridecane is eluted with 4 ml of hexane. The $[1\text{-}^{14}C]$tetradecanonitrile is eluted from the column with 4 ml of dichloromethane.
$[1\text{-}^{14}C]$tetradecanonitrile is eluted from the column with 4 ml of dichloromethane.

The nitrile is hydrolyzed to the corresponding carboxylic acid by reaction with 10 mg of NaOH in a mixture of water (0.1 ml) and ethanol (1 ml) for 16 hr at 100°C in a screw-cap vial. Water (1 ml) is added, and the reaction mixture is washed with hexane to remove any unreacted $[1\text{-}^{14}C]$tetradecanonitrile. The aqueous layer is acidified with H_2SO_4 (2 drops in 1 ml of water), and $[1\text{-}^{14}C]$tetradecanoic acid is extracted with hexane.

Conversion of $[1\text{-}^{14}C]$tetradecanoic acid to the corresponding alcohol is carried out by evaporating the hexane solution of the acid to apparent dryness in a screw-cap vial with nitrogen, and adding 0.5 ml Red-Al [sodium bis(2-methoxyethoxy)aluminum hydride, 3.4 M in toluene, Aldrich Chemical Co.] to the neat acid. The reaction is immediate. Excess hydride reagent is destroyed by adding 2 M NaOH (2 ml) until the mild fizzing stops. The $[1\text{-}^{14}C]$tetradecan-1-ol is extracted twice with hexane (1 ml each). The hexane solution is washed twice with water in a 4-ml vial (1 ml each) and evaporated to apparent dryness with a nitrogen stream, and the product is taken up in 1 ml dichloromethane.

Synthesis of [1-^{14}C]bromotetradecane from the alcohol is accomplished with triphenylphosphine dibromide (Wiley *et al.*, 1964). Triphenylphosphine dibromide is prepared by adding bromine dropwise with shaking to a solution of triphenylphosphine (50 mg) in dichloromethane (1 ml) until the yellow color persists, and then adding more triphenylphosphine until the solution loses the yellow tint. The dichloromethane solution of [1-^{14}C]tetradecan-1-ol is added to the triphenylphosphine dibromide solution. The reaction is immediate. The solution is reduced nearly to dryness with nitrogen, and hexane (1 ml) is added, precipitating unreacted triphenylphosphine dibromide. The solution is filtered through a small wad of Kimwipe in a Pasteur pipette and reduced to apparent dryness with nitrogen, and hexane (1 ml) is added. This solution is applied to the top of a small chromatograph column made from a Pasteur pipette half-filled with a slurry of Florisil in hexane. Elution of [1-^{14}C]bromotetradecane from the column is carried out with 4 ml of hexane, leaving behind any unreacted alochol.

Nonradioactive KCN is used to add a single carbon to [1-^{14}C]bromotetradecane as described above. Hydrolysis of the nitrile produces [2-^{14}C]pentadecanoic acid. Reduction of the acid, bromination of the resulting alcohol, addition of KCN, and hydrolysis of the nitrile then complete the synthesis of [3-^{14}C]hexadecanoic acid. Purity can be checked by preparing a small amount of methyl [3-^{14}C]hexadecanoate with diazomethane (Fieser and Fieser, 1967), collecting fractions by GLC, and analyzing the fractions with scintillation counting.

b. Synthesis of Tritium-Labeled Fatty Acids. Synthesis of a fatty acid labeled with tritium on the terminal carbon atom can be carried out with sodium borotritiide (NaB^{3}H$_4$). For example, the synthesis of [16-^{3}H](Z)-11-hexadecenoic acid can be carried out as follows (Bjostad and Roelofs, 1983). The tetrahydropyranyl ether of 5-bromopentan-1-ol was prepared as described in Henrick (1977), and 5-tetrahydropyranyloxy-pentanal was prepared from the bromide with pyridine *N*-oxide as described by Stowell (1970). Methyl 11-bromoundecanoate was also prepared, as described by Scheme 15 in Henrick (1977), and was refluxed with triphenylphosphine in benzene to generate the phosphonium salt. Sodium bis(trimethylsilyl)amide was added to a solution of the phosphonium salt in dry hexamethylphosphoramide, and to the deep red solution was added 5-tetrahydropyranyloxy-pentanal (Bestmann and Vostrowsky, 1979). The product methyl 16-tetrahydropyranyloxy-(Z)-11-hexadecenoate was treated with HCl in methanol to remove the tetrahydropyranyl protecting group, and the resulting alcohol was converted to the tosylate (Fieser and Fieser, 1967). The tosylate was purified by AgNO$_3$–TLC (Bjostad and Roelofs, 1981). Methyl [16-^{3}H](Z)-11-hexadecenoate was prepared by adding the tosylate to a dimethyl sulfoxide solution of NaB^{3}H$_4$ (Amersham). After 24 hr the reaction mixture was extracted twice with hexane, and this was washed twice with water. Base hydrolysis of the methyl ester with 10 mg of NaOH in a mixture of water (0.1 ml) and ethanol (1 ml) was conducted to produce $[16-^3H](Z)$-11-hexadecenoic acid. Alternative routes for tritium-labeling of fatty acids and their derivatives are described by Prestwich (Chapter 14, this volume).

2. Application to Pheromone Glands

Labeled compounds to be evaluated as pheromone precursors can be tested *in vivo* by applying a dimethyl sulfoxide solution of a labeled compound to the pheromone glands of adult females. For species with normally eversible glands, such as *A. velutinana* and *T. ni*, the ovipositor and pheromone glands are everted by clamping the tip of the abdomen with a microalligator clip with smooth jaws. The jaws of each clip are bent so that a gap remains between them when the clip is closed, holding the gland everted without harming the female. A 10-μl gas-tight syringe mounted on a micromanipulator is filled with a solution of a labeled compound, and 0.2 μl of the solution is applied topically to the pheromone gland of each female. The syringe should be cleaned with a detergent solution immediately after use, because radioactive residues have proved difficult to remove with organic solvents alone. The applied droplet absorbs into the pheromone gland in about 1 hr, and at this time the gland can be dissected from the ovipositor as described above, or the clip can be removed from the female if the gland is to be dissected at a later time. When the clip is removed, the female cannot retract her gland immediately, but is usually able to do so within an hour, and will exhibit normal pheromone release behavior by the appropriate time in her circadian rhythm the next day, if the clip has caused no damage.

3. Evaluation of Incorporation

Incorporation of a radiolabeled compound into various lipid classes in the pheromone gland of a moth species can be determined by TLC of the crude lipid extract as described above. Fractions can be scraped from the plate onto glassine paper and tapped into 7-ml scintillation vials containing a solution of 2,5-diphenyloxazole (PPO) in toluene (5 g/liter) for scintillation counting (see Fig. 1).

Incorporation of radiolabel into the fatty acyl groups of each glycerolipid class can be determined by GLC with a polar packed column, such as 10% XF-1150. This column packing allows adequate separation of geometric isomers of most pheromone complements and their precursors, and also allows separation of the common fatty acyl groups that are constituents of membranes and lipid deposits in most organisms, including palmitate, palmitoleate, stearate, oleate, linoleate, and linolenate. The TLC fraction that includes a given lipid class is scraped from the plate, and the lipid is extracted for 16 hr at 4°C with 2 : 1 chloroform : methanol in a screw-cap vial. The extract is filtered through a small Kimwipe wad in a broken Pasteur pipette to remove TLC powder and is evaporated to apparent dryness with nitrogen. Methanolysis with acid or base is conducted on the recovered lipid as described above to prepare methyl esters from the fatty acyl groups of the glycerolipid.

After derivatization by methanolysis (and acetylation, for a pheromone blend that includes acetate components), the products can be separated and collected by GLC (Fig. 3). An aliquot of a nonradioactive derivatized gland extract is analyzed by FID on the GLC to determine the retention times of the compounds of interest. The end of the GLC column is then disconnected from the detector, to allow collection in 30-cm glass capillary tubes. The derivatized radioactive ex-

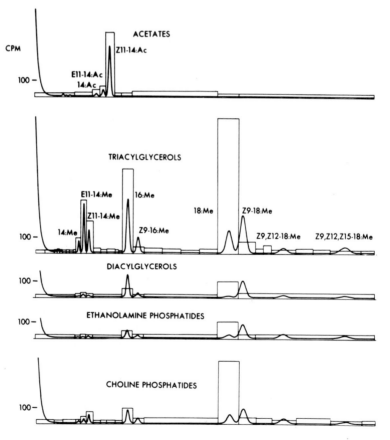

Fig. 3. Incorporation of [1-^{14}C]acetate into *A. velutinana* sex pheromone gland lipids after a 4 hr incubation. Histogram of counts per minute in each GLC fraction is superimposed on GLC peaks detected by flame ionization. Ac, Acetate; Me, methyl ester. Reproduced from Bjostad and Roelofs (1984a), by permission of Plenum Publishing Corp.

tract is injected onto the column, and collection tubes are sequentially replaced to collect all compounds of interest as indicated by their retention times in the FID run. A small piece of dry ice may be used on each collection tube to enhance recovery of the compounds. About 30 collection tubes are usually adequate for a single GLC collection. At the end of the collection, the contents of each collection tube are rinsed into a different scintillation vial with a PPO solution in toluene (described above), and radioactivity is determined with a scintillation counter.

C. Stable Isotope Labeling Studies

The method of choice for studying sex pheromone biosynthesis involves the use of candidate precursors that are multiply labeled with the stable isotopes carbon-13 or deuterium and analysis of the perhomone gland lipids with chemical ionization mass spectrometry in the selected ion monitoring mode (GLC–SIM–CI–MS). Because a compound that contains several stable isotopes is "mass-labeled," it is possible to analyze a series of compounds in a GLC trace for incorporation of a mass-labeled compound by using a GLC–MS program that specifies a set of mass filters. Each GLC peak consists of a mixture of mass-labeled and unlabeled isotopomers, and, prior to emergence of the GLC peak into the source of the mass spectrometer, the GLC–MS program is changed to scan only for the masses of the chemically ionized unlabeled and mass-labeled compounds in the GLC peak. A pair of mass-filtered GLC traces is generated by each injected sample, one showing unlabeled compounds and one showing mass-labeled compounds for the specified increment in mass. By using one of the unlabeled compounds in the sample as an internal standard, the pair of mass-filtered GLC traces from pheromone glands incubated with a mass-labeled compound can be compared with the pair of traces from unincubated control glands, and degree of incorporation can readily be determined (Bjostad and Roelofs, 1986).

This technique offers several important advantages over radiolabeling techniques. First, the health hazard associated with radiosynthesis is avoided. Second, the likelihood of misleading results because of recycling of acetyl-CoA from mitrochondrial degradation of the labeled precursor is greatly reduced. For example, although mitochondrial degradation of the multiple-labeled precursor [1,2,3,4-^{13}C]tetradecanoic acid would produce [1,2-^{13}C]acetyl-CoA, incorporation of only one of these labeled acetyl-CoA molecules would produce a molecule of [1,2-^{13}C](Z)-11-tetradecenoate in *A. velutinana,* which would not be detected as a compound with four additional mass units (it has two additional mass units). Exactly two [1,2-^{13}C]acetyl-CoA molecules would have to be incorporated in order to mislead the investigator, but the probability that two would enter the same (Z)-11-tetradecenoate is very tiny (the square of the probability

It seemed reasonable that biosynthetic processes found in one species would probably occur in many others.

Although it appeared to us that fatty acyl precursors would be involved in the biosynthesis of the sex pheromone components because of their similarity of structure, we were pessimistic that such precursors could be isolated from the gland. It seemed likely that fatty acyl precursors would only exist fleetingly in the gland, undergoing efficient conversion to the sex pheromone components as soon as they were generated. Nevertheless, we were hopeful that trace amounts might be found, and that these might serve as guides in interpreting the results of experiments with radiolabeled precursors.

We extracted pheromone glands with 2 : 1 chloroform : methanol and performed acid methanolysis on the crude lipid extract to generate methyl esters from whatever derivatives of the fatty components might exist in the gland. GLC of the methanolyzed gland extract showed that the expected fatty acyl precursors 14 : Acyl, Z11-14 : Acyl, and E11-14 : Acyl were abundant in the gland, present in even larger amounts than the pheromone components themselves (Bjostad et al., 1981). Other common fatty acyl groups were also present, including palmitate (16 : Acyl), palmitoleate (Z9-16 : Acyl), stearate (18 : Acyl), oleate (Z9-18 : Acyl), linoleate (Z9,Z12-18 : Acyl), and linolenate (Z9,Z12,Z15-18 : Acyl), all of which are common components of membranes and lipid deposits in most animal tissues. The pheromone fatty acyl precursors were found only in the sex pheromone gland and, like the pheromone components themselves, were absent from the gland at adult emergence, increasing to a maximum over the first 4 days of adult life.

We had anticipated that if Z and E11-14 : Acyl groups occurred in the sex pheromone gland, that they would occur in the 91 : 9 $Z : E$ ratio observed for the corresponding pheromone components. It was puzzling to find that the E fatty acyl groups occurred in larger amounts in the gland than the Z components, in the proportions 42 : 58 $Z : E$. Thin-layer chromatography of a crude lipid extract of pheromone glands was performed to find out if several lipid classes might contain these two components, where only one or a few of the lipid classes might contain them in a 91 : 9 $Z : E$ ratio. Methanolysis of TLC fractions indicated that apart from the pheromone components, which are acetates, four lipid classes are abundant in the gland, including triacylglycerols, diacylglycerols, ethanolamine phosphatides, and choline phosphatides. Triacylglycerols contained most of the Z and E11-14 : Acyl groups, in the proportions 39 : 61 $Z : E$. Only trace amounts of these acyl groups occurred in the diacylglycerols, but they occurred in the same proportions as in the triacylglycerols. The choline phosphatides and ethanolamine phosphatides contained smaller amounts of these fatty acyl groups, and in both a 69 : 31 $Z : E$ ratio was found. This ratio was intermediate between the 39 : 61 $Z : E$ ratio of the triacylglycerols and the 91 : 9 $Z : E$ ratio of the pheromone components themselves (Bjostad et al., 1981).

The presence of several lipid classes with differing proportions of the Z and E11-14 : Acyl groups seemed to implicate them in sex pheromone biosynthesis, but it was curious that the 91 : 9 proportion of the pheromone components themselves was found in none of the lipid classes. The possibility that particular stereospecific positions in the glycerolipids might harbor the 91 : 9 ratio did not seem unreasonable, but proved not to be the case. The choline phosphatides were analyzed with phospholipase A_2, and the Z and E11-14 : Acyl groups were found only at the *sn*-2 position. The triacylglycerols were analyzed with lipase, and these fatty acyl groups were not found to be preferentially distributed at particular positions on the glycerol backbone (Bjostad *et al.*, 1981).

The structural information in the experiments cited above did not offer a simple mechanism for regulation of the pheromone blend, nor for the biosynthetic steps involved. A series of experiments with precursors labeled with radioactive or stable isotopes was initiated to attack the problem from a different direction.

1. Carbon Skeleton and Chain Length

Because Jones and Berger (1978) had shown with radioactive acetate that the cabbage looper *Trichoplusia ni* can biosynthesize its main sex pheromone component *de novo*, we first wished to know if *A. velutinana* was also able to do so. Glands were incubated *in vivo* with a dimethyl sulfoxide solution of sodium [1-^{14}C]acetate. We found that radiolabel was incorporated into the pheromone components, and we found in addition that radiolabel was incorporated into the Z and E11-14 : Acyl groups and into tetradecanoate, hexadecanoate, and octadecanoate with similar specific activities (Fig. 4). It was striking that the longer unsaturated fatty acyl groups palmitoleate, oleate, linoleate, and linolenate did not incorporate appreciable amounts of radiolabel (Bjostad and Roelofs, 1981). This suggested that the only lipid synthesis taking place in the pheromone gland of the adult female was involved in production of the sex pheromone components.

Having established that the biosynthesis of the sex pheromone components proceeded from acetate, we wished to know how the chain length was established. Two quite different mechanisms had precedent in the literature. In some insects, a long-chain fatty acid is chain-shortened to generate smaller fatty acids. Octadecanoate is chain-shortened to hexadecanoate in *Anthonomus grandis* (Lambremont *et al.*, 1976), and hexadecanoate is chain-shortened to tetradecanoate in *Drosophila melanogaster* (Keith, 1967). A second pathway has been found in the pea aphid *Acyrthosiphon pisum*, in which a special thioesterase hydrolyzes fatty acyl chains from fatty acid synthase when they have reached a chain length of 14 carbon atoms (Ryan *et al.*, 1982).

We incubated sex pheromone glands of *A. velutinana* with the uniformly labeled precursor [U-^{14}C]hexadecanoic acid and compared the results with those

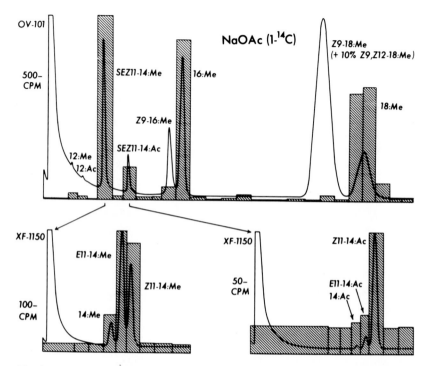

Fig. 4. Incorporation of radiolabel from topically applied sodium [1-¹⁴C]acetate into pheromone components and fatty acyl groups in sex pheromone glands of female *A. velutinana.* Ac, Acetate; Me, methyl ester; S, saturated; E, (*E*); Z, (*Z*). Reproduced from Bjostad and Roelofs (1981), by permission of *The Journal of Biological Chemistry.*

of a second experiment in which glands were incubated with [1-¹⁴C]hexadecanoic acid. We expected that if tetradecanoate was produced by chain shortening of hexadecanoate, radiolabel would be incorporated into tetradecanoate from [U-¹⁴C]hexadecanoic acid but not from [1-¹⁴C]hexadecanoic acid. We found that the specific activity of tetradecanoate in glands incubated with [1-¹⁴C]hexadecanoic acid was about half that observed for lgands incubated with [U-¹⁴C]hexadecanoic acid, indicating that tetradecanoate did arise by chain shortening in *A. velutinana,* but also indicating that some radiolabeled hexadecanoate was metabolized to acetate in both experiments and was used in *de novo* synthesis of tetradecanoate (Fig. 5).

Incubation of glands *in vivo* with [16,16,16-²H]hexadecanoic acid and analysis by GLC–SIM–CI–MS indicated the biosynthesis of trideuterated 14:Acyl, Z11-14:Acyl, E11-14:Acyl, 14:Ac, Z11-14:Ac, and E11-14:Ac by the glands (Fig. 6). This is consistent with our previous experiment showing that [U-¹⁴C]hexadecanoic acid is incorporated into these compounds and verifies that

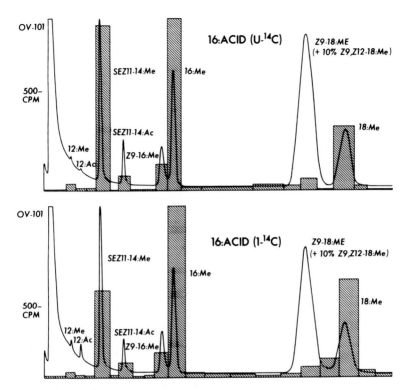

Fig. 5. Incorporation of radiolabel from topically applied [U-14C]hexadecanoic acid and [1-14C]hexadecanoic acid into pheromone components and fatty acyl groups in sex pheromone glands of female *A. velutinana*. Ac, Acetate; ME or Me, methyl ester; S, saturated; E, *(E)*; Z, *(Z)*. Reproduced from Bjostad and Roelofs (1981), by permission of *The Journal of Biological Chemistry*.

hexadecanoate is a distal precursor in the pathway. Incorporation of three extra mass units into palmitoleate, oleate, linoleate, and linolenate was not observed, indicating that these are not produced in the pheromone gland after adult emergence (Bjostad and Roelofs, 1986).

Experiments with cell-free preparations of pheromone glands from the related species *A. citrana* provided more rigorous evidence for chain shortening. Only 0.01% incorporation of radiolabel into 14-carbon fatty acyl intermediates was observed with [1-14C]hexadecanoic acid as a precursor, but 0.96% incorporation was observed with [U-14C]hexadecanoic acid and 0.84% incorporation was observed with [9,10-3H]hexadecanoic acid. Incubation of pheromone glands with [3-14C]hexadecanoic acid provided even more compelling evidence for chain shortening, because decarboxylation of the recovered 14-carbon fatty acyl intermediates showed that 80% of the radiolabel was in the first carbon (Wolf and Roelofs, 1983).

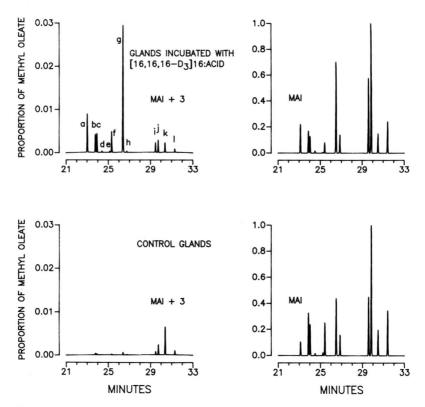

Fig. 6. Incorporation of [16,16,16-²H]hexadecanoic acid into pheromone components and fatty acyl groups in sex pheromone glands of female *A. velutinana*. a, Methyl tetradecanoate; b, methyl (*E*)-11-tetradecenoate; c, methyl (*Z*)-11-tetradecenoate; d, 1-tetradecyl acetate; e, (*E*)-11-tetradecen-1-yl acetate; f, (*Z*)-11-tetradecen-1-yl acetate; g, methyl hexadecanoate; h, methyl (*Z*)-9-hexadecenoate; i, methyl octadecanoate; j, methyl (*Z*)-9-octadecenoate; k, methyl (*Z,Z*)-9,12-octadecadienoate; l, methyl (*Z,Z,Z*)-9,12,15-octadecatrienoate. MAI, Most abundant ion of most abundant isotopomer. Reproduced from Bjostad and Roelofs (1986), by permission of Plenum Publishing Corp.

2. Double Bond Position and Desaturation

The construction of double bonds in fatty acids of most eukaryote species is due to desaturases, enzymes that place the double bond at a particular position in a saturated fatty acid (Wakil, 1970). Pheromone glands incubated with [1-¹⁴C]tetradecanoic acid prepared in our laboratory showed excellent incorporation into Z and E11-14 : Acyl groups, indicating desaturase activity (Fig. 7). Fatty acyl groups with 16 or 18 carbon atoms incorporated almost no radiolabel, verifying that recycling of radiolabel from the breakdown products of the starting material had not occurred.

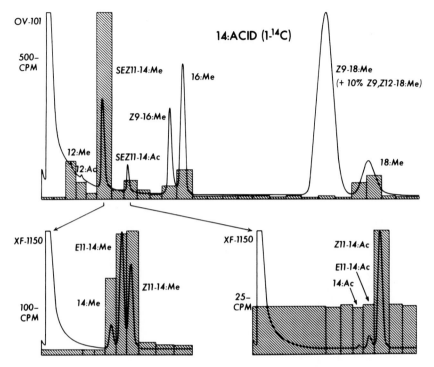

Fig. 7. Incorporation of radiolabel from topically applied [1-^{14}C]tetradecanoic acid into pheromone components and fatty acyl groups in sex pheromone glands of female *A. velutinana*. Ac, Acetate; Me, methyl ester. Reproduced from Bjostad and Roelofs (1981), by permission of *The Journal of Biological Chemistry*.

In a separate set of experiments, glands were incubated with [1,2,3-^{13}C]tetradecanoic acid or with [1,2,3,4-^{13}C]tetradecanoic acid. Incubation of glands with the first compound resulted in incorporation of three extra mass units into 14:Acyl, Z11-14:Acyl, E11-14:Acyl, 14:Ac, Z11-14:Ac, and E11-14:Ac, and incubation with the second compound resulted in incorporation of four extra mass units into the same compounds, as indicated by GLC–SIM–CI–MS (Fig. 8). Incorporation into unsaturated fatty acyl groups with 16 or 18 carbon atoms was not observed. These experiments verified that (Z)-11 and (E)-11 desaturation of tetradecanoate takes place in the gland (Bjostad and Roelofs, 1986).

Because E desaturases are uncommon in nature, we wished to rule out the possibility that an isomerase might exist in the gland. For example, retinene isomerase catalyzes the isomerization of all-(E)-retinal to form the 11-(Z)-retinal chromophore of the visual pigment rhodopsin (Hubbard, 1956). An isomerase that can interconvert geraniol (the E isomer) and nerol (the Z isomer) has also been characterized (Shine, 1973). Both geometric isomers [1-^{14}C](Z)-11-

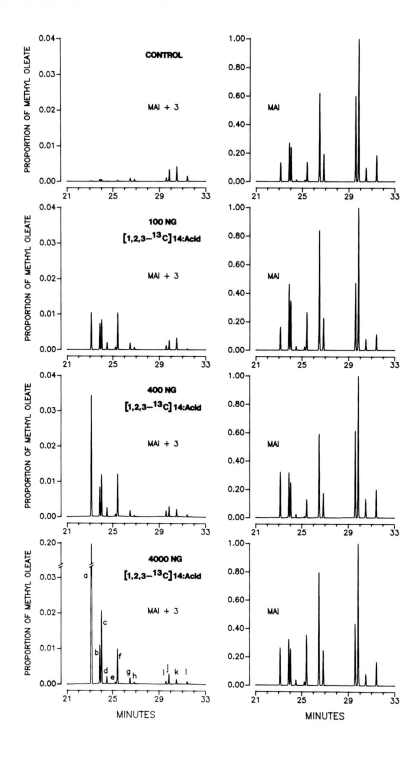

tetradecenoic acid and [1-^{14}C](E)-11-tetradecenoic acid were synthesized, and each was incubated *in vivo* with sex pheromone glands. The corresponding acetate pheromone component was produced in both cases, but in neither case was the opposite fatty acyl geometric isomer produced, indicating that isomerases do not occur in the gland. The same results were obtained when glands were incubated with the stable isotopomers [1,2,3,4-^{13}C](Z)-11-tetradecenoic acid or [1,2,3,4,-^{13}C](E)-11-tetradecenoic acid, as indicated by analysis with GLC–SIM–CI–MS.

3. Roles of Glycerolipid Classes

The information from the labeling studies discussed above indicated that the sequence of fatty acyl intermediates in biosynthesis of the sex pheromone components Z and E11-14 : Ac proceeds as shown in Fig. 9. Because the fatty acyl groups are components of glycerolipids, the function of each of the glycerolipid classes was examined next.

a. *Time Course of [1-^{14}C]Acetate Incorporation.* Pheromone glands were incubated with sodium [1-^{14}C]acetate for different times, and incorporation into the fatty acyl components was determined for the different glycerolipid classes in the gland. We anticipated that for brief incubations, the radiolabel found in early intermediates in the pathway would represent a larger proportion of the total than in longer incubations. Hexadecanoate is postulated to be an early intermediate in the pathway, and we found that the relative proportion of radiolabel in this fatty acyl group was much greater after 8 min incubation (Fig. 10) than after 15, 40, or 240 min incubations (Fig. 11), consistent with our hypothesis. This was true within the triacylglycerols and also within the choline phosphatides. Tetradecanoate is postulated to be a subsequent intermediate in the pathway, and we found that the proportion of radiolabel in tetradecanoate relative to the proportions in E and Z11-14 : Acyl groups was greater after 8 min incubation than after longer incubations, consistent with the view that it is an intermediate in the production of the unsaturated compounds (Bjostad and Roelofs, 1984a).

We hypothesized initially that radiolabel would first appear in E and Z11-14 : Acyl in the glycerolipids and after a time lag would appear in the pheromone components. We found instead that even for the shortest incubation

---

Fig. 8. Incorporation of [1,2,3-^{13}C]tetradecanoic acid into pheromone components and fatty acyl groups in sex pheromone glands of female *A. velutinana*. a, Methyl tetradecanoate; b, methyl (E)-11-tetradecenoate; c, methyl (Z)-11-tetradecenoate; d, 1-tetradecyl acetate; e, (E)-11-tetradecen-1-yl acetate; f, (Z)-11-tetradecen-1-yl acetate; g, methyl hexadecanoate; h, methyl (Z)-9-hexadecenoate; i, methyl octadecanoate; j, methyl (Z)-9-octadecenoate; k, methyl (Z,Z)-9,12-octadecadienoate; l, methyl (Z,Z,Z)-9,12,15-octadecatrienoate. MAI, Most abundant ion of most abundant isotopomer. Reproduced from Bjostad and Roelofs (1986), by permission of Plenum Publishing Corp.

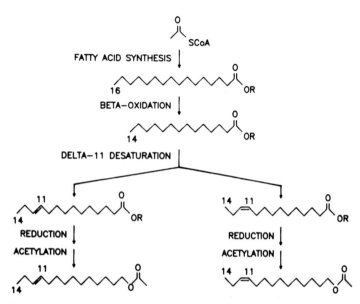

Fig. 9. Sequence of fatty acyl intermediates in biosynthesis of sex pheromone components of *A. velutinana*. Reproduced from Roelofs and Bjostad (1984), by permission of Academic Press, Inc.

practical (8 min), a large proportion of the incorporated radiolabel was found in the pheromone components. It appears that once hexadecanoate has been biosynthesized, the subsequent steps occur in close succession, including chain shortening, desaturation, reduction, and acetylation. Hexadecanoate is presumably produced by fatty acid synthase in the cytosol (Volpe and Vagelos, 1976), which may account for a delay in its availability to the enzymes involved in subsequent steps, which are likely to be membrane bound (Bell and Coleman, 1980; Holub and Kuksis, 1978) and may exist in close association with one another.

We also hypothesized that the sequence of glycerolipid intermediates could be determined by observing the order of appearance of radiolabeled E and Z11-14:Acyl in each lipid class. We found that the triacylglycerols contained most of the radiolabeled fatty acyl groups for all incubation times, indicating that the enzymes involved in fatty acyl transfer may be closely associated with one another.

b. Triacylglycerols. Because the triacylglycerols contain most of E and Z11-14:Acyl groups in the gland, we wished to know if this class served as an acyl donor in the production of the corresponding pheromone components. We synthesized 1-palmitoyl-2-[1-^{14}C]tetradecanoyl-3-palmitoyl-*sn*-glycerol and ap-

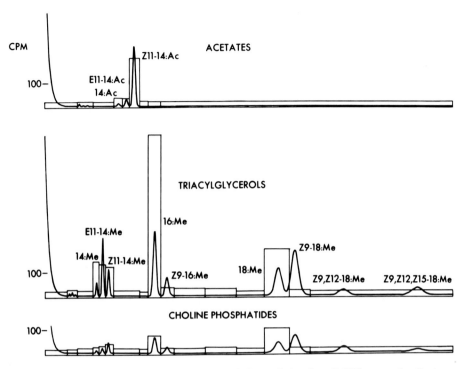

Fig. 10. Incorporation of radiolabel from topically applied sodium [1-¹⁴C]acetate after 8 min incubation in pheromone gland of *A. velutinana*. Ac, Acetate; Me, methyl ester. Reproduced from Bjostad and Roelofs (1984a), by permission of Plenum Publishing Corp.

plied this topically to pheromone glands in dimethyl sulfoxide. No radiolabeled E or Z11-14 : Acyl compounds were produced at all, nor was radiolabel incorporated into the pheromone components. In contrast, incorporation of radiolabel into all these compounds was observed when glands were incubated with [1-¹⁴C]tetradecanoic acid. Tetradecanoate in the synthetic triacylglycerol was clearly not a substrate for the desaturases in the gland, nor could it serve as an acyl donor. This indicates that the desaturases act on one of the early tetradecanoyl intermediates in the pathway, probably a CoA thioester or a phospholipid, and there is precedent for both in the literature (Pugh and Kates, 1979).

In a second set of experiments with synthetic triacylglycerols, pheromone glands were incubated with a 50 : 50 mixture of 1-oleoyl-2-[1,2,3,4-¹³C](Z)-11-tetradecenoyl-3-oleoyl-*sn*-glycerol and 1-oleoyl-2-[1,2,3,4-¹³C](E)-11-tetradecenoyl-3-oleoyl-*sn*-glycerol prepared in our laboratory. The methanolysis–acetylation derivatives of the gland extract were analyzed by GLC–SIM–CI–MS as described above. No incorporation of the labeled E or Z11-14 : Acyl groups into

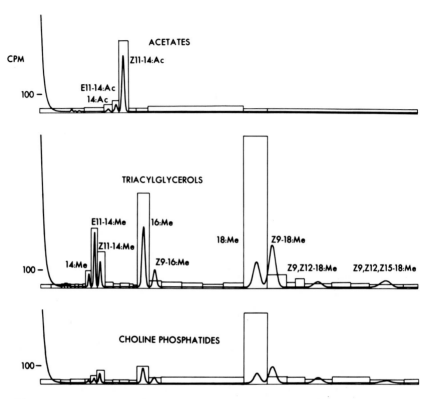

Fig. 11.   Incorporation of radiolabel from topically applied sodium [1-¹⁴C]acetate after 240 min incubation in pheromone gland of *A. velutinana*. Ac, Acetate; Me, methyl ester. Reproduced from Roelofs and Bjostad (1984), by permission of Academic Press, Inc.

the pheromone components was observed. In a second experiment, a triacylglycerol with different acyl groups at the *sn*-1 and *sn*-3 positions were tested to see if oleate had been a determinant in the first experiment. Pheromone glands were incubated with 1-palmitoyl-2-[1,2,3,4-¹³C](Z)-11-tetradecenoyl-3-palmitoyl-*sn*-glycerol, but no incorporation into Z11-14 : Ac was observed (Bjostad and Roelofs, 1986). In all these experiments, the triacylglycerols did not serve as acyl donors in the production of the pheromone components, despite the fact that the labeled fatty acyl groups in each case were incorporated readily into the pheromone components when presented to the gland as the free fatty acids.

c.   Choline and Ethanolamine Phosphatides.   We have little information concerning the roles of the ethanolamine phosphatides and choline phosphatides in the gland. It is possible that they are early intermediates in the pathway. The substrates for desaturases are conventionally regarded to be fatty acyl-CoA esters, but there is evidence that phospholipids themselves can be substrates for desaturases (Pugh and Kates, 1979). If this is true in *A. velutinana*, the $E:Z$ ratio in the phosphatides in the gland may reflect the relative activities of (Z)-11 and (E)-11 desaturases that determine the initial availabilities of Z and E11-14:Acyl groups. In either case, Z and E11-14:Acyl groups in the choline phosphatides and ethanolamine phosphatides may be released by the action of phospholipase A_2 in the membrane, as part of the ongoing deacylation–reacylation cycles that normally occur in membranes of cell organelles (Bell and Coleman, 1980), and these fatty acyl groups would then be available for production of intermediates in the biosynthesis of triacylglycerols.

From simple bookkeeping with respect to the amounts of Z and E isomers in the triacylglycerols, the choline phosphatides, the ethanolamine phosphatides, and the pheromone components themselves, it is apparent that the sum of the picomoles of E isomers in the triacylglycerols and in the pheromone complement is about half the sum of the picomoles of the Z isomers in the triacylglycerols and in the pheromone complement. This $1:2$ ratio is the same as the $E:Z$ ratio in the choline phosphatides and in the ethanolamine phosphatides and implies that the phosphatides may provide the pool of E and Z11-14:Acyl groups used to biosynthesize the triacylglycerols and the pheromone components.

d.   Implications with Respect to $Z:E$ Blend Regulation.   Both the Z and E fatty acyl precursors are biosynthesized in large amounts, but the selection of Z precursors for conversion to pheromone components is 10 times that of E precursors. As the E precursor accumulates, it might be expected that the $E:Z$ ratio of the pheromone components would increase as well, but this does not occur. One way the gland could achieve this would be to select fatty acyl groups from one of the glycerolipid intermediates in pheromone biosynthesis (perhaps the choline or ethanolamine phosphatides), and simply allow the remainder to be converted to triacylglycerols. If this were the case, the triacylglycerols in the gland could function as a chemical dump, assuring that selection would always be made from a fresh pool of the glycerolipid intermediate. A pathway of this sort is consistent with our observation that labeled fatty acyl groups in synthetic triacylglycerols are not incorporated into sex pheromone components.

4.   Multicomponent Pheromone Blend

In the course of determining the biosynthetic pathway involved in the production of the main pheromone components Z and E11-14:Ac, it became apparent that additional acetates were present in small amounts. Behavioral tests showed that these were additional pheromone components, including 12:Ac, E9-12:Ac, Z9-12:Ac, 11-12:Ac, and 14:Ac (Bjostad *et al.*, 1985). The biosynthesis of all these compounds can be accounted for on the basis of (Z)-11 desaturation of

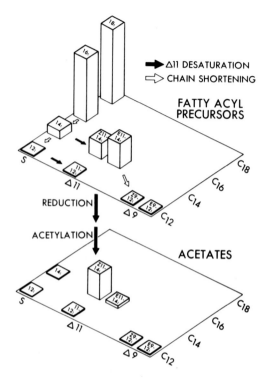

Fig. 12. Proposed biosynthetic routes for additional pheromone components in *A. velutinana.* Heights of blocks are proportional to amounts of compounds in pheromone glands. Reproduced from Bjostad *et al.* (1985), by permission of Walter de Gruyter, Inc.

tetradecanoate and dodecanoate, in conjunction with chain shortening of Z11-14 : Acyl groups and 14 : Acyl groups (Fig. 12).

B. *Trichoplusia ni*

1. Carbon Skeleton and Chain Length

By analogy with what we had found with *A. velutinana,* we expected that hexadecanoate would be an early precursor in the biosynthesis of Z7-12 : Ac by *Trichoplusia ni.* If hexadecanoate underwent chain shortening by two cycles of β-oxidation, dodecanoate would be produced. Desaturation of dodecanoate by a (Z)-7 desaturase could produce Z7-12 : Acyl, which could be reduced and acetylated to produce the main pheromone component Z7-12 : Ac. The biosynthetic pathway for this compound proved to be completely different. The expected precursor Z7-12 : Acyl was present (Fig. 13), but a large amount of another

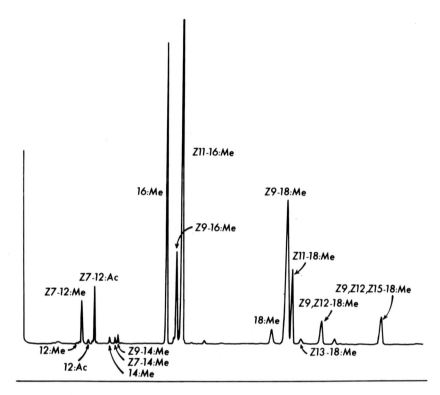

Fig. 13. GLC trace on polar capillary column of fatty acyl complement and pheromone components in the sex pheromone gland of *Trichoplusia ni*. Reproduced from Bjostad and Roelofs (1983). Copyright © 1983 by the AAAS.

uncommon fatty acyl group, Z11-16:Acyl, was also present (Bjostad and Roelofs, 1983).

The large amount of Z11-16:Acyl suggested a pathway in which desaturation occurs early in the pathway, generating Z11-16:Acyl from hexadecanoate. Chain shortening could then generate Z9-14:Acyl and Z7-12:Acyl in turn, as intermediates in the biosynthesis of Z7-12:Ac. Sex pheromone glands of *T. ni* were incubated *in vivo* with [16-^{3}H](Z)-11-hexadecenoic acid prepared in our laboratory. Radiolabel was incorporated into Z9-14:Acyl, into Z7-12:Acyl groups, and into Z7-12:Ac. Ozonolysis of the radiolabeled Z7-12:Ac was conducted to break the molecule into two aldehydes at the double bond. More stable benzyloxime derivatives were prepared from the aldehyde fragments and were separated by GLC. Analysis of the GLC fractions with scintillation counting showed that radiolabel occurred only at the methyl end of the molecule. In contrast, Z7-12:Ac produced by glands incubated with sodium [1-^{14}C]acetate were shown to contain radiolabel throughout the molecule. This verified that chain shortening of Z11-16 : Acyl groups is a key step in the biosynthesis of the pheromone (Bjostad and Roelofs, 1983).

2. Double Bond Position and Desaturation

Having established that Z11-16 : Acyl was a biosynthetic intermediate in the production of Z7-12 : Ac, we wished to verify that the double bond is produced by a (Z)-11 desaturase acting on hexadecanoate. In an initial experiment, glands of *T. ni* were incubated *in vivo* with 16-fluorohexadecanoic acid prepared in our laboratory from 16-fluoro-(E)-9-hexadecenol (a gift from Dr. Glenn Prestwich, Chemistry Dept., State University of New York, Stony Brook). Methanolysis–acetylation derivatives of the gland extract were analyzed by GLC–SIM–CI–MS. The glands produced (16-F)Z11-16 : Acyl, indicating (Z)-11 desaturation of hexadecanoate, and the glands also produced (14-F)Z9-14 : Acyl, (12-F)Z7-12 : Acyl, and (12-F)Z7-12 : Ac (Fig. 14).

A more rigorous study of the desaturase has been completed by Wolf and Roelofs (1986), who showed by incubation of cell-free extracts that the (Z)-11 desaturase is microsomal, will accept [1-^{14}C]hexadecanoyl CoA or [1-^{14}C]octadecanoyl CoA (but not [1-^{14}C]tetradecanoyl CoA), and occurs only in the sex pheromone gland. Unlike the (Z)-9 desaturases that occur in other organisms (Wang *et al.*, 1982, and references therein), the (Z)-11 desaturase requires NADH instead of NADPH and has a pH optimum of 7.4–7.8 instead of 6.8–7.2.

3. Roles of Glycerolipid Classes

The information from the labeling studies discussed above indicated that the sequence of fatty acyl intermediates in biosynthesis of the sex pheromone component Z7-12 : Ac proceeds as shown in Fig. 15. No work has been done with labeled glycerolipids in *T. ni*. As in *A. velutinana*, most of the fatty acyl groups in the gland occur in the triacylglycerols, and much smaller amounts occur in 1,2-diacylglycerols, choline phosphatides, and ethanolamine phosphatides (Bjostad and Roelofs, 1983). The glycerolipid classes contained the maximal amount of Z11-16 : Acyl groups the first day of female emergence, and this changed little over the first 4 days of adult life. In contrast, the pheromone component Z7-12 : Ac was absent at female emergence, and levels rose day by day until it reached a maximum on the fourth night (about 800 ng per gland). Sex pheromone production in *A. velutinana* differed in that the pheromone components and their fatty acyl precursors were absent at adult emergence and increased day by day to a maximum on the fourth night.

4. Multicomponent Pheromone Blend

In the course of determining the biosynthetic pathway involved in the production of the main pheromone component Z7-12 : Ac, it became apparent that

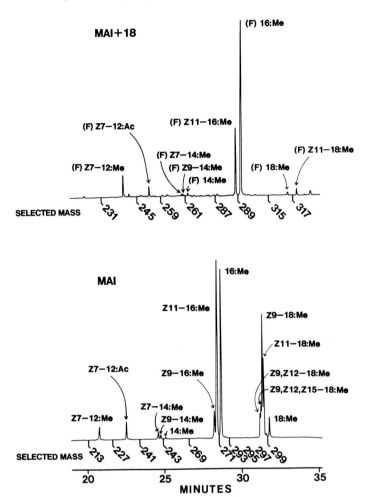

Fig. 14. Incorporation of 16-fluorohexadecanoic acid into fatty acyl complement and pheromone components in sex pheromone gland of *T. ni*. MAI, Most abundant ion of most abundant isotopomer.

additional acetates were present in small amounts. Behavioral tests showed that these were additional pheromone components, including 12 : Ac, Z5-12 : Ac, Z11-12 : Ac, Z7-14 : Ac, and Z9-14 : Ac (Bjostad *et al.*, 1984). The biosynthesis of all these compounds (Fig. 16) can be accounted for on the basis of (Z)-11 desaturation of hexadecanoate, octadecanoate, and dodecanoate, in conjunction with chain shortening of A11-16 : Acyl and Z11-18 : Acyl groups (Bjostad *et al.*, 1985).

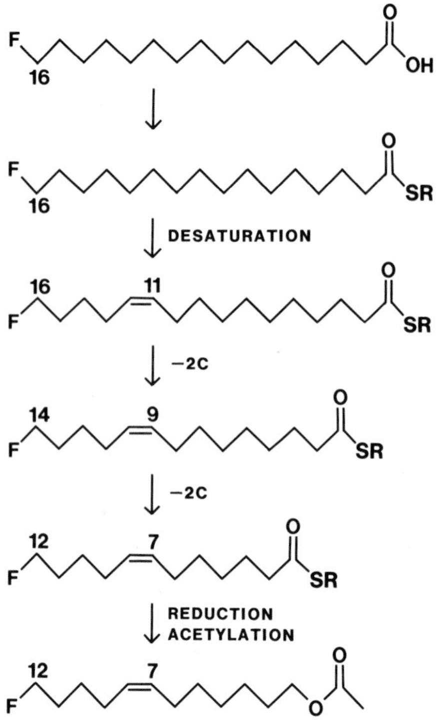

Fig. 15. Sequence of fatty acyl intermediates in biosynthesis of sex pheromone components of *T. ni.*

C. *Bombyx mori*

1. Fatty Acyl Biosynthetic Intermediates

The origins of the pheromone components in *A. velutinana* and in *T. ni* could all be attributed to (Z)-11 desaturation of saturated fatty acids. *Bombyx mori* was of interest because there was no obvious way that the conjugated double bond system in the main pheromone component bombykol, E10,Z12-16:OH, could arise from a (Z)-11 fatty acyl precursor. Nevertheless, Yamaoka and Hayashiya (1982) reported that Z11-16:Acyl groups occurred in silkmoth pheromone glands in large amounts. This report was puzzling in that the GLC traces presented did not indicate the presence of E10,Z12-16:Acyl groups. the expected fatty acyl precursor of bombykol.

It seemed possible that the silkmoth might use a very different means of sex pheromone biosynthesis than *A. velutinana* or *T. ni,* but an alternative explanation occurred to us when we noticed that bombykol itself was also absent from

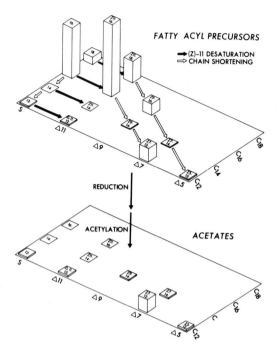

Fig. 16. Proposed biosynthetic routes for additional pheromone components in *T. ni.* Reproduced from Bjostad *et al.* (1985), by permission of Walter de Gruyter, Inc.

the GLC traces. Acid methanolysis had been used to prepare methyl esters from the fatty acyl groups in the gland, and compounds with conjugated double bond systems tend to be destroyed under acidic conditions. We separated the glycerolipids in silkmoth pheromone gland extracts by TLC and performed base methanolysis on the purified glycerolipid classes (Bjostad and Roelofs, 1984b). We found that the expected E10,Z12-16: Acyl precursors were present in large amounts in the gland (Fig. 17), in addition to the Z11-16: Acyl groups reported by Yamaoka and Hayashiya (1982), occurring in the triacylglycerols, choline phosphatides, and ethanolamine phosphatides (but in very tiny amounts in the diacylglycerols). We also verified that acid methanolysis destroys bombykol and E10,Z12-16: Acyl groups but does not degrade fatty acyl groups in the gland that lack conjugated double bonds.

2. Sequence of Desaturations

The presence of Z11-16: Acyl groups in large amounts in the pheromone gland, distributed among the glycerolipid classes in the same approximate proportions as E10,Z12-16: Acyl groups, is circumstantial evidence that the Z-11

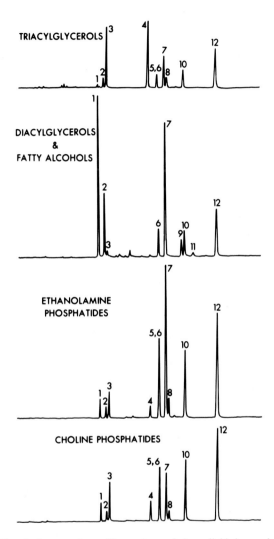

Fig. 17. GLC analysis on a polar capillary column of glycerolipids in sex pheromone glands of *Bombyx mori* after base methanolysis and treatment with acetyl chloride. 1, Methyl hexadecanoate; 2, methyl (Z)-9-hexadecenoate; 3, methyl (Z)-11-hexadecenoate; 4, methyl (E,Z)-10,12-hexadecadieno-ate; 5, methyl (E,E)-10,12-hexadecadienoate; 6, methyl octadecanoate; 7, methyl (Z)-9-octadeceno-ate; 8, methyl (Z)-11-octadecenoate; 9, (E,Z)-10,12-hexadecadien-1-yl acetate; 10, methyl (Z,Z)-9, 12-octadecadienoate; 11, (E,E)-10,12-hexadecadien-1-yl acetate; 12, methyl (Z,Z,Z)-9,12.15- octa-decatrienoate. Reproduced from Bjostad and Roelofs (1984b), copyright 1984, Pergamon Press, Ltd.

double bond is undergoes a 1,4-desaturation to generate the conjugated double bond system. The nature of the enzyme system required to effect such a 1,4-desaturation is not known.

3. Glycerolipid Classes

No experiments have been done to determine the role of the glycerolipid classes in *B. mori*. The unusual fatty acyl groups Z11-16 : Acyl and E10,Z12-16 : Acyl are apparently involved in the biosynthesis of the pheromone component, E10,Z12-16 : OH, and occur mainly in the triacylglycerols, in smaller amounts in the choline phosphatides and ethanolamine phosphatides, and are nearly absent from the diacylglycerols. This pattern of distribution is strikingly similar to that observed for the pheromone biosynthetic precursors in *A. velutinana* and *T. ni*, which have been studied more intensively. In *A. velutinana* the fatty acyl precursors Z and E11-14 : Acyl are similarly most abundant in the triacylglycerols, less so in the phospholipids, and nearly absent from the diacylglycerols. In *T. ni*, the fatty acyl precursors Z11-16 : Acyl, Z9-14 : Acyl, and Z7-12 : Acyl occur principally in the triacyclglycerols, in smaller amounts in the phospholipids, and in trace amounts in the diacylglycerols.

It is not yet known what role each of the glycerolipid classes plays in pheromone biosynthesis of any of these three species. These three species occur in three different families of Lepidoptera. yet in all three species the fatty acyl biosynthetic precursors predominate in the triacylglycerols, are less abundant in the choline phosphatides and ethanolamine phosphatides, and are nearly absent from the diacylglycerols.

REFERENCES

Arai, K., Ando, T., Tatsuki, S., Usui, K., Ohguchi, Y., Kurihara, M., Fukami, J., and Takahashi, N. (1984). The biosynthetic pathway of (Z)-11-hexadecenal, the sex pheromone component of the rice stem borer, *Chilo suppressalis*. *Agric. Biol. Chem.* **48**, 3165–3168.

Bell, R. M., and Coleman, R. A. (1980). Enzymes of glycerolipid synthesis in eukaryotes. *Annu. Rev. Biochem.* **49**, 459–487.

Berger, R. S. (1966). Isolation, identification, and synthesis of the sex attractant of the cabbage looper, *Trichoplusia ni*. *Ann. Entomol. Soc. Am.* **59**, 767–771.

Beroza, M., and Bierl, B. A. (1966). Apparatus for ozonolysis of microgram to milligram amounts of compound. *Anal. Chem.* **38**, 1976–1977.

Bestmann, H. J., and Vostrowsky, O. (1979). Synthesis of pheromones by stereoselective carbonyl olefination: a unitised construction principle. *Chem. Phys. Lipids* **24**, 335–389.

Biemann, K. (1962). "Mass Spectrometry." McGraw-Hill, New York.

Bierl, B. A., Beroza, M., and Collier, C. W. (1970). Potent sex attractant of the gypsy moth: Its isolation, identification, and synthesis. *Science* **170**, 87–89.

Bjostad, L. B., and Roelofs, W. L. (1981). Sex pheromone biosynthesis from radiolabeled fatty acids in the redbanded leafroller moth. *J. Biol. Chem.* **256**, 7936–7940.

Bjostad, L. B., and Roelofs, W. L. (1983). Sex pheromone biosynthesis in *Trichoplusia ni:* Key steps involve Δ^{11} desaturation and chain shortening. *Science* **220,** 1387–1389.

Bjostad, L. B., and Roelofs, W. L. (1984a). Biosynthesis of sex pheromone components and glycerolipid precursors from sodium [1-^{14}C]acetate in redbanded leafroller moth. *J. Chem. Ecol.* **10,** 681–691.

Bjostad, L. B., and Roelofs, W. L. (1984b). Sex pheromone biosynthetic precursors in *Bombyx mori. Insect Biochem.* **14,** 275–278.

Bjostad, L. B., and Roelofs, W. L. (1986). Sex pheromone biosynthesis in the redbanded leafroller moth, studied by mass-labeling with stable isotopes and analysis with mass spectrometry. *J. Chem. Ecol.* **12,** 431–450.

Bjostad, L. B., Wolf, W. A., and Roelofs, W. L. (1981). Total lipid analysis of the sex pheromone gland of the redbanded leafroller moth, *Argyrotaenia velutinana,* with reference to pheromone biosynthesis. *Insect Biochem.* **11,** 73–79.

Bjostad, L. B., Linn, C. E., Du, J. W., and Roelofs, W. L. (1984). Identification of new sex pheromone components in *Trichoplusia ni,* predicted from biosynthetic precursors. *J. Chem. Ecol.* **10,** 1309–1323.

Bjostad, L. B., Linn, C. E., Du, J. W., and Roelofs, W. L. (1985). Identification of new sex pheromone components in *Trichoplusia ni* and *Argyrotaenia velutinana,* predicted from biosynthetic precursors. *In* ''Semiochemicals: Flavors and Pheromones'' (T. E. Acree and D. M. Soderlund, eds.), pp. 223–237. American Chemical Society, Washington, D.C.

Blomquist, G. J., and Ries, M. K. (1979). The enzymatic synthesis of wax esters by a microsomal preparation from the honeybee *Apis mellifera. Insect Biochem.* **9,** 183–188.

Brockerhoff, H. (1975). Determination of the positional distribution of fatty acids in glycerolipids. *In* ''Methods in Enzymology'' (J. M. Lowenstein, ed.), Vol. 35, pp. 315–325. Academic Press, New York.

Butenandt, A., Beckman, R., Stamm, D., and Hecker, E. (1959). Uber den Sexuallockstoff des Seidenspinner *Bombyx mori,* Reidarstellung und Konstitution. *Z. Naturforsch. B* **14,** 283–284.

Carson, R. (1964). ''Silent Spring.'' Fawcett, Greenwich, Connecticut.

Feng, K. C., and Roelofs, W. L. (1977). Sex pheromone gland development in redbanded leafroller moth, *Argyrotaenia velutinana,* pupae and adults. *Ann. Entomol. Soc. Am.* **70,** 721–732.

Fieser, L. F., and Fieser, M. (1967). ''Reagents, for Organic Synthesis.'' Wiley, New York.

Folch, J., Lees, M., and Sloane-Stanley, G. (1957). A simple method for the isolation and purification of total lipids from animal tissues. *J. Biol. Chem.* **226,** 497–509.

Hassner, A., and Alexanian, V. (1978). Direct room temperature esterification of carboxylic acids. *Tetrahedron Lett.* **46,** 4475–4478.

Henrick, C. A. (1977). The synthesis of insect sex pheromones. *Tetrahedron* **33,** 1845–1889.

Hill, A. S., and Roelofs, W. L. (1981). Sex pheromone of the saltmarsh caterpillar moth *Estigmene acrea. J. Chem. Ecol.* **7,** 655–668.

Holub, B. J., and Kuksis, A. (1978). Metabolism of molecular species of diacylglycerophospholipids. *Adv. Lipid Res.* **16,** 1–125.

Hubbard, R. (1956). Retinene isomerase. *J. Gen. Physiol.* **39,** 935–962.

Inoue, S., and Hamamura, Y. (1972). The biosynthesis of bombykol, sex pheromone of *Bombyx mori. Proc. Jpn. Acad.* **48,** 323–326.

Jones, I. G., and Berger, R. S. (1978). Incorporation of [1-^{14}C]acetate into *cis*-7-dodecenyl acetate, a sex pheromone in the cabbage looper. *Environ. Entomol.* **7,** 666–669.

Jones, I. G., Berger, R. S., and Hargis, J. H. (1982). Unsuitability of carbon-13 nuclear magnetic resonance for studying pheromone biosynthesis in the cabbage looper moth. *J. Agric. Food Chem.* **30,** 1002–1004.

Kasang, G., and Schneider, D. (1974). Biosynthesis of the sex pheromone disparlure by olefin-epoxide conversion. *Naturwissenschaften* **61,** 130–131.

Keith, A. D. (1967). Fatty acid metabolism in *Drosophila melanogaster:* Interaction between dietary fatty acids and *de novo* synthesis. *Comp. Biochem. Physiol.* **21**, 587–600.

Klun, J. A., and Brindley, T. A. (1970). *cis*-11-Tetradecenyl acetate. a sex stimulant of the European corn borer. *J. Econ. Entomol.* **63**, 779–780.

Klun, J. A., Plimmer, J. R., Bieerl-Leonhardt, B. A., Sparks, A. N., Primiani, M., Chapman, O. L., Lee, G. H., and Lepone, G. (1980). Sex pheromone chemistry of the female corn earworm moth, *Heliothis zea. J. Chem. Ecol.* **6**, 165–175.

Kolattukudy, P. E., and Rogers, L. (1978). Biosynthesis of fatty alcohols, alkane-1,2-diols and wax esters in particulate preparations from the uropygial glands of white-crowned sparrows. *Arch. Biochem. Biophys.* **191**, 244–258.

Lambremont, E. N., and Wykle, R. L. (1979). Wax synthesis by an enzyme system from the honeybee. *Comp. Biochem. Physiol.* **63B**, 131–135.

Lambremont, E. N., Ernst, N. R., Ferguson, J. R., and Dial, P. F. (1976). Lipid metabolism of insects: Chain shortening of a long-chain dietary fatty acid. *Comp. Biochem. Physiol. B* **54**, 167–169.

Litchfield, C. (1972). "Analysis of Triglycerides." Academic Press, New York.

Mangold, H. (1969). *In* "Thin-Layer Chromatography: A Laboratory Handbook" (E. Stahl, ed.), pp. 363–421. Springer, New York.

Miller, J. R., and Roelofs, W. L. (1980). Individual variation in sex pheromone component ratios in two populations of the redbanded leafroller moth, *Argyrotaenia velutinana. Environ. Entomol.* **9**, 359–363.

Morse, D., and Meighen, E. (1984). Aldehyde pheromones in Lepidoptera: Evidence for an acetate ester precursor in *Choristoneura fumiferana. Science* **226**, 1434–1436.

Morse, D., and Meighen, E. (1986). Pheromone biosynthesis and role of functional groups in pheromone specificity. *J. Chem. Ecol.* **12**, 335–351.

Nichols, B. W., Haris, R. V., and James, A. T. (1965). The lipid metabolism of blue-green algae. *Biochem. Biophys. Res. Commun.* **20**, 256–262.

Percy, J. (1979). Development and ultrastructure of sex pheromone gland cells in females of the cabbage looper moth, *Trichoplusia ni. Can. J. Zool.* **57**, 220–236.

Prestwich, G. D., Plavcan, K. A., and Melcer, M. J. (1981a). Synthesis of fluorolipids: 1-*O*-Alkyl-2,3-*O*-diacylglycerols as targeted insecticides. *J. Agric. Food Chem.* **29**, 1018–1022.

Prestwich, G. D., Melcer, M. J., and Plavcan, K. A. (1981b). Fluorolipids as targeted termiticides and biochemical probes. *J. Agric. Food Chem.* **29**, 1023–1027.

Pugh, E. L., and Kates, M. (1979). Membrane-bound phospholipid desaturases. *Lipids* **14**, 159–165.

Rock, C. D., Fitzgerald. V., and Snyder, F. (1978). Coupling of the biosynthesis of fatty acids and fatty alcohols. *Arch. Biochem. Biophys.* **186**, 77–83.

Roelofs, W. L., and Bjostad, L. B. (1984). Biosynthesis of lepidopteran pheromones. *Bioorg. Chem.* **12**, 279–298.

Roelofs, W. L., and Brown, R. L. (1982). Pheromones and evolutionary relationships of Tortricidae. *Ann. Rev. Ecol. Syst.* **13**, 395–422.

Roelofs, W., Hill, A., and Carde, R. (1975). Sex pheromone components of the redbanded leafroller, *Argyrotaenia velutinana. J. Chem. Ecol.* **1**, 83–89.

Ryan, R. O., De Renobales, M., Dillwith, J. W., Heisler, C. R., and Blomquist, G. J. (1982). Biosynthesis of myristate in an aphid: Involvement of a specific acylthioesterase. *Arch. Biochem. Biophys.* **213**, 26–36,

Schlosser, M. (1978). Introduction of fluorine into organic molecules: Why and how. *Tetrahedron* **34**, 3–17.

Shine, W. (1973). Trans–cis isomerization of geraniol and geranyl phosphate by cell-free enzymes from higher plants. Ph.D. dissertation in Biochemistry, Oregon State University, Corvallis.

Shorey, H. H., Gaston, L. K., and Saario, C. A. (1967). Sex pheromones of noctuid moths. XIV. Feasibility of behavioral control by disrupting pheromone communication in cabbage loopers. *J. Econ. Entomol.* **60,** 1541–1545.

Steck, W., Underhill, E. W., and Chisholm, M. D. (1982). Structure–activity relationships in sex attractants for North American moths. *J. Chem. Ecol.* **8,** 731–754.

Stowell, M. (1970). A short synthesis of the sex pheromone of the pink bollworm moth. *J. Org. Chem.* **35,** 244–254.

Tamaki, Y. (1985). Sex pheromones. *In* "Comprehensive Insect Physiology, Biochemistry, and Pharmacology" (G. A. Kerkut and L. I. Gilbert, eds.), Chap. 9. Pergamon, New York.

Volpe, J. J., and Vagelos, P. R. (1976). Mechanisms and regulation of biosynthesis of saturated fatty acids. *Physiol. Rev.* **56,** 339–417.

Wakil, S. J. (1970). "Lipid Metabolism." Academic Press, New York.

Wang, D. L., Dillwith, J. W., Ryan, R. O., Blomquist, G. J., and Reitz, R. C. (1982). Characterization of the acyl-CoA desaturase in the housefly, *Musca domestica. Insect Biochem.* **12,** 545–555.

Weatherston, J., Roelofs, W., Comeau, A., and Sanders, C. J. (1971). Studies of physiologically active arthropod secretions. X. Sex pheromone of the eastern spruce budworm, *Choristoneura fumiferana. Can. Entomol.* **103,** 1741–1747.

Wiley, G. A., Hershkowitz, R. L., Rein, B. M., and Chung, B. C. (1964). Studies in organophosphorus chemistry. I. Conversion of alchols and phenols to halides by tertiary phosphine dihalides. *J. Am. Chem. Soc.* **86,** 964–965.

Wolf, W. A., and Roelofs, W. L. (1983). A chain-shortening reaction in orange tortrix moth sex pheromone biosynthesis. *Insect Biochem.* **13,** 375–379.

Wolf, W. A., and Roelofs, W. L. (1986). Properties of the Δ^{11} desaturase enzyme used in cabbage looper moth sex pheromone biosynthesis. *Arch. Insect Biochem. Physiol.* **3,** 45–52.

Yamaoka, R., and Hayashiya, K. (1982). Daily changes in the characteristic fatty acid (Z)-11-hexadecenoic acid of the pheromone gland of silkworm pupa and moth, *Bombyx mori. Jpn. J. Appl. Entomol. Zool.* **26,** 125–130.

Yamaoka, R., Taniguchi, Y., and Hayashiya, K. (1984). Bombykol biosynthesis from deuterium-labeled (Z)-11-hexadecenoic acid. *Experientia* **40,** 80–81.

4

Pheromone Biosynthesis: Enzymatic Studies in Lepidoptera

DAVID MORSE[1]
EDWARD MEIGHEN
Department of Biochemistry
McGill University
McIntyre Medical Sciences Building
Montreal, Quebec, Canada H3G 1Y6

I. INTRODUCTION

Although the characterization of the chemical structures of insect pheromones has advanced very rapidly since 10,12-hexadecadienol was identified as the major component of the sex pheromone of the silkworm moth, *Bombyx mori (Butenandt et al.,* 1959), studies on the pathways and mechanisms for pheromone biosynthesis have been very limited (Weaver, 1978; Blomquist and Dillwith, 1983). The paucity of biochemical studies on insect pheromones can be at least partially traced to the low amounts of material available and the absence of suitable techniques for measuring the synthesis and degradation of pheromones. Knowledge of the biochemical pathways for pheromone production and their regulation is important for understanding the signal-generating mechanism used for communication by insect species.

The pheromones of the Lepidoptera are generally a blend of long chain unsaturated aldehydes (**I**), alcohols (**II**), and acetate esters (**III**) (Inscoe, 1982). Specificity in the pheromone signal is achieved by variation in the chain length, the

[1]Present address: Biological Laboratories, Harvard University, Cambridge, Massachusetts 02138.

Pheromone Biochemistry

$$\text{CH}_3\text{—(CH}_2)_x\text{—CH=CH—(CH}_2)_y\text{—}\overset{\overset{\displaystyle O}{\|}}{\text{C}}\text{—H}$$
I

$$\text{CH}_3\text{—(CH}_2)_x\text{—CH=CH—(CH}_2)_y\text{—CH}_2\text{OH}$$
II

$$\text{CH}_3\text{—(CH}_2)_x\text{—CH=CH—(CH}_2)_y\text{—CH}_2\text{O}\overset{\overset{\displaystyle O}{\|}}{\text{C}}\text{—CH}_3$$
III

number, location, and isomeric nature of the double bond(s), the nature of the functional group, and by the blending together of several compounds (pheromone components) in a precise ratio. Consequently, investigation of the mechanisms of fatty acid biosynthesis, desaturation, and reduction and characterization of the pathways for interconversion of the aldehydes, alcohols, and acetate esters in Lepidoptera are essential for understanding the control of pheromone biosynthesis in these insects.

The pheromone of the eastern spruce budworm, *Choristoneura fumiferana*, is a blend of (*E*)-11-tetradecenal (**IV**) and (*Z*)-11-tetradecenal (**V**) in a 96 : 4 ratio (Sanders and Weatherston, 1976). The pheromone, which attracts male moths of the same species, is secreted from a specialized gland located at the end of the abdomen of the female moth (see Percy-Cunningham and MacDonald, Chapter 2, this volume). The levels of aldehyde pheromone in the gland are relatively low compared to the amount of acetate ester in the gland or the amount of pheromone released each night (Silk *et al.*, 1980; Morse *et al.*, 1982), suggesting a precursor–product relationship between the acetate ester and the aldehyde.

$$
\begin{array}{ccc}
\text{H} & (\text{CH}_2)_9\text{—}\overset{\overset{\displaystyle O}{\|}}{\text{CH}} & \\
\diagdown & \diagup & \\
& \text{C=C} & \\
\diagup & \diagdown & \\
\text{CH}_3\text{CH}_2 & \text{H} & \\
& \textbf{IV} &
\end{array}
\qquad
\begin{array}{ccc}
\text{H} & \text{H} & \\
\diagdown & \diagup & \\
& \text{C=C} & \\
\diagup & \diagdown & \\
\text{CH}_3\text{CH}_2 & (\text{CH}_2)_9\text{—}\overset{\overset{\displaystyle O}{\|}}{\text{CH}} & \\
& \textbf{V} &
\end{array}
$$

Interest in the metabolic pathways leading to the formation of insect pheromones has expanded in the past few years. Although *in vivo* labeling studies have been performed on a number of insect species, identification and *in vitro* analysis of specific enzymes in the pheromone biosynthetic pathway have only recently been accomplished (Morse and Meighen, 1984a, 1987; Wolf and Roelofs, 1986). The present chapter focuses on the biosynthesis of fatty aldehydes, alcohols, and acetate esters in Lepidoptera with particular attention to the characterization and analysis of enzymes involved in the metabolic pathway leading to the synthesis of the spruce budworm pheromone.

II. BIOSYNTHESIS OF LONG CHAIN ACETATE ESTER, ALCOHOL, AND ALDEHYDE PHEROMONES

A. Fatty Acid Biosynthesis

1. Reaction Pathways

Acetyl-CoA and malonyl-CoA are the basic building blocks used for the *de novo* biosynthesis of fatty acids in living organisms (Volpe and Vagelos, 1973, 1976). Acetyl-CoA normally arises in the cell as a product of the glycolytic cycle or by β-oxidation of fatty acids in the mitochondria. In addition, acetyl-CoA can also be formed by direct esterification of acetate in the cytoplasm by acetyl-CoA synthetases [reaction (1)]. The synthesis of malonyl-CoA is catalyzed by acetyl-CoA carboxylases [reaction (2)] which condense carbon dioxide with acetyl-CoA

$$CH_3COO^- + CoASH + ATP \longrightarrow CH_3-\overset{\overset{\displaystyle O}{\|}}{C}-SCoA + ADP + P_i \qquad (1)$$

$$CH_3-\overset{\overset{\displaystyle O}{\|}}{C}-SCoA + CO_2 (HCO_3^-) + ATP \longrightarrow {}^-OOC-CH_2-\overset{\overset{\displaystyle O}{\|}}{C}-SCoA + ADP + P_i \qquad (2)$$

in an ATP-dependent reaction. Fatty acids are then synthesized by condensation of two-carbon units from malonyl-CoA with a growing fatty acyl chain covalently linked to fatty acid synthase (X) in eukaryotic systems [reaction (3)] or

$$R-\overset{\overset{\displaystyle O}{\|}}{C}-X + {}^-OOC-CH_2-\overset{\overset{\displaystyle O}{\|}}{C}-SCoA \longrightarrow R-\overset{\overset{\displaystyle O}{\|}}{C}-CH_2-\overset{\overset{\displaystyle O}{\|}}{C}-X + CO_2 (HCO_3^-) + CoASH \qquad (3)$$

attached to the acyl carrier protein in prokaryotic systems; the release of carbon dioxide provides the driving force for the condensation reaction. The β-ketoacyl derivative is reduced, dehydrated, and reduced again to form the fatty acyl derivative two carbons longer [reaction (4)]. The cycle is then repeated with

$$R-\overset{\overset{\displaystyle O}{\|}}{C}-CH_2-\overset{\overset{\displaystyle O}{\|}}{C}-X + 2\ NADPH \longrightarrow R-(CH_2)_2-\overset{\overset{\displaystyle O}{\|}}{C}-X + 2\ NADP^+ + H_2O \qquad (4)$$

condensation of another malonyl-CoA molecule with the elongated fatty acyl chain. Biosynthesis of palmitic acid by fatty acid synthase thus involves sequential condensation of seven malonyl-CoA residues with an acetyl-CoA primer and the oxidation of 14 molecules of NADPH [reaction (5)]. Seven different activities are involved in the reaction catalyzed by fatty acid synthases. These

$$\begin{array}{c} \text{O} \\ \parallel \\ \text{CH}_3\text{—C—SCoA} \end{array} + 7\ \begin{array}{c} \text{O} \\ \parallel \\ ^-\text{OOC—CH}_2\text{—C—SCoA} \end{array} + 14\ \text{NADPH} \longrightarrow$$

$$\begin{array}{c} \text{O} \\ \parallel \\ \text{CH}_3\text{—(CH}_2)_{14}\text{—C—OH} \end{array} + 14\ \text{NADP}^+ + 7\ \text{CoASH} + 7\ \text{CO}_2\ (\text{HCO}_3^-) + 6\ \text{H}_2\text{O} \qquad (5)$$

activities are located on different polypeptides in a multienzyme complex in prokaryotic systems or in different domains on a single polypeptide chain of a multifunctional protein in eukaryotic systems (Wakil *et al.*, 1983).

2. *In Vivo* Incorporation of Labeled Acetate

Reactions (1)–(5) account for the direct incorporation of exogenous radiolabeled acetate into fatty acids by insects. Fatty acid biosynthesis can be assayed directly in cells by injection with aqueous solutions of labeled acetate into the abdomen of the insect (Jones and Berger, 1978), topical application of the labeled substrate in dimethyl sulfoxide (DMSO) (Bjostad and Roelofs, 1981), or by placing excised tissue pieces into aqueous solutions containing the radiolabeled compound (Dillwith *et al.*, 1981). Lipids containing the labeled material (e.g., fatty acids) can be extracted from the insect with organic solvents. There are no apparent differences, at least qualitatively, in the labeled products, using the three different techniques for *in vivo* incorporation of labeled acetate into the lipids of the spruce budworm. Approximately 0.5–1% of [1-^{14}C]acetate topically applied to the spruce budworm gland as a solution in DMSO is incorporated into lipids after a 2 hr incubation period. This technique gives a higher degree of labeling of lipids than the other two methods, in which the incorporation of label into glandular lipid is typically 10- to 100-fold lower (for excised tissue and injection into the abdomen, respectively).

Incorporation of radioactivity into lipids of the spruce budworm gland from acetate labeled with tritium (^{3}H) is lower than that from acetate labeled with carbon-14 (^{14}C) (Table I). This result is expected since a portion of the tritium atoms would be lost from acetate during formation of malonyl-CoA [reaction (2)] as well as during the dehydration step in fatty acid biosynthesis [reaction (4)]. One-third of the radiolabel in [^{3}H]acetate is lost during formation of malonyl-CoA, and at least another one-third is lost during the dehydration step (Fig. 1). In contrast, label would not be lost from [1-^{14}C]acetate in these reactions. Thus the maximum amount of tritium which could end up in a fatty acid containing n carbons compared to the amount of carbon-14 label is $(n + 4)/3n$, assuming that the specific activity of the labeled pools of acetyl-CoA and malonyl-CoA are identical *in vivo*. This assumption seems likely since the biosynthesis of malonyl-CoA is believed to be the rate-limiting step in fatty acid biosynthesis and thus the pool of malonyl-CoA in cells would be relatively low. Consequently, the max-

TABLE I

Incorporation of [¹⁴C]- and [³H]Acetate into Lipids of the Spruce Budworm Moth[a]

Precursor	Incorporation (%)
[1-¹⁴C]Acetate	0.51
(56 mCi/mmol)	0.54
[³H]Acetate	0.18
(2.8 Ci/mmol)	0.11
	0.24

[a]Radiolabeled acetate solutions (1 μl, 0.7 nmol) in DMSO were topically applied to the pheromone-producing glands of 20 *Choristoneura fumiferana*. After a 2 hr incubation the glands were excised and extracted in hexane containing 10% acetone, and the radioactivity was determined by scintillation counting. The percent of the applied radioactivity extracted into hexane is given for five independent experiments.

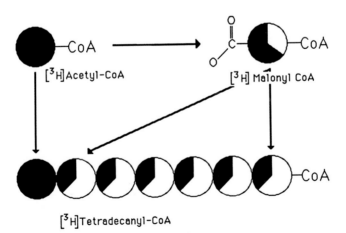

Fig. 1. Loss of tritium label during fatty acid synthesis. Acetate molecules labeled with tritium are shown as filled circles. The relative loss of tritium during biosynthesis of a fatty acyl chain from acetyl-CoA is represented by the change from filled to unfilled circles. The terminal acetate is incorporated directly whereas the internal acetate molecules are incorporated via malonyl-CoA.

imum amount of radioactivity incorporated into tetradecanoic acid from [³H]ace-
tate would be three-sevenths of that incorporated from the equivalent amount of
[1-¹⁴C]acetate (Fig. 1). If tritium exchange occurs with the medium during
biosynthesis then the ratio of tritium to carbon-14 would be even lower.

The major lipid products can rapidly be separated by thin-layer chromatography and the labeled material detected by autoradiography as shown in Fig. 2 for
extracts from the abdomen and the gland of the spruce budworm moth. Incorporation of acetate into glandular lipid reaches a plateau within 2 hr followed by a
decline in the amount of label in lipids that turn over more rapidly [e.g., tetradecenyl acetate, (TDA)]. Differences in the labeled lipid products extracted from
different tissues permit identification of compounds specifically synthesized in
one tissue or the other. Hence, long-chain fatty acid derivatives specifically
synthesized in the pheromone-producing gland (e.g., TDA) can be readily
identified.

3. In Vitro Fatty Acid Synthase Activity

Fatty acid synthase activity can be measured in vitro in extracts from the
spruce budworm gland. The in vitro reaction requires acetyl-CoA, malonyl-
CoA, and NADPH. By using labeled acetyl-CoA or malonyl-CoA, the synthesis

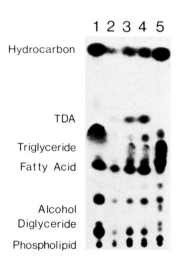

Fig. 2.   Incorporation of [1-¹⁴C]acetate into the lipids of the spruce budworm moth. Auto-
radiogram of a thin-layer chromatogram (TLC) of lipids labeled with [1-¹⁴C]acetate and extracted from
the spruce budworm moth. Radiolabeled acetate was topically applied in DMSO to the abdomen for 2
hr (lane 1) or to the gland for 15 min, 1 hr, 2 hr, or 20 hr (lanes 2–5, respectively) before extraction
with hexane and chromatography in hexane : diethyl ether : acetic acid (90 : 10 : 2) on silica gel. Each
lane contains the extract from eight insects with each insect exposed to approximately 0.06 μCi (1
nmol) of [1-¹⁴C]acetate. TDA, Tetradecanyl acetate or 11-tetradecenyl acetate.

of fatty acids can easily be followed by the incorporation of radiolabel into material extractable into hexane (Fig. 3). The relative incorporation (in moles) of malonyl-CoA and acetyl-CoA ($\sim$8:1) into lipid provides a rapid method for estimating the average chain length of the fatty acids synthesized *in vitro*. Analysis of the product by silver nitrate thin-layer chromatography has shown that only saturated and not unsaturated fatty acids are synthesized in this system.

The final product of the fatty acid synthase reaction *in vitro* is a free rather than an activated (esterified) fatty acid due to the presence of a thioesterase activity which in eukaryotic systems is an integral part of the fatty acid synthase enzyme [reaction (6)]. The esterase is relatively specific for acyl chains containing 16

$$\underset{R-C-X}{\overset{O}{\parallel}} + H_2O \longrightarrow \underset{R-C-OH}{\overset{O}{\parallel}} + X \tag{6}$$

carbons, resulting in the specific release of palmitic acid in most biological systems (Wakil *et al.*, 1983). Several cases are known, however, where the predominant fatty acid released has a shorter chain length. In the aphid, over 90% of the fatty acid released is tetradecanoic acid, due to the presence of a

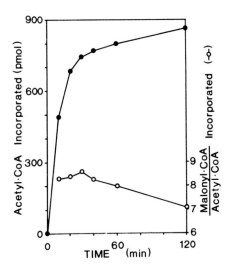

Fig. 3. *In vitro* fatty acid synthase activity in extracts of the female spruce budworm gland. The increase in the number of moles of acetyl-CoA or malonyl-CoA (given as a ratio) is shown as a function of time for a reaction mixture containing 15 μM [^{3}H]acetyl-CoA (200 mCi/mmol), 10 μM [2-^{14}C]malonyl-CoA (48 mCi/mmol), 500 μM NADPH, and 2 μg of a pheromone gland homogenate from the spruce budworm in 1.0 ml of 50 mM phosphate buffer (pH 7.0) with 1 mM dithiothreitol at 37°C. The number of moles of each molecule incorporated into fatty acid was calculated from the specific radioactivity of the substrate and the increase of ^{14}C or ^{3}H label extracted into hexane.

distinct thioesterase in this insect with specificity for acyl chains of shorter chain length (Ryan *et al.*, 1982). Although the thioesterase activity is not involved in pheromone biosynthesis in this species, it does, however, suggest a potential mechanism for producing pheromones derived from fatty acids with less than 16 carbons.

The possibility that the product of the fatty acid synthase reaction *in vivo* is an esterified rather than a free fatty acid should be considered. For example, an enzyme with acyltransferase activity could simply transfer the fatty acyl group from the fatty acid synthase enzyme to an acceptor other than water (Knudsen and Grunnet, 1982). This system could be advantageous in some cases since the fatty acyl group would still be in an activated (esterified) state and could there-fore be further metabolized without the necessity for reesterification of the car-boxyl group by the fatty acid activating enzymes (Groot *et al.*, 1976). However, only free fatty acids have been found *in vitro* as the product of fatty acid synthesis in insect extracts (Municio *et al.*, 1972; Ryan *et al.*, 1982).

B. Desaturation and Chain Shortening

1. Reaction Pathways

The majority of lepidopteran pheromones (77%) are monounsaturated acetate esters, alcohols, and aldehydes with long-chain carbon backbones between 10 and 16 carbons in length (Inscoe, 1982). In Fig. 4, the number of species attracted to a specific compound is given in the vertical dimension for different combinations of chain length, double bond position and configuration, and func-tional group. The horizontal and oblique axes define the chain length and the double bond position with respect to either the terminal carbon atom of the chain (ω^1) or the carbon containing the functional group (Δ^1).

A close metabolic relationship exists between the components on the ω axis. Once the double bond is introduced into the carbon chain, its position relative to the terminal carbon (ω value) will be fixed as the processes of chain shortening or elongation occur at the functional Δ^1 carbon. The position of insertion of a double bond into a fatty acyl chain, if inserted by a mechanism similar to that for mammalian desaturases, is dictated by its distance from the functional carbon (Δ^1) (James, 1977; Jeffcoat, 1979). Thus an enzyme with the same specificity [reaction (7)] as the mammalian Δ^9-desaturase acting on a 14-carbon fatty acyl-

$$CH_3(CH_2)_{12}\!\!-\!\!\overset{\displaystyle O}{\overset{\displaystyle \|}{C}}\!\!-\!\!SCoA + NADPH + O_2 \longrightarrow$$

$$CH_3(CH_2)_3\!\!-\!\!CH\!\!=\!\!CH\!\!-\!\!(CH_2)_7\!\!-\!\!\overset{\displaystyle O}{\overset{\displaystyle \|}{C}}\!\!-\!\!SCoA + NADP^+ + 2\,H_2O \tag{7}$$

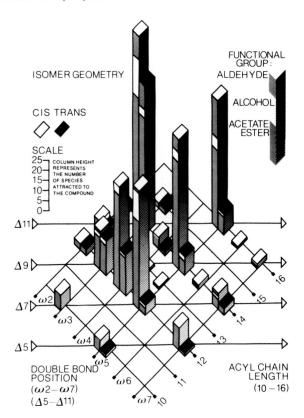

Fig. 4. Common lepidopteran sex attractants. Data from a recent listing of insect sex attractants by Inscoe (1982) are plotted to illustrate the frequency of use of different sex attractants for the Lepidoptera. All attractants listed are long-chain monounsaturated aldehydes, alcohols, and acetate esters, with the position of the double bond and the length of the acyl chain backbone defined by the axes. The heights of the columns are proportional to the number of species attracted to the particular compound defined by the horizontal axes. Almost four-fifths of the known lepidopteran sex attractants are included in this plot. From Morse and Meighen (1986).

CoA derivative would produce an ω^5 double bond. All the other unsaturated acyl derivatives with a ω^5 double bond (Fig. 4) can then be produced by chain elongation or shortening mechanisms.

A Δ^9 desaturase has been measured in extracts of the housefly and appears to be required for biosynthesis of the (Z)-9-tricosene pheromone (Wang *et al.*, 1982). Δ^9 Desaturation of stearic acid would produce oleic acid with a ω^9 double bond. Chain elongation followed by decarboxylation leads to the formation of the alkene pheromone with the double bond still located nine carbons from the end of the chain.

2. Δ^{11} Desaturation

Recent experiments by Roelofs and co-workers have provided evidence that unique Δ^{11} desaturases are responsible for the introduction of the double bonds into pheromones from several species of Lepidoptera (see Bjostad *et al.*, Chapter 3, this volume). The pheromone of the cabbage looper moth, *Trichoplusia ni*, contains as its major component (Z)-7-dodecenyl acetate, with the double bond located at the ω^5 position. Using long-chain acyl-CoAs as substrates, it has been demonstrated that extracts from the glands of the cabbage looper moth specifically catalyzed the synthesis of Δ^{11}-unsaturated acyl-CoAs with a high specificity for palmitoyl-CoA (and stearoyl-CoA) to form an unsaturated derivative with the requisite ω^5 double bond (Wolf and Roelofs, 1986). The net reaction for desaturation appears to be similar to that observed for mammalian Δ^9 desaturases [reaction (7)], except NADH rather than NADPH is the preferred nicotinamide cofactor for this reaction.

A chain shortening process has been implicated in biosynthesis of the cabbage looper pheromone. Label from [16-^{3}H](Z)-11-hexadecenoic acid is incorporated exclusively into the ω terminal of (Z)-7-dodecenyl acetate providing support for a mechanism involving desaturation followed by chain shortening (Bjostad and Roelofs, 1983). Evidence for chain shortening has also been provided by *in vitro* studies on *Argyrotaenia citrana*. Extracts from this insect were able to catalyze formation of labeled tetradecanoic acid from [U-^{14}C]palmitate but not from [1-^{14}C]palmitate (Wolf and Roelofs, 1983).

Evidence for a Δ^{11} desaturase has also been provided by studies on the red-banded leafroller moth (Bjostad and Roelofs, 1981). This insect produces a blend of (Z)- and (E)-11-tetradecenyl acetates with an isomeric ratio of 91 : 9 $Z : E$ as its pheromone. Radiolabeling studies *in vivo* using tetradecanoic acid indicated that this compound could be directly desaturated as the pheromone was labeled to a greater extent with [1-^{14}C]tetradecanoic acid than with [1-^{14}C]acetate whereas the reverse was the case for labeling of the 16- and 18-carbon fatty acids. However, some degree of caution must be exercised in interpretation of these data as [U-^{14}C]palmitate and [1-^{14}C]palmitate incorporated label into the pheromone components to the same extent. These results do not support a mechanicm involving chain shortening followed by Δ^{11} desaturation since the label in [1-^{14}C]palmitate should be lost in this mechanism.

The presence of an unique Δ^{11} desaturase in insects coupled with a chain shortening mechanism could account for the biosynthesis of the majority of the Lepidoptera pheromones which contain monounsaturated carbon chains with ω^3 and ω^5 double bonds. A Δ^{11} desaturase that functions specifically with palmitoyl-CoA could produce all the compounds with a ω^5 double bond (see Fig. 4). Similarly, a Δ^{11} desaturase with specificity for tetradecanoyl-CoA could produce the pheromones with ω^3 double bonds. It is interesting to note that very few pheromones have 16-carbon backbones with ω^3 double bonds, indicating that elongation of Δ^{11}-tetradecenoic acid does not readily occur in insects. As palmitic acid is the most abundant fatty acid in most species, it also appears likely that Δ^{13} desaturases are not present in insects. The data compiled in Fig. 4 suggest that most species with pheromones containing ω^5 double bonds have desaturases that preferentially synthesize the Z isomer, analogous to the mammalian Δ^9 desaturases, whereas species containing pheromones with ω^3 double bonds have an equal probability of having the Z or E compound as the predominant unsaturated isomer.

3. Other Desaturation Mechanisms

A number of pheromones contain carbon chains in which the double bonds are located at positions other than the ω^3 and ω^5 positions (Fig. 4). At present the mechanism of their synthesis is unknown, although a Δ^{10} desaturase coupled with a chain shortening mechanism has been proposed to explain the biosynthesis of the Δ^8-tetradecenyl acetate pheromones of the Olethreutinae (Roelofs and Brown, 1982). In two species of this subfamily, the pheromone glands contained high levels of Δ^{10}-hexadecenoic acid in addition to the Δ^8-tetradecenyl acetate ester pheromone (Lofstedt and Roelofs, 1985).

Many insect pheromones are also composed of components with two double bonds in their carbon chain backbones. The most well-known example is bombykol [(E,Z)-10,12-hexadecadienol], the major component of the pheromone of the silkworm moth. Recent studies show that (Z)-11-hexadecenoic acid can be incorporated directly into the pheromone, indicating that an enzyme system may exist that catalyzes the conversion of the monounsaturated precursor into the conjugated diene (Yamaoka *et al.*, 1984).

Chain elongation may also be required for the biosynthesis of some pheromones as over 60 insect species are attracted to pheromones with diunsaturated (Δ^3,Δ^{13}) 18-carbon chains (Inscoe, 1982). The Δ^3 double bond in these compounds could be introduced by a mechanism similar to that found for bacterial β-hydroxyacyl dehydrogenase in which a Δ^3 rather than a Δ^2 double bond is introduced during chain elongation and will thus not be reduced (Kass *et al.*, 1967; Brock *et al.*, 1967). For example, desaturation of palmitic acid to Δ^{11}-hexadecenoic acid followed by chain elongation and desaturation by a β-hydroxylacyl dehydrogenase during the elongation process would produce a Δ^3,Δ^{13}-octadecadienoic acid.

C. Fatty Acid Reduction

1. Reaction Pathways

Very little is known about the pathway in insects for reduction of fatty acids to the corresponding aldehydes and alcohols, although fatty acid reductase and acyl-CoA reductase activities have been identified in extracts from different biological systems (Riendeau and Meighen, 1985). In these latter systems, highest activities were usually obtained on reduction of the saturated acyl chains, although in one case a more efficient reduction of the unsaturated isomer was obtained (Griffith *et al.*, 1981). The reduction of fatty acids in extracts from eukaryotes is generally catalyzed by the microsomal fraction.

The requirements for fatty acid reduction have been elucidated for a multienzyme complex isolated from luminescent bacteria [reaction (8)]. In this reac-

$$\underset{\substack{\| \\ R-COH}}{O} + ATP + NADPH \longrightarrow \underset{\substack{\| \\ R-C-H}}{O} + AMP + PP_i + NADP^+ \qquad (8)$$

tion, the fatty acid is activated with ATP to form an acyl-AMP intermediate (Rodriguez and Meighen, 1985). The acyl group is then transferred to the enzyme and reduced with NADPH to generate the fatty aldehyde (Riendeau *et al.*, 1982; Rodriguez *et al.*, 1983).

In most systems, aldehyde reductases (i.e., alcohol dehydrogenases) are also present that catalyze the reduction of the fatty aldehyde to form the corresponding alcohol [reaction (9)]. Consequently, fatty alcohols and not fatty aldehydes are the

$$\underset{\substack{\| \\ R-C-H}}{O} + NAD(P)H \longrightarrow RCH_2OH + NAD(P)^+ \qquad (9)$$

major products arising from the reduction of fatty acids as aldehyde reductases appear to be associated with the fatty acid reductases presumably to prevent accumulation of the relatively reactive aldehyde (Riendeau and Mieghen, 1985).

2. Fatty Acid Reductase

In vitro evidence for fatty acid reductase activity in insects has so far been obtained only for extracts from *A. citrana*. Tetradecenyl acetates were formed from both palmitic acid and tetradecanoyl-CoA, showing that the fatty acid had been reduced to the fatty alcohol *in vitro* (Wolf and Roelofs, 1983). Information on the specificity of this activity has not yet been obtained. *In vivo* labeling studies of the redbanded leafroller moth also indicated that the fatty acid could be reduced directly to form the 11-tetradecenyl acetate pheromone. This conclusion was supported by the formation of acetate esters labeled with [1-^{14}C](*E*)-11-tetradecenoic acid with a higher *E*:*Z* ratio (0.5) than the naturally occurring isomeric ratio (0.1) observed on labeling with [1-^{14}C]acetate (Bjostad and Roelofs, 1981).

The specificity of the reductase system for unsaturated fatty acids will be important in controlling the ratio of the *E* and *Z* isomers in the final pheromone blend. In a study of 10 lepidopteran species, the ratio of isomers $(Z:E)$ of unsaturated fatty acyl derivatives in the gland was often found to differ significantly from the $Z:E$ ratio of the pheromone (Wolf et al., 1981). Interestingly, the ratios were different when the major pheromone component was the Z isomer but not when the major pheromone component was the E isomer. It appears that the desaturase and reductase systems must function in concert to control the final ratio of isomers in the pheromone blend.

3. Aldehyde Reductase

Aldehyde reductase activity [reaction (9)], but not fatty acid reductase activity [reaction (8)], has been detected in extracts of the gland of the spruce budworm (Morse and Meighen, 1986). In this assay, the labeled aldehyde substrate is produced in situ by a purified fatty acid reductase from luminescent bacteria [reaction (8)]. In the presence of NAD(P)H and the gland homogenate, the aldehyde can be reduced to fatty alcohol. The relative amounts of the product can be determined by scintillation counting after separation by thin-layer chromatography on silica gel. Unfortunately, this assay can not be used to characterize the aldehyde reductase system since the observed properties reflect those of the coupled system. An alternate coupled assay system involving conversion of the alcohol product to a labeled acetate ester with [³H]acetyl-CoA (Morse and Meighen, 1987) has also shown that aldehyde can be reduced by gland extracts.

D. Formation of Acetate Esters by an Acetyl-CoA : Fatty Alcohol Acetyltransferase

1. In Vivo Labeling of Acetate Esters

Acetate esters of long-chain fatty alcohols are the most abundant type of pheromones found in Lepidoptera (Inscoe, 1982). In addition, relatively large amounts of acetate esters may be found in the pheromone-producing glands of most insects that secrete fatty alcohols or aldehydes as their major pheromone components. For example, in the spruce budworm moth the levels of the acetate ester in the gland are 20–40 times greater than the levels of aldehyde pheromone (Silk et al., 1980). However, in some Lepidoptera with aldehyde pheromones, acetate esters have not yet been detected in pheromone gland extracts (Teal and Tumlinson, 1986).

By topical application of radiolabeled acetate in DMSO to the spruce budworm it can be demonstrated that tetradecenyl acetate is specifically synthesized in the pheromone-producing gland (see Fig. 1). Alternatively, if radiolabeled tetradecanol is topically applied to the budworm gland, formation of tetradecyl acetate (the saturated analog of the glandular ester) is observed (Fig. 5). The formation of the saturated acetate indicates that the fatty alcohol can be directly

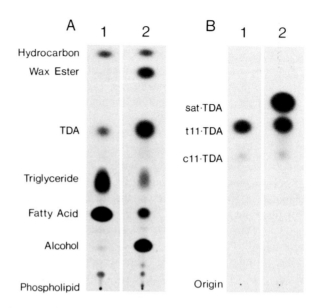

Fig. 5. *In vivo* labeling of the acetate ester of the female spruce budworm moth. (A) Auto-radiogram of a silica gel TLC of lipids from the spruce budworm moth radiolabeled with [1-^{14}C]tetra-decanoic acid (lane 1) or [1-^{14}C]tetradecanol (lane 2). Groups of 16 moths were labeled for 90 min by topical application in DMSO of 1–2 nmol of the radiolabeled compound (31 mCi/mmol). (B) The labeled tetradecenyl acetate (TDA) was extracted with diethyl ether from the chromatogram in A and run on a silica gel TLC impregnated with silver nitrate. The autoradiogram shows that the acetate ester labeled with tetradecanoic acid is composed of unsaturated 11-tetradecenyl acetate esters (lane 1) whereas large amounts of the saturated tetradecanyl acetate are present in the acetate ester sample labeled with tetradecanol (lane 2). t11-TDA, E11-14: Ac; c11-TDA, Z11-14: Ac. From Morse and Meighen (1987), copyright 1987, Pergamon Journals, Ltd.

incorporated into the acetate ester. In contrast, the labeling experiments with labeled sodium acetate or even tetradecanoic acid resulted primarily in the forma-tion of labeled acetate esters which are unsaturated with an isomeric ratio $Z:E$ corresponding to that observed for the aldehyde pheromone. These results indi-cate that tetradecanoic acid topically applied to the gland of the budworm cannot be directly reduced *in vivo* to form the saturated fatty alcohol.

2. *In Vitro* Acetyltransferase Activity

Analysis of extracts of the budworm gland for enzymes responsible for the incorporation of fatty alcohols into acetate esters has demonstrated the presence of an acetyl-CoA: fatty alcohol acetyltransferase [reaction (10)] that catalyzes

$$CH_3\!-\!\overset{\overset{\textstyle O}{\|}}{C}\!-\!SCoA + CH_3(CH_2)_nCH_2OH \longrightarrow CH_3\!-\!\overset{\overset{\textstyle O}{\|}}{C}\!-\!OCH_2(CH_2)_nCH_3 + CoASH \quad (10)$$

the reaction of acetyl-CoA with long-chain alcohols (Morse and Meighen, 1987). This activity can easily be followed using radiolabeled acetyl-CoA since the labeled lipid product (an ester) can readily be extracted in organic solvents and separated from acetyl-CoA. Consequently, the amount of radioactivity extracted into hexane with time provides a simple and convenient measurement of the rate of the enzyme reaction (Fig. 6).

The transfer of the acetyl group to saturated alcohols is specific for long-chain fatty alcohols with chain lengths of 12–15 carbons. The enzyme also prefers monounsaturated fatty alcohols over the saturated isomers although no significant distinction can be made between compounds with unsaturation at the Δ^9 and Δ^{11} positions or between the Z and E isomers (Table II). Higher activities are obtained with the unsaturated tetradecenols than with the longer chain hexadecenols and octadecenols.

The acetyltransferase obeys Michaelis–Menten kinetics as illustrated by the linear Lineweaver–Burk plots in Fig. 7. The enzyme has a K_m of 12 μM for acetyl-CoA and 2 μM for (E)-11-tetradecenol under these assay conditions. No significant difference could be observed in specificity with respect to the K_m values for other 14-carbon alcohols [i.e., (Z)-11-tetradecenol and tetradecanol].

The acetyltransferase activity is found almost exclusively in extracts from the pheromone-producing gland with a specific activity (picomoles per minute per microgram protein) at least 100-fold greater than that from extracts of other

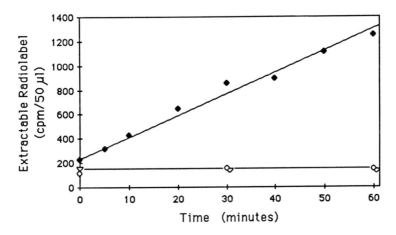

Fig. 6. Kinetics of acetate ester formation in extracts of the spruce budworm gland. Reaction mixtures containing 8 μg gland homogenate, 31 μM [³H]acetyl-CoA, and 10 μM (E)-11-tetradecenol in 1.0 ml 50 mM phosphate buffer (pH 7) were extracted with 1.0 ml hexane at the indicated times, and the radioactivity in a 50-μl aliquot was determined by scintillation counting ($\blacklozenge$). An increase in extractable radioactivity was not observed in the absence of either gland extract ($\triangledown$) or fatty alcohol ($\diamond$). From Morse and Meighen (1987), copyright 1987, Pergamon Journals, Ltd.

TABLE II

Substrate Specificity of
Acetyl-CoA : Fatty Alcohol
O-Acetyltransferase

Alcohol substrate		Enzyme activity[a]
	10 : 0	0.3
	12 : 0	3.3
	13 : 0	3.3
	14 : 0	2.7
	15 : 0	3.3
	16 : 0	0.5
	18 : 0	0.2
(Z)-11	14 : 1	7
(E)-11	14 : 1	5
(Z)-9	16 : 1	2.7
(Z)-11	16 : 1	3
(Z)-9	18 : 1	1.5
(E)-9	18 : 1	1.2

[a]Acetyltransferase activity, given in picomoles acetate ester formed per minute, was measured in reaction mixtures containing 10 μg of
protein from a spruce budworm moth gland homogenate, 10 μM long-chain alcohol substrate,
and 31 μM [^{3}H]acetyl-CoA (200 mCi/mmol).
The amount of ester formed was calculated from
the specific activity of the radiolabeled substrate
and the amount of radiolabel in a hexane extract
after a 60 min reaction.

tissues of the budworm. Furthermore, the activity in extracts from developing glands excised from the pupae is much lower than in extracts of glands excised from the adult moth.

The existence of an acetyl-CoA : fatty alcohol acetyltransferase has not been previously noted in other biological systems, perhaps reflecting the evolution of specific pheromone communication systems in insects. This enzyme may be located in the microsomes in insect glands since centrifugation of budworm extracts at 100,000 g resulted in a pellet which contained the majority of the activity with an increase in specific activity of almost 30-fold (Table III). The possibility that this enzyme is present in other Lepidoptera should be given serious consideration in view of the large number of insects using long-chain acetate esters as pheromones. By *in vitro* analysis of gland extracts from other Lepidoptera, it will be possible to ascertain whether this activity represents a common step in pheromone biosynthesis. Of particular interest would be the

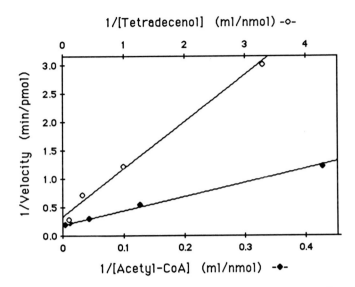

Fig. 7. Lineweaver–Burk plots for acetyl-CoA : fatty alcohol acetyltransferase. Dependence of the reciprocal of the initial reaction rate on the reciprocal of the acetyl-CoA and (E)-11-tetradecenol concentrations. Assays were conducted in 1.0 ml of 50 mM phosphate (pH 7.0) containing 8 μg of protein from a gland homogenate with a fixed concentration of either (E)-11-tetradecenol (10 μM) or [³H]acetyl-CoA (31 μM).

analysis of gland extracts of *Heliothis virscens* and *H. zea* in which acetate esters have not yet been detected (Teal and Tumlinson, 1986). If the acetyltransferase is specifically located in the microsomes, then analysis for this activity should be increased in sensitivity and accuracy after a high-speed centrifugation step to enrich for this enzyme.

TABLE III
Differential Centrifugation of Glandular Enzymes

Fraction[a]	Specific activity (pmol/min/μg protein)		
	Acetyltransferase	Acetate esterase	Alcohol oxidase
Homogenate	0.19	3.7	0.9
Supernatant	0.11	5.3	0.8
Pellet	4.6	0.7	0.15

[a]Fifty glands from female spruce budworm moths were extracted in 5 ml of 50 mM phosphate buffer (pH 7) and cellular debris eliminated by low speed centrifugation. The supernatant and pellet fractions were obtained by centrifugation of the homogenate at 105,000 g for 90 min.

E. Conversion of Acetate Esters to Alcohol and Aldehyde Pheromones

1. *In Vivo* Analysis

Ester hydrolysis occurs during the synthesis and degradation of pheromones by insects (see Prestwich, Chapter 14, this volume; Prestwich *et al.*, 1986; Ding and Prestwich, 1986). Although esterases, in general, appear to be rather non-specific, it is possible that enzymes with high specificity might be involved in the hydrolysis of acetate esters (Vogt *et al.*, 1985). For example, in *Drosophila melanogaster*, the pheromone, (Z)-11-octadecenol, is transferred from the males in the form of the acetate ester. The males also transfer an esterase to the female which hydrolyzes the ester to form the alcohol pheromone and inhibits further mating by the females (Mane *et al.*, 1983). Apparently, esterases in the female cannot efficiently hydrolyze the (Z)-11-octadecenyl acetate.

An esterase capable of hydrolyzing the acetate ester to fatty alcohol has been implicated in the biosynthesis of the aldehyde pheromone in the spruce bud-worm. After *in vivo* labeling of tetradecenyl acetate in the moth by injection of labeled acetate into the abdomen, radioactive aldehyde pheromone was found to be released by the insect. Radiolabeled acetate is introduced here by injection instead of the more efficient topical application of labeled acetate in DMSO to the gland as this latter procedure interferes with the subsequent release of al-dehyde pheromone in the scotophase. The amount of labeled aldehyde phe-romone released by budworm moths in the scotophase decreases with time, and parallels the decrease in labeled tetradecenyl acetate levels inside the gland during the same period (Fig. 8). This correlation suggests that the acetate ester is a precursor to the aldehyde pheromone. Topical application of labeled tetradec-anyl acetate to the budworm showed that this compound was readily hydrolyzed *in vivo* with a higher conversion on application to the glands than the heads or abdomens (Morse and Meighen, 1984a).

2. *In Vitro* Acetate Esterase Activity

The acetate esterase activity from the budworm gland can be measured *in vitro* by using a luminescence coupled assay after conversion of the fatty alcohol product to the corresponding fatty aldehyde as depicted in reactions (11)–(13).

$$CH_3-(CH_2)_{12}CH_2-O-\overset{\overset{\displaystyle O}{\|}}{C}-CH_3 \xrightarrow{\text{esterase}} CH_3COOH + CH_3(CH_2)_{12}-CH_2OH \quad (11)$$

$$CH_3-(CH_2)_{12}-CH_2OH + NAD^+ \xrightarrow{\text{HLAD}} CH_3-(CH_2)_{12}-\overset{\overset{\displaystyle O}{\|}}{C}-H + NADH \quad (12)$$

$$FMNH_2 + O_2 + CH_3-(CH_2)_{12}-\overset{\overset{\displaystyle O}{\|}}{C}-H \xrightarrow{\text{luciferase}}$$

$$FMN + H_2O + CH_3-(CH_2)_{12}-\overset{\overset{\displaystyle O}{\|}}{C}OH + \text{light (490 nm)} \tag{13}$$

Reactions are initiated by mixing the acetate ester [e.g., (E)-11-tetradecenyl acetate] and the glandular homogenate in buffer at pH 8.0. At the appropriate time intervals, the reaction mixture is mixed with horse liver alcohol dehydrogenase (HLAD) and NAD^+ for a few seconds to convert the fatty alcohol to the corresponding aldehyde. The HLAD-catalyzed reaction is very rapid and surprisingly unselective toward different alcohol substrates. The sample is then injected into an assay mixture containing bacterial luciferase and $FMNH_2$ in an enclosed chamber exposed to a photomultiplier tube. The maximum light emission, which reaches a peak in less than a second, is proportional to the amount of aldehyde in the injected sample (Meighen et al., 1982). Some caution must be exercised in application of these coupled assays as high concentrations of either protein or the lipid substrates will result in inhibition of light production. The release of fatty

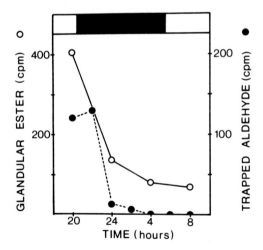

Fig. 8. Temporal relation between acetate ester degradation and aldehyde release. Adult spruce budworm moths were injected in the abdomen with ~18 nmol of [1-^{14}C]acetate in 50 mM phosphate buffer (pH 7) at 1600 hr. Trapping began at 1800 hr in a small wind tunnel with a Porapak Q trap at the outlet. The trap was extracted with ether at 2 hr intervals, and the aldehyde pheromone was purified by TLC on silica gel before analysis of the amount of radioactivity incorporated. Glandular levels of labeled acetate ester were determined after extraction of the glands with hexane and separation by TLC. From Morse and Meighen (1984b). Copyright 1984 by the AAAS.

alcohol from the acetate ester is linear with time (up to 20 min) (Fig. 9) and protein concentration in the assay (up to 5 µg/ml) (Fig. 10). Rates as low as 4 pmol/min can be measured, making this assay system approximately 100 times more sensitive than most spectrophotometric assays.

The dependence of activity on acetate ester concentration follows Michaelis–Menten kinetics. Tetradecyl acetate and the 11-unsaturated derivatives (Z or E) have similar K_m values and are hydrolyzed at comparable rates. A K_m of 0.4 µM for (E)-11-tetradecenyl acetate can be measured from the Lineweaver–Burk plot given in Fig. 11. However, specificity studies using this assay system are limited since the relative responses can be affected by all enzymes in this coupled assay system.

The esterase activity cannot be sedimented even under a centrifugal field of 100,000 g for 90 min, indicating that it is a soluble enzyme (see Table III). This activity can be detected in all tissues, with slightly higher specific activities in extracts of the gland compared to other body parts (Morse and Meighen, 1984a). Partial purification of the esterase by anion-exchange chromatography has indicated that there are multiple molecular forms (Fig. 12) whereas gel filtration

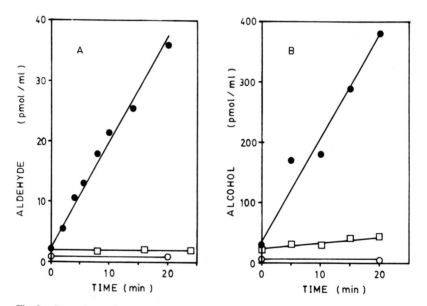

Fig. 9. Dependence of product formation on time for the alcohol oxidase and the acetate esterase of the spruce budworm. The product formed by incubation of 2 µg of gland extract with (E)-11-tetradecenol (A) or (E)-11-tetradecenyl acetate (B) is given by the filled circles, and was calculated as picomoles product from the luminescent response. In the latter assay, the alcohol product is converted to aldehyde by horse liver alcohol dehydrogenase before analysis. No reaction occurred in the absence of substrate (○) or extract (□) in either assay. From Morse and Meighen (1984a).

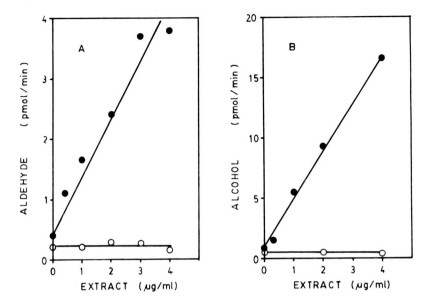

Fig. 10. Dependence of reaction velocity on enzyme concentration for the alcohol oxidase and the acetate esterase of the spruce budworm. Complete reaction mixtures (●) contained the gland extract and either 1 μM (E)-11-tetradecenol (A) or 1 μM (E)-11-tetradecenyl acetate (B). The control curves (○) are in the absence of substrate. From Morse and Meighen (1984a).

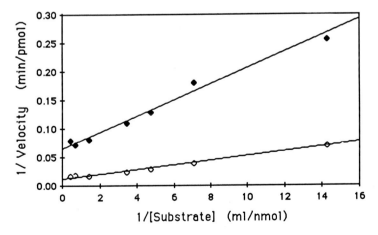

Fig. 11. Lineweaver–Burk plots for the alcohol oxidase and acetate esterase of the spruce budworm. Dependence of the reciprocal of the initial reaction rate on the inverse of the concentration of (E)-11-tetradecenyl acetate (◇) and (E)-11-tetradecenol (◆) in assays at pH 8.0 and 7.0, respectively, for the acetate esterase and the alcohol oxidase. Reaction mixtures contained 2 μg protein of gland extract in 1.0 ml of 50 mM phosphate buffer.

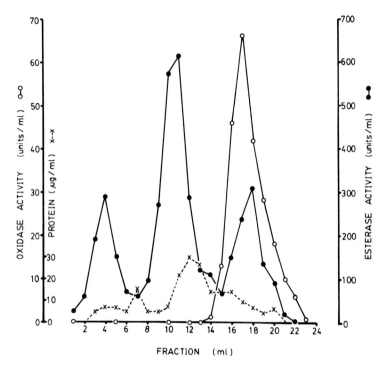

Fig. 12. Ion-exchange chromatograph of alcohol oxidase and acetate esterase. The extract from 60 female budworm glands, after centrifugation at 105,000 g for 90 min, was loaded onto 1.0 ml of DEAE-Sepharose CL6B preequilibrated with 1 mM phosphate (pH 7.0). The gel was washed with 2 ml of the same buffer and eluted with a 20 ml linear gradient from 1 to 100 mM phosphate (pH 7.0). From Morse and Meighen (1984a).

gives a single peak with a size equivalent to a molecular mass of approximately 90 kDa (Fig. 13). Individual variation in esterase isozymes has been found in antennal tissues of *Antheraea polyphemus* (Vogt, Chapter 12, this volume).

3. *In Vitro* Alcohol Oxidase Activity

Two distinct types of enzymes in terms of reaction mechanism can be involved in the oxidation of alcohols to aldehydes in biological systems. The dehydrogenases use cofactors such as NAD(P) to accept electrons whereas oxidases use molecular oxygen directly as the electron acceptor. This latter class of enzyme usually contains a metal ion or tightly bound flavin cofactor to mediate the reduction of the oxygen molecule.

For the spruce budworm, conversion of the fatty alcohol to the aldehyde appears to be catalyzed by an alcohol oxidase as represented in reaction (14). The peroxide will then be broken down or further utilized in other metabolic reac-

$$CH_3(CH_2)_{12}-CH_2OH + O_2 \xrightarrow{\text{oxidase}} CH_3(CH_2)_{12}-\overset{\overset{\displaystyle O}{\|}}{C}-H + H_2O_2 \qquad (14)$$

tions. By replacing most of the oxygen in the reaction mixture with nitrogen, the reaction rate is significantly reduced; activity is restored when the solution is again exposed to the atmosphere (Fig. 14). Neither nicotinamide (NAD, NADP) nor other electron acceptors stimulated the activity, further supporting the proposal that oxygen is the immediate electron acceptor and an oxidase is responsible for formation of the aldehyde pheromone. A similar alcohol oxidase activity also appears to be responsible for the biosynthesis of the aldehyde pheromone of *Heliothis virescens* (Ding and Prestwich, 1986; Teal and Tumlinson, 1986).

The *in vitro* activity of alcohol oxidase in gland extracts is determined by the luminescence response of bacterial luciferase to the aldehyde product [reaction (13)] as described in the previous subsection. The production of fatty aldehyde is linear with time (up to 20 min) (see Fig. 9) and extract concentration (up to 5 μg/ml) (Fig. 10). The sensitivity of this assay is even higher than the acetate esterase assay described in the previous subsection as the product of the alcohol oxidase (fatty aldehyde) can be measured directly in the luminescence assay. A reaction velocity producing as low as 0.1 pmol/min of aldehyde can be measured.

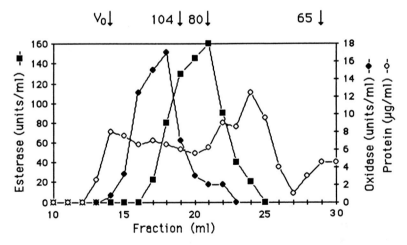

Fig. 13. Gel filtration of the acetate esterase and alcohol oxidase of the spruce budworm. An extract of 20 female budworm glands was centrifuged at 105,000 g and the supernatant applied to an AcA44 gel filtration column (0.9 × 50 cm). The column was eluted with 50 m*M* phosphate buffer (pH 7.0), and fractions were analyzed for acetate esterase and alcohol oxidase activities. The positions of the void volume (*V*₀) and different molecular weight markers [in kilodaltons (kDa)] are indicated.

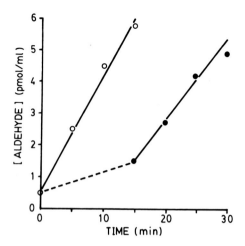

Fig. 14. Dependence of alcohol oxidase activity on oxygen. Reaction mixtures were prepared by adding 2 μg gland homogenate and 1 μM (E)-11-tetradecenol to 5 ml 50 mM phosphate buffer (pH 7.0) that had been purged of oxygen by boiling and then cooled under nitrogen. The reaction mixture was either immediately exposed to the atmosphere (○) or kept under nitrogen for 15 min before exposure to the air (●). Aldehyde production was monitored using a luminescence coupled assay as described in the text. From Morse and Meighen (1984a).

A Lineweaver–Burk plot for the dependence of reaction velocity on the concentration of (E)-11-tetradecenol is given in Fig. 11. The E and Z isomers of 11-tetradecenol and tetradecanol have similar K_m values (0.1–0.2 μM), with the reaction velocity being up to twofold higher with the E isomer.

The alcohol oxidase, like the acetate esterase, did not sediment under high-speed centrifugation, indicating that it is also a soluble enzyme (see Table III). On both ion-exchange chromatography (see Fig. 12) and gel filtration (Fig. 13), the alcohol oxidase activity eluted as one major peak. The distribution of the alcohol oxidase activity in extracts of different tissues indicated that this enzyme was specifically located in the gland with a specific activity at least sevenfold higher in extracts of the gland compared to those of the head, abdomen, legs, or thorax.

III. CRITERIA FOR IDENTIFICATION OF ENZYMES IN PHEROMONE BIOSYNTHESIS

Identification of the metabolic pathway or even a specific step in the reaction pathway leading to the synthesis of an essential metabolite in a biological system requires a combination of *in vivo* and *in vitro* experimental approaches. Among the more critical experiments are the demonstration of *de novo* biosynthesis of the specific metabolite, establishment of precursor–product relationships *in vivo* for the different steps in the metabolic pathway, and *in vitro* identification and characterization of the appropriate enzyme functions responsible for individual steps. Only in the rare case will a single experimental approach provide data that unambiguously associate a specific step with the biosynthetic pathway. Rather, in many instances, the results may provide only indirect evidence or the experiment cannot be accomplished for theoretical or practical reasons. In these cases, additional experimental evidence may be necessary including data on the morphological location, specificity, and regulation of the enzyme activities and whether these properties are consistent with the control and function of the biological system under investigation. The object of this section is to analyze some of the criteria used to implicate specific enzymes in pheromone biosynthesis in Lepidoptera with particular attention to the pheromone biosynthetic pathway in the spruce budworm leading to the formation of long-chain acetate esters, alcohols, and aldehydes. As these components represent the most common type of pheromones found in Lepidoptera, the results and approaches may be generally applicable to the characterization of the pathways for pheromone biosynthesis in other insects.

A. *De Novo* Biosynthesis

Insect pheromones can either be synthesized *de novo* or derived from more complex molecules present in the natural environment of the insect. The bark beetles from the order Coleoptera use as aggregation pheromones chemicals in the host tree oleoresin either directly or after modification (Vanderwel and Oehlschlager, Chapter 6, this volume; Fish *et al.*, 1979; Hughes, 1974). In the latter case, microbial symbionts in the gut of the insect have been directly implicated in the biosynthetic process (Brand *et al.*, 1975; Byers and Wood, 1981; Hoyt *et al.*, 1971). Similarly, precursors to the pheromone components of the boll weevil are normal constituents of cotton buds, the primary source of nutrition for this insect, and can be very efficiently incorporated into the pheromone blend (Thompson and Mitlin, 1979). However, the boll weevil can also synthesize its pheromone *de novo* (Mitlin and Hedin, 1974), making it necessary to decide which route is operative under normal conditions. In contrast, the sex pheromones of the Lepidoptera appear to be produced exclusively by *de novo* biosynthesis in all insects examined to date. In only one instance has it been suggested that a lepidopteran sex attractant was derived from the food of the insect (Hendry *et al.*, 1975), and a subsequent examination of different food sources revealed that this was not the case (Miller *et al.*, 1976; Hindenlang and Wichmann, 1977). The site of sex pheromone production in female Lepidoptera is believed to be a specialized gland located at the tip of the abdomen.

Evidence for *de novo* biosynthesis of sex pheromones in Lepidoptera is based on the *in vivo* incorporation of radiolabeled acetate into their pheromone components. Analysis of the acetate ester pheromone in gland extracts of a number of insects has demonstrated that acetate is incorporated into their long-chain carbon backbones (Bjostad and Roelofs, 1981; Jones and Berger, 1978; Schmidt and Monroe, 1976). In extracts of the spruce budworm gland, the aldehyde pheromone labeled *in vivo* with acetate could not be detected due to the relatively low levels of the aldehyde pheromone compared to the abundance of other fatty acid derivatives (e.g., acetate esters) synthesized *de novo* in the gland. This problem can be avoided by analysis of pheromone released by the insect into the atmosphere as has been demonstrated for the pheromone (nonanal, undecanal) of the greater wax moth (Schmidt and Monroe, 1976). By trapping of pheromone released from spruce budworm moths that had been injected with labeled acetate it could be demonstrated that the aldehyde pheromone was synthesized *de novo* (see Fig. 8).

B. Pheromone Precursors

1. Identification

A number of strategies are possible to identify precursors in the *de novo* pheromone biosynthetic pathway in Lepidoptera. One common strategy involves addition of a labeled intermediate to the insect to determine if it can be efficiently incorporated into the pheromone. A second approach involves establishing a temporal relationship between levels of a putative precursor and the product under investigation. Both experimental approaches have been applied to identify precursors to components on the pheromone biosynthetic pathway in the spruce budworm.

Fatty alcohol has been shown to be the immediate precursor to the long-chain acetate ester in the spruce budworm since topical application of labeled tetradecanol to the gland resulted in incorporation of high levels of radiolabel into the saturated tetradecanyl acetate ester (see Fig. 5). In contrast, the unsaturated *E* and *Z* isomers of 11-tetradecenyl acetate and not the saturated acetate ester are formed during *de novo* synthesis from acetate. Topical application of labeled tetradecanoic acid to the budworm gland also resulted in preferential incorporation of label into the unsaturated 11-tetradecenyl acetate esters with the extent of labeling being similar to that with acetate and fatty acids of different chain lengths (lauric and palmitic acid), suggesting that the fatty acid is degraded before being incorporated into the acetate ester. Similar experiments with other insect species have indicated that β-oxidation of the fatty acid to acetyl-CoA followed by resynthesis of the long-chain fatty acids may be a major route for incorporation of radiolabel into pheromone in many instances (Bjostad and Roelofs, 1981).

Direct evidence for the degradation of the fatty acid followed by resynthesis can be obtained by comparing the incorporation of label into acetate esters from ^{14}C- and ^{3}H-labeled tetradecanoic acid. The relative amounts of ^{14}C and ^{3}H label in the acetate ester should be identical if the fatty acid is directly incorporated into the long-chain carbon backbone. In contrast, if the fatty acid is first degraded to acetyl-CoA and the long-chain backbone resynthesized, then most of the ^{3}H label would be lost (Fig. 15). *In vivo* labeling of the acetate ester of the budworm moth shows that the relative incorporation from [^{3}H]tetradecanoic acid is approximately fivefold lower than from [1-^{14}C]tetradecanoic acid, indicating that a substantial proportion of the labeled fatty acid is degraded (Table IV).

2. Stored Precursors

The levels of aldehyde pheromone (11-tetradecenal) in the gland of the spruce budworm moth are very low compared to the amount of 11-tetradecenyl acetate

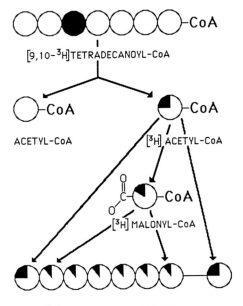

Fig. 15. Loss of tritium from fatty acid on β-oxidation. Two-carbon units, formed from acetate, are represented by circles in the acyl-CoA molecule with the relative amount of tritium label given by the shaded area. After β-oxidation to acetyl-CoA, three-quarters of the tritium label is lost to the medium. The two-carbon units from acetyl-CoA are incorporated directly into the terminals of the acetate ester without loss of tritium, whereas the internal two carbon units, also derived from acetyl-CoA, must pass through a malonyl-CoA intermediate and undergo further loss of tritium (see Fig. 1).

TABLE IV

**Differential Incorporation of ^{14}C and ^{3}H
Labels from Tetradecanoic Acid into
Acetate Esters**[a]

	Incorporation into 11-tetradecenyl acetate isomers (%)	
	Trans	Cis
[^{14}C]Tetradecanoic acid	0.31 ± 0.06	0.03 ± 0.007
[^{3}H]Tetradecanoic acid	0.07 ± 0.01	0.006 ± 0.002
$^{3}H/^{14}C$ ratio	0.2 ± 0.08	0.2 ± 0.12

[a]Each spruce budworm moth gland was treated with 1–2 nmol (~0.05 μCi) in DMSO of either [1-^{14}C]tetradecanoic acid or [9,10- ^{3}H]tetradecanoic acid for 90 min. Three groups of 15–20 insects were used per experiment, and the ester product was purified on silica gel before resolution of the unsaturated esters (trans/cis) on silver nitrate TLC and analysis for the amount of radioactivity (given as the percent applied to the gland).

in the gland and the amount of pheromone released by the insect each day (Silk *et al.*, 1980; Grant *et al.*, 1982; Morse *et al.*, 1982). These results have indicated that the acetate ester may be a stored precursor of the pheromone of the spruce budworm. This proposal is supported by the temporal relation between the decrease of labeled acetate ester in the gland and the release of radiolabeled pheromone (Morse and Meighen, 1984b). Storage of the pheromone as the less reactive acetate ester would be advantageous to the insect as it allows the biosynthetic steps which require large expenditures of energy to occur continuously and not simply during the period of pheromone release. In addition, accumulation of high levels of the aldehyde pheromone, which may be toxic to the cell, can now be avoided. A related mechanism for aldehyde pheromones, involving storage of the alcohol precursor with "activation" by an alcohol oxidase, has been described for *Heliothis* species (Teal and Tumlinson, 1986; Tumlinson and Teal, Chapter 1, this volume).

Pheromone precursors may be stored in forms other than acetate esters in different insects. In the silkworm, *Bombyx mori,* the hexadecadienol pheromone (bombykol) has been found in pupal hemolymph esterified to lineolate (Yamaoka *et al.*, 1985). If this wax ester is in fact a storage form of the pheromone, then it will be of interest to determine the exact site of pheromone biosynthesis in this insect as fatty acids with the same double bond distribution as the pheromone are found only in the gland (Bjostad and Roelofs, 1984a).

A glycoside rather than an ester has been reported as a storage form for the phenylethyl alcohol pheromone of *Mamestra configurata* (Clearwater, 1975;

Weatherston and Percy, 1976). In this case, the alcohol is stored as a β-glycoside in the gland, possibly to overcome the problems of the insolubility and toxicity of the pheromone. A β-glycosidase activity, which can catalyze the release of the aromatic alcohol pheromone, has been found in the abdominal hairpencils leading from the gland.

It has also been suggested that triglycerides may be stored intermediates on the pathway leading to formation of lepidopteran pheromones (Bjostad and Roelofs, 1984b). This proposal is based on the presence in the insect of triglycerides containing fatty acids with double bonds in the same position as found in the final pheromone product. However, as synthetic radiolabeled triacylglycerols could not be used as acyl donors for pheromone biosynthesis (Bjostad and Roelofs, 1986; Bjostad *et al.*, Chapter 3, this volume), it appears more likely that triglycerides do not serve as direct precursors to the insect pheromone.

C. Enzyme Properties

1. *In Vitro* Assays

Characterization of a specific enzyme function provides the opportunity to relate its kinetic properties to the behavioral, physiological, and biological properties of the organism *in vivo*. Perhaps of most importance for this comparison is the establishment of an *in vitro* assay that quantitates the level of the enzyme function in question. It is therefore essential to establish experimental conditions in which the rate of formation of the product is linearly dependent on the concentration of extract (i.e., protein) in the assay. Since extracts from different sources may contain material (e.g., lipids) inhibitory to the assay system, it may be necessary to analyze different amounts of each extract to establish that the specific activity (units activity per unit protein) remains constant from a given source. Demonstrating whether or not the activity of a mixture of two extracts is the sum of the activity of its components also provides an independent check for the presence of inhibitors to one extract or the other.

The formation of product should also be linear with time in most assay systems so that the initial rate of reaction can easily be established. If possible, it is generally advantageous to work at substrate concentrations above their respective K_m values in the enzyme-catalyzed reaction. Under these conditions, the rate of the reaction will be constant even if a substantial proportion of the substrate has been converted to product. If it is necessary to work at substrate concentrations below the K_m, then the formation of product will be linear only for the short period of time in which no significant change has occurred in the initial substrate concentration. Alternatively, an integrated form of the Michaelis–Menten equation can be used to obtain the initial rate of the reaction (Morse and Meighen, 1984a).

The *in vitro* assay systems for the acetyltransferase, acetate esterase, and

alcohol oxidase enzymes of the spruce budworm fulfill most of these requirements although there are certain limitations. For the acetate esterase and alcohol
oxidase assays, the extract and substrate (i.e., lipid) concentrations must be
limited to prevent inhibition of the luminescence coupled assays. As direct
measurement of the acetate ester product is possible in the acetyltransferase
assay, higher extract and substrate concentrations could be used in this case. In
general, however, substrate concentrations must still be relatively low in assays
involving lipid-metabolizing enzymes as the substrates not only can function as
detergents and inactivate the enzymes but also form micelles at higher concentrations. Consequently, application of highly sensitive techniques (radioactivity,
luminescence) to measure the reaction products is generally a prerequisite for *in
vitro* analyses of most enzyme activities involved in pheromone metabolism. In
this regard, the assays which have been developed to investigate the function and
regulation of the acetyltransferase, acetate esterase, and alcohol oxidase enzymes
of the spruce budworm should be applicable to the study of pheromone metabolism in other Lepidoptera.

2. Substrate Specificity

Since pheromones are precise blends of volatile compounds used specifically
for communication, it might be predicted that enzymes with unique specificities
would be involved in the biosynthetic pathway. Two enzymes that fulfill this
criterion are the Δ^{11} desaturase detected in gland extracts of the cabbage looper
moth (Wolf and Roelofs, 1986) and the acetyl-CoA : fatty alcohol acetyltransferase found in extracts of the spruce budworm gland (Morse and Meighen, 1987).
The possibility that the aldehyde reductase, alcohol oxidase, or the acetate esterase found in spruce budworm extracts also have unique functional properties is
not yet known since the studies on specificity are still limited due to the application of coupled assay systems to measure these enzyme activities.

3. Regulation

Coordinate regulation of an enzyme function and the synthesis or release of the
pheromone product provides direct evidence for its involvement in the biosynthetic pathway. For example, the levels of activity of the acetyltransferase in the
gland are dependent on the age of the moth, rising to a maximum at roughly 2
days after emergence of the moth from the pupa (Table V). This change in
specific activity contrasts with the level of acetate esterase and alcohol oxidase
activities which are independent of age and have high levels even in the pupal
glands. The acetyltransferase activity closely parallels the levels of the aldehyde
pheromone extracted from the gland (Fig. 16), suggesting that the activity of this
enzyme is closely connected with the development of the pheromone biosynthetic system in the gland. In this regard, two neurohormones (juvenile hormone and
β-ecdysone) have also been found to have increased levels in other insects during

TABLE V

**Dependence of Acetyltransferase
Activity on Insect Age**

Age of adult spruce budworms[a]	Acetyltransferase activity[b] (pmol/min/μg)
−2	0.009
−1	0.03
0	0.05
2	0.15
4	0.16

[a]Insect ages before eclosion (negative values) are given relative to the time when the majority of moths emerged from the pupae.

[b]Activities were measured in gland homogenates of female budworm moths and represent the average of at least 12 separate analyses.

the early adult stages of gland development (Riddiford and Truman, 1978), raising the possibility that these hormones might control the development of the system responsible for pheromone biosynthesis (Raina and Khun, 1984). Interestingly, the Δ^{11} desaturase from the cabbage looper moth also appears to have a similar dependence on insect age, with the maximum levels of activity

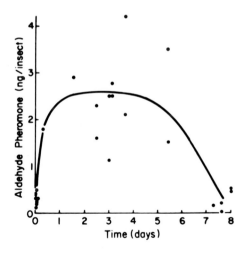

Fig. 16. Dependence of aldehyde pheromone levels in extracts of the glands of female budworms on time after emergence from pupae. Insects were maintained on continuous light, and the gland was excised between 1200 and 1700 hr. Each point represents the average value for analysis of four to seven individual female moths. From Grant *et al.* (1982).

TABLE VI
Tissue Distribution of Enzyme Activities in the
Spruce Budworm Moth

Body tissue	Enzyme activity (pmol/min/µg)		
	Acetyltransferase	Acetate esterase	Alcohol oxidase
Gland	0.12	4.2	1.1
Head	0.0008	1.5	0.14
Abdomen	0.0003	1.7	0.15
Leg	0.001	1.0	0.07
Thorax	0.0003	1.4	0.14

found at 2 days of age (Wolf and Roelofs, 1986). A detailed discussion of neural regulation of pheromone production in Lepidoptera can be found in this volume (Raina and Menn, Chapter 5, this volume).

4. Morphological Location

The location of an enzyme specifically in the tissue (i.e., gland) responsible for pheromone production provides strong support for its involvement in the metabolic pathway. As shown in Table VI, the acetyltransferase enzyme responsible for synthesis of the long-chain acetate ester in the spruce budworm moth is found exclusively in extracts of the gland with insignificant activities (<1%) in other tissues of the budworm. A similar tissue specificity has been reported for the Δ^{11} desaturase of the cabbage looper moth (Wolf and Roelofs, 1986).

In contrast, acetate esterase and alcohol oxidase activities, believed to be responsible for conversion of the long-chain acetate ester into the aldehyde pheromone, are present in all tissues with specific activities two- and sevenfold higher, respectively, in extracts of the gland (Morse and Meighen, 1984a). The tissue distribution of these functions may reflect the existence of more than one enzyme or molecular form with the respective activity (see Figs. 12 and 13). Although the tissue distribution of the alcohol oxidase indicates that this enzyme plays a role in pheromone biosynthesis, the distribution of the acetate esterase in the budworm does not provide strong evidence to link this enzyme to the pheromone biosynthetic pathway.

IV. PATHWAY FOR PHEROMONE BIOSYNTHESIS IN THE SPRUCE BUDWORM MOTH

The tetradecenal pheromone of the spruce budworm moth appears to be synthesized via a tetradecenyl acetate precursor. This conclusion is supported by the observation that the ester is synthesized *de novo* specifically in the pheromone-producing gland (see Fig. 2) and is turned over during the period of pheromone release (Fig. 8). In addition, a unique acetyl-CoA : fatty alcohol acetyltransferase activity catalyzing the biosynthesis of the acetate ester can be found exclusively in extracts of the pheromone gland, and its activity appears to be coordinately regulated with the increase in pheromone levels in the gland just as the female moths emerge from the pupae.

The proposed pathway for pheromone biosynthesis in the spruce budworm moth in Fig. 17 incorporates the results described on the budworm and other Lepidoptera into a framework consistent with biochemical observations in other biological systems. The pathway begins with fatty acid synthesis in the cytoplasm resulting in the formation of either a free or an activated (esterfied) fatty acid. This acyl derivative would then undergo desaturation and reduction in the microsomes. This fraction contains the smooth endoplasmic reticulum which is involved in lipid metabolism and is present in large amounts in the gland cells (Percy, 1974). The Δ^{11} desaturase from the cabbage looper moth has been found in the microsomal fraction (Wolf and Roelofs, 1986) as have all mammalian desaturases (James, 1977; Jeffcoat, 1979). Similarly, the reduction of fatty acids is believed to be catalyzed in the microsomes (Riendeau and Meighen, 1985).

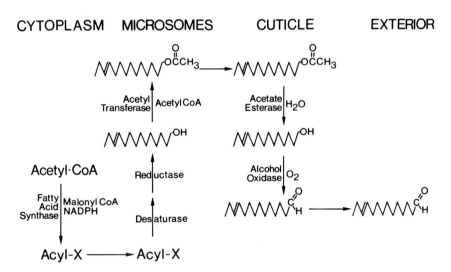

Fig. 17. Pheromone biosynthesis in the spruce budworm. The pathway for pheromone biosynthesis is proposed to begin with fatty acid synthesis in the cytoplasm. Fatty acids are further metabolized in the microsomes to form acetate esters. Although the acetate ester may be released directly as pheromone in some insects, the budworm further metabolizes this compound to form the aldehyde pheromone. These latter steps may occur in the cuticle as no cellular energy or metabolic cofactors are needed for the last two steps except O_2 and H_2O. From Morse and Meighen (1986).

Subcellular fractionation by differential centrifugation of the gland extract from the spruce budworm also clearly demonstrated that the acetyltransferase was present in the microsomes (see Table III). Consequently, in this model, all the pheromone biosynthetic activities involved in converting the fatty acid into long-chain acetate ester are proposed to be located in the same cellular compartment. As the smooth endoplasmic reticulum is also associated with the storage and secretion of material, this result is consistent with the high levels of acetate ester in the gland and secretion of this compound to form the aldehyde pheromone.

The acetate esterase and the alcohol oxidase, in contrast, are soluble enzymes and cannot be sedimented by high-speed centrifugation. The soluble nature of these two enzymes is consistent with the alcohol oxidase and acetate esterase being physically separated in the cell from enzymes involved in the formation of the acetate ester, which appear to be associated with the endoplasmic reticulum. It is possible that the acetate esterase and alcohol oxidase are exterior to the gland cells in the cuticle since ultrastructural studies of the gland of the budworm have revealed the presence of pore canals which in other insects have been shown to contain oxidase and esterase activity (Locke and Krishnan, 1971; Locke, 1961). The location of these enzymes in the cuticle would be advantageous as it would clearly separate the pathways of ester synthesis and degradation which pass through a common 11-tetradecenol intermediate. Furthermore, metabolic energy and cellular cofactors are not necessary for conversion of the acetate ester to the aldehyde pheromone, only water and oxygen.

V. CONCLUSIONS

The identification and characterization of enzymes involved in pheromone metabolism are important steps leading to the understanding of the mechanism and regulation of pheromone biosynthesis in insects. Based on *in vivo* and *in vitro* experiments, a general pathway has been proposed for the biosynthesis of long-chain acetate ester, alcohol, and aldehyde pheromones. The specificity, regulation, and morphological location of an acetyl-CoA : fatty alcohol acetyltransferase in the spruce budworm has provided critical evidence for an acetate ester as a precursor storage form in the pathway leading to the aldehyde pheromone. Acetate esterase and alcohol oxidase enzymes can then catalyze the conversion of the acetate ester to the corresponding long-chain aldehyde without the need for additional energy or cellular cofactors. Since many of the Lepidoptera have long-chain acetate esters, alcohols, and aldehydes as pheromones, the pathway leading to formation of the spruce budworm pheromone may serve as a general model for pheromone biosynthesis in other insects.

ACKNOWLEDGMENTS

We would like to express our appreciation to Dr. Gary Grant, Forest Pest Management Institute, Sault Saint Marie, for his support and advice during the authors' studies on the enzymes involved in pheromone biosynthesis in the spruce budworm. Our thanks also go to Rose Szittner for her assistance in many of these experiments and to Maureen Caron for typing the manuscript. The research on the spruce budworm was supported by a grant from the Medical Research Council of Canada (MT-4314).

REFERENCES

Bjostad, L. B., and Roelofs, W. L. (1981). Sex pheromone biosynthesis from radiolabeled fatty acids in the redbanded leafroller. *J. Biol. Chem.* **256,** 7936–7940.

Bjostad, L. B., and Roelofs, W. L. (1983). Sex pheromone biosynthesis in *Trichoplusia ni:* Key steps involve Δ^{11} desaturation and chain shortening. *Science* **220,** 1387–1389.

Bjostad, L. B., and Roelofs, W. L. (1984a). Sex pheromone biosynthetic precursors in *Bombyx mori. Insect Biochem.* **14,** 275–278.

Bjostad, L. B., and Roelofs, W. L. (1984b). Biosynthesis of sex pheromone components and glycerolipid precursors from sodium acetate in the redbanded leafroller moth. *J. Chem. Ecol.* **10,** 681–691.

Bjostad, L. B., and Roelofs, W. L. (1986). Sex pheromone biosynthesis in the redbanded leafroller moth, studied by mass labelling with stable isotopes and analysis with mass spectrometry. *J. Chem. Ecol.* **12,** 431–450.

Blomquist, G. J., and Dillwith, J. W. (1983). Pheromones: Biochemistry and physiology. *In* "Endocrinology of Insects" (R. G. Downer and H. Laufer, eds.), pp. 527–542. Alan R. Liss, New York.

Brand, J. M., Bracke, J. W., Markovitz, A. J., Wood, D. L., and Browne, L. E. (1975). Production of verbenol pheromone by a bacterium isolated from bark beetles. *Nature (London)* **254,** 136–137.

Brock, D. J. H., Kass, L. R., and Bloch, K. (1967). β-Hydroxydecanoyl thioester dehydrase. II. Mode of action. *J. Biol. Chem.* **24,** 4431–4440.

Butenandt, A., Beckmann, R., Stamm, D., and Hecker, E. (1959). Uber den Sexual-Lockstoff des Seidenspinners *Bombyx mori*. Reindarstellung und Konstitution. *Z. Naturforsch.* **B14,** 283–284.

Byers, J. A., and Wood, D. L. (1981). Antibiotic induced inhibition of pheromone synthesis in a bark beetle. *Science* **213,** 763–764.

Clearwater, J. R. (1975). Synthesis of a pheromone precursor in the male noctuid moth *Mamestra configurata. Insect Biochem.* **5,** 737–746.

Dillwith, J. W., Blomquist, G. J., and Nelson, D. R. (1981). Biosynthesis of the hydrocarbon components of the sex pheromone of the housefly, *Musca domestica. Insect Biochem.* **11,** 247–253.

Ding, Y.-S., and Prestwich, D. G. (1986). Metabolic transformation of tritium labeled pheromone by tissues of *Heliothis virescens* moths. *J. Chem. Ecol.* **12,** 411–429.

Fish, R. H., Browne, L. E., Wood, D. L., and Hendry, L. B. (1979). Pheromone biosynthetic pathways: Conversion of deuterium labelled ipsdienol with sexual and enantioselectivity in *Ips paraconfusus. Tetrahedron Lett.* **17,** 1565–1568.

Grant, G. G., Slessor, K. N., Szittner, R. B., Morse, D., and Meighen, E. A. (1982). Development of a bioluminescence assay for aldehyde pheromones of insects. II. Analysis of the pheromone glands. *J. Chem. Ecol.* **8**, 923–933.

Griffith, T. W., Sand, D. M., and Schlenk, M. (1981). Reduction of fatty acids to alcohols in roe of gourami (*Trichogaster cosby*). *Biochim. Biophys. Acta* **665**, 34–39.

Groot, P. H. E., Scholte, R. H., and Hulsmann, W. C. (1976). Fatty acid activation: Specificity, localization and function. *Adv. Lipid Res.* **14**, 75–126.

Hendry, L. B., Wichmann, J. K., Hindenlang, D. M., Mumma, R. D., and Anderson, M. E. (1975). Evidence for origin of insect sex pheromones: Presence in food plants. *Science* **188**, 59–63.

Hindenlang, D. M., and Wichmann, J. K. (1977). Reexamination of tetradecenyl acetates in oakleafroller sex pheromone and in plants. *Science* **195**, 86–89.

Hoyt, C. P., Osborne, G. O., and Mulcock, A. P. (1971). Production of an insect sex attractant by symbiotic bacteria. *Nature (London)* **230**, 472–473.

Hughes, P. R. (1974). Myrcene: A precursor of pheromones in *Ips* beetles. *J. Insect Physiol.* **20**, 1271–1275.

Inscoe, M. N. (1982). Insect attractants, pheromones and related compounds. *In* "Insect Suppression with Controlled Release Pheromone Systems" (A. F. Kydoneus and M. Beroza, eds.), pp. 201–295. CRC Press, Boca Raton, Florida.

James, A. T. (1977). The specificity of mammalian desaturases. *Adv. Exp. Med. Biol.* **83**, 51–74.

Jeffcoat, R. (1979). The biosynthesis of unsaturated fatty acids and its control in mammalian liver. *Essays Biochem.* **15**, 1–36.

Jones, I. F., and Berger, R. S. (1978). Incorporation of acetate into *cis*-7-dodecenyl acetate, a sex pheromone in the cabbage looper *Trichoplusia ni*. *Environ. Entomol.* **7**, 666–669.

Kass, L. R., Brock, D. J. H., and Bloch, K. (1967). β-Hydroxydecanoyl thioester dehydrase. I. Purification and properties. *J. Biol. Chem.* **242**, 4418–4431.

Knudsen, J., and Grunnet, I. (1982). Transacylation as a chain-termination mechanism in fatty acid synthesis by mammalian fatty acid synthase. *Biochem. J.* **202**, 139–143.

Locke, M. (1961). Pore canals and related structures in insect cuticle. *J. Biophys. Biochem. Cytol.* **10**, 598–618.

Locke, M., and Krishnan, N. (1971). The distribution of phenoloxidase and polyphenols during cuticle formation. *Tiss. Cell.* **3**, 103–126.

Lofstedt, C., and Roelofs, W. L. (1985). Sex pheromone precursors in two primitive New Zealand tortricid moth species. *Insect Biochem.* **15**, 729–734.

Mane, S. D., Tompkins, L., and Richmond, R. C. (1982). Male esterase 6 catalyzes the synthesis of a sex pheromone in *Drosophila melanogaster* females. *Science* **222**, 419–421.

Meighen, E. A., Slessor, K. N., and Grant, G. G. (1982). Development of a bioluminescence assay for aldehyde pheromones of insects. I. Sensitivity and specificity. *J. Chem. Ecol.* **8**, 911–921.

Miller, J. R., Baker, T. C., Cardé, R. T., and Roelofs, W. L. (1976). Reinvestigation of oakleafroller sex pheromone components and the hypothesis that they vary with diet. *Science* **192**, 140–143.

Mitlin, N., and Hedin, P. A. (1974). Biosynthesis of grandlure, the pheromone of the boll weevil, from acetate, mevalonate and glucose. *J. Insect Physiol.* **20**, 1825–1831.

Morse, D., and Meighen, E. A. (1984a). Detection of pheromone biosynthetic and degradative enzymes *in vitro*. *J. Biol. Chem.* **259**, 475–480.

Morse, D., and Meighen, E. A. (1984b). Aldehyde pheromones in Lepidoptera: Evidence for an acetate ester precursor in *Choristoneura fumiferana*. *Science* **226**, 1434–1436.

Morse, D., and Meighen, E. A. (1986). Pheromone biosynthesis and the role of functional groups in pheromone specificity. *J. Chem. Ecol.* **12**, 335–351.

Morse. D., and Meighen, E. A. (1987). Biosynthesis of the acetate ester precursor of the spruce budworm sex pheromone by an acetyl-CoA:alcohol acetyltransferase. *Insect Biochem.* **17**, 53–59.

Morse, D., Szittner, R. B., Grant, G. G., and Meighen, E. A. (1982). Rate of pheromone release by individual spruce budworm moths. *J. Insect Physiol.* **28**, 863–866.

Municio, A. M., Odriozola, J. M., Pinero, A., and Ribera, A. (1972). *In vitro* elongation and desaturation of fatty acids during development of insects. *Biochim. Biophys. Acta* **280**, 248–257.

Percy, J. E. (1974). Ultrastructure of sex pheromone gland cells and cuticle before and during release of pheromone in female spruce budworm, *Choristoneura fumiferana. Can. J. Zool.* **52**, 695–705.

Prestwich, G. D., Vogt, R. G., and Riddiford, L. M. (1986). Binding and hydrolysis of radiolabelled pheromone and several analogs by male-specific antennal proteins of the moth *Antheraea polyphemus. J. Chem. Ecol.* **12**, 323–333.

Raina, A. K., and Khun, J. A. (1984). Brain factor control of sex pheromone production in the female corn earworm moth. *Science* **225**, 531–533.

Riddiford, L. M., and Truman, J. W. (1978). Biochemistry of insect hormones and insect growth regulators. *In* "Biochemistry of Insects" (M. Rockstein. ed.), pp. 307–357. Academic Press, New York.

Riendeau, D., and Meighen, E. A. (1985). Enzymatic reduction of fatty acids and acyl-CoAs to long chain aldehydes and alcohols. *Experientia* **41**, 707–713.

Riendeau, D., Rodriguez, A., and Meighen, E. (1982). Resolution of the fatty acid reductase from *Photobacterium phosphoreum* into acyl protein synthase and acyl-CoA reductase activities. *J. Biol. Chem.* **257**, 6908–1915.

Rodriguez, A., and Meighen, E. (1985). Fatty acyl-AMP as an intermediate in fatty acid reduction to aldehyde in luminescent bacteria. *J. Biol. Chem.* **260**, 771–774.

Rodriguez, A., Wall, L., Riendeau, D., and Meighen, E. (1983). Fatty acid acylation of proteins in bioluminescent bacteria. *Biochemistry* **22**, 5604–5611.

Roelofs, W. L., and Brown, R. L. (1982). Pheromones and evolutionary relationships of Tortricidae. *Annu. Rev. Ecol. Syst.* **13**, 395–422.

Ryan, R. D., deRenobales, M., Dillwith, J. W., Heisler, C. R., and Blomquist, G. J. (1982). Biosynthesis of myristate in an aphid: Involvement of a specific acylthioesterase. *Arch. Biochem. Biophys.* **213**, 26–36.

Sanders, C. J., and Weatherston, J. (1976). Sex pheromone of the eastern spruce budworm (Lepidoptera: Tortricidae): Optimum blend of *trans-* and *cis*-11-tetradecenal. *Can. Entomol.* **108**, 1285–1290.

Schmidt, S. P., and Monroe, R. E. (1976). Biosynthesis of the waxmoth sex attractants. *Insect Biochem.* **6**, 377–380.

Silk, P. J., Wiesner, C. J., Tan, S. H., Ross, R. J., and Lonergan, G. (1980). Sex pheromone chemistry of the eastern spruce budworm *Choristoneura fumiferana. Environ. Entomol.* **9**, 640–644.

Teal, P. E. A., and Tomlinson, J. H. (1986). Terminal steps in pheromone biosynthesis by *Heliothis virescens* and *H. zea. J. Chem. Ecol.* **12**, 353–366.

Thompson, A. C., and Mitlin, P. A. (1979). Biosynthesis of the sex pheromone of the male boll weevil from monoterpene precursors. *Insect Biochem.* **9**, 293–294.

Vogt, R. G., Riddiford, L. M., and Prestwich, G. D. (1985). Kinetic properties of a sex pheromone degrading enzyme: The sensillar esterase of *Antheraea polyphemus. Proc. Natl. Acad. Sci. U.S.A.* **82**, 8827–8831.

Volpe, J. J., and Vagelos, P. R. (1973). Saturated fatty acid synthesis and its regulation. *Annu. Rev. Biochem.* **42**, 21–60.

Volpe, J. J., and Vagelos, P. R. (1976). Mechanisms and regulation of biosynthesis of saturated fatty acids. *Physiol. Rev.* **56**, 339–417.

Wakil, S. J., Stoops, J. K., and Joshi, Y. C. (1983). Fatty acid synthesis and its regulation. *Annu. Rev. Biochem.* **52**, 537–579.

Wang, D. L., Dillwith, J. W., Ryan, R. O., Blomquist, G. J., and Reitz, R. C. (1982). Characterization of the acyl-CoA desaturase in the housefly *Musca domestica* L. *Insect Biochem.* **12**, 545–551.

Weatherston, J., and Percy, J. E. (1976). The biosynthesis of phenylethyl alcohol in the male bertha armyworm *Mamestra configurata*. *Insect Biochem.* **6**, 413–417.

Weaver, N. (1978). Chemical control of insects—intraspecific. *In* ''Biochemistry of Insects'' (M. Rockstein, ed.), pp. 359–389. Academic Press, New York.

Wolf, W. A., and Roelofs, W. L. (1983). A chain shortening reaction in orange tortrix moth sex pheromone biosynthesis. *Insect Biochem.* **13**, 375–379.

Wolf, W. A., and Roelofs, W. L. (1986). Properties of the Δ^{11} desaturase enzyme used in cabbage looper moth sex pheromone biosynthesis. *Arch. Insect Biochem. Physiol.* **3**, 45–52.

Wolf, W. A., Bjostad, L. B., and Roelofs, W. L. (1981). Correlation of fatty acid and pheromone component structures in sex pheromone glands of ten lepidopteran species. *Environ. Entomol.* **10**, 943–946.

Yamaoka, R., Taniguchi, Y., and Hayashiya, K. (1984). Bombykol biosynthesis from deuterium labelled *cis*-11-hexadecenoic acid. *Experientia* **40**, 80–81.

Yamaoka, R., Nakayama, Y., and Hayashiya, K. (1985). Identification of bombykol lineolate in the haemolymph of the female silkworm pupae *Bombyx mori*. *Insect Biochem.* **15**, 73–76.

5

Endocrine Regulation of Pheromone Production in Lepidoptera

ASHOK K. RAINA*
JULIUS J. MENN†
*Insect Chemical Ecology Laboratory
†National Program Staff
Agricultural Research Service
U.S. Department of Agriculture
Beltsville, Maryland 20705

I. INTRODUCTION

A. Role of Sex Pheromones in Reproduction

Most species of moths produce and release discrete chemicals that act as messengers to solicit a mate. Research to date has shown that these chemical messengers, or sex pheromones, are usually produced by the females in glands typically located in the terminal abdominal segments. The chemicals volatilize from the gland surface during the act of calling (rhythmic extension of the ovipositor to expose the pheromone gland surface) and are dispersed by the wind. When conspecific males encounter the pheromone, they follow the plume to the release source, sometimes over great distances, and mating ensues. Pheromones for about 350 insect species have been identified, and the majority (~70%) of these are sex pheromones for Lepidoptera (Ridgway et al., 1986). Evidence is mounting to suggest that some males, on landing near a female,

Pheromone Biochemistry

release a pheromone that differs from that of the female and acts as a female arrestant and/or as an aphrodisiac (Birch, 1974; Baker and Cardé, 1979; Hirai, 1980). Sex pheromones function not only to bring conspecific sexes together but also to maintain reproductive isolation among closely related species that share a common ecological niche. (Lanier, 1970; Roelofs and Cardé, 1974).

B. Barth's Hypothesis on Endocrine Control of Pheromone Production

In insects, pheromonal communication may be regulated by the neuroendocrine systems in the producer of the signal, the receiver, or both. Thus hormones and/or neurotransmitters may regulate the biosynthesis or release of the pheromone and may also mediate the response to the pheromone. Barth (1965) proposed that ''neuroendocrine control of mating behavior would occur only in those insects which are long-lived as adults and which have repeated reproductive cycles containing periods during which mating is not appropriate and perhaps not even possible. In insects which are short-lived as adults, which possess mature oocytes at eclosion and which lay them and die within a few days, the female must attract a male within a brief time span'' (quoted in Barth and Lester. 1973). He further postulated that in Lepidoptera that do not feed as adults, one would not expect to find a neuroendocrine control mechanism influencing the production of sex pheromone. Barth's conclusion was based on experiments with several species of cockroaches and two species of moths: a saturniid, *Antheraea pernyi*, and a pyralid, *Galleria mellonella*.

C. Importance of Endocrine Control of Sex Pheromone Production in Lepidoptera

Among Lepidoptera, reproductive activity is probably never distributed evenly over a day but instead peaks at or is restricted to a few hours during the photophase or scotophase. The timing for the female of a species to release the sex pheromone has coevolved with male flight activity and maximal responsiveness to pheromonal signals. Such a coordination of mating activity provides the species with a high probability of mate finding and reproductive isolation. In nocturnal species of moths, reproductive activity is usually gated and follows an endogenous rhythm that is modified by environmental cues (Cardé and Webster, 1980). Circadian endogenous rhythms of pheromone production and calling behavior have been reported in several species of moths. Examples include *Trichoplusia ni* (Sower *et al.*, 1970), *Platyptilia carduidactyla* (Haynes *et al.*, 1983), and *Heliothis zea* (Pope *et al.*, 1984; Raina *et al.*, 1986). These studies have demonstrated a diel periodicity of pheromone titer and calling, with peak pheromone production and calling in each species taking place during a specific period in the scotophase.

Some mechanism of hormonal or neuroendocrine control appears to be essential to maintain such a periodicity of pheromone production. Although Riddiford and Williams first suggested neurohormonal control of pheromone release in the Lepidoptera, as early as 1971, it was not until 1984 that the first experimental evidence was reported (Raina and Klun, 1984) for such control of pheromone production in a lepidopteran species. Since results published to date on the endocrine control of pheromone production in the Lepidoptera pertain only to moths, our discussion is confined to this group.

II. PREVIOUS RESEARCH FINDINGS

A. Role of Corpora Allata in Pheromone Production

An example of the role of corpora allata (CA) in sex pheromone production came from Barth's (1961) study of the cockroach *Byrsotria fumigata*. He reported that adult female cockroaches failed to produce sex pheromone if their CA were removed shortly after the imaginal molt. Implantation of CA into allatectomized females restored pheromone production. By contrast, in the lepidopterans *G. mellonella* (Roller *et al.*, 1963; Barth, 1965), *A. pernyi* (Barth, 1965), *Hyalophora cecropia, A. polyphemus* (Riddiford and Williams, 1971), and *Manduca sexta* (Sasaki and Riddiford, 1984), removal of the CA had no effect on calling behavior; however, pheromone production was not directly assessed. *Heliothis zea* females ligated between head and thorax failed to produce sex pheromone, and pheromone production was not restored by the injection of CA homogenates (Raina and Klun, 1984). Hollander and Yin (1985) reported that in the gypsy moth, *Lymantria dispar*, CA were not involved with either calling behavior or pheromone release.

These reports indicate that the CA may not play a role in the regulation of sex pheromone production in the lepidopteran species studied thus far. However, indirect and contrary evidence has been reported by Chang *et al.* (1979) and Webster and Cardé (1984). Application of sublethal amounts of precocene II [anti-juvenile hormone (AJH)] to virgin females of diamondback moth, *Plutella xylostella,* reduced their sex attractancy (Chang *et al.*, 1979); Webster and Cardé (1984) reported that the application of a juvenile hormone (JH) analog, hydroprene (ZR-512), to *Platynota stultana* virgin females blocked pheromone production. Webster and Cardé speculated that JH might be involved in the switchover from virgin behavior to mated behavior (increased rate of oviposition) in this species. However, it is not clear from these studies whether the AJH or JH analogs had a direct effect on pheromone biosynthesis or acted indirectly by promoting egg laying and in turn suppressing calling.

B.   Role of Corpora Cardiaca in Pheromone Production

Riddiford and Williams (1971) proposed that calling in *H. cecropia* and *A. polyphemus* is induced by environmental cues processed by the brain, which in turn stimulates release of a hormone from the intrinsic cells of the corpora cardiaca (CC). Removal of the CC–CA complex or severance of the nervi corporis cardiaci (NCC) I and II reduced the proportion of females calling from over 70% to less than 20%. These results indicated that the release of a "calling hormone" was controlled neurally by the brain. The same authors, however, reported that removal of the CC from females of *A. pernyi* did not disrupt normal mating behavior in this species. Riddiford (1974) reported induction of calling in females of *A. polyphemus* by transfusion of blood from actively calling females and suggested that calling was triggered by a CC-released neurosecretory hormone in the blood.

Sasaki *et al.* (1983) reevaluated the role of CC in the calling behavior of *H. cecropia* and *A. polyphemus* and reported that CC played no essential role in the calling behavior of the virgin females. In their study, a blood-tight ligature between the third and fourth abdominal segments, excluding the ventral nerve cord, had no effect on the calling behavior. They speculated that a humoral factor from the anterior end was not necessarily involved and that only an intact nervous connection between the brain and the terminal abdominal ganglion was necessary for normal calling behavior. Similarly in *M. sexta* females, removal of the CC–CA complex had no effect on calling behavior (Sasaki and Riddiford, 1984; Itagaki and Conner, 1986). However, these studies did not determine if calling was accompanied by pheromone release. Hollander and Yin (1985), working with the gypsy moth, reported that removal of the CC–CA complex did not interfere with calling or pheromone release.

By contrast, Raina and Klun (1984) reported that injection of CC homogenates into ligated females of *H. zea* caused pheromone production, even though the resultant pheromone titer was significantly lower than that produced after injection of a brain–suboesophageal ganglion (SOG) homogenate. As indicated earlier. this was the first experimental evidence linking an endocrine organ with pheromone production in Lepidoptera.

C.   Role of Brain–Suboesophageal Ganglion
in Pheromone Production

Cardé and Webster (1980) reported a decline in pheromone titer of decapitated *P. stultana* females even though such females did not call. They speculated that the decline in titer was due to enzymatic degradation of the pheromone and/or presumably a lack of active neural or neurohormonal regulation of pheromone biosynthesis. Hollander and Yin (1982) suggested that the anterior portion of the nervous system, including the brain, was involved in the control of pheromone release in female gypsy moths. They speculated that a humoral factor from the brain, coupled with direct neural control, were involved in pheromone release. Subsequently, Hollander and Yin (1985) reported that the presence of brain was not a prerequisite for calling in gypsy moth. However, removal of the brain or disconnecting it from the rest of the nervous system eliminated pheromone release. They further speculated that the intact nerve connections rather than the presence of brain humoral factors were indispensable for normal pheromone release. Recently Itagaki and Conner (1986) reported that calling behavior in *M. sexta* females was controlled by the neural output from the brain and/or the SOG; however, they did not examine pheromone titers in the females.

Raina and Klun (1984) provided conclusive evidence of the involvement of a brain factor in pheromone production in *H. zea* females. The female sex pheromone of *H. zea* has four components: 92% (Z)-11-hexadecenal (Z11-16 : Al), 1.7% (Z)-9-hexadecenal (Z9-16 : Al), 1.1% (Z)-7-hexadecenal (Z7-16 : Al), and 4.4% hexadecanal (16 : Al) (Klun *et al.*, 1979). Females produce and release pheromone only during the scotophase, and the pheromone titer of a 3-day-old female in the middle of the scotophase is about 130 ng. A 3-day-old female in the photophase has less than 5 ng of the pheromone (Raina *et al.*, 1986). Ligation of a female between head and thorax prevents pheromone production (Raina and Klun, 1984). A simple and very sensitive assay was developed to detect the hormonal activity. Homogenates of the neuroendocrine complex or its fractions are injected into the abdomen of a ligated female during the scotophase at least 3 hr after ligation. The ovipositor of the injected female is excised 3 hr after injection and extracted in heptane containing an internal standard; then, the quantity of Z11-16 : Al is determined by open tubular capillary gas chromatography. Using this assay, Raina and Klun (1984) demonstrated that the hormonal factor was present in the brain in both the scotophase and photophase but was released into the hemolymph to stimulate pheromone production only during the scotophase.

III. CURRENT RESEARCH

A. Hormonal Control of Pheromone Production in *Heliothis zea*

1. Origin of the Neurohormone

In adult Lepidoptera, the circumoesophageal connectives are reduced and the brain and SOG are fused. For this reason the pheromontropic activity was reported as a brain factor by Raina and Klun (1984) although it was, in fact, derived from the brain–SOG complex. Subsequently, when brain and SOG (Fig. 1) were separated at their approximate junction, the activity was found to be associated with the SOG (Raina *et al.*, 1987). This finding was further confirmed in tests with ligated *H. zea* females injected with larval brains and SOGs (in the

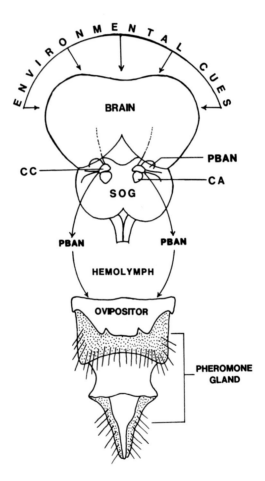

Fig. 1. Diagrammatic representation of the neuroendocrine complex of *Heliothis zea*, showing the area in the suboesophageal ganglion (SOG), where the pheromone biosynthesis–activating neuropeptide (PBAN) is produced. In response to environmental cues, PBAN is released via the corpora cardiaca (CC) into the hemolymph to initiate pheromone biosynthesis in the pheromone gland, located in the terminal abdominal segments. CA, Corpus allatum.

larvae, brain and SOG are morphologically distinct and separable because they are connected by relatively long circumoesophageal connectives). The tests showed that although the pheromontropic activity was very low in the larvae, it was always associated with the SOG rather than the brain.

2. Purification of the Neurohormone

Brain–SOGs were dissected from adult *H. zea* in physiological saline (Meyer and Miller, 1969) and stored in Bennett's buffer (Bennett *et al.*, 1980) at $-90°C$. Batches of 100 brain–SOGs in 250 μl buffer were homogenized with a Polytron homogenizer, and each homogenate was centrifuged at 4,000 rpm at 5°C for 30 min. The supernatant was passed through a prepared Sep-Pak C_{18} cartridge and the cartridge rinsed with 0.1% trifluoroacetic acid (TFA). The peptides were eluted with an 80 : 20 (v/v) solution of acetonitrile and 0.1% TFA, and the eluate was extracted three times with ethyl acetate. Residual ethyl acetate in the extracted eluate was removed in a Speed-Vac. The eluate was then filtered and fractionated by reverse phase high-performance liquid chromatography (HPLC) as described by Jaffe *et al.* (1986). Aliquots from each HPLC fraction were dried in a Speed-Vac. The dried fractions were dissolved in 50 μl sucrose–phosphate buffer (0.35 *M* sucrose in 20 m*M* sodium phosphate buffer, pH 6.8) and assayed for pheromonotropic activity. The remainder of the fractions were also dried and stored at $-90°C$ until further use. After two more HPLC runs of the most active combined fractions, a purified peptide with very high biological activity was obtained (Fig. 2).

3. Biological and Biochemical Characteristics of the Neurohormone

When the hormone was injected into ligated females, immediate induction of pheromone production occurred. The pheromone titer attained a maximal level 4 hr after injection and then declined to the preinjection level in the next 4 hr (Raina *et al.*, 1987). Since the ligated females were not observed to call and presumably did not release the pheromone, the drop in pheromone titer after 4 hr was interpreted to mean that the supply of the hormone was exhausted and that the existing pheromone had been enzymatically degraded (cf. Ding and Prestwich, 1986). The hormone was stable at 37°C and retained most of its activity after 4 hr of incubation at this temperature. Incubation with immobilized carboxypeptidase Y, which removed amino acids sequentially from the COOH terminus of a peptide, completely destroyed the activity. This result indicates that the hormone is a peptide. High-performance size-exclusion chromatography of brain–SOG homogenate and subsequent assays of the fractions for biological activity indicated that the hormone is a 2000- to 3000-dalton peptide. Amino acid analysis and sequence of this peptide are being pursued.

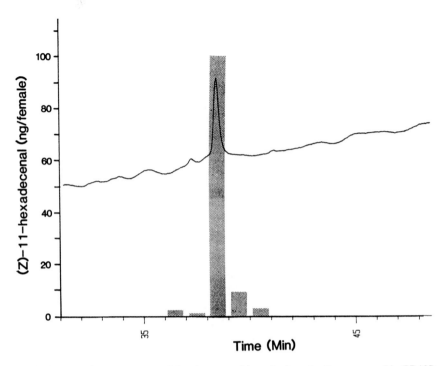

Fig. 2. HPLC chromatogram of the pheromone biosynthesis–activating neuropeptide (PBAN) on a Zorbax C-8 150SP column, using a linear gradient from 10 to 50% acetonitrile (0.1% v/v trifluoroacetic acid) against 0.1% aqueous trifluoroacetic acid, over 1 hr at 0.4 ml/min ($0.035A_{215}$ full scale). Histogram: Assay was conducted by injection of $\frac{1}{80}$ of the material collected in each fraction into a ligated *Heliothis zea* female, and pheromone (measured as nanograms of (Z)-11-hexadecenal) was extracted 3 hr later and quantified by internal standard gas chromatographic analysis.

B. Neuroregulatory Model

Presence of pheromonotropic activity in both the SOG and CC of *H. zea* and the established course for the release of other insect neurohormones indicate that the hormone controlling pheromone production is probably synthesized in the SOG and released into the hemolymph via the CC. The hormone is detectable in the SOG during the scotophase and photophase, and its titer is highest during the photophase. However, its titer is higher in the CC during the scotophase than in the photophase. Indications are that the hormone is continually produced in the SOG and transferred, via the neurosecretory axons, into the CC, which photoperiodically gates the release of the hormone into the hemolymph (Fig. 3). Temperature could be an additional factor modulating the release of the neurohormone. *Platynota stultana,* for example, began calling earlier at lower tem-

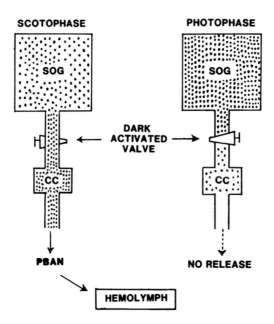

Fig. 3. Diagrammatic representation of origin and release of the pheromone biosynthesis–activating neuropeptide (PBAN). Note that the titer of PBAN in the suboesophageal ganglion (SOG) is higher during photophase, apparently because there is no release. In contrast, the hormone titer in the corpus cardiacum (CC) is higher during the scotophase.

peratures than at higher temperatures (Webster and Cardé, 1982). Release of the hormone from the CC could be controlled by aminergic synapses, the control mechanism hypothesized by Orchard and Loughton (1981) for the adipokinetic hormone in *Locusta migratoria*.

After its release into the hemolymph, the neurohormone may activate specific enzymes, which in turn convert the pheromone procursors to the sex pheromone (Fig. 4) (for chemical and enzymological studies, see Prestwich, Chapter 14, this volume; Morse and Meighen, Chapter 4). The sex attractants for most noctuid moths studied thus far are straight-chain (Z)-alkenols, -alkenals, or -alkenyl acetates of even carbon number (Steck *et al.*, 1982). Bjostad and Roelofs (1983) and Bjostad *et al.* (Chapter 3, this volume) reported that the majority of lepidopteran sex pheromones can be derived biosynthetically from the combined action of Δ^{11} desaturase and chain shortening enzymes. For example, they suggest that in *T. ni*, Δ^{11} desaturase converts the fatty acid precursor hexadecanoate to (Z)-11-hexadecenoate. This in turn undergoes chain shortening by two cycles of β-oxidation to produce (Z)-7-dodecenoate which is reduced and acetylated to give rise to (Z)-7-dodecenyl acetate, the primary component of *T. ni* sex pheromone. Based on the preceding assumptions, we propose to designate the pep-

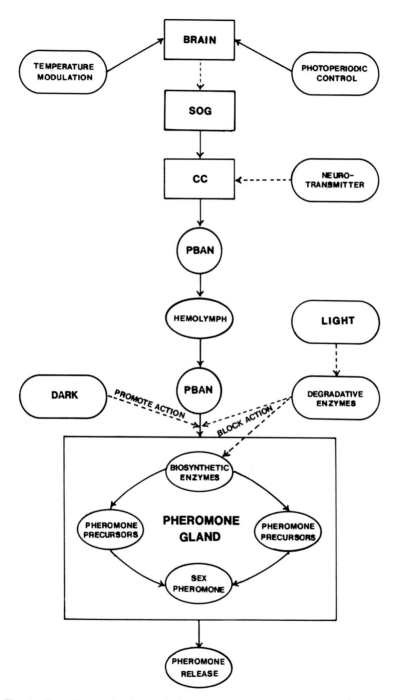

Fig. 4. Flow diagram showing production, release, and possible mode of action of the pheromone biosynthesis–activating neuropeptide (PBAN). Dashed arrows indicate speculative interactions that have not been experimentally tested.

tide neurohormone involved in controlling pheromone production as "pheromone biosynthesis–activating neuropeptide" (PBAN).

Preliminary experiments have indicated that the injection of PBAN into females during the photophase does not induce pheromone production (A. K. Raina, unpublished results). This finding suggests the possibility of light-activated degradative enzyme(s) that may inactivate PBAN and/or metabolize any pheromone that is produced. Similar extreme photoperiod dependence of the esterase, alcohol oxidase, and aldehyde dehydrogenases of *Heliothis virescens* glands has not been observed (Ding and Prestwich, 1986; Yu-S. Ding and G. D. Prestwich, unpublished results). The aldehyde is produced from stored alcohols by cuticular alcohol oxidases (Teal and Tumlinson, 1986; Tumlinson and Teal, Chapter 1, this volume), implicating alcohol availability as the limiting step in aldehyde production.

IV. FUTURE RESEARCH

A. Identification of Pheromone Biosynthesis–Activating Neuropeptide(s) in Other Lepidopteran Species and Mechanisms Controlling Specificity of Pheromone Composition

The effectiveness of the procedure (Section III,A,2) to purify the neuropeptide and the work presently underway to determine its amino acid composition and sequence indicate that in one lepidopteran species, we are on the verge of having a fully identified and sequenced PBAN. Cross-reactivity has been demonstrated with brain–SOG homogenates from several species of Lepidoptera representing five families and a species of cockroach (Raina and Klun, 1984; Raina *et al.,* 1987). Thus, when brain–SOG homogenate from any one of these species was injected into a ligated *H. zea,* the female produced the pheromone having a normal blend of its components, even though the pheromonal composition of the donor species was very different from that of *H. zea.* These results indicate that such species may have a hormone similar or identical to PBAN of *H. zea;* thus, PBAN may occur widely, at least among Lepidoptera. Obviously, we need to isolate and identify PBAN from several other species belonging to different families before we can confirm this.

An important question that remains to be answered is, What controls the specificity of the pheromonal composition in a species? Preliminary research (A. K. Raina, unpublished results) with the European cornborer, *Ostrinia nubilalis,* indicates that the neurohormone is not responsible for specificity of the pheromone. In *O. nubilalis* there are three genotypes categorized by the composition of their sex pheromone blends. Phenotypically they produce 11-tetradecenyl acetate in the isomeric $(Z:E)$ ratios of 3 : 97, 40 : 60, and 97 : 3 (Klun and Maini, 1979). When brain–SOG homogenates from the Z type were injected into ligated females of the E type, the recipient produced its own specific pheromone.

B. Biosynthesis, Release, and Degradation of Neurohormones

Based on the identified and partially characterized invertebrate neurohormones (Cook and Holman, 1985; Menn, 1985; O'Shea, 1985), the evidence is that most insect neurohormones are peptides. Most likely, insect neuropeptides are derived from posttranslational proteolytic cleavage of larger neuropeptide precursors. This has been shown to be the case with vertebrate neuropeptides (Krieger, 1983). Such a cleavage could be catalyzed by processing enzymes believed to be present in the lumen of the endoplasmic reticulum and in secretory granules (O'Shea, 1985). To date, no insect neuropeptide precursors have been discovered; consequently, we lack knowledge pertaining to the regulation of neuropeptide biosynthesis, actual presence and characteristics of processing enzymes, and peptide release mechanisms. Furthermore, information is also lacking regarding the degradative events terminating the action of the neuropeptides.

In a study reported by Quistad et al. (1984), proctolin was degraded by proteolytic enzymes within minutes of addition of proctolinergic tissues and hemolymph. The rapid degradation of proctolin is analogous to the facile hydrolysis of enkephalins in the brain by enkephalinases (Schwartz et al., 1981).

V. PROSPECTS AND STRATEGIES FOR EXPLOITING NEUROHORMONAL REGULATION IN INSECTS

The exciting discovery of PBAN in *H. zea* and the demonstration that brain extracts of other lepidopteran species can elicit a response similar to that produced by PBAN (Raina and Klun, 1984) provide us with bright prospects for developing novel strategies to control insect behavior and, ultimately, reproduction. Although research on PBAN and other such insect neurohormones is still embryonic, several control strategies have already been outlined and discussed, in general terms, by Menn and Henrick (1985), Menn (1985), and O'Shea (1985). Research efforts can focus on these strategies, once the structures of the hormones become known.

A. Blocking Processing Enzymes

The formation of PBAN may involve a scission reaction similar to that by which active angiotensin I (formed from a prohormone) is converted to active angiotensin II. The conversion takes place by scission of two amino acid residues from angiotensin I and is mediated by a truncating protease. This scission reaction can be effectively blocked by the proline derivative captopril, a potent inhibitor of the protease (Ondetti *et al.*, 1977). If a processing enzyme is, in fact, associated with PBAN formation, potent nonpeptide antagonists might be developed to block its action also.

B. Blocking the Mechanisms Involved in Triggering Neuropeptide Release

Neurotransmitters may be involved in releasing PBAN from the SOG and CC (see Fig. 4). Orchard and Loughton (1981) have reported suggestive evidence that octopamine can trigger the release into the hemolymph of adipokinetic hormone from the locust CC. Linn and Roelofs (1986) reported that octopamine potentiates the sensitivity of male moths to the female pheromone. By learning how neurotransmitters interact with neurohormones, researchers may be able to develop chemicals which can serve as agonists and/or antagonists in the release process of neurohormones.

C. Interfering with Neuropeptide Binding

Presently nothing is known concerning receptors for insect neuropeptides. Receptor binding assays should, therefore, be developed so that exogenous receptor ligands to block neurohormone binding may be discovered. Such ligands could serve as models for researchers to snythesize inhibitors with control potential.

D. Using Antagonists or Agonists of Peptide-Degrading Enzymes

Human pharmacological studies have shown that the degrading enzyme enkephalinase A is inhibited by the drug thiorphan ($K_i = 4 \times 10^{-9} M$) (Roques *et al.*, 1980). Conceivably, by analogy, an enzyme-degrading antagonist that would prolong the action of PBAN-like neurohormones or an agonist that would shorten the action of the peptide might be discovered. In either case, such nonpeptide compounds might be used as control agents, as both substances would be potentially harmful to the moths, interfering with their normal behavior pattern.

E. Using Synthetic Peptide Analogs

Using synthetic peptide-like analogs that interfere with the native neuropeptide is an attractive control strategy. The analogs would be modeled after identified neuropeptides and should preferably be small-chain compounds. They may need lipophilic substituents to facilitate penetration and transport to the active sites; highly effective bioassays would be needed for their evaluation. Furthermore, particular attention would have to be directed at the economics of producing such compounds.

Undoubtedly, other strategies will evolve during accelerated research in this fertile field. Indeed there is an opportunity and challenge to devote human and financial resources to behavioral neuropeptide research with the potential of developing totally new approaches to insect control.

ACKNOWLEDGMENTS

We thank the following individuals of the U.S. Department of Agriculture, Agricultural Research Service: Howard Jaffe (Livestock Insects Laboratory), for providing unpublished information on the purification of PBAN of *Heliothis zea;* Jerome Klun (Insect Chemical Ecology Laboratory), for critically reviewing the manuscript; and Alice Kunishi (Information Staff), for editorial comments.

REFERENCES

Baker, T. C., and Cardé, R. T. (1979). Courtship behavior of the oriental fruit moth (*Grapholitha molesta*): Experimental analysis and consideration of the role of sexual selection in the evolution of courtship pheromones in the Lepidoptera. *Ann. Entomol. Soc. Am.* **72,** 173–188.

Barth, R. H., Jr. (1961). Hormonal control of sex attractant production in the Cuban cockroach. *Science* **133,** 1598–1599.

Barth, R. H., Jr. (1965). Insect mating behavior: Endocrine control of a chemical communication system. *Science* **149,** 882–883.

Barth, R. H., and Lester, R. J. (1973). Neurohormonal control of sexual behavior in insects. *Ann. Rev. Entomol.* **18,** 445–472.

Bennett, H. P. J., Browne, C. A., Goltzman, D., and Solomon, S. (1980). Isolation of peptide hormones by reversed-phase high pressure liquid chromatography. *In* "Proceedings of the 6th American Peptide Symposium" (E. Gross and J. Maenhofer, eds.), pp. 121–124. Pierce Chem. Co., Rockford, Illinois.

Birch, M. C. (1974). Aphrodisiac pheromones in insects. *In* "Pheromones" (M. C. Birch, ed.), pp. 115–134. North-Holland, Amsterdam.

Bjostad, L. B., and Roelofs, W. L. (1983). Sex pheromone biosynthesis in *Trichoplusia ni:* Key steps involve Δ^{11} desaturation and chain-shortening. *Science* **220,** 1387–1389.

Cardé, R. T., and Webster, R. P. (1980). Endogenous and exogenous factors controlling insect sex pheromone production and responsiveness, particularly among Lepidoptera. *In* "Regulation of Insect Development and Behaviour," No. 22, 2, pp. 991–997. Sci. Papers Inst. Organic and Physical Chemistry, Wroclaw Tech. Univ., Karpacz, Poland.

Chang, F., Kou, R.. and Chow, Y.-S. (1979). The effect of precocene II on sex attractancy in the diamondback moth, *Plutella xylostella. Proc. Natl. Sci. Counc. Repub. China.* **3,** 67–76.

Cook, B. J., and Holman, G. M. (1985). Peptides and kinins. *In* "Comprehensive Insect Physiology, Biochemistry, and Pharmacology" (G. A. Kerkut and L. I. Gilbert, eds.), Vol. 11, pp. 531–593. Pergamon, Oxford, New York.

Ding, Yu-S., and Prestwich, G. D. (1986). Metabolic transformation of tritium-labelled pheromone by tissues of *Heliothis virescens* moths. *J. Chem. Ecol.* **12**, 411–429.

Haynes, K. F., Gaston, L. K. Pope, M. M., and Baker, T. C. (1983). Rate and periodicity of pheromone release from individual female artichoke plume moths, *Platyptilia carduidactyla* (Lepidoptera: Pterophoridae). *Environ. Entomol.* **12**, 1597–1600.

Hirai, K. (1980). Behavioral function of male scent in moths (Lepidoptera: Noctuidae). *Bull. Chugoku Natl. Agric. Exp. Stn., Ser. E* **16**, 132.

Hollander, A. L., and Yin, C.-M. (1982). Neurological influences on pheromone release and calling behaviour in the gypsy moth, *Lymantria dispar*. *Physiol. Entomol.* **7**, 163–166.

Hollander, A. L., and Yin, C.-M. (1985). Lack of humoral control in calling and pheromone release by brain, corpora cardiaca, corpora allata and ovaries of the female gypsy moth, *Lymantria dispar* (L.). *J. Insect Physiol.* **31**, 159–163.

Itagaki, H., and Conner, W. E. (1986). Physiological control of pheromone release behaviour in *Manduca sexta* (L.). *J. Insect Physiol.* **32**, 657–664.

Jaffe, H., Raina, A. K., Riley, C. T. Fraser, B. A., Holman, G. M., Wagner, R. M., Ridgway, R. L., and Hayes, D. K. (1986). Isolation and primary structure of a peptide from the corpora cardiaca of *Heliothis zea* with adipokinetic activity. *Biochem. Biophys. Res. Commun.* **135**, 622–628.

Klun, J. A., and Maini, S. (1979). Genetic basis of an insect chemical communication system: The European corn borer. *Environ. Entomol.* **8**, 423–426.

Klun, J. A., Plimmer, J. R., Bierl-Leonhardt, B. A., Sparks, A. N., and Chapman, O. L. (1979). Trace chemicals: The essence of sexual communication systems in *Heliothis* species. *Science* **204**, 1328–1330.

Krieger, D. T. (1983). Brain peptides: What, where, why? *Science* **222**, 975–985.

Lanier, G. N. (1970). Sex pheromone: Abolition of specificity in hybrid bark beetles. *Science* **169**, 71–72.

Linn, C. E., and Roelofs, W. L. (1986). Modulatory effects of octopamine and serotonin on male sensitivity and periodicity of response to sex pheromone in the cabbage looper moth, *Trichoplusia ni*. *Arch. Insect. Biochem. Physiol.* **3**, 161–171.

Menn, J. J. (1985). New research horizons in insect control. *J. Pestic. Sci. 10 (Special Issue)*, 372–376.

Menn, J. J., and Henrick, C. A. (1985). Newer chemicals for insect control. *In* "Agricultural Chemicals of the Future" (J. L. Hilton ed.), pp. 247–265 (Beltsville Agric. Res. Ctr. Symp. No. 8). Rowman & Allanheld, Ottawa.

Meyer, J., and Miller, T. (1969). Starvation induced activity in cockroach Malpighian tubules. *Ann. Entomol. Soc. Am.* **62**, 725–729.

Ondetti, M. A., Rubin, B., and Cushman, D. W. (1977). Design of specific inhibitors of angiotensin-converting enzyme: New class of orally active antihypertensive agents. *Science* **196**, 441–444.

Orchard, I., and Loughton, B. G. (1981). Is octopamine a transmitter mediating hormone release in insects? *J. Neurobiol.* **12**, 143–153.

O'Shea, M. (1985). Neuropeptides in insects: Possible leads to new control methods. *In* "Approaches to New Leads for Insecticides" (H. C. Von Keyserlingk, A. Jager, and Ch. von Szczepanski, eds.), pp. 133–151. Springer-Verlag, Berlin, Heidelberg, New York.

Pope, M. M., Gaston, L. K., and Baker, T. C. (1984). Composition, quantification, and periodicity of sex pheromone volatiles from individual *Heliothis zea* females. *J. Insect Physiol.* **12**, 943–945.

Quistad, G. B., Adams, M. E., Scarborough, R. M., Carney, R. L., and Schooley, D. A. (1984). Metabolism of proctolin. A pentapeptide neurotransmitter in insects. *Life Sci.* **34**, 569–576.

Raina, A. K., and Klun, J. A. (1984). Brain factor control of sex pheromone production in the female corn earworm moth. *Science* **225**, 531–533.

Raina, A. K., Klun, J. A., and Stadelbacher, E. A. (1986). Diel periodicity and effect of age and mating on female sex pheromone titer in *Heliothis zea* (Lepidoptera: Noctuidae). *Ann. Entomol. Soc. Am.* **79**, 128–131.

Raina, A. K., Jaffe, H., Klun, J. A., Ridgway, R. L., and Hayes, D. K. (1987). Characteristics of a neurohormone that controls sex pheromone production in *Heliothis zea*. *J. Insect Physiol.* (in press).

Riddiford, L. M. (1974). The role of hormones in the reproductive behavior of female wild silk moths. *In* "Experimental Analysis of Insect Behaviour" (L. B. Browne, ed.), pp. 278–285. Springer-Verlag, New York.

Riddiford, L. M., and Williams, C. M. (1971). Role of corpora cardiaca in the behavior of saturniid moths. I. Release of sex pheromone. *Biol. Bull.* **140**, 1–7.

Ridgway, R. L., Leonhardt, B. A., and Inscoe, M. N. (1986). Cooperative development and expanding uses of delivery systems for insect attractants. *Proc. Abst. 13th Intl. Symp. Controlled Release Bioactive Materials, Norfolk, Virginia Aug. 3–6, 1986,* pp. 100–101.

Roelofs, W. L., and Cardé, R. T. (1974). Sex pheromones in the reproductive isolation of lepidopterous species. *In* "Pheromones" (M. C. Birch, ed.), pp. 96–114. North-Holland, Amsterdam.

Roller, H., Piepho, H., and Holz, I. (1963). The problem of hormone dependency of copulation behaviour in insects. Studies of *Galleria mellonella* (L.). *J. Insect Physiol.* **9**, 187–194.

Roques, B. P., Fournie-Zaluski, M. C., Soroca, E., LeConte, J. M., Malfroy, B., Lorenz, C., and Schwartz, J. C. (1980). The enkephalinase inhibitor thiorphan shows antinociceptive activity in mice. *Nature (London)* **228**, 286–288.

Sasaki, M., and Riddiford, L. M. (1984). Regulation of reproductive behavior and egg maturation in the tobacco hawk moth, *Manduca sexta. Physiol. Entomol.* **9**, 315–327.

Sasaki, M., Riddiford, L. M., Truman, J. W., and Moore, J. K. (1983). Reevaluation of the role of corpora cardiaca in calling and oviposition behaviour of giant silk moth. *J. Insect Physiol.* **29**, 695–705.

Schwartz, J. C., Malfroy, B., and DeLaBaume, S. (1981). Biological inactivation of enkephalins and the role of enkephalin–dipeptidylcarboxypeptidase ("enkephalinase") neuropeptidase. *Life Sci.* **29**, 1715–1740.

Sower, L. L., Shorey, H. H., and Gaston, L. K. (1970). Sex pheromones of noctuid moths. XXI. Light: dark cycle regulation and light inhibition of sex pheromone release by females of *Trichoplusia ni. Ann. Entomol. Soc. Am.* **63**, 1090–1092.

Steck, W., Underhill, E. W., and Chisholm, M. D. (1982). Structure–activity relationships in sex attractants for North American noctuid moths. *J. Chem. Ecol.* **8**, 731–754.

Teal, P. E. A., and Tumlinson, J. H. (1986). Terminal steps in pheromone biosynthesis of *Heliothis virescens* and *H. zea. J. Chem. Ecol.* **12**, 353–366.

Webster, R. P., and Cardé, R. T. (1982). Relationship among pheromone titer, calling and age in the omnivorous leafroller moth (*Platynota stultana*). *J. Insect Physiol.* **28**, 925–933.

Webster, R. P., and Cardé, R. T. (1984). The effect of mating, exogenous juvenile hormone and a juvenile hormone analogue on pheromone titer, calling and oviposition in the omnivorous leafroller moth (*Platynota stultana*). *J. Insect Physiol.* **30**, 113–118.

6

Biosynthesis of Pheromones and Endocrine Regulation of Pheromone Production in Coleoptera

DÉSIRÉE VANDERWEL
A. CAMERON OEHLSCHLAGER
Department of Chemistry
Simon Fraser University
Burnaby, British Columbia, Canada V5A 1S6

I. INTRODUCTION

Interest in coleopteran pheromones has been aroused both by academic curiosity and by the potential for these behavior-modifying chemicals to be used for the detection and manipulation of pest populations. These investigations have revealed a surprising complexity in the pheromone bouquets of many coleopterans. Not only are the messages encoded by a diverse group of chemicals, but their meanings can be drastically altered simply through variation of the quantity, the relative proportion, and/or the chirality of each pheromone that is emitted. Moreover, the type and quantity of pheromone released by an individual may vary in response to a variety of environmental and/or physiological stimuli. In this chapter we have attempted to summarize current knowledge and speculation about the biochemical mechanisms that lie behind these fascinating variations.

Pheromone Biochemistry

II. MECHANISMS OF PRODUCTION

Coleopterans are known to utilize several types of pheromone biosynthetic pathways. Many pheromones are obtained through simple modifications of dietary components, while others are synthesized *de novo* from simple biogenic precursors. Symbiotic microorganisms may be involved in the biosynthesis of some pheromones, but as yet the significance of this contribution is not well understood. In this section, the mechanisms of coleopteran pheromone biosynthesis will be examined in more detail.

A. Sequestration of Host Compounds

Both sexes of the Douglas-fir beetle, *Dendroctonus pseudotsugae,* release limonene with their aggregation pheromones when stimulated by acoustic signals from the opposite sex (Rudinsky *et al.,* 1977). Limonene, a major constituent of Douglas-fir oleoresin, acts synergistically with the aggregation pheromones to facilitate mass attack (Rudinsky *et al.,* 1966). It is not known if Douglas-fir beetles simply sequester host limonene in their hindguts during larval and maturation feeding or if they synthesize it *de novo* (Rudinsky *et al.,* 1977). As some form of the host monoterpene α-pinene is sequestered by pupae of the southern pine beetle, *Dendroctonus frontalis* (Hughes, 1975), it is possible that other host monoterpenes, such as limonene, could be likewise stored.

B. Modification of Host Compounds

1. Terpene-Derived Pheromones

a. *Boll Weevil.* Grandlure, the sex pheromone of the male boll weevil, *Anthonomus grandis,* is comprised of four monoterpenoid components: (+)-*cis*-2-isopropenyl-1-methylcyclobutaneethanol (grandisol, **I**); (Z)-3,3-dimethyl-$\Delta^{1,\beta}$-cyclohexaneethanol (**II**); (Z)-3,3-dimethyl-$\Delta^{1,\alpha}$-cyclohexaneacetaldehyde (**III**); and (E)-3,3-dimethyl-$\Delta^{1,\alpha}$-cyclohexaneacetaldehyde (**IV**) (Fig. 1) (Tumlinson *et al.,* 1969). The observation that weevils feeding on their natural food source (cotton buds) exhibited enhanced pheromone production (Hardee, 1970; Hedin *et al.,* 1975) led to the hypothesis that plant-derived constituents are utilized for pheromone production. Tumlinson *et al.* (1970) proposed a biosynthetic route from monoterpene alcohols to the pheromones, through an intermediate such as γ-isogeraniol (**V**, see Fig. 1). Subsequent studies demonstrated that the host-contained geraniol (**VI**) and nerol (**VII**) (Hedin *et al.,* 1971) could serve as pheromone precursors (Thompson and Mitlin, 1979). Male boll weevils exposed to a mixture of tritiated geraniol and nerol incorporated the tritium label into all four pheromone components. Boll weevils can also synthesize their

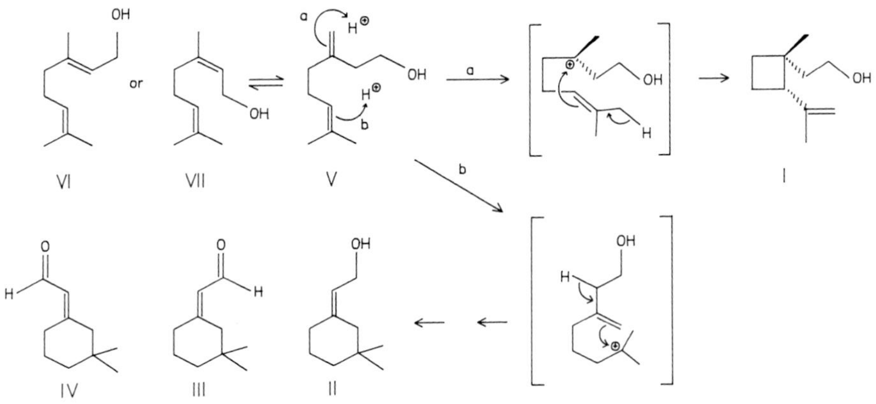

Fig. 1.   Biosynthesis of boll weevil sex pheromones from geraniol (**VI**) or nerol (**VII**).

pheromones *de novo* (Mitlin and Hedin, 1974), but the relative contribution of each pathway to pheromone biosynthesis is not yet known (see Section II,C).

  b.   Bark Beetles.   Bark beetles in the family Scolytidae are known to use both kairomones and pheromones in the location and colonization of host trees. Primary host selection may or may not be guided by host-produced monoter-penes (Rudinsky, 1966; Moeck *et al.*, 1981, and references cited therein), while mass attack and colonization are usually facilitated by beetle-produced aggrega-tion pheromones (Borden, 1985, and references cited therein). These largely consist of bicyclic ketals and secondary alcohols. The cyclic ketals are of uncer-tain biosynthetic origin (Section II,E,1), but most secondary alcohols appear to be derived from host monoterpenes. The biosynthesis of these pheromones from host monoterpenes primarily involves allylic oxidation or hydration, but may be accompanied by secondary reactions such as further oxidation, hydrogenation, or rearrangement of the carbon skeleton (Francke and Vite, 1983).

  Many monoterpenes found in host trees have been shown to be toxic to the beetles that feed on them (Smith, 1961, 1965a,b; Coyne and Lott, 1976; Raffa *et al.*, 1985). It is widely suspected that scolytids must possess effective mecha-nisms for monoterpene detoxification in order to survive extensive exposure to monoterpenes (Hughes, 1973a; White *et al.*, 1980; Francke and Vite, 1983). The prevailing biochemical strategy appears to involve the oxidation of the hydro-phobic toxicants to more polar derivatives, thus facilitating transportation and elimination (Dowd *et al.*, 1983; Ahmad, 1986). Some of the volatile products of this detoxification process may have been secondarily adopted for use as phe-romones (Hughes, 1973a; White *et al.*, 1980; Francke and Vite, 1983).

  Studies in which the males and/or females of a scolytid species were exposed to one host monoterpene are summarized in Table I. The compounds which

TABLE I

Metabolism of Specific Host Monoterpenes by Scolytid Beetles

PRECURSORS		myrcene			*alpha*-pinene						*beta*-pinene			camphene	3-carene	PRECURSORS
SPECIES \ PRODUCTS		ipsdienol	ipsenol	myrcenol	*cis*-verbenol	*trans*-verbenol	verbenone	myrtenol	*cis*-3-pinen-2-ol	4-methyl-2-pentanol	*trans*-pinocarveol	pinocarvone	myrtenol	camphenol	1-methyl-5-(*alpha*-hydroxyisopropyl)cyclohexa-1,3-diene	PRODUCTS / REFERENCES
Dendroctonus brevicomis	(♂♂)	+		+		P			+					+		Hughes, 1973a; Renwick et al., 1976c; Byers, 1983a,b
	(♀♀)	−		+		P			+					+		Hughes, 1973a; Renwick et al., 1976c; Byers, 1983a,b
D. frontalis	(♂♂)				+	P	P	P		+	+	+	P	+		Hughes, 1973a,1975; Renwick and Hughes, 1975; Renwick et al., 1973, 1976c
	(♀♀)				+	P			+	+	+		P	+		Hughes,1973a; Renwick et al, 1973, 1976c; Renwick and Hughes, 1975
D. valens	(♂♂)	+			+	+		+	+		+	+				Hughes, 1973a
D. ponderosae	(♂♂)	+		+	+	P			+		+	+				Hughes, 1973a,b; Hunt et al., 1986
	(♀♀)			+	+	P										Hughes, 1973a,b; Hunt et al., 1986
D. pseudotsugae	(♂♂)	+														Hughes, 1973a

Table (rotated 90° on page). Column headers (compound names) are not present on this page. Symbols: + = produced, – = not produced, tr = only produced in trace quantities, P = produced and is a known pheromone of the species.

Species	Sex						Reference
Ips amitinus	(♂♀)				+	+	Klimetzek and Francke, 1980
I. avulsus	(♂♂)			–	P		Hughes, 1974
I. calligraphus	(♂♂)			–	P		Hughes, 1974
I. cembrae	(♂♂)			P	P		Renwick and Dickens, 1979
	(♀♀)			tr	tr		Renwick and Dickens, 1979
I. grandicolis	(♂♂)		+	+	+		Hughes, 1974
I. paraconfusus	(♂♂)	+	+	P	P	+	Hughes, 1974; Renwick et al., 1976b,c; Hughes and Renwick, 1977a; Byers et al., 1979; Hendry et al., 1980; Byers, 1981b, 1983b
	(♀♀)		+	–			Renwick et al., 1976b; Byers et al., 1979; Hendry et al., 1980; Byers, 1981b, 1983b
I. pini	(♂♀)	+			P		Renwick et al, 1976c
I. typographus	(♂♀)			P	P	+	Klimetzek and Francke, 1980
Pityokteines curvidens	(♂♂)			–	+	+	Harring, 1978
	(♀♀)			–	+	+	Harring, 1978
P. spinidens	(♂♂)			+	+	+	Harring, 1978
	(♀♀)			–	+	+	Harring, 1978
P. voronizovi	(♂♂)			P	+	+	Harring, 1978
	(♀♀)			–	+	+	Harring, 1978

+ = produced
– = not produced
tr = only produced in trace quantities
P = produced and is a known pheromone of the species

179

appeared after the monoterpene treatment were found primarily to be the corresponding allylic alcohols (White *et al.*, 1980; Francke and Vite, 1983). It is likely that the oxidation of host monoterpenes is performed by mixed-function oxidases (MFOs) present in the insect's microsomal enzyme system. Originally, this process may have functioned to metabolize toxicants associated with the insect's diet (Dowd *et al.*, 1983), but MFOs in scolytids may have become specialized to deal with host tree resin. Indeed, the microsomal cytochrome *P*-450 isolated from *Dendroctonus terebrans* exhibits an unusually high specificity for the *in vitro* oxidation of the host monoterpene α-pinene (White *et al.*, 1979).

The allylic oxidation of monoterpenes during detoxification does not appear to be as nonspecific as originally proposed (Hughes, 1973a; Renwick and Hughes, 1975). The metabolic products of most host monoterpenes were determined in a detailed study of the volatiles of female *Dendroctonus ponderosae* feeding in its natural hosts lodgepole and ponderosa pine (Libbey *et al.*, 1985; H. D. Pierce *et al.*, 1987). To account for the alcohol derivatives of the host monoterpenes encountered, three metabolic pathways were proposed (H. D. Pierce *et al.*, 1987). One pathway apparently facilitates the oxidation of any vinyl methyl group which is *E* to an allylic methylene (see Fig. 2). This system does not discriminate between substrates, as judged from the relative proportions of monoterpene precursors in the host oleoresin and the corresponding alcohol products. The second oxidation system is specific for the hydroxylation of allylic

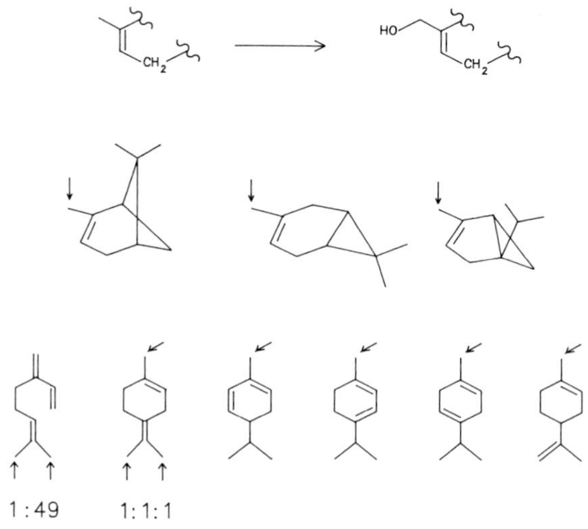

Fig. 2. Regiospecific oxidation of monoterpenes to primary alcohols in female *Dendroctonus ponderosae* (H. D. Pierce *et al.*, 1987).

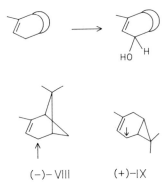

(−)− VIII   (+)−IX

Fig. 3. Stereospecific oxidation of bicyclic monoterpenes to *trans*-alcohols in female *D. ponderosae* (H. D. Pierce *et al.*, 1987).

methylenes *E* to vinyl methyl groups (see Fig. 3) in bicyclic monoterpenes such as α-pinene (**VIII**) and 3-carene (**IX**). An aggregation pheromone of *D. ponderosae*, (−)-*trans*-verbenol (McKnight, 1979; Libbey *et al.*, 1985; Borden *et al.*, 1987), is produced by this system, which appears to be enantioselective for (−)-α-pinene [(−)-**VIII**] (H. D. Pierce *et al.*, 1987). The third enzymatic system revealed in *D. ponderosae* does not appear to be an allylic MFO, but rather mediates the anti-Markovnikov hydration of the major host monoterpene, (−)-β-phellandrene [(−)-**X**], to give largely the trans product (**XI**). As shown in Fig. 4, an 8 : 1 ratio of trans : cis (**XI : XII**) product was observed. This system is apparently specific for **X** since hydration products of other host monoterpenes (such as β-pinene) were not detected in *D. ponderosae* volatiles (H. D. Pierce *et al.*, 1987).

There is evidence that, at least in those cases where the oxidation products have been adopted for use as pheromones, the metabolism of host monoterpenes can be highly stereo- and enantioselective (Renwick *et al.*, 1976b; Harring,

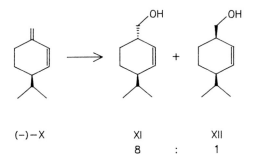

(−)−X   XI   XII
                          8   :   1

Fig. 4. Anti-Markovnikov hydration of β-phellandrene (**X**) in female *D. ponderosae*.

1978; Fish *et al.*, 1979; Renwick and Dickens, 1979; Klimetzek and Francke, 1980; Byers, 1983a). Due to the pheromonal activity of *cis*- and *trans*-verbenols in several *Dendroctonus* and *Ips* species, the oxidation of α-pinene to these allylic alcohols has been extensively investigated. As discussed below, the varying selectivities of the oxidase systems of different species of beetles give rise to different isomeric mixtures of *trans*- (**XIII**) and *cis*-verbenol (**XIV**) (see Fig. 5).

Ips species (*I. amitinus, I. typographus,* and *I. paraconfusus*) stereospecifically replace the pro-(4*S*) hydrogen of α-pinene (**VIII**) with a hydroxyl group. Thus, as shown in Fig. 5, (+)-α-pinene [(+)-**VIII**] is oxidized to (+)-(1*R*,4*S*,5*R*)-*trans*-verbenol [(+)-**XIII**], while (−)-α-pinene [(−)-**VIII**] is

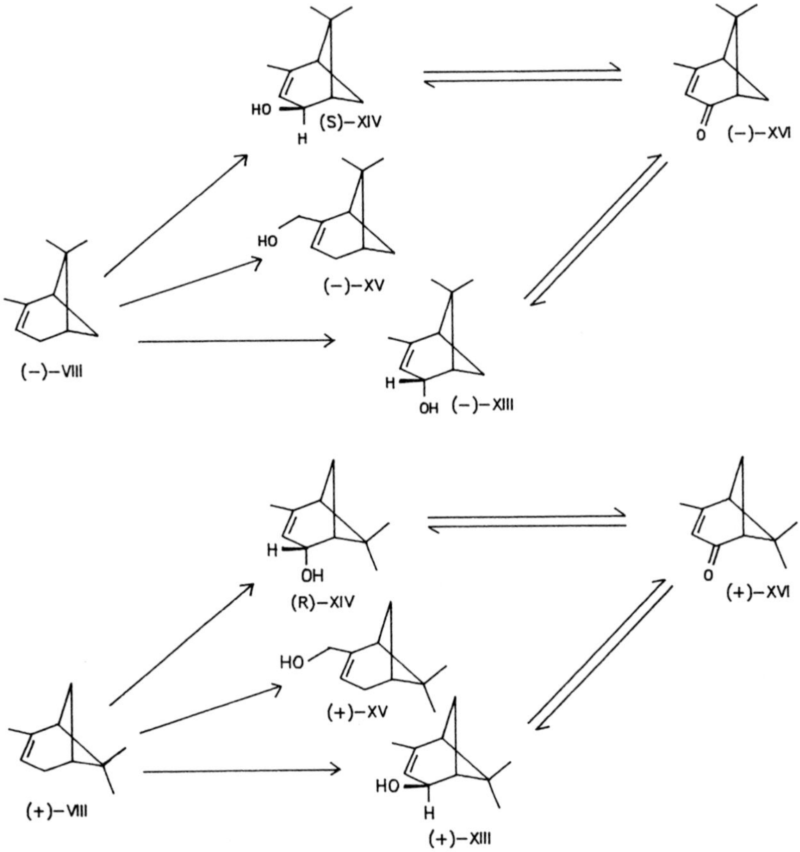

Fig. 5.   Oxidation of α-pinene (**VIII**) enantiomers to *cis*- (**XIV**) and *trans*-verbenol (**XIII**), verbenone (**XVI**), and mrytenol (**XV**).

converted to $(1S,4S,5S)$-*cis*-verbenol $[(S)$-**XIV**$]^1$ (Renwick *et al.*, 1976b; Klimetzek and Francke, 1980). Many *Ips* species use (S)-*cis*-verbenol $[(S)$-**XIV**] as an aggregation pheromone (Borden, 1985, and references cited therein). The production of this pheromone is thus dependent on the enantiomeric ratio of α-pinene contained in the host tree oleoresin—a unique insect–host relationship (Renwick *et al.*, 1976b; Klimetzek and Francke, 1980).

A 1:1 mixture of *cis*- and *trans*-verbenol was produced by *Ips paraconfusus* (Renwick *et al.*, 1976b), *I. typographus*, and *I. amitinus* beetles exposed to racemic α-pinene (Klimetzek and Francke, 1980). Thus, the oxidase(s) of these *Ips* species must be fairly tolerant of the location of the bulky *gem*-dimethyl group. In contrast, *Dendroctonus brevicomis* converts the $(+)$ and $(-)$ enantiomers of α-pinene to $(+)$-$(1R,4S,5R)$- $[(+)$-**XIII**] and $(-)$-$(1S,4R,5S)$-*trans*-verbenol $[(-)$-**XIII**], respectively (Byers, 1983a). Little, if any, *cis*-verbenol (**XIV**) is produced, indicating that in this species the enzymes are more sensitive to steric effects in the substrate. These differences in the enzyme systems help to reduce interspecific competition. Since *D. brevicomis* and *I. paraconfusus* are sympatric, it would be disadvantageous for one species to produce a compound that attracts the other species. At the same time, it is not surprising that both species would derivatize a major component of the host oleoresin and use the products as pheromones. Thus, male *D. brevicomis* produce $(-)$-*trans*- instead of (S)-*cis*-verbenol and use it to inhibit the response of female *D. brevicomis* to aggregation pheromones (apparently to reduce intraspecific competition) (Bedard *et al.*, 1980; Byers, 1983a). Neither *D. brevicomis* nor the *Ips* species seem to use $(+)$-*trans*-verbenol as a pheromone (Borden, 1985, and references cited therein).

Pityokteines species, which are not known to use the verbenols as pheromones, exhibit less stereoselectivity than *Ips* or *Dendroctonus* species in the derivatization of α-pinene. Although the $(-)$ enantiomer was apparently the favored substrate, *P. spinidens, P. curvidens,* and *P. vorontzovi* produced both *cis*- and *trans*-verbenol on exposure to either $(+)$- or $(-)$-α-pinene (Harring, 1978). However, since only a small quantity of *cis*-verbenol was produced when the insects were exposed to $(+)$-α-pinene, one cannot rule out the possibility that it was derived from $(-)$-α-pinene present as an impurity in the $(+)$-α-pinene.

Other oxidation products of α-pinene that are utilized as pheromones include myrtenol (**XV**) and verbenone (**XVI**) (Fig. 5). Myrtenol is formed through the oxidation of the allylic methyl group of α-pinene, as described for *D. ponderosae* in Fig. 2. Renwick *et al.* (1973) noted that *D. frontalis* produced myr-

---

[1]A phenomenon which has caused some confusion in the literature is that the optical rotation of $(4S)$-*cis*-verbenol can be either $(+)$ or $(-)$, depending on the solvent (Mori *et al.*, 1976). Therefore we will refer to $(1S,4S,5S)$-*cis*-verbenol as (S)-*cis*-verbenol and to its $(1R,4R,5R)$-enantiomer as (R)-*cis*-verbenol.

tenol (in addition to other oxidation products) on exposure to α-pinene. Similarly, *I. paraconfusus* produced (+)- and (−)-myrtenol after exposure to the corresponding enantiomers of α-pinene (Renwick *et al.*, 1976b). While myrtenol has no known pheromonal activity in *Ips* species, it is a multifunctional pheromone of *D. frontalis* (Rudinsky *et al.*, 1974) and has been identified as an aggregation pheromone of *Dryocoetes confusus* (Borden *et al.*, 1986b).

Verbenone, a multifunctional pheromone utilized by several scolytid species (Borden, 1985, and references cited therein), is considered to be derived from α-pinene through oxidation of the verbenols. Although Hughes (1975) provided circumstantial evidence for this route, with the demonstration that *D. frontalis* males exposed to α-pinene contained about twice as much verbenone as unexposed males, other such studies have failed to corroborate this relationship (Renwick *et al.*, 1973; Byers, 1983a,b). However, any attempt to correlate verbenone production by adult beetles with α-pinene exposure is complicated by the possibility that the precursor may be carried over from earlier developmental stages. Hughes (1975) demonstrated that *D. frontalis* pupae do not complete the metabolism of α-pinene to the known oxidation products but likely store the terpene as a conjugated intermediate. This intermediate is metabolized to yield the pheromones *trans*-verbenol and verbenone once the insect becomes a mature adult.

An additional source of α-pinene-derived semiochemicals that should be considered is from the autooxidation of α-pinene. On exposure to air, α-pinene autooxidizes to a variety of compounds (Moore *et al.*, 1966), which include *cis*- and *trans*-verbenol and, in turn, verbenone (Borden *et al.*, 1986). It is possible that biologically significant quantities of these behavior-modifying chemicals are formed when the host tree exudes resin in response to attack (Borden *et al.*, 1986). The possibility that α-pinene-derived semiochemicals are produced independently of insect metabolism has interesting implications on the dynamics of host colonization (Borden *et al.*, 1986).

Myrcene (**XVII**), the only prominent acyclic monoterpene in pine oleoresin, is oxidized at three different allylic positions by *Dendroctonus* and *Ips* species. Both allylic methyl groups are oxidized, producing (*E*)- or (*Z*)-myrcenol [(*E*)-**XVIII** and (*Z*)-**XVIII**] (Figs. 2 and 6), while only one of the allylic methylenes is oxidized, leading to ipsdienol (**XIX**) and ipsenol (**XXI**) (Figs. 6 and 7). On exposure to myrcene vapors female *D. ponderosae* produce both (*E*)- and (*Z*)-myrcenol ($E:Z = 49:1$) but no ipsdienol (**XIX**) (Hunt *et al.*, 1986). Males, however, produce approximately equal amounts of (+)-ipsdienol [(+)-**XIX**, >97% e.e. (enantiomeric excess)] and (*E*)- and (*Z*)-myrcenol ($E:Z = 9:1$) (Hunt *et al.*, 1986). Male and female *D. brevicomis* also convert myrcene to (*E*)-myrcenol (Renwick *et al.*, 1976b). It is of interest that the oxidations of the C-1 methyl group, C-3, and C-6 of 1-methylcyclohexene (**XX**) in male *D. frontalis* (Renwick and Hughes, 1975) occur in approximately the same ratio as oxidation of the corresponding allylic positions of myrcene by male *D. ponderosae* (Fig. 6).

While the myrcenols have no known pheromonal activity, ipsdienol and ipsenol are commonly used as pheromones in the genus *Ips* (Borden, 1985, and references cited therein). Male beetles oxidize myrcene to either or both of the (+) and (−) enantiomers of ipsdienol [(+)- and (−)-**XIX**], but will reduce only (−)-ipsdienol to (−)-ipsenol [(−)-**XXI**] (Fig. 7). Initial evidence for the conversion of myrcene to ipsdienol and ipsenol was provided by Hughes (1974) and by Hughes and Renwick (1977a), who showed that *I. paraconfusus* males could produce ipsdienol and ipsenol when exposed to myrcene vapors. Ipsenol was produced when these insects were treated topically with ipsdienol. More conclusive evidence was supplied by Hendry *et al.* (1980), who demonstrated the conversion of deuterium-labeled myrcene to labeled ipsdienol and ipsenol by male *I. paraconfusus*. Fish *et al.* (1979) demonstrated the *in vivo* conversion of deuterated ipsdienol to deuterated ipsenol. Stereoselective reduction of (−)-, but not (+)-, ipsdienol to ipsenol was noted by Renwick and Dickens (1979) in *Ips cembrae* and by Fish *et al.* (1979) in *I. paraconfusus*.

It has been suggested that an alternate pathway to (−)-ipsenol, involving an oxidation–reduction equilibrium between ipsdienol and its ketone, ipsdienone (**XXII**), is present in *I. paraconfusus* (Fish *et al.*, 1979). This alternative was originally proposed to account for the loss of deuterium observed when male beetles were exposed to racemic deuterated ipsdienol (64% D, labeled at the carbinol carbon). The deuterium contents of the recovered ipsdienol and ipsenol

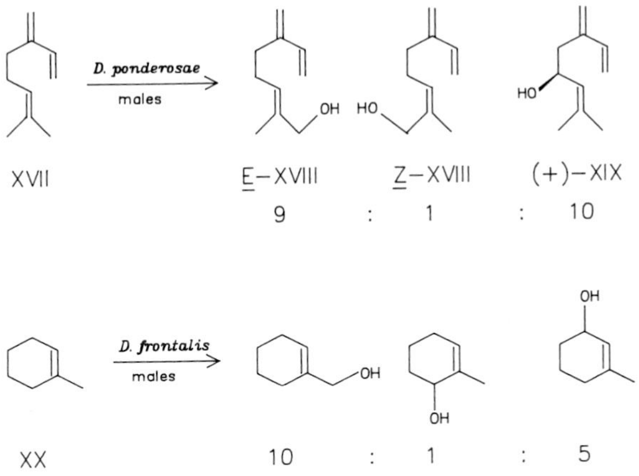

Fig. 6. Allylic oxidation of myrcene (**XVII**) and 1-methylcyclohexene (**XX**) in *Dendroctonus* species.

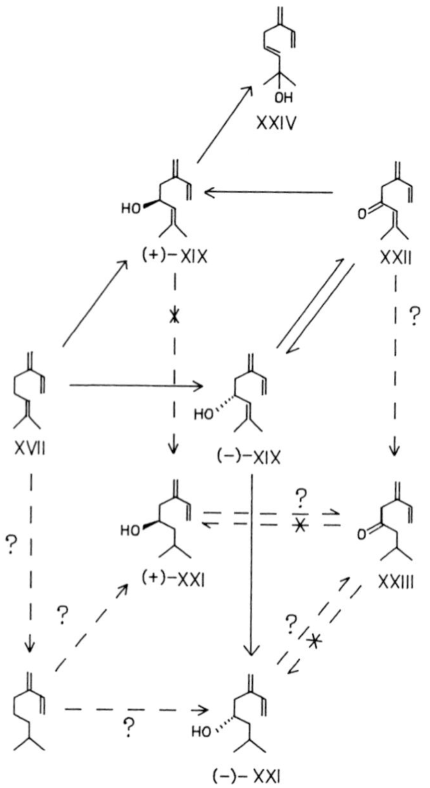

Fig. 7. Oxidation of myrcene (**XVII**) to ipsdienol (**XIX**), ipsenol (**XXI**), amitinol (**XXIV**), and the corresponding ketones. Dashed lines represent possible conversions which have not been conclusively disproved.

were reduced to 59 and 25%, respectively (Fish *et al.,* 1979). In subsequent experiments, male beetles converted exogenous ipsdienone to (+)- and (−)-ipsdienol (in a 36 : 64 ratio) and (−)-ipsenol (86% e.e.) (Fish *et al.,* 1984). These results suggest that (−)-ipsenol can be generated indirectly, through the oxidation of ipsdienol to ipsdienone, reduction back to both (+)- and (−)-ipsdienol, and, finally, through the reduction of the thus formed (−)-ipsdienol (see Fig. 7). Ipsenone (**XXIII**) does not appear to be involved, since no ipsenol was detected when the males were exposed to ipsenone (Fish *et al.,* 1984). Furthermore, although not directly demonstrated, the oxidation of ipsdienol is apparently enantioselective, in that only the (−) enantiomer of ipsdienol is converted to ipsdienone. If this were not the case, beetles exposed to (+)-ipsdienol could form (−)-ipsenol through ipsdienone. This, in fact, does not occur (Fish *et al.,*

1979). The implications of this alternate route to ipsenol are discussed in Section III.

c. *Stored-Product Beetles.* While the biosynthesis of terpenoid pheromones by scolytid beetles has been investigated in some depth, the production of such pheromones by beetles in other families has been virtually neglected. Preliminary work with one of the macrolide aggregation pheromones (**XXV**) (Fig. 8) produced by males of the rusty grain beetle, *Cryptolestes ferrugineus,* has confirmed earlier expectations (H. D. Pierce *et al.,* 1984) that this pheromone was of terpenoid origin. When beetles were allowed to feed on oats coated with 1-deutero-(*E,E*)-farnesol ([D]-**XXVI**), the macrolide **XXV** produced was enriched with deuterium at C-10 [as determined by single ion monitoring/gas chromatography–mass spectrometry (SIM/GC–MS) and nuclear magnetic resonance (NMR)] (D. Vanderwel, H. D. Pierce, Jr.,[2] and A. C. Oehlschlager, unpublished work), indicating that (*E,E*)-farnesol can serve as a precursor. The biosynthetic transformation is presumed to involve oxidative cleavage of the terminal double bond (generating a hydroxy acid intermediate, **XXVII**) followed by cyclization, as shown in Fig. 8. As discussed in Section II,C the beetle can utilize either dietary farnesol or terpenes produced *de novo* (perhaps via the juvenile hormone pathway) as the pheromone precursor.

As shown in Fig. 8, the lactonization reaction to form **XXV** could conceivably occur in either of two directions. In order to distinguish between the two, *C. ferrugineus* was exposed to 1-deutero-(*E,E*)-farnesol that was also enriched for ^{18}O at C-1. The macrolide **XXV** produced by the insect was enriched for both deuterium and ^{18}O (D. Vanderwel, H. D. Pierce, Jr., and A. C. Oehlschlager, unpublished work). Thus the lactonization reaction leading to **XXV** apparently proceeds with retention of the hydroxyl oxygen (at C-10 of intermediate **XXVII**) and therefore cannot proceed by mechanisms which involve loss of this oxygen (such as through the pyrophosphate intermediate shown in Fig. 8).

Although terpenes are believed to serve as pheromone precursors in other stored-product beetles (see Section II,E,1), as yet no supporting experimental evidence has been offered.

2. Fatty Acid–Derived Pheromones

Males of other cucujids in the genera *Cryptolestes* and *Oryzaephilus* have been found to produce several macrolide aggregation pheromones[3] (**XXVIII** through

---

[2]Present address: Department of Chemistry, Simon Fraser University, Burnaby, British Columbia, Canada V5A 1S6.

[3]Macrolides **XXVII** and **XXVIII** were also identified in the secretion of the metasternal gland of *Phoracantha synonyma* (Moore and Brown, 1976) but were not determined to be pheromones of this species.

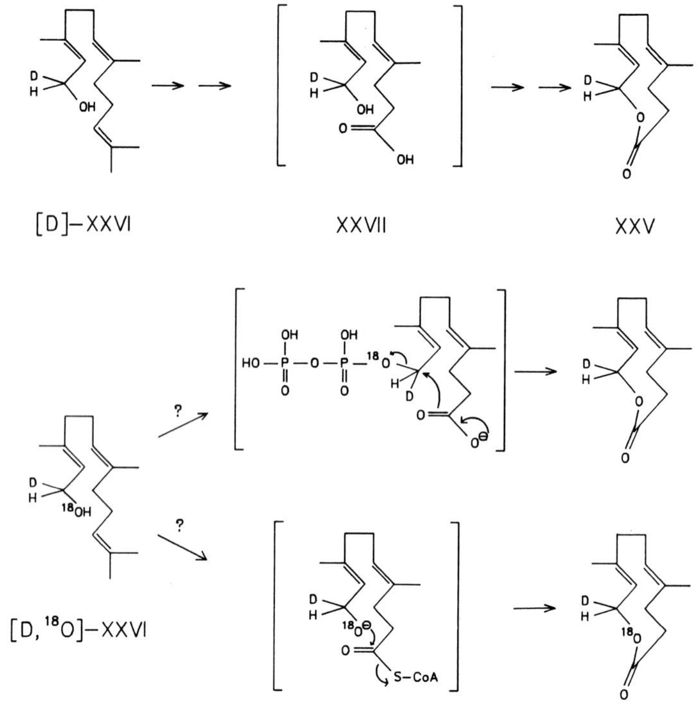

Fig. 8. Proposed biosynthesis of macrolide pheromone **XXV** of *Cryptolestes ferrugineus* from farnesol (**XXVI**), showing two possible mechanisms of lactonization. (See text regarding incorporation of [D]- and [D, ^{18}O]- labeled farnesol into **XXV**).

XXXIII) (Fig. 9) (H. D. Pierce *et al.*, 1984; A. M. Pierce *et al.*, 1985). The position (6–7 and/or 9–10 from the terminal carbon) and *Z* geometry of the double bond(s) suggest that these compounds are derived from fatty acids (such as oleate and linoleate) (H. D. Pierce *et al.*, 1984). After release of the fatty acids from the phospholipids or triglycerides by hydrolysis, a plausible biosynthetic route from the fatty acids to the macrolide lactones would involve (i) two (or three) cycles of β-oxidation, (ii) hydroxylation at the terminal (or penultimate) carbon, and (iii) cyclization of the hydroxy acid intermediate to form the macrolide lactone (Fig. 9). Steps (i) and (ii) could conceivably occur in any order. Chain shortening of fatty acids through partial β-oxidation is known to be involved in the biosynthesis of many lepidopteran pheromones (Roelofs and Bjostad, 1984; also see Bjostad *et al.*, Chapter 3, this volume), while the terminal oxidation of fatty acids has been reported to occur in termites (Prestwich *et al.*, 1985). Preliminary investigations indicate that the biosynthesis of the macrolide pheromones does indeed proceed essentially as shown in Fig. 9. *Cryp-*

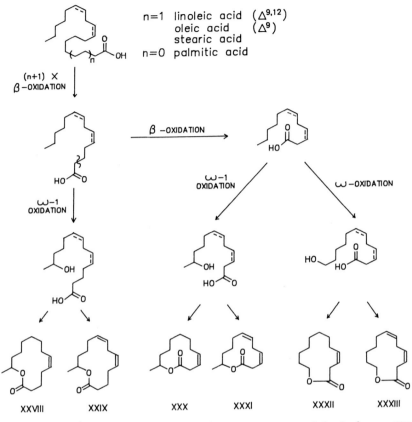

Fig. 9. Proposed biosynthesis of macrolide pheromones of cucujid grain beetles from representative fatty acids. Note: "ω" is meant to represent the terminal carbon, while "ω−1" is meant to represent the penultimate carbon.

tolestes ferrugineus, allowed to feed on oats coated with radiolabeled oleic, linoleic, and palmitic acids, incorporated radiolabel into the appropriate macrolides (D. Vanderwel, H. D. Pierce, Jr., and A. C. Oehlschlager, unpublished work). The insects could also produce the macrolides through *de novo* synthesis, as discussed in the following section.

C. De Novo Biosynthesis

To our knowledge, *de novo* biosynthesis of pheromones has been demonstrated to occur in only two coleopteran species, although no doubt many more such examples remain to be discovered. Boll weevils were shown by Mitlin and

Hedin (1974) to incorporate radiolabeled acetate, mevalonate, and D-glucose into all four components of grandlure. Similarly, it was shown using radiolabeled precursors that *C. ferrugineus* could incorporate acetate into the fatty acid-derived pheromone, **XXX,** and could incorporate both acetate and mevalonate into the terpenoid pheromone, **XXV** (D. Vanderwel, H. D. Pierce, Jr., and A. C. Oehlschlager, unpublished work). These species apparently can produce their pheromones through either (or both) of two routes: through the derivatization of dietary components or through *de novo* synthesis. The relative proportion of pheromone that is contributed by the *de novo* pathway when host precursors are readily available is as yet unknown.

In most species studied, feeding enhances or triggers pheromone production. This does not necessarily indicate the requirement for a specific component from the diet as a precursor. For example, *C. ferrugineus,* when fed rolled oats, produces about 27 times more macrolide **XXV** than when food is absent (H. D. Pierce *et al.,* 1984), yet can produce this pheromone *de novo* (D. Vanderwel, H. D. Pierce, Jr., and A. C. Oehlschlager, unpublished work). The mechanisms by which insects might regulate pheromone production are discussed in Section IV.

D. Role of Microorganisms

The ability of coleopterans to colonize their host is, in many cases, augmented by their association with microorganisms. For example, attacking scolytids distribute pathogenic fungi which help to render the host incapable of impairing beetle development (Graham, 1967). Symbiotic microorganisms may also play a role in the production or degradation of chemicals involved in mediating coleopteran behavior.

Examination of the metabolites of coleopteran symbionts has revealed that, in some cases, the microorganisms produce the same compounds that are utilized as pheromones by their host. Such symbionts include bacteria isolated from the grass grub beetle, *Costelytra zealandica* (Hoyt *et al.,* 1971), a *Serratia* species isolated from the bark beetle *Phloeosinus armatus* (Chararas *et al.,* 1980), and a *Bacillus cereus* strain isolated from *I. paraconfusus* (Brand *et al.,* 1975). This is not surprising since microorganisms, exposed to many of the same compounds as their hosts, could by coincidence metabolize some of these compounds to the same end products. In order to assess the importance of the microbial contribution to overall pheromone production, some studies have attempted to ascertain the metabolic capability of insects made as devoid as possible of their natural endo- (intracellular) and exo- (extracellular) symbionts. The surface sterilization of eggs, followed by axenic rearing to adulthood on aseptic host material, has been the technique most often used to obtain adults free of readily culturable exosymbionts (Whiteney and Spanier, 1982). The populations of endosymbionts have been reduced by administration of membrane-permeable antibiotics to wild (contaminated) adults (Chararas, 1980; Byers and Wood, 1981).

Experiments with *I. paraconfusus* and *D. ponderosae* have been conducted utilizing these techniques (Conn *et al.*, 1984; D. W. A. Hunt,[4] personal communication). The males of both species convert myrcene (**XVII**) to ipsdienol (**XIX**) (Fig. 7). After wild male *I. paraconfusus* were fed a host phloem diet containing streptomycin for 96 hr, the production of ipsdienol from myrcene was inhibited (Byers and Wood, 1981). Near normal levels of ipsdienol, however, were produced by axenically reared male *I. paraconfusus* as well as by axenically reared and streptomycin-treated male *D. ponderosae* (Conn *et al.*, 1984; D. W. A. Hunt, personal communication). Thus both insect and microbial involvement are indicated in ipsdienol production by male *I. paraconfusus*, but there is apparently no significant microbial involvement in the production by male *D. ponderosae*.

These results help in some way to resolve the dilemma posed by earlier work on a *B. cereus* strain isolated from *I. paraconfusus*. Brand *et al.* (1975) reported that this microorganism was capable of the oxidation of α-pinene to *cis*- and *trans*-verbenol. Subsequent experiments by Byers and Wood (1981) indicated that streptomycin sulfate, to which *B. cereus* is susceptible, did not reduce the production of *cis*-verbenol by *I. paraconfusus*. These results are not necessarily conflicting, however, as the relative contributions by both symbiont and insect to overall pheromone production must be considered.

Both sexes of *I. paraconfusus* and *D. ponderosae* metabolize α-pinene (**VIII**) to *cis*- (**XIV**) and *trans*-verbenol (*XIII*) and myrtenol (**XV**) (Fig. 5). Axenically reared male *I. paraconfusus* and female *D. ponderosae* contain significantly more α-pinene metabolites than wild beetles, whereas axenically reared female *I. paraconfusus* contain near normal levels of α-pinene metabolites (Conn *et al.*, 1984; D. W. A. Hunt, personal communication). Similarly, both sexes of wild *D. ponderosae* contained up to six times more α-pinene metabolites after ingestion of a host phloem diet containing streptomycin sulfate (D. W. A. Hunt, personal communication). Thus, in both species studied, reduction of the symbiont populations does not reduce pheromone content, and may actually result in its increase.

These observations parallel those on boll weevils by Gueldner *et al.* (1977); weevils that were relatively free of bacteria produced significantly more pheromone than those that were heavily contaminated. Increased pheromone production in microbe-suppressed insects could simply be due to healthier insects (Gueldner *et al.*, 1977). Alternatively the symbionts present in wild (contaminated) insects could decrease pheromone content through competition with the

[4]Present address: Centre for Pest Mangement, Department of Biological Sciences, Simon Fraser University, Burnaby, British Columbia, Canada V5A 1S6.

beetle for substrate or through use of the beetle-produced pheromone as a substrate (Conn et al., 1984). Such activities could, under natural conditions, serve to regulate pheromone levels (Conn et al,, 1984).

In an extension of this idea, it has been suggested that microorganisms may also be involved in converting aggregation pheromones to compounds that inhibit attraction (Leufven et al., 1984). Evidence supporting this role of microorganisms is provided by studies of the ability of various symbiont isolates to metabolize α-pinene-derived pheromones. Several yeast isolates of the spruce bark beetle, *Ips typographus,* were shown to interconvert the chiral isomers of *cis-* (**XIV**) and *trans*-verbenol (**XIII**) with the respective verbenones (**XVI**) (Leufven et al., 1984). Mycangial fungi of *D. frontalis* perform the same verbenol to verbenone conversion as well as oxidation of seudenol (**XXXIV**), an aggregation pheromone of *D. pseudotsugae,* to 2-methyl-3-cyclohexen-1-one (2,3-MCH) (**XXXV**) (Fig. 10) (Brand et al., 1976), an antiaggregation pheromone of this species. The conversion of scolytid aggregation pheromones to antiaggregation pheromones by symbionts could play a significant role in terminating the attack of a successfully colonized host (Raffa and Berryman, 1983; Leufven et al., 1984; Borden et al., 1987).

E. Pheromones of Uncertain Origin

Although the biosynthetic pathways of most coleopteran pheromones have not been extensively investigated, they have been the object of much speculation. The following is an attempt to summarize most of the ideas and evidence that have accumulated in the quest to determine the origin of these "neglected" coleopteran pheromones. This discussion is, of necessity, largely speculative, and the major headings describe merely the presumed biosynthetic origins.

1.   Terpenoid Origin

Several low molecule weight alcohols and ketones used as pheromones by the bark and ambrosia beetles are derivatives of isoprene (**XXXVI**). These include the five-carbon alcohols 2-methyl-3-buten-2-ol (**XXXVII**), 3-methyl-3-buten-1-ol (**XXXVIII**) and 3-methyl-1-butanol (**XXXIX**), respectively utilized by *I. typographus* (Bakke et al., 1977), *I. cembrae* (Stoakley et al., 1978), and the

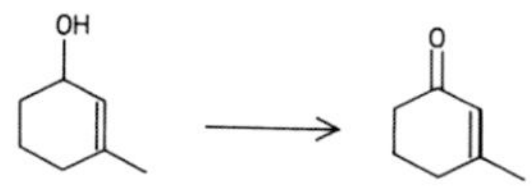

XXXIV   XXXV

Fig. 10.   Oxidation of seudenol (**XXXIV**) to 2-methyl-3-cyclohexen-1-one (**XXXV**).

ambrosia beetle, *Platypus flavicornis* (Renwick *et al.*, 1977); and the ketone 3-hydroxy-3-methylbutan-2-one (**XL**) (Fig. 11), emitted by *Trypodendron domesticum* (Francke and Heemann, 1974; Francke *et al.*, 1974). It is unknown if these pheromones are insect or microorganism produced, or whether they arise as degradation products of host monoterpenes or from *de novo* terpene biosynthetic pathways. Microbial origins are possible since yeasts isolated from *I. tyographus* (Leufven *et al.*, 1984), and a yeast (Brand *et al.*, 1977) and a basidiomycete (Brand and Barras, 1977) associated with *D. frontalis,* produce 3-methylbutanol *in vitro*. However, since the production of these pheromones is known to be under hormonal control in *I. typographus* (Hackstein and Vite, 1978) and *I. cembrae* (Renwick and Dickens, 1979) (see Section IV), the relative contribution of microorganism metabolism to overall pheromone production may not be significant. It would be difficult to envision a mechanism by which the insect could hormonally regulate production by microorganisms.

The structures of callosbruchusic acid (**XLI**) (Fig. 11), a component of the copulation release pheromone of the azuki bean weevil, *Callosbruchus chinensus* (Mori *et al.*, 1983), and *trans,trans*-farnesyl acetate (**XLII**), a component of the sex pheromone of the click beetle, *Agriotis ponticus* (Kovalev *et al.*, 1985), strongly suggest that they are terpenoid. Similarly, sulcatol (**XLIII**), an aggregation pheromone of *Gnathotrichus sulcatus* and *G. retusus* (Borden *et al.*, 1980), and 6-methyl-5-hepten-2-one (**XLIV**), believed to be an antiaggregant of

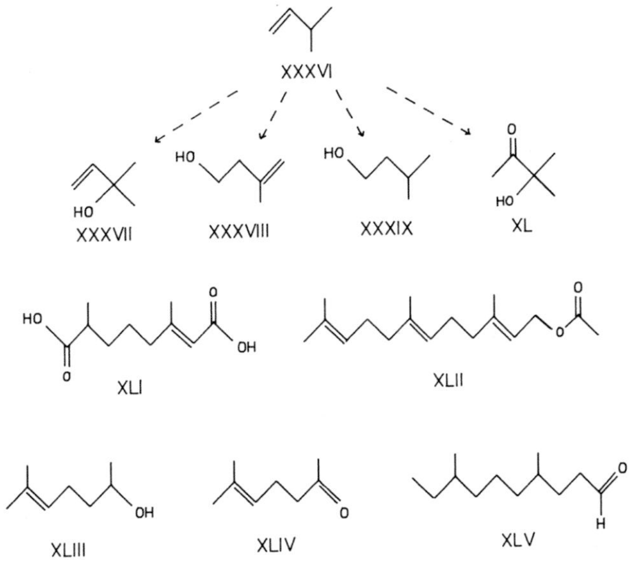

Fig. 11. Coleopteran pheromones of possible terpenoid origin.

D. pseudotsugae (Ryker *et al.*, 1979), are probably monoterpenoid. Plausible biosynthetic routes to **XLIV** involve oxidative cleavage of the 2,3 double bond of geraniol (**VI**) or retroaldol reaction of geranial. Reduction of the thus formed 6-methyl-5-hepten-2-one would give sulcatol (as shown in Fig. 12). It is possible that microorganisms play an important role in the genesis of these two compounds: both are produced by a basidiomycete associated with *D. frontalis* (Brand and Barras, 1977).

Although Bradshaw (1985) has suggested that 4,8-dimethyldecanal (**XLV**) (Fig. 11), the male-produced aggregation pheromone of the flour beetles, *Tribolium castaneum* and *T. confusum* (Suzuki, 1980; Suzuki and Sugawara, 1979), is derived from substituted long-chain fatty acids, one could also envision a terpenoid origin. The carbon skeleton of this pheromone is identical to that of the oxidation product of farnesol (**XXVII**) leading to the terpenoid macrolide **XXV** described in Section II,B,1. Conversion of this intermediate to the pheromone **XLV** would involve reductive removal of the allylic hydroxyl, hydrogenation of the double bonds, and reduction of the carboxylic acid to an aldehyde.

Francke and Vite (1983) have suggested that the host terpenes sabinene (**XLVI**) and α-thujene (**XLVII**) might be precursors of (4R)-(−)-terpinen-4-ol [(−)-**XLVIII**], a male-produced aggregation pheromone of *Polygraphus poligraphus* (Kohnle *et al.*, 1985). Markovnikov hydration of either terpene would give *cis*- (**XLIX**) and *trans*-4-thujanol (**L**), which on rearrangement (with concomitant cleavage of the three-membered ring) would produce terpinen-4-ol (Francke and Vite, 1983) (see Fig. 13). The putative thujanol intermediates have been detected in male *P. poligraphus* hindguts (Francke and Vite, 1983). Chararas *et al.* (1980) have also reported the conversion of sabinene to terpinen-4-ol and α-terpineol (**LI**), attractants of the bark beetle *Phloeosinus armatus*. Bacteria isolated from the hindguts produced both alcohols when allowed to ferment commercial grade limonene. The authors observed the disappearance of sabinene, present as an impurity in the limonene, during the fermentation. The roles of other obvious precursors of α-terpineol and (−)-terpinen-4-ol, such as the host monoterpenes limonene (**LII**) (Francke and Vite, 1983) and terpinolene (**LIII**) (Fig. 13), respectively, remain to be examined.

Despite much deliberation, very little is known about the biosynthesis of bicyclic ketal and tricyclic acetal pheromones. These compounds are produced mainly by the bark and ambrosia beetles, and include frontalin (**LIV**), *exo*- (**LV**)

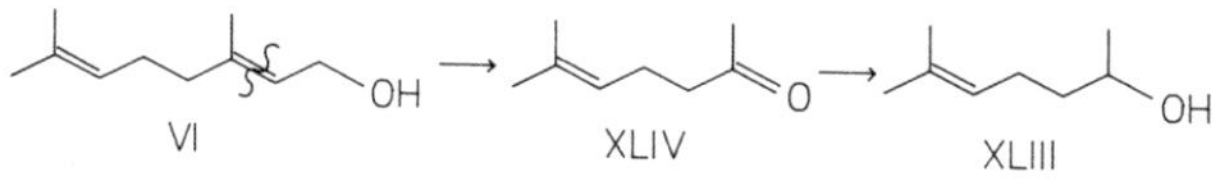

Fig. 12. Proposed biosynthesis of sulcatol (**XLIII**) from geraniol (**VI**).

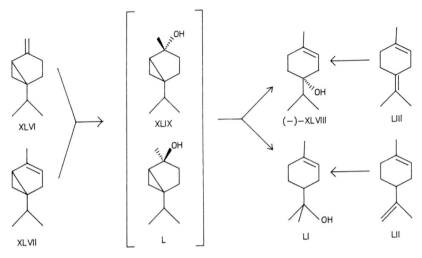

Fig. 13. Proposed biosynthesis of (−)-terpinen-4-ol [(−)-**XLVIII**] and α-terpineol (**LI**) from host monoterpenes.

and *endo*-brevicomin (**LVI**), multistriatin (**LVII**), lineatin (**LVIII**), chalcogran (**LIX**), and (*E*)-7-methyl-1,6-dioxaspiro[4.5]decane (**LX**) (Fig. 14). The possibility that multistriatin, chalcogran, and **LX** are derived through the cyclization of acetogenins is discussed in Section II,E,3. White *et al.* (1980) have speculated that frontalin, *exo*-, and *endo*-brevicomin are biosynthesized through specialization of a hormone type of metabolic pathway. Silverstein (according to White *et al.*, 1980) speculated that the biosynthetic pathways may, alternatively, be similar to laboratory routes to these pheromones which utilize short-chain dihydroxy ketones (e.g., **LXI** and **LXII**) as precursors. The logical biosynthetic precursor of the intermediate in the case of frontalin (Fig. 14) is 6-methyl-6-hepten-2-one (**LXIII**), which could in turn be derived from 6-methyl-5-hepten-2-one (**XLIV**) and sulcatol (**XLIII**) (Brand *et al.*, 1979). The latter two precursors are present in volatiles of the Douglas-fir beetle (Butterfield, 1984; Madden *et al.*, 1987). Brand *et al.* (1979) suggested that microbial symbionts may supply beetles with biosynthetic precursors to frontalin, since mycangial fungi of female *D. frontalis* produce **XLIV** (Brand and Barras, 1977).

Information concerning the origin of the tricyclic acetal lineatin is also vague. Francke and Vite (1983) pointed out the structural similarity between lineatin and monoterpenoid compounds such as myrcene (**XVII**) and grandisol (**I**). It is conceivable that lineatin is indeed derived through oxidation and cyclization of a monoterpenoid precursor such as nerol (**VII**) (Fig. 14), but as yet no supporting evidence for such a route has been offered.

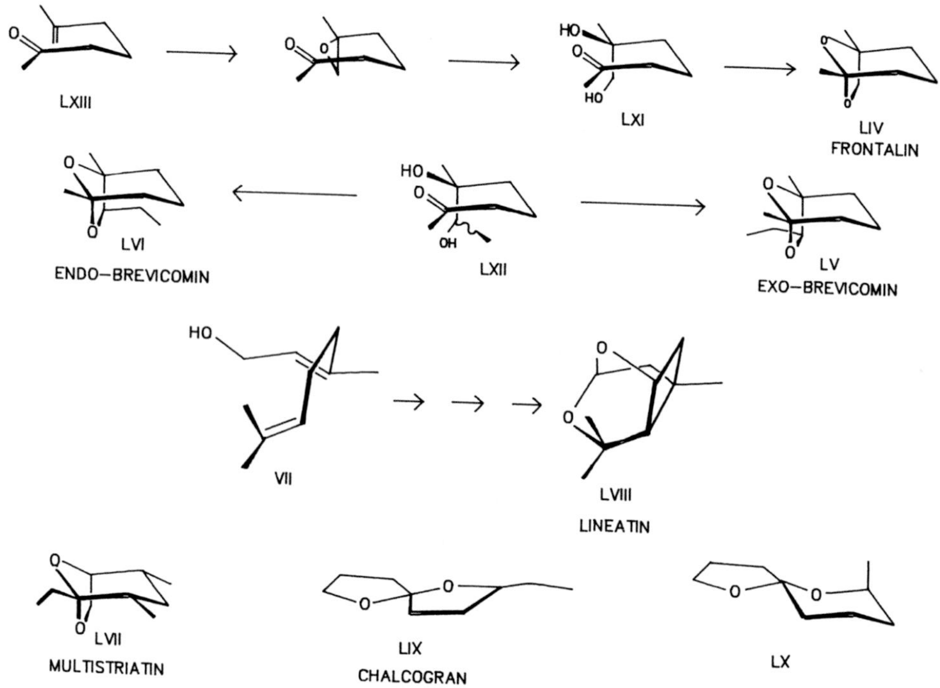

Fig. 14. Proposed biosynthetic routes to ketal and acetal pheromones. See text for explanation.

2. Fatty Acid Origin

Coleopteran pheromones include a large number and variety of long-chain compounds generally assumed to be derived from substituted fatty acids (Bradshaw, 1985). Examples include (E)- and (Z)-14-methyl-8-hexadecen-1-ol (**LXIV**), along with the corresponding aldehydes (**LXV**) and methyl esters (**LXVI**), which are utilized by dermestid beetles of the genus *Trogoderma* (Rodin *et al.*, 1969; Yarger *et al.*, 1975; Cross *et al.*, 1976; Greenblatt *et al.*, 1977) (see Fig. 15). Similarly the western corn rootworm, *Diabrotica virgifera virgifera,* and the southern corn rootworm, *Diabrotica undecimpunctata,* utilize 8-methyl-2-decyl propionate (**LXVII**) (Guss *et al.*, 1982) and 10-methyl-2-tridecanone (**LXVIII**) (Guss *et al.*, 1983), respectively.

The pheromone of the dried bean beetle, *Acanthoscelides obtectus,* is (−)-methyl (E)-2,4,5-tetradecatrienoate (**LXIX**) (Horler, 1970), is one of the few allenic compounds to be isolated from insects. Although the mechanism of the biosynthesis of the allene functionality is unknown, this pheromone is otherwise very similar to those of *Attagenus* spp., which use fatty acid–derived (Bradshaw,

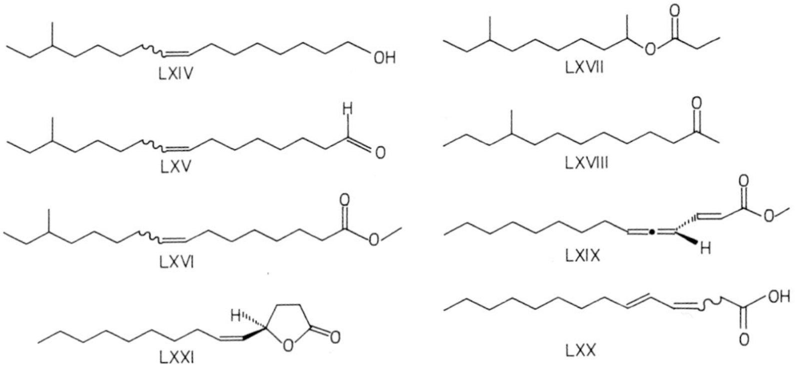

Fig. 15. Coleopteran pheromones of possible fatty acid origin.

1985) (E)-3,(Z)-5- or (Z)-3,(Z)-5-tetradecadienoic acid (**LXX**) (Fukui *et al.*, 1977; Silverstein *et al.*, 1967).

The structures of some beetle pheromones are very similar to those of the cucujid macrolide pheromones discussed in Section II,B,2 and, hence, may similarly be derived from fatty acids. For example, virgin female Japanese beetles, *Popillia japonica,* produce (R)-(Z)-5-(1-decenyl)dihydro-2-(3H)-furanone (**LXXI**) (Tumlinson *et al.*, 1977). Biosynthesis from oleic acid would involve two cycles of β-oxidation, an allylic oxidation, and cyclization.

3. Polyketide Origin

The structure of a number of coleopteran pheromones fit the oxygenation and substitution pattern expected for acetogenins (Chuman *et al.*, 1983; Phillips *et al.*, 1985). Although normally these compounds arise through the condensation of acetyl coenzyme A with a variable number of malonyl units, other acids (such as propionic acid) may be involved in either chain initiation or chain propagation. The factor distinguishing acetogenin biosynthesis from fatty acid biosynthesis is that reduction of the β-keto ester intermediates does not necessarily occur in acetogenin biosynthesis. The resulting enzyme-bound β-polyketo thiol ester intermediates may undergo a variety of reactions, including substitution by methyl, isopentyl, or hydroxyl at an activated methylene position; reduction of a keto group to an alcohol, which may be followed by dehydration; and terminal decarboxylation (since the compounds are β-keto acids) (Hendrickson, 1973; Money, 1973).

The male-produced aggregation pheromones sitophilure (**LXXII**) (emitted by the rice and maize weevils, *Sitophilus oryzae* and *S. zeamais*, respectively) (Phillips *et al.*, 1985) and 4-methyl-3,5-heptanedione (**LXXIII**) (produced by the pea and bean weevil, *Sitona lineatus*) (Blight *et al.*, 1984) exhibit the typical 1,3-oxygenation pattern expected for polyketides (see Fig. 16). If these pheromones are acetogenin derived, the polyketide chain would have been derived from propionic acid, acting as the chain initiator and terminator, and acetic acid, acting as the chain elongator. Further modifications would have included methylation at the activated methylene carbon, decarboxylation at the terminal action, and, in the case of sitophilure, reduction at one of the keto groups.

The structurally related compound, 4-methyl-3-heptanol (**LXXIV**) (Fig. 16), an aggregation pheromone of the elm bark beetles, could similarly be derived from acetogenins, through the propionate pathway (Phillips *et al.*, 1985). Unmated female *Scolytus multistriatus* produce the (3*S*,4*S*)-(−) isomer (Pearce *et al.*, 1975; Mori, 1977) whereas male *S. scolytus* emit both the (3*S*,4*S*)-(−) and

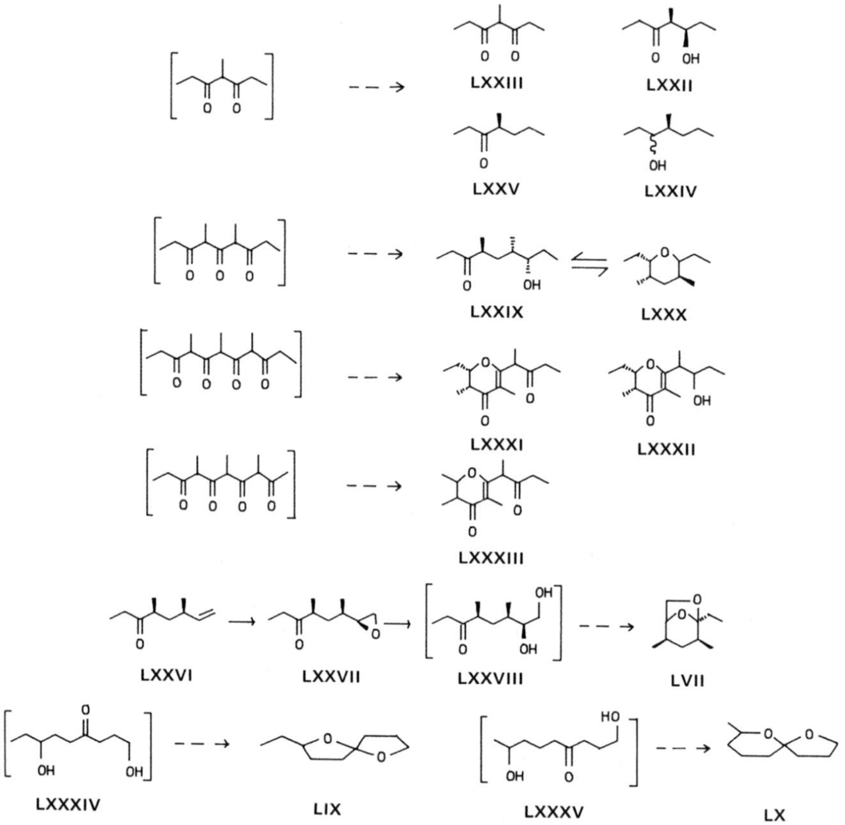

Fig. 16. Coleopteran pheromones of possible acetogenin origin. See text for explanation.

the $(3R,4S)$-$(-)$ isomers (Blight *et al.*, 1978, 1979a). Blight *et al.* (1983) observed that boring female *S. multistriatus* and male *S. scolytus* also produced $(4S)$-4-methyl-3-heptanone (**LXXV**), which was suggested to be an intermediate in the biosynthesis of 4-methyl-3-heptanol and/or a pheromone itself. There has been speculation that 4-methyl-3-heptanol is fatty acid derived (Bradshaw, 1985), but one can see in Fig. 16 that both this compound and its ketone exhibit a typical polyketide oxidation and substitution pattern.

Another elm bark beetle pheromone, the bicyclic ketal multistriatin, might also be derived from acetogenins (Phillips *et al.*, 1985). Gore *et al.* (1977) proposed that 3,5-dimethyl-1-octen-5-one (**LXXVI**) and 3,5-dimethyl-1,2-epoxyoctan-6-one (**LXXVII**) were intermediates in the biosynthesis. This hypothesis seems especially viable since the epoxidation of **LXXVI** to give **LXXVII**, followed by acid-catalyzed rearrangement of the latter, gives multistriatin (Pearce *et al.*, 1975; Gore *et al.*, 1977). However, neither **LXXVI** nor **LXXVII** could be detected in extracts of emergent or boring female *S. multistriatus* (Gore *et al.*, 1977). It is possible either that these intermediates are present at very low levels, and were simply not detected, or that they are not directly involved in the biosynthesis of multistriatin. A closely related structure such as 3,5-dimethyl-1,2-dihydroxyocta-6-one (**LXXVIII**), as suggested by Phillips *et al.* (1985), might be the actual *in vivo* precursor.

It has also been suggested that acetogenins play a crucial role in the biosynthesis of the sex pheromones of the tobacco beetle, *Lasioderma serricorne* (Chuman *et al.*, 1983; Phillips *et al.*, 1985). As shown in Fig. 16, the structures of $(4S,6S,7S)$-serricornin (**LXXIX**), $(4S,6S,7S)$-anhydroserricornin (**LXXX**) (the cyclic hemiacetal form of serricornin) (Mori *et al.*, 1984), 2,3-*cis*-serricorone (**LXXXI**), and 2,3-*cis*-serricorole (**LXXXII**) all follow the polyketide pattern. Although anhydroserricornin is present with serricornin in solvent extracts of adult females (Levinson *et al.*, 1981; Mochizuki *et al.*, 1986), its biological role is not clear. Reports that anhydroserricornin had pheromonal activity (Levinson *et al.*, 1981, 1982) have been disputed by other studies (Chuman *et al.*, 1982a,b; Mochizuki *et al.*, 1986). Compound **LXXXIII**, the sex pheromone of both the drugstore beetle, *Stegobium paniceum* (Kuwahara *et al.*, 1978), and the furniture beetle, *Anobium punctatum* (White and Birch, 1986), is structurally very similar to 2,3-*cis*-serricorone (**LXXXI**) and likewise could be derived from polyketides.

Bradshaw (1985) proposed that chalcogran (**LIX**), the spiroketal aggregation pheromone of *Pityogenes chalcographus* (Francke *et al.*, 1977), is formed through the internal condensation of an acetogenin precursor. Spiroketals have been shown to be derived from acetogenins in microorganisms, and could be similarly derived in insects (Bradshaw, 1985). As shown in Fig. 16, the polyketide precursor (**LXXXIV**) of chalcogran could be formed from three propionic acid units. Similarly, (E)-7-methyl-1,6-dioxaspiro[4.5]decane (**LX**), an antiaggregation pheromone of the ash bark beetle, *Leperisinus various* (Francke *et al.*, 1979), could be derived from the polyketide precursor **LXXXV**.

4. Miscellaneous Hydrocarbon Origin

Investigation of the aggregation pheromones of *Dendroctonus jeffreyi* revealed that the major compounds present in the hindguts of attacking females were 1- and 2-heptanol (Renwick and Pitman, 1979). 1-Heptanol was shown to be an aggregation pheromone of this species, but the behavioral role of 2-heptanol was unclear (Renwick and Pitman, 1979). Renwick and Pitman (1979) suggested that these compounds were derived through the oxidation of heptane, present at an unusually high level in the resin of the host tree species, *Pinus jeffreyi*. Similarly, 1- and 2-heptanol were found in the hindguts of *Dendroctonus vitei* attacking another heptane-containing host, *Pinus maximinoi,* but the biological role(s) of these compounds for this species is not understood (Renwick *et al.*, 1975).

5. Unknown Origin

Several low molecular weight scolytid pheromones are of more obscure origins than those previously discussed. A plausible but unverified route to 1- and 2-phenylethanol (**LXXXVI** and (**LXXXVII**) (Fig. 17), pheromones of *D. vitei* (Renwick *et al.*, 1975) and *I. paraconfusus* (Renwick *et al.*, 1976a), respectively, involves the decarboxylation of the amino acids tyrosine or phenylalanine (Bradshaw, 1985). Evidence for two sites of 2-phenylethanol biosynthesis exists.

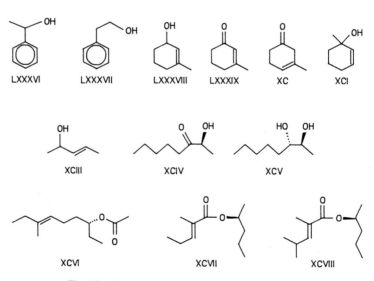

Fig. 17.   Coleopteran pheromones of unknown origin.

Yeasts isolated from *D. frontalis* (Brand *et al.*, 1977) and from *I. typographus* (Leufven *et al.*, 1984) produce 2-phenylethanol *in vitro*. However, in *I. para-confusus* the biosynthesis of 2-phenylethanol appears to be hormonally controlled (Hughes and Renwick, 1977a) (see Section IV), and thus this pheromone is likely largely insect derived.

Dendroctonus pseudotsugae produces several structurally related pheromones of uncertain origin, including seudenol, 3-methyl-2-cyclohexen-1-one (3,2-MCH), 3-methyl-3-cyclohexen-1-one (3,3-MCH) (Borden, 1985, and references cited therein) and 1-methyl-2-cyclohexen-1-ol (1,2-MCH-ol) (Libbey *et al.*, 1983) (compounds **LXXXVIII** through **XCI**, Fig. 17). Seudenol, 1,2-MCH-ol, and 3,2-MCH were detected in *D. frontalis* exposed to vapors of 1-methyl-1-cyclohexene (Renwick and Hughes, 1975). *Dendroctonus pseudotsugae* may also be capable of performing these oxidations, but since 1-methyl-1-cyclohexene is not known to be a component of the host tree, the relevance of this route to the *in vivo* situation is not clear. It is conceivable that 3,2-MCH and seudenol are derived from hepta-2,6-dione (**XCII**) (Fig. 18) (H. D. Pierce, Jr., personal communication), which could possibly be formed through the polyketide pathway. The origin of (*E*)-pent-3-en-2-ol (**XCIII**) (Fig. 17), also an aggregation pheromone of *D. pseudotsugae* (Borden, 1985, and references cited therein), is likewise not known.

Stored-product beetle pheromones of unknown origin include the sex pheromones of the grape borer, *Xylotrechus pyrrhoderus*, (2*S*)-hydroxy-3-octanone (**XCIV**) and (2*S*,3*S*)-octanediol (**XCV**) (Sakai *et al.*, 1984); the aggregation pheromone of the square-necked grain beetle, *Cathartus quadricollis,* (*E*)-3-methyl-(7*R*)-acetoxy-3-nonene (**XCVI**) (Johnston and Oehlschlager, 1986; H. D. Pierce, Jr., personal communication); and Dominicalures 1 and 2 (**XCVII** and **XCVIII**), components of the aggregation pheromone of the lesser grain borer, *Rhizopertha dominica* (Williams *et al.*, 1981). The square-necked grain beetle pheromone (**XCVI**) could conceivably arise via oxidative degradation of metabolites possessing JH I-related structures. The structures of the carboxyl-containing moieties of Dominicalures 1 and 2 are most consistent with an acetogenin origin.

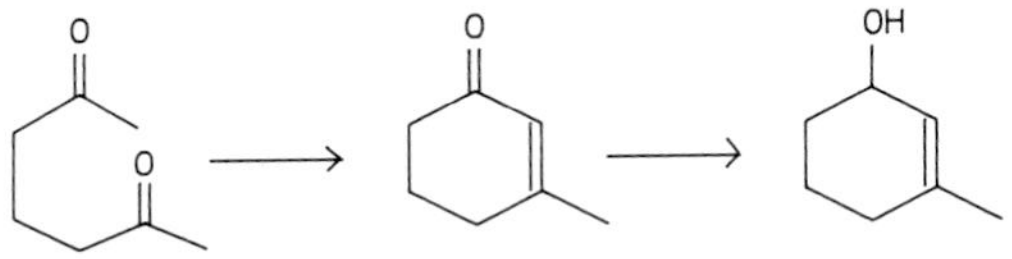

XCII   LXXXIX   LXXXVIII

Fig. 18. Proposed biosynthesis of 3-methyl-2-cyclohexen-1-one (**LXXXIX**) and seudenol (**LX-XXVIII**) from **XCII**.

III.   MANIPULATION OF PHEROMONE CHIRALITY

Though the widespread use of common pheromones among closely related species would seem to preclude their effectiveness for species-specific communication, attraction can be limited to conspecifics through variation in the number of pheromones involved in a given message as well as variation in component ratios and chirality. Chiral-specific activity has been well documented in scolytids (Borden, 1985, and references cited therein) and cucujids (Oehlschlager et al., 1987; A. M. Pierce et al., 1987).

Within the genus Ips, maintenance of species specificity in semiochemical messages is effected, in part, through variations in the chirality of ipsdienol (**XIX**) (Fig. 7) and in the relative proportions of ipsenol (**XXI**) that are emitted by the males. In the case of I. amitinus, where the males use (−)-ipsdienol [(−)-**XIX**] as a pheromone, but produce only traces of ipsenol (**XXI**), it has been suggested that the reduction of (−)-ipsdienol is blocked and that (+)-ipsdienol is enantioselectively rearranged to amitinol (**XXIV**) (Fig. 7) (Francke and Vite, 1983).

Both inter- and intrapopulational variation of ipsdienol chirality have been noted in the pine engraver, Ips pini. Populations of I. pini in Idaho (Plummer et al., 1976) and California (Birch et al., 1980) produce primarily (−)-ipsdienol, while New York populations produce a 65 : 35 mixture of (+)- : (−)-ipsdienol (Lanier et al., 1980). Slessor et al. (1985) reported significant differences in the chirality of ipsdienol produced by different individuals within an I. pini population. On inspection of Fig. 7 (discussed in Section II,B,1,b), two possible mechanisms for this biological resolution of (+)-ipsdienol become apparent. Different individuals might simply oxidize myrcene to different ratios of (+)- : (−)-ipsdienol. Alternatively, the enantioselective interconversion between ipsdienol and ipsdienone (Fish et al., 1984) might be involved in "fine-tuning" the chirality of ipsdienol. As discussed in Section II,B,1,b, in I. paraconfusus only the (−) enantiomer of ipsdienol is converted to the ketone, while both the (+) and the (−) enantiomers of ipsdienol are formed on reduction. If this oxidation–reduction equilibrium exists in bark beetle species other than I. paraconfusus, it could conceivably affect the chirality of the ipsdienol that they emit: the greater the extent of the interconversion, the more (+)-ipsdienol that would be formed [at the expense of the (−) enantiomer].

IV.   ENDOCRINE REGULATION
OF PHEROMONE PRODUCTION

To our knowledge, there are no cases in which coleopterans continuously emit their full complement of pheromones. Pheromone production and/or release is usually coordinated with a variety of physiological and environmental factors.

For example, the production of aggregation pheromones may be greatly enhanced in the presence of food (Hedin *et al.*, 1975; Burkholder, 1982; Millar *et al.*, 1985). Aggregation and sex pheromones are not generally released until insects attain reproductive maturity (Byers, 1983b; A. M. Pierce *et al.*, 1984). Once release is initiated, production of attractants may decrease (or the release of antiattractants may increase) in response to situations such as the presence of a potential mate (Nijholt, 1970; Rudinsky *et al.*, 1973; Hedin, 1977; Byers, 1981a; Birgersson *et al.*, 1984), increased population density (A. M. Pierce *et al.*, 1984), or the successful subjugation of a host tree (Francke and Vite, 1983).

Vite *et al.* (1972) proposed that pheromones involved in bark beetle aggregation be functionally classified as "contact" and "frass" pheromones. Contact pheromones are produced and/or released on "contact" with the host, without the necessity for prior feeding, while frass pheromones are released more gradually in the frass, only after a period of feeding (Vite *et al.*, 1972). The aggregation of aggressive species of bark beetles is generally facilitated by contact pheromones: in order to overcome a vigorous, living host it is advantageous to initiate mass attack without delay (Vite *et al.*, 1972; Borden, 1985). Less aggressive species, which would not gain an advantage from rapid pheromone release, generally indicate host suitability with frass pheromones (Vite *et al.*, 1972; Borden, 1985).

In some cases, the production of contact pheromones may be regulated by the availability of essential biosynthetic precursors present in the host resin. For example, *D. ponderosae* and *D. brevicomis* produce substantial quantities of their pheromone *trans*-verbenol when exposed to α-pinene (Hughes, 1973a). Newly emerged *I. cembrae* males exposed to myrcene vapor produced ipsenol and ipsdienol at levels comparable to those found during a natural attack (Renwick and Dickens, 1979). However, stimulation of contact pheromone production on arrival at a new host can usually not be explained in terms of an obligate dependence of production on host precursors. Some contact pheromones, such as frontalin in *D. frontalis* (Coster and Vite, 1972; Rudinsky *et al.*, 1974), are already present in emergent beetles and are simply released when required (Borden 1985, and references therein). Other contact pheromones may be produced from monoterpenes sequestered from the host during developmental stages. For example (as discussed in Section II,B,1,b), *trans*-verbenol is absent in emergent *D. frontalis* but is synthesized from a sequestered α-pinene intermediate on arrival at a new host (Hughes, 1975). The production and/or release of "frass" pheromones is, likewise, not stimulated simply by the availability of appropriate precursors but requires a period of feeding on a suitable host (Vite *et al.*, 1972). In many cases, the insects' endocrine system plays a central role in coordinating the production and/or release of these pheromones.

Reports that pheromone production by certain species of moths and cockroaches was under endocrine control (Barth, 1965; Roth and Barth, 1964), and the observation that the periods of pheromone production by many bark beetles appeared to coincide with periods of juvenile hormone (JH) release, led Borden *et al.* (1969) to the hypothesis that JH might be involved in the regulation of pheromone production and/or release by scolytids. The hindguts of male *I. paraconfusus* treated topically with synthetic JH III (10,11-epoxyfarnesenic acid methyl ester) were found to be attractive to females (Borden *et al.*, 1969). Subsequent experiments by Hughes and Renwick (1977a) with male *I. paraconfusus* confirmed that the conversion of myrcene to the aggregation pheromones ipsenol and ipsdienol was indeed stimulated by treatment with JH III. Furthermore, pheromone production by *I. paraconfusus* males boring in ponderosa pine was almost completely inhibited after topical treatment with precocene II (Kiehlmann *et al.*, 1982). Though their effects in Coleoptera are not well understood (Staal, 1986), the precocenes are known to antagonize JH-mediated events in some insects through irreversible damage to their corpora allata (CA) (Bowers, 1983).

The involvement of JH in the regulation of pheromone production and/or release has since been demonstrated in numerous other coleopterans, including the yellow mealworm (*Tenebrio molitor*) (Menon, 1970), *D. brevicomis* (Hughes and Renwick, 1977b), *I. typographus* (Hackstein and Vite, 1978), the European fir engraver beetles (*Pityokteines curvidens, P. spinidens,* and *P. vorontzovi*) (Harring, 1978), *Scolytus scolytus* (Blight *et al.*, 1979b), *I. cembrae* (Renwick and Dickens, 1979), *D. frontalis* (Bridges, 1982), *Anthonomus grandis* (Hedin *et al.*, 1982), and *D. ponderosae* (Conn *et al.*, 1984). Following the suggestion of Gerken and Hughes (1976) that stimulation of pheromone production by JH might facilitate the isolation of new pheromones, Francke *et al.* (1977) identified the bicyclic ketal chalcogran from *Pityogenes chalcographus* using a JH analog.

A. Stimulation of JH Action by Feeding

The mechanisms by which JH mediates pheromone biosynthesis are not well understood. In *Pityokteines* spp. (*P. curvidens, P. spinidens,* and *P. vorontzovi*), *D. brevicomis,* and *I. paraconfusus,* the JH effect is apparently initiated by feeding. In a study of male *I. paraconfusus* by Hughes and Renwick (1977a), it was demonstrated that the JH III stimulation of pheromone production could be prevented by decapitation. Pheromone biosynthesis was effectively restored only when corpora cardiaca (CC) (either alone or in combination with the CA) were implanted into the insects. Furthermore, the stimulatory effects of feeding or JH III treatment could be mimicked by distention of the gut with air. These observations led Hughes and Renwick (1977a) to propose the following sequence of events: (1) distention of the gut through feeding removes the neural inhibition of the CA present in unfed males; (2) JH, released from the CA, stimulates the production and/or release of brain hormone (BH) from the CC or the brain neurosecretory cells: (3) BH then acts directly to stimulate pheromone biosynthesis, presumably by stimulating synthesis or activity of pheromone-producing enzymes. BH has also been implicated in the control of lepidopteran pheromone release (see Raina and Menn, Chapter 5, this volume).

Results obtained in a study of the mechanism of regulation of pheromone production by the *Pityokteines* species (Harring, 1978) indicate that a similar control mechanism operates in the European fir engravers. Additional observations by Harring (1978) have interesting implications for the mechanism of sex-specific production of aggregation pheromones by scolytids. Treatment of unfed female *Pityokteines* beetles with a JH analog stimulated the conversion of myrcene to ipsdienol and ipsenol, and of ipsdienol to ipsenol. These conversions are not normally performed by the females, nor could they be induced by prefeeding or by distention of the gut with air, but evidently this is not due to a lack of the necessary enzymes.

Pheromone production in *D. brevicomis* is also initiated by feeding, and can be induced by JH III. Large quantities of the pheromone *exo*-brevicomin were found in the hindguts of female western pine beetles treated topically with JH III (in the absence of exogenous precursors) (Hughes and Renwick, 1977b). Stimulation of pheromone production by JH III was not prevented by decapitation, and the stimulatory effect could not be mimicked by implantations of the CA–CC complex from pheromone-producing females or by artificial distention of the gut. However, *exo*-brevicomin production was stimulated by the ingestion of a polar constituent of the host phloem. Apparently, then, ingestion of this constituent triggers JH release, which acts directly (i.e., not through BH) to regulate pheromone production (Hughes and Renwick, 1977b).

B. Stimulation of JH Action by Unknown Factor(s)

The onset of pheromone biosynthesis by *D. frontalis* is apparently also mediated by JH. Topical treatment of teneral adults with either JH II or methoprene [a structural analog of natural JH (Sehnal, 1983)] stimulated the production of *trans*-verbenol in both sexes, and *endo*-brevicomin in males, in the absence of exogenous precursors (Bridges, 1982). The stimulus initiating pheromone synthesis in *D. frontalis* is apparently neither ingestion of a dietary component nor distention of the gut through feeding, since the process of feeding is not required to initiate production. The stimulus could conceivably be distention of the gut due to air swallowing during flight (J. H. Borden,[5] personal communication). This phenomenon has been reported in *D. pseudotsugae* (Bennet and Borden, 1971) and *Trypodendron lineatum* (Graham, 1961).

Production of sex pheromone by the female yellow mealworm, *Tenebrio*

[5]Present address: Centre for Pest Management, Department of Biological Sciences, Simon Fraser University, Burnaby, British Columbia, Canada V5A 1S6.

molitor, also appears to be under endocrine control (Menon, 1970). Pheromone production by females was prevented by allatectomy, by removal of the brain, or by decapitation. Pheromone production could not be restored by reimplantation of the brain or CA, but it was restored by injection of JH analogs. These observations suggest pheromone production was directly controlled by JH and that an intact brain–CA axis was necessary for normal production. The stimulus initiating JH release is unknown, but ovariectomy had no effect on sex pheromone production.

C. Applications

The ability to manipulate pheromone production, through application of knowledge of the insects' regulatory systems, is a potentially useful tool for the control of pest populations. Enhancement of pheromone production was observed in four stored-product coleopterans (*Oryzaephilus surinamensis, O. mercator, Cryptolestes ferrugineus,* and *Tribolium castaneum*) allowed to feed on methoprene-treated oats (A. M. Pierce *et al.,* 1986). As pointed out by the authors, the addition of methoprene to traps baited with aggregation pheromones could greatly increase trap effectiveness. The methoprene would not only cause the trapped insects to function as enhanced pheromone sources, and thus facilitate the aggregation of endemic pest populations, but would also serve to inhibit reproduction of the aggregated populations.

V. CONCLUDING REMARKS

Despite the astounding structural diversity of coleopteran pheromones, most do not appear to be formed through unique biosynthetic pathways. Rather, the production of most coleopteran pheromones can be explained in terms of either specializations of detoxification mechanisms or modifications of existing fatty acid, terpenoid, or acetogenin biosynthetic pathways. It is easy to envision a scenario where volatiles produced through normal insect metabolism were secondarily adopted to serve as pheromones.

Much more remains to be discovered about the biosynthesis of coleopteran pheromones. As discussed, the origins of many pheromones are known only through speculation. The biosynthetic mechanism(s) by which organisms of closely related species, presumably with similar biosynthetic pathways, can manipulate the chirality of their pheromone is not well understood. Moreover, little is known of the mechanisms by which pheromone production is regulated.

A greater understanding of these areas is desirable for both academic and practical reasons. First, this knowledge could help to clarify the evolutionary relationships between different coleopteran species. For example, more primitive species of scolytids seem to simply oxidize host terpenes to a relatively non-specific array of volatiles, while more advanced species have evolved specialized enzyme systems for the production of unique pheromone blends (White *et al.*, 1980). Second, greater knowledge of the regulation of pheromone production would be of significant strategic value in the management of pest populations. For example, the use of methoprene to manipulate the insects' regulatory systems has shown great promise for the design of more effective traps. The discovery of unique pheromone biosynthetic pathways could also allow the rational design of latent, highly specific pesticides. Last, further investigation in this area would lead to a greater appreciation of the remarkable subtleties of chemical-mediated communication.

ACKNOWLEDGMENTS

We wish to thank Simon Fraser University and the Natural Sciences and Engineering Council of Canada for sponsoring our work. We are also indebted to Professors J. H. Borden and K. N. Slessor, as well as Dr. A. M. Pierce, Dr. H. D. Pierce, Jr., Dr. D. W. A. Hunt, and Mr. D. R. Miller, for permission to cite unpublished work and for valuable suggestions.

REFERENCES

Ahmad, S. (1986). Enzymatic adaptations of herbivorous insects and mites to phytochemicals. *J. Chem. Ecol.* **12**, 533–560.

Bakke, A., Froyen, P., and Skattebol, L. (1977). Field response to a new pheromonal compound isolated from *Ips typographus. Naturwissenschaften* **64**, 98–99.

Barth, Jr., R. H. (1965). Insect mating behavior: Endocrine control of a chemical communication system. *Science* **149**, 882–883.

Bedard, W. D., Tilden, P. E., Lindahl, K. Q., Wood, D. L., and Rauch, P. A. (1980). Effects of verbenone and *trans*-verbenol on the response of *Dendroctonus brevicomis* to natural and synthetic attractant in the field. *J. Chem. Ecol.* **6**, 997–1013.

Bennett, R. B., and Borden, J. H. (1971). Flight arrestment of tethered *Dendroctonus pseudotsugae* and *Trypodendron lineatum* (Coleoptera: Scolytidae) in response to olfactory stimuli. *Ann. Entomol. Soc. Am.* **64**, 1273–1286.

Birch, M. C., Light, D. M., Wood, D. L., Browne, L. E., Silverstein, R. M. Bergot, B. J., Ohloff, G., West, J. R., and Young, J. C. (1980). Pheromone attraction and allomonal interruption of *Ips pini* in California by the two enantiomers of ipsdienol. *J. Chem. Ecol.* **6**, 703–717.

Birgersson, G., Schlyter, F., Lofqvist, J., and Bergstrom, G. (1984). Quantitative variation of pheromone components in the spruce bark beetle *Ips typographus* from different attack phases. *J. Chem. Ecol.* **10**, 1029–1055.

Blight, M. M., Wadhams, L. J., and Wenham, M. J. (1978). Volatiles associated with unmated *Scolytus scolytus* beetles on English elm: differential production of α-multistriatin and 4-methyl-3-heptanol, and their activities in a laboratory bioassay. *Insect Biochem.* **8**, 135–142.

Blight, M. M., Wadhams, L. J., and Wenham, M. J. (1979a). The stereoisomeric composition of the

4-methyl-3-heptanol produced by *Scolytus scolytus* and the preparation and biological activity of the four synthetic stereoisomers. *Insect Biochem.* **9**, 525–533.

Blight, M. M., Wadhams, L. J., and Wenham, M. J. (1979b). Chemically mediated behavior in the large elm bark beetle, *Scolytus scolytus. Bull. Entomol. Soc. Am.* **25**, 122–124.

Blight, M. M., Henderson, N. C,, and Wadhams, L. J. (1983). The identification of 4-methyl-3-heptanone from *Scloytus scolytus* (F.) and *S. multistriatus* (Marsham). Absolute configuration, laboratory bioassay and electrophysiological studies on *S. scolytus. Insect Biochem.* **13**, 27–38.

Blight, M. M., Pickett, J. A., Smith, M. C., and Wadhams, L. J. (1984). An aggregation pheromone of *Sitona lineatus:* Identification and initial field studies. *Naturwissenschaften* **71**, 480.

Borden, J. H. (1985). Aggregation pheromones. *In* ''Comprehensive Insect Physiology, Biochemistry, and Pharmacology'' (G. A. Kerkut and L. I. Gilbert, eds.), Vol. 9, pp. 257–285. Pergamon, Oxford.

Borden, J. H., Nair, K. K., and Slater, C. E. (1969). Synthetic juvenile hormone: Induction of sex pheromone production in *Ips confusus. Science* **166**, 1626–1627.

Borden, J. H., Handley, J. R., McLean, J. A., Silverstein, R. M., Chong, L., Slessor, K. N., Johnston, B. D., and Schuler, H. R. (1980). Enantiomer-based specificity in pheromone communication by two sympatric *Gnathotrichus* species (Coleoptera: Scolytidae). *J. Chem. Ecol.* **6**, 445–446.

Borden, J. H., Hunt, D. W. A., Miller, D. R., and Slessor, K. N. (1986a). Orientation in forest Coleoptera: An uncertain outcome of responses by individual beetles to variable stimuli. *In* ''Mechanisms of Perception and Orientation: Insect Olfactory Signals'' (T. L. Payne, M. C. Birch, and C. E. J. Kennedy, eds.), pp. 97–109. Clarendon Press, Oxford.

Borden, J. H., Pierce, A. M., Pierce, H. D., Jr., Chong, L. J., Stock, A. J., and Oehlschlager, A. C. (1987). Semiochemicals produced by the western balsam bark beetle, *Dryocoetes confusus* Swaine (Coleoptera: Scolytidae). *J. Chem. Ecol.* **13**, 823–836.

Borden, J. H., Ryker, L. C., Chong, L. J., Pierce, H. D., Jr., Johnston, B. D., and Oehlschlager, A. C. (1987). Response of the mountain pine beetle, *Dendroctonus ponderosae* Hopkins (Coleoptera: Scolytidae), to five semiochemicals in British Columbia lodgepole pine forests. *Can. J. For. Res.* **17**, 118–128.

Bowers, W. S. (1983). The precocenes. *In* ''Endocrinology of Insects'' (R. G. H. Downer and H. Laufer, eds.), pp. 517–523. Alan R. Liss, New York.

Bradshaw, J. W. S. (1985). Insect natural products—compounds derived from acetate, shikimate and amino acids. *In* ''Comprehensive Insect Physiology, Biochemistry, and Pharmacology'' (G. A. Kerkut and L. I. Gilbert, eds.), Vol. 11, pp. 655–703. Pergamon, Oxford.

Brand, J. M., and Barras, S. J. (1977). The major volatile constituents of a basidiomycete associated with the southern pine beetle. *Lloydia* **40**, 398–400.

Brand, J. M., Bracke, J. W., Markovetz, A. J., Wood, D. L., and Browne, L. E. (1975). Production of verbenol pheromone by a bacterium isolated from bark beetles. *Nature (London)* **254**, 136–137.

Brand, J. M., Bracke, J. W., Britton, L. N., Markovetz, A. J., and Barras, S. J. (1976). Bark beetle pheromones: Production of verbenone by a mycangial fungus of *Dendroctonus frontalis. J. Chem. Ecol.* **2**, 195–199.

Brand, J. M., Schultz, J., Barras, S. J., Edson, L. J., Payne, T. L., and Hedden, R. L. (1977). Bark-beetle pheromones. Enhancement of *Dendroctonus frontalis* (Coleoptera: Scolytidae) aggregation pheromones by yeast metabolites in laboratory bioassays. *J. Chem. Ecol.* **3**, 657–666.

Brand, J. M., Young, J. C., and R. M. Silverstein. (1979). Insect pheromones: A critical review of recent advances in their chemistry, biology and application. *Fortschr. Chem. Org. Naturst.* **37**, 1–190.

Bridges, J. R. (1982). Effects of juvenile hormone on pheromone synthesis in *Dendroctonus frontalis. Environ. Entomol.* **11**, 417–418.

Burkholder, W. E. (1982). Reproductive biology and communication among grain storage and warehouse beetles. *J. Georgia Entomol. Soc., Second Suppl.* **17**, 1–10.

Butterfield, A. (1984). Pheromone production and control mechanisms in *Dendroctonus pseudotsugae* Hopkins. Master of Pest Management Professional Paper, Simon Fraser Univ., Burnaby, British Columbia.

Byers, J. A. (1981a). Effect of mating on terminating aggregation during host colonization in the bark beetle, *Ips parconfusus. J. Chem. Ecol.* **7**, 1135–1147.

Byers, J. A. (1981b). Pheromone biosynthesis in the bark beetle, *Ips parconfusus,* during feeding or exposure to vapours of host plant precursors. *Insect Biochem.* **11**, 563–569.

Byers, J. A. (1983a). Bark beetle conversion of a plant compound to a sex-specific inhibitor of pheromone attraction. *Science* **220**, 624–626.

Byers, J. A. (1983b). Influence of sex, maturity and host substances on pheromones in the guts of the bark beetles, *Ips paraconfusus* and *Dendroctonus brevicomis. J. Insect Physiol.* **29**, 5–13.

Byers, J. A., and Wood, D. L. (1981). Antibiotic-induced inhibition of pheromone synthesis in a bark beetle. *Science* **213**, 763–764.

Byers, J. A., Wood, D. L., Browne, L. E., Fish, R. H., Piatek, B., and Hendry, L. B. (1979). Relationship between a host plant compound, myrcene and pheromone production in the bark beetle, *Ips paraconfusus. J. Insect Physiol.* **25**, 477–482.

Chararas, C. (1980). Physiologie des invertebres—Attraction primaire et secondaire chez trois especes de Scolytidae (*Ips*) et mecanisme de colonisation. *C. R. Acad. Sci. Paris, Ser. D.* **290**, 375–378.

Chararas, C., Riviere, J., Ducauze, C., Rutledge, D., Delpui, G., and Cazelles, M.-T. (1980). Bioconversion d'un compose terpenique sous l'action d'une Bacterie du tube digestif de *Phloeosinus armatus* (Coleoptera, Scolytidae). *C. R. Acad. Sci. Paris, Ser. D.* **291**, 299–302.

Chuman, R., Mochizuki, K., Mori, M., Kohno, M., Ono, M., Onishi, I., and Kato, K. (1982a). The pheromone activity of (+/−)-serricornins for male cigarette beetle (*Lasioderma serricorne* F.). *Agric. Biol. Chem.* **46**, 593–595.

Chuman, R., Mochizuki, K., Mori, M., Kohno, M., Kato, K., Nomi, H., and Mori, K. (1982b). Behavioral and electroantennogram responses of male cigarette beetle (*Lasioderma serricorne* F.) to optically active serricornins. *Agric. Biol. Chem.* **46**, 3109–3112.

Chuman, T., Mochizuki, K., Kato, K., Ono, M., and Okubo, A. (1983). Serricorone and serricorole. New sex pheromone components of cigarette beetle. *Agric. Biol. Chem.* **47**, 1413–1415.

Conn, J. E., Borden, J. H., Hunt, D. W. A., Holman, J., Whitney, H. S., Spanier, O. J., Pierce, H. D., Jr., and Oehlschlager, A. C. (1984). Pheromone production by axenically reared *Dendroctonus ponderosae* and *Ips paraconfusus* (Coleoptera: Scolytidae). *J. Chem. Ecol.* **10**, 281–290.

Coster, J. E., and Vite, J. P. (1972). Effects of feeding and mating on pheromone release in the southern pine beetle. *Ann. Entomol. Soc. Am.* **65**, 263–266.

Coyne, J. F., and Lott, L. H. (1976). Toxicity of substances in pine oleoresin to southern pine beetle. *J. Georgia Entomol. Soc.* **11**, 301–305.

Cross, J. H., Byler, R. C., Cassidy, R. F., Silverstein, R. M., Greenblatt, R. E., Burkholder, W. E., Levinson, A. R., and Levinson, H. Z. (1976). Porapak Q collection of pheromone components and isolation of (*Z*)- and (*E*)-14-methyl-8-hexadecanal, potent sex attracting components from the females of four species of *Trogoderma* (Coleoptera: Dermestidae). *J. Chem. Ecol.* **2**, 457–468.

Dowd, P. F., Smith, C. M., and Sparks, T. C. (1983). Detoxification of plant toxins by insects. *Insect Biochem.* **13**, 453–468.

Fish, R. H., Browne, L. E., Wood, D. L., and Hendry, L. B. (1979). Pheromone biosynthetic pathways: Conversions of deuterium-labelled ipsdienol with sexual and enantioselectivity in *Ips paraconfusus. Tetrahedron Lett.* **17**, 1465–1468.

Fish, R. H., Browne, L. E., and Bergot, B. J. (1984). Pheromone biosynthetic pathways: Conversion of ipsdienone to (−)-ipsdienol, a mechanism for enantioselective reduction in the male bark beetle, *Ips paraconfusus. J. Chem. Ecol.* **10,** 1057–1064.

Francke, W., and Heemann, V. (1974). Lockversuche bei *Xyloterus domesticus* L. und *X. lineatus* Oliv. (Coleoptera: Scolytidae) mit 3-hydroxy-3-methylbutan-2-on. *Z. Angew. Entomol.* **75,** 67–72.

Francke, W., and Vite, J. P. (1983). Oxygenated terpenes in pheromone systems of bark beetles. *Z. Angew. Entomol.* **96,** 146–156.

Francke, W., Heeman, V., and Heyns, K. (1974). Fluchtige inhaltstoffe von Ambrosiakafern (Coleoptera: Scolytidae). *Z. Naturforsch.* **29C,** 243–245.

Francke, W., Heeman, V., Gerken, B., Renwick, J. A. A., and Vite, J. P. (1977). 2-Ethyl-1,6-dioxaspiro[4.4]nonane, principal aggregation pheromone of *Pityogenes chalcographus* (L.). *Naturwissenschaften* **64,** 590–591.

Francke, W., Hindorf, G., and Reith, W. (1979). Alkyl-1,6-dioxaspiro[4.5]decanes—A new class of pheromones. *Naturwissenschaften* **66,** 618–196.

Fukui, H., Matsumura, F., Barak, A. V., and Burkholder, W. E. (1977). Isolation and identification of a major sex-attracting component of *Attagenus elongatus* (Casey) (Coleoptera: Dermestidae). *J. Chem. Ecol.* **3,** 539–548.

Gerken, V. B., and Hughes, P. (1976). Hormonale stimulation der biosynthese geschlectsspezifischer duftstoffe bei borkenkafern. *Z. Angew. Entomol.* **82,** 108–110.

Gore, W. E., Pearce, G. T., Lanier, G. N., Simeone, J. B., Silverstein, R. M., Peacock, J. W., and Cuthbert, R. A. (1977). Aggregation attractant of the European elm bark beetle, *Scolytus multistriatus.* Production of individual components and related aggregation behaviour. *J. Chem. Ecol.* **3,** 429–446.

Graham, K. (1961). Air swallowing: a mechanism in photic reversal of the beetle *Trypodendron. Nature (London)* **191,** 519–520.

Graham, K. (1967). Fungal–insect mutualism in trees and timber. *Annu. Rev. Entomol.* **12,** 105–127.

Greenblatt, R. E., Burkholder, W. E., Cross, J. H., Cassidy, R. F., Silverstein, R. M., Levinson, A. R., and Levinson, H. Z. (1977). Chemical basis for interspecific responses to sex pheromones of *Trogoderma* species. *J. Chem. Ecol.* **3,** 337–347.

Gueldner, R. C., Sikorowski, P. P., and Wyatt, J. M. (1977). Bacterial load and pheromone production in the boll weevil, *Anthonomus grandis. J. Invest. Pathol.* **29,** 397–398.

Guss, P. L., Tumlinson. J. H., Sonnet, P. E., and Proveaux, A. T. (1982). Identification of a female-produced sex pheromone of the western corn rootworm. *J. Chem. Ecol.* **8,** 545–556.

Guss, P. L., Tumlinson, J. H., Sonnet, P. E., and Proveaux, A. T. (1983). Identification of a female-produced sex pheromone from the southern corn rootworm, *Diabrotica undecimpunctata howardi* Barber. *J. Chem. Biol.* **9,** 1363–1375.

Hackstein, E., and Vite, J. P. (1978). Pheromone biosynthese und Reizkett in der Besiedlung von Fichten durch den Buchdrucker *Ips typographus. Mitt. Dtsch. Ges. Allg. Angew. Entomol.* **1,** 185–188.

Hardee, D. D. (1970). Pheromone production by male boll weevils as affected by food and host factors. *Contr. Boyce Thompson Inst. Plant Res.* **24,** 315–322.

Harring, C. M. (1978). Aggregation pheromones of the European fir engraver beetles *Pityokteines curvidens, P. spinidens* and *P. vorontzovi* and the role of juvenile hormone in pheromone biosynthesis. *Angew. Entomol.* **85,** 281–317.

Hedin, P. A. (1977). A study of factors that control biosynthesis of the compounds which comprise the boll weevil pheromone. *J. Chem. Ecol.* **3,** 279–283.

Hedin, P. A., Thompson, A. C., Gueldner, R. A., and Minyard, J. P. (1971). Malvaceae: Constituents of the cotton bud. *Phytochemistry* **10,** 3316–3318.

Hedin, P. A., Rollins, C. S., Thompson, A. C., and Gueldner, R. C. (1975). Pheromone production of male boll weevils treated with chemosterilants. *J. Econ. Entomol.* **68,** 587–591.

Hedin, P. A., Lindig, O. H., and Wiygul, G. (1982). Enhancement of boll weevil *Anthonomus grandis* Boh. (Coleoptera: Curculionidae) pheromone biosynthesis with JH III. *Experientia* **38,** 375–376.

Hendrickson, J. B. (1973). Biogenesis of natural products. *In* "The Molecules of Nature" (R. Breslow, ed.), pp. 12–57. Benjamin, New York.

Hendry, L. B., Piatek, B., Browne, L. E., Wood, D. L., Byers, J. A., Fish, R. H., and Hicks, R. A. (1980). *In vivo* conversion of a labelled host plant chemical to pheromones of the bark beetle *Ips paraconfusus. Nature (London)* **284,** 485.

Horler, D. (1970). (−)-Methyl *n*-tetradeca-(*E*)-2,4,5-trienoate, an allenic ester produced by the male dried bean beetle, *Acanthoscelides obtectus* (Say). *J. Chem. Soc. C,* 859–862.

Hoyt, C. P., Osborne, G. O., and Mulcock, A. P. (1971). Production of an insect sex attractant by symbiotic bacteria. *Nature (London)* **230,** 472–473.

Hughes, P. R. (1973a). *Dendroctonus:* Production of pheromones and related compounds in response to host monoterpenes. *Z. Angew. Entomol.* **73,** 294–312.

Hughes, P. R. (1973b). Effect of α-pinene exposure on *trans*-verbenol synthesis in *Dendroctonus ponderosae. Naturwissenschaften* **60,** 261–262.

Hughes, P. R. (1974). Myrcene: A precursor of pheromones in *Ips* beetles. *J. Insect Physiol.* **20,** 1271–1275.

Hughes, P. R. (1975). Pheromones of *Dendroctonus:* Origin of α-pinene oxidation products present in emergent adults. *J. Insect Physiol.* **21,** 687–691.

Hughes, P. R., and Renwick, J. A. A. (1977a). Neural and hormonal control of pheromone biosynthesis in the bark beetle, *Ips parconfusus. Physiol. Entomol.* **2,** 117–123.

Hughes, P. R., and Renwick, J. A. A. (1977b). Hormonal and host factors stimulating pheromone synthesis in female western pine beetles, *Dendroctonus brevicomis. Physiol. Entomol.* **2,** 289–292.

Hunt, D. W. A., Borden, J. H., Pierce, H. D., Jr., Slessor, K. N., King, G. G. S., and Czyzewska, E. (1986). Sex-specific production of ipsdienol and myrcenol by *Dendroctonus ponderosae* (Coleoptera: Scolytidae) exposed to myrcene vapors. *J. Chem. Ecol.* **12,** 1579–1586.

Johnston, B. D., and Oehlschlager, A. C. (1986). Synthesis of the aggregation pheromone of the square-necked grain beetle, *Catharthus quadricollis. J. Org. Chem.* **51,** 760–764.

Kiehlmann, E., Conn, J. E., and Borden, J. H. (1982). 7-Ethoxy-6-methoxy-2,2-dimethyl-2*H*-1-benzopyran. *Org. Prep. Proc. Int.* **14,** 337–342.

Klimetzek, D., and Francke, W. (1980). Relationship between the enantiomeric composition of α-pinene in host trees and the production of verbenols in *Ips* species. *Experientia* **36,** 1343–1345.

Kohnle, U., Francke, W. and Bakke, A. (1985). *Polygraphus poligraphus* (L.): Response to enantiomers of beetle specific terpene alcohols and a bicyclic ketal. *Z. Angew. Entomol.* **100,** 5–8.

Kovalev, B. G., Vrkoch, J., Streinz, L., Filippov, N. A., Fedoseev, N. Z., Nesterov, E. A., and Avdeeva, L. A. (1985). Isolation and identification of a component of the sex pheromone of *Agriotis ponticus. Khim. Prir. Soedin.* **2,** 278–279 [via Chem. Abstr. search (1985) **103,** 35074z].

Kuwahara, Y., Fukami, H., Howard, R., Ishii, S., Matsumura, F., and Burkholder, W. E. (1978). Chemical studies on the Anobiidae: Sex pheromone of the drugstore beetle, *Stegobium paniceum* (L.) (Coleoptera). *Tetrahedron* **34,** 1769–1774.

Lanier, G. N., Classon, A., Stewart, T., Piston, J. J., and Silverstein, R. M. (1980). *Ips pini:* The basis for interpopulational differences in pheromone biology. *J. Chem. Ecol.* **6,** 677–687.

Leufven, A., Bergstom, G., and Falsen, E. (1984). Interconversion of verbenols and verbenone by identified yeasts isolated from the spruce bark beetle *Ips typographus. J. Chem. Ecol.* **10,** 1349–1361.

Levinson, H. Z., Levinsin, A. R., Francke, W., Mackenroth, W., and Heeman, V. (1981). The pheromonal activity of anhydroserricornin and serricornin for male cigarette beetles (*Lasioderma serricorne* F.). *Naturwissenschaften* **68**, 148–149.

Levinson, H. Z., Levinsin, A. R., Francke, W., Mackenroth, W., and Heeman, V. (1982). Suppressed pheromone responses of male tobacco beetles to anhydroserricornin in presence of serricornin. *Naturwissenschaften* **69**, 454–455.

Libbey, L. M., Oehlschlager, A. C., and Ryker, L. C. (1983). 1-Methylcyclohex-2-en-1-ol as an aggregation pheromone of *Dendroctonus pseudotsugae. J. Chem. Ecol.* **9**, 1533–1541.

Libbey, L. M., Ryker, L. C., and Yandell, K. L. (1985). Laboratory and field studies of volatiles released by *Dendroctonus ponderosae. Z. Angew. Entomol.* **100**, 381–392.

McKnight, R. C. (1979). Differences in response among populations of *Dendroctonus ponderosae* (Hopkins to its pheromone complex. M.Sci. Thesis, University of Washington, Seattle.

Madden, J. L., Pierce, H. D., Jr., and Borden, J. H. (1987). Sites of production and occurrence of volatiles in the Douglas-fir beetle, *Dendroctonus pseudotsugae* Hopkins. *J. Chem. Ecol.* (in press).

Menon, M. (1970). Hormone–pheromone relationships in the beetle, *Tenebrio molitor. J. Insect Physiol.* **16**, 1123–1139.

Millar, J. G., Pierce, Jr., H. D., Pierce, A. M., Oehlschlager, A. C., Borden, J. H., and Barak, A. V. (1985). Aggregation pheromones of the flat grain beetle, *Cryptolestes pusillus* (Coleoptera: Cucujidae). *J. Chem. Ecol.* **11**, 1053–1070.

Mitlin, N., and Hedin, P. A. (1974). Biosynthesis of grandlure, the pheromone of the boll weevil, *Anthonomus grandis,* from acetate, mevalonate, and glucose. *J. Insect Physiol.* **20**, 1825–1831.

Mochizuki, K., Mori, M., Chuman, T., Kohno, M., Ohnishi, A., Watanabe, H., and Mori, K. (1986). Reinvestigations of anhydroserricornin, (2*S*,3*S*)-2,6-diethyl-3,5-dimethyl-3,4-dihydro-2H-pyran, as a sex pheromone component for male cigarette beetle. *J. Chem. Ecol.* **12**, 179–186.

Moeck, H. A., Wood, D. L., and Lindahl, K. Q., Jr. (1981). Host selection behavior of bark beetles (Coleoptera: Scolytidae) attacking *Pinus ponderosae,* with special emphasis on the Western pine beetle, *Dendroctonus brevicomis. J. Chem. Ecol.* **7**, 49–83.

Money, T. (1973). Biosynthesis of polyketides. *In* "Specialist Periodical Reports: Biosynthesis" (T. A. Giessman, Senior Reporter), Vol. 2, pp. 183–214. The Chemical Society, London.

Moore, B. P., and Brown, W. V. (1976). The chemistry of the metasternal gland secretion of the eucalypt longicorn *Phoracantha synonyma* (Coleoptera: Cerambycidae). *Aust. J. Chem.* **29**, 1365–1374.

Moore, R. N., Golumbic, C., and Fisher, G. S. (1956). Autoxidation of α-pinene. *J. Am. Chem. Soc.* **78**, 1173–1176.

Mori, K. (1977). Absolute configuration of (−)-4-methylheptan-3-ol, a pheromone of the smaller European elm bark beetle, as determined by the synthesis of its (3*R*,4*R*)-(+)- and (3*S*,4*R*)-(+)-isomers. *Tetrahedron* **33**, 289–294.

Mori, K., Mizumachi, N., and Matsui, M. (1976). Synthesis of optically pure (1*S*,4*S*,5*S*)-2-pinen-4-ol (*cis*-verbenol) and its antipode, the pheromone of *Ips* bark beetles. *Agric. Biol. Chem.* **40**, 1611–1615.

Mori, K., Ito, T., Tanaka, K., Honda, H., and Yamamoto, I. (1983). Synthesis and biological activity of optically active forms of (*E*)-3,7-dimethyl-2-octen-1,8-dioic acid (callosbruchusic acid). *Tetrahedron* **39**, 2303–2306.

Mori, K., Chuman, T., and Kato, K. (1984). Cyclic hemiacetal and acyclic chain—the two forms of serricornin. *Tetrahedron Lett.* **25**, 2553–2556.

Nijholt, W. W. (1970). The effect of mating and the presence of the male ambrosia beetle, *Trypodendron lineatum,* on "secondary" attraction. *Can. Entomol.* **102**, 894–897.

Oehlschlager, A. C., King, G. G. S., Pierce, H. D., Jr., Pierce, A. M., Slessor, K. N., and Borden, J. H. (1987). The chirality of macrolide pheromones of grain beetles in the genera *Oryzaephilus* and *Cryptolestes* and its implications for species specificity. *J. Chem. Ecol.* **13**, 1543–1553.

Pearce, G. T. Gore, W. E., Silverstein, R. M., Peacock, J. W., Cuthbert, R. A., Lanier, G. N., and Simeone, J. B. (1975). Chemical attractants for the smaller European elm bark beetle, *Scolytus multistriatus* (Coleoptera: Scolytidae) *J. Chem. Ecol.* **1**, 115–124.

Phillips, J. K., Walgenbach, C. A., Klein, J. A., Burkholder, W. E., Schmuff, N. R., and Fales, H. M. (1985). (*R**,*S**)-5-hydroxy-4-methyl-3-heptanone: male produced aggregation pheromone of *Sitophilus oryzae* (L.) and *S. zeamais* Motsch. *J. Chem. Ecol.* **11**, 1263–1274.

Pierce, A. M., Pierce, H. D., Jr., Millar, J. G., Borden, J. H., and Oehlschlager, A. C. (1984). Aggregation pheromones in the genus *Oryzaephilus* (Coleoptera: Cucujidae). *Proc. Third Intl. Working Conf. Stored-Prod. Entomol.*, Manhattan, Kansas, 107–120.

Pierce, A. M., Pierce, H. D., Jr., Oehlschlager, A. C., and Borden, J. H. (1985). Macrolide aggregation pheromones in *Oryzaephilus surinamensis* and *Oryzaephilus mercator* (Coleoptera: Cucujidae). *J. Agric. Food Chem.* **33**, 848–852.

Pierce, A. M., Pierce, H. D., Jr., Borden, J. H., and Oehlschlager, A. C. (1986). Enhanced production of aggregation pheromones in four stored-product coleopterans feeding on methoprene-treated oats. *Experientia* **42**, 164–165.

Pierce, A. M., Pierce, H. D., Jr., Oehlschlager, A. C., Czyzewska, E., and Borden, J. H. (1987). Influence of pheromone chirality on response by *Oryzaephilus surinamensis* and *O. mercator* (Coleoptera: Cucujidae). *J. Chem. Ecol.* **13**, 1525–1542.

Pierce, H. D., Jr., Pierce, A. M., Millar, J. G., Wong, J. W., Verigin, V. G., Oehlschlager, A. C., and Borden, J. H. (1984). Methodology for isolation and analysis of aggregation pheromones in the genera *Cryptolestes* and *Oryzaephilus* (Coleoptera: Cucujidae). *Proc. Third Intl. Working Conf. Stored-Prod. Entomol.*, Manhattan, Kansas, 121–137.

Pierce, H. D.. Jr., Conn, J. E., Borden, J. H., and Oehlschlager, A. C. (1987). Monoterpene metabolism in female mountain pine beetles, *Dendroctonus ponderosae* Hopkins, attacking lodgepole and ponderosa pines. *J. Chem. Ecol.* **13**, 1455–1480.

Plummer, E. L., Stewart, T. F., Byrne, K., Pearce, G. T., and Silverstein, R. M. (1976). Determination of enantiomeric composition of several insect pheromone alcohols. *J. Chem. Ecol.* **2**, 307–331.

Prestwich, G. D., Yamaoka, R., and Carvalho, J. F. (1985). Metabolism of tritiated ω-fluorofatty acids and alcohols in the termite *Reticulitermes flavipes* (Kollar) (Isoptera, Rhinotermitidae). *Insect Biochem.* **15**, 205–209.

Raffa, K. F., and Berryman, A. A. (1983). The role of host plant resistance in the colonization behavior and ecology of bark beetles (Coleoptera: Scolytidae). *Ecol. Monogr.* **53**, 27–49.

Raffa, K. F., Berryman, A. A., Simasko, J., Teal, W., and Wong, B. L. (1985). Effects of grand fir monoterpenes on the fir engraver, *Scolytus ventralis* (Coleoptera: Scolytidae), and its symbiotic fungus. *Environ. Entomol.* **14**, 552–556.

Renwick, J. A. A., and Dickens, J. C. (1979). Control of pheromone production in the bark beetle, *Ips cembrae. Physiol. Entomol.* **4**, 377–381.

Renwick, J. A. A., and Hughes, P. R. (1975). Oxidation of unsaturated cyclic hydrocarbons by *Dendroctonus frontalis. Insect. Biochem.* **5**, 459–463.

Renwick, J. A. A., and Pitman, G. B. (1979). An attractant isolated from female Jeffrey pine beetles, *Dendroctonus jeffreyi. Environ. Entomol.* **8**, 40–41.

Renwick, J. A. A., Hughes, P. R.. and Ty, T. D. (1973). Oxidation products of pinene in the bark beetle, *Dendroctonus frontalis. J. Insect Physiol.* **19**, 1735–1740.

Renwick. J. A. A., Hughes, P. R., and Vite, J. P. (1975). The aggregation pheromone system of a *Dendroctonus* bark beetle in Guatemala. *J. Insect Physiol.* **21**, 1097–1100.

Renwick, J. A. A., Pitman, G. B., and Vite, J. P. (1976a). 2-Phenylethanol isolated from bark beetles. *Naturwissenschaften* **63**, 198.

Renwick, J. A. A., Hughes, P. R., and Krull, I. S. (1976b). Selective production of *cis*- and *trans*-verbenol from (−)- and (+)-α-pinene by a bark beetle. *Science* **191**, 199–200.

Renwick, J. A. A., Hughes, P. R., Pitman, G. B., and Vite, J. P. (1976c). Oxidation products of terpenes identified from *Dendroctonus* and *Ips* bark beetles. *J. Insect Physiol.* **22**, 725–727.

Renwick, J. A. A., Vite, J. P., and Billings, R. F. (1977). Aggregation pheromones in the ambrosia beetle, *Platypus flavicornis*. *Naturwissenschaften* **64**, 226.

Rodin, J. O., Silverstein, R. M., Burkholder, W. E., and Gorman, J. E. (1969). Sex attractant of the female dermestid beetle, *Trogoderma inclusum* LeConte. *Science* **165**, 904–906.

Roelofs, W., and Bjostad, L. (1984). Biosynthesis of lepidopteran pheromones. *Bioorg. Chem.* **12**, 279–298.

Roth, L. M., and Barth, R. H. (1964). The control of sexual receptivity in female cockroaches. *J. Insect Physiol.* **10**, 965–975.

Rudinsky, J. A. (1966). Scolytid beetles associated with Douglas fir: Response to terpenes. *Science* **152**, 218–219.

Rudinsky, J. A., Morgan, M., Libbey, L. M., and Michael, R. R. (1973). Sound production in Scolytidae: 3-methyl-2-cyclohexen-1-one released by the female Douglas fir beetle in response to male sonic signal. *Environ. Entomol.* **2**, 505–509.

Rudinsky, J. A., Morgan, M. E., Libbey, L. M., and Putnam, T. B. (1974). Antiaggregative-rivalry pheromone of the mountain pine beetle, and a new arrestant of the southern pine beetle. *Environ. Entomol.* **3**, 90–98.

Rudinsky, J. A., Morgan, M. E., Libbey, L. M., and Putnam, T. B. (1977). Limonene released by the scolytid beetle *Dendroctonus pseudotsugae*. *Z. Angew. Entomol.* **82**, 376–380.

Ryker, L. C., Libbey, L. M., and Rudinsky, J. A. (1979). Comparison of volatile compounds and stridulation emitted by the Douglas-fir beetle from Idaho and western Oregon populations. *Environ. Entomol.* **8**, 789–798.

Sakai, T., Nakagawa, Y., Takahashi, J., Iwabuchi, K. and Ishii, K. (1984). Isolation and identification of the male sex pheromone of the grape borer *Xylotrechus pyrrhoderus* Bates (Coleoptera: Cerambycidae). *Chem. Lett.*, 263–264.

Sehnal, F. (1983). Juvenile hormone analogues. *In* "Endocrinology of Insects" (R. G. H. Downer and H. Laufer, eds.), pp. 657–672. Alan R. Liss, New York.

Silverstein, R. M., Rodin, J. O., Burkholder, W. E., and Gorman, J. E. (1967). Sex attractant of the black carpet beetle. *Science* **157**, 85–87.

Slessor, K. N., King, G. G. S., Miller, D. R., Winston, M. L., and Cutforth, T. L. (1985). Determination of chirality of alcohol or latent alcohol semiochemicals in individual insects. *J. Chem. Ecol.* **11**, 1659–1667.

Smith, R. H. (1961). The fumigant toxicity of three pine resins to *Dendroctonus brevicomis* and *D. jeffreyi*. *J. Econ. Entomol.* **54**, 365–369.

Smith, R. H. (1965a). A physiological difference among beetles of *Dendroctonus ponderosae* (= *D. monticolae*) and *D. ponderosae* (= *D. jeffreyi*). *Ann. Entomol. Soc. Am.* **58**, 440–442.

Smith, R. H. (1965b). Effect of monoterpene vapors on the western pine beetles. *J. Econ. Entomol.* **58**, 509–510.

Staal, G. B. (1986). Anti juvenile hormone agents. *Annu. Rev. Entomol.* **31**, 391–429.

Stoakley, J. T., Bakke, A., Renwick, J. A. A., and Vite, J. P. (1978). The aggregation pheromone system of the larch bark beetle *Ips cembrae*. *Z. Angew. Entomol.* **86**, 174–177.

Suzuki, T. (1980). 4,8-Dimethyldecanal: The aggregation pheromone of the flour beetles, *Tribolium castaneum* and *T. confusum* (Coleoptera: Tenebrionidae). *Agric. Biol. Chem.* **11**, 2519–2520.

Suzuki, T., and Sugawara, R. (1979). Isolation of aggregation pheromone from the flour beetle, *Tribolium castaneum* and *T. confusum* (Coleoptera: Tenebrionidae). *Appl. Entomol. Zool.* **14**, 228–230.

Thompson, A. C., and Mitlin, N. (1979). Biosynthesis of the sex pheromone of the male boll weevil from monterpene precursors. *Insect Biochem.* **9**, 293–294.

Tumlinson, J. H., Hardee, D. D., Gueldner, R. C., Thompson, A. C., Hedin, P. A., and Minyard, J. P. (1969). Sex pheromones produced by male boll weevil: Isolation, identification, and synthesis. *Science* **166**, 1010–1012.

Tumlinson, J. H., Gueldner, R. C., Hardee, D. D., Thompson, A. C., Hedin, P. A., and Minyard, J. P. (1970). The boll weevil sex attractant. *In* "Chemicals Controlling Insect Behavior" (M. Beroza, ed.), pp. 41–59. Academic Press, New York.

Tumlinson, J. H., Klein, M. G., Doolittle, R. E., Ladd, T. L., and Proveaux, A. T. (1977). Identification of the female Japanese beetle sex pheromone: Inhibition of male response by an enantiomer. *Science* **197**, 789–792.

Vite, J. P., Bakke, A., and Renwick, J. A. A. (1972). Pheromones in *Ips* (Coleoptera: Scolytidae): Occurrence and production. *Can. Entomol.* **104**, 1967–1975.

White, P. R., and Birch, M. C. (1986). How do boring males find the right mate?: Sex pheromones of anobiid beetles. *Third Annu. Mtg. Intl. Soc. Chem. Ecol.* Univ. California, Berkeley, California.

White, R. A., Franklin, R. T., and Agosin, M. (1979). Conversion of α-pinene to α-pinene oxide by rat liver and the bark beetle *Dendroctonus terebrans* microsomal fractions. *Pest. Biochem. Physiol.* **10**, 233–242.

White, R. A., Jr., Agosin, M., Franklin, R. T., and Webb, J. W. (1980). Bark beetle pheromones: Evidence for physiological synthesis mechanisms and their ecological implications. *Z. Angew. Entomol.* **90**, 254–274.

Whitney, H. S., and Spanier, O. J. (1982). An improved method for rearing axenic mountain pine beetles, *Dendroctonus ponderosae* (Coleoptera: Scolytidae). *Can. Entomol.* **114**, 1095–1100.

Williams, H. J., Silverstein, R. M., Burkholder, W. E., and Khorramshahi, A. (1981). Dominicalure 1 and 2: Components of aggregation pheromone from male lesser grain borer *Rhyzopertha dominica* (F.) (Coleoptera: Bostrichidae). *J. Chem. Ecol.* **7**, 759–780.

Yarger, R. G., Silverstein, R. M., and Burkholder, W. E. (1975). Sex pheromone of the female dermestid beetle *Trogoderma glabrum* (Herbst). *J. Chem. Ecol.* **1**, 323–334.

7

Biosynthesis and Endocrine Regulation of Sex Pheromone Production in Diptera

GARY J. BLOMQUIST
Department of Biochemistry
University of Nevada
Reno, Nevada 89557

JACK W. DILLWITH
Department of Entomology
Oklahoma State University
Stillwater, Oklahoma 74078

T. S. ADAMS
Metabolism and Radiation Research Laboratory
Agricultural Research Service
U.S. Department of Agriculture
Fargo, North Dakota 58105

I. INTRODUCTION: DIPTERAN PHEROMONES—AN OVERVIEW

A. Dipteran Pheromones

In Diptera, as in other insects, gamete fertilization is the end result of a complex series of behaviors that are released by taste, touch, sound, smell, and sight. Sex pheromones have been demonstrated in 43 species of Diptera, both male and female, and have been chemically identified in 17 species (Table I)[1].

[1]Table I is arranged to provide the following information: (1) classification of Diptera that produce pheromones, (2) sex that produces pheromone, (3) distance over which the pheromone is active and type of system used to evaluate this, (4) close range effects of the pheromone, (5) effect of the pheromone on contact, (6) source of the pheromone and whether pheromone release is controlled or uncontrolled, and (7) chemical composition of the pheromone.

217

TABLE I

Characteristics of Dipteran-Produced Sex Pheromones[a]

Family	Species	Pheromone range and action					Chemical composition	References
		Sex	Distance[b]	Close	Contact	Source		
Culicidae	Culiseta inornata	F	+/−	−	SR, CP	Legs (UC)	?	Lang, 1977; Lang and Foster, 1976; Kliewer et al., 1966
	Deinocerites cancer	F	FL, 10 cm	+	CP	Pupal case (UC)	?	Downes, 1966
	Aedes albopictus	F	−	?	SR, CP	Cuticle (UC)	?	Nijhout and Craig, 1971
	Culex pipiens	M	OL, 15 cm	?	?	?	?	Gjullin et al., 1967
	Culex tarsalis	M	OL, 15 cm	?	?	?	?	Gjullin et al., 1967
	Culex quinquefasciatus	M	OL, 15 cm	?	?	?	?	Gjullin et al., 1967
Cecidomyiidae	Mayetiola destructor	F	OL, 19 cm	?	?	Ovipositor (CN)	?	McKay and Hatchett, 1984
Sciaridae	Lycoriella mali	F	OL	?	?	Cuticle (UC)	n-Heptadecane	Kostelc et al., 1975, 1979, 1980; Girard et al., 1974
	Bradysia impatiens	F	OL, 1 m	?	?	Legs (UC)	?	Alberts et al., 1981
	Bradysia tritici	F	OL, 10 cm	?	?	?	?	Casartelli et al., 1971
Ceratopogonidae	Culicoides nubeculosus	F	OL, 30 cm	?	CP	Abdomen, oenocytes (UC)	?	Kremer et al., 1979; Ismail, 1982; Ismail and Kremer, 1982; Ismail and Zachary, 1984
	Culicoides melleus	F	?	?	CP	Cuticle (UC)	?	Linley and Carlson, 1978; Linley, 1983

218

Family	Species							Reference
Syrphidae	Microdon cothurnatus	F	FL	?	?	?	?	Akre et al., 1973
Tephritidae	Dacus oleae	F	OL, 30 cm FL, >1 m	?	?	Rectal glands (CN)	1,7-Dioxaspiro[5,5]undecane	Baker et al., 1980; Haniotakis et al., 1977; Haniotakis, 1974; Mazomenos, 1984; Mazomenos and Haniotakis, 1981
	Dacus opiliae	M	?	CT	OP	Rectal glands (CN)	?	Fitt, 1981
	Dacus jarvasi	M	?	CT	OP	Rectal glands (CN)	?	Fitt, 1981
	Dacus aquilonis	M	?	CT	OP	Rectal glands (CN)	?	Fitt, 1981
	Dacus tryoni	M	FL	CT	OP	Rectal glands (CN)	?	Tychsen, 1977; Fletcher and Giannakakis, 1973
	Dacus dorsalis	M	FL	?	?	Rectal glands (CN)	?	Ohinata et al., 1982
	Dacus cucurbitae	M	FL	?	?	Rectal glands (CN)	?	Ohinata et al., 1982
	Rhagoletis pomonella	M	FL, 2 m	?	?	Rectal glands (CN)	?	Prokopy, 1982
	Rhagoletis cerasi	M	FL, 2 m	?	?	Rectal glands (CN)	?	Katsoyannos 1976, 1982
	Ceratitis capitata	M	OL, 27 cm	?	?	Rectal glands (CN)	E6-9 : Acid, E6-9 : OH	Jacobson et al., 1973; Feron, 1959; Chang and Hsu, 1982; Chang et al., 1984

(continued)

219

TABLE I (*Continued*)

Family	Species	Pheromone range and action					Chemical composition	References
		Sex	Distance[b]	Close	Contact	Source		
	Anastrepha suspensa	M	OL, 20 cm	CT	PP	Rectal glands (CN), abdominal pouch	?	Nation 1972, 1981
	Rioxa pornia	M	CG, 20 cm	CT	AR	Abdominal epithelium, salivary gland (CN)	?	Pritchard, 1967
Chloropidae	*Hippelates collusor*	F	OL, 15 cm	CT	?	Cuticle (UC)	?	Adams and Mulla, 1968
Drosophilidae	*Drosophila melanogaster*	F	–	CT	?	Cuticle (UC)	Heptacosadiene	Antony and Jallon, 1982a,b; Shorey and Bartell, 1970; Spieth, 1974; Averhoff and Richardson, 1976; Tompkins and Hall, 1981
	Drosophila melanogaster	M	?	AP	?	Male ejaculatory bulb	Z11-18 : Ac Z11-18 : OH	Tompkins and Hall, 1981; Jallon et al., 1981; Mane et al., 1983; Zawistowski and Richmond, 1986
	Drosophila pseudoobscura	F	?	CT	?	Cuticle (UC)	?	Sloane and Spiess, 1971
	Drosophila grimshawi	M	+	CT	?	Intraanal lobes (CN)	?	Spieth, 1966; Hodosh et al., 1979

220

Family	Species							Reference
Calliphoridae	*Lucilia cuprina*	F	—	ST	CP	Cuticle (UC)	?	Bartell et al., 1969
	Cochliomyia hominivorax	F	—	ST	CP	Cuticle (UC)	?	Mackley and Broce, 1981; Hammack, 1986
Sarcophagidae	*Sarcophaga bullata*	M	OL, 45 cm	?	?	?	Hexanal	Girard et al., 1979; Girard and Burdis, 1975
Muscidae	*Musca domestica*	F	OL, 75 cm	ST, SR	AR, CP	Cuticle (UC)	(Z)-9-Tricosene (Z)-14-Tricosen-10-one (Z)-9,10-Epoxytricosane Methylalkanes	Rogoff et al., 1964, 1973, 1980; Carlson et al., 1971; Uebel et al., 1976, 1978a; Adams et al., 1984a; Adams and Holt, 1986
	Musca autumnalis	F	OL, 40 cm	ST	?	Cuticle (UC)	(Z)-14-Nonacosene (Z)-13-Nonacosene (Z)-13-Heptacosene	Chaudhury et al., 1972; Sonnet et al., 1976; Uebel et al., 1975b
	Stomoxys calcitrans	F	OL, 50 cm	ST	?	Cuticle (UC)	(Z)-9-Hentriacontene (Z)-9-Tritriacontene 13-Methyl-1-hentriacontene 13-Methyl-1-tritriacontene	Harris et al., 1966, 1976; Muhammed et al., 1975; Sonnet et al., 1977; Uebel et al., 1975a
	Haematobia irritans	F	?	ST	AR, CP	Cuticle (UC)	(Z)-5-Tricosene (Z)-9-Pentacosene (Z)-9-Heptacosene	Bolton et al., 1980
	Fannia canicularis	F	?	ST	?	Cuticle (UC)	(Z)-9-Pentacosene	Uebel et al., 1977

(continued)

221

TABLE I (*Continued*)

Family	Species	Pheromone range and action[a]					Chemical composition	References
		Sex	Distance[b]	Close	Contact	Source		
	Fannia femoralis	F	?	ST	CP	Cuticle (UC)	(Z)-11-Hentriacontene	Uebel *et al.*, 1978b
	Fannia pusio	F	?	ST	?	Cuticle (UC)	(Z)-11-Hentriacontene	Uebel *et al.*, 1978b
Glossinidae	*Glossina morsitans morsitans*	F	—	—	AR, CP	Cuticle (UC)	15,19,23-Trimethylheptatriacontane, 17,21-Dimethylheptatriacontane, 15,19-Dimethylheptatriacontane	Carlson *et al.*, 1978; Huyton *et al.*, 1980a; Langley *et al.*, 1975
	Glossina austeni	F	—	—	AR, CP	Cuticle (UC)	15,19-Dimethyltritriacontane (?)	Huyton *et al.*, 1980b
	Glossina palpalis	F	?	?	CP	Cuticle (UC)	?	Offori *et al.*, 1981
	Glossina pallidipes	F	—	—	AR, CP	Cuticle (UC)	13,23-Dimethylpentatriacontane	Carlson *et al.*, 1984

[a] Abbreviations used in the table: AP, antipheromone (antiaphrodisiac); AR, arrestant, increases contact time; CG, cage tests in field or laboratory; CN, pheromone release is controlled and occurs during calling behavior; CP, pheromone induces copulatory attempts; CT, pheromone induces courtship behavior; F, pheromone produced by female; FL, pheromone is an attractant and was active in field tests; M, pheromone produced by males; OL, pheromone was an attractant and was active in laboratory olfactometer bioassay; OP, pheromone induces ovipositor probing; PP, pheromone induces probing with proboscis; SR, pheromone acts as a sex recognition factor; ST, pheromone induces male mating strike behavior; UC, pheromone release is uncontrolled; ?, no information available; —, no activity when tested; +, active when tested; +/−, conflicting reports on activity.

[b] Numbers indicate effective distance of pheromone when assayed.

These pheromones may be active at a distance, at close range, or only on contact (Table I). The female-produced sex attractant in *Dacus oleae* has an effective range of several meters (Haniotakis, 1974; Haniotakis *et al.*, 1977). Other dipteran pheromones have an effective range of only several centimeters and release courtship behavior, as in *Hippelates collusor* (Adams and Mulla, 1968), *Lucilla cuprina* (Bartell *et al.*, 1969), and *Drosophila melanogaster* (Shorey and Bartell, 1970), or increase mating strike activity as in *Musca domestica* (Rogoff *et al.*, 1964, 1973), *Haematobia irritans* (Bolton *et al.*, 1980), and *Cochliomyia hominovorax* (Mackley and Broce, 1981). The pheromones of the tsetse flies, *Glossina* species, are effective only on contact and release copulatory attempts and increase the amount of contact time (arrestants) (Carlson *et al.*, 1978, 1984).

Diptera vary considerably as to the sites of pheromone production (Table I). Pheromone is synthesized in the rectal glands of tephritids, in the intraanal lobes in *Drosophila grimshawi,* and in epidermal tissue in the housefly and tsetse fly (Table I). The pheromone biosynthetic sites have not been identified for the remaining Diptera, although the oenocytes have been suggested as a synthetic site for pheromones in *Culicoides nubeculosus* (Ismail and Zachary, 1984). The site of pheromone biosynthesis in the housefly and tsetse fly are discussed in more detail in Section V of this chapter.

B. Timing of Production/Release

Tephritids (Fletcher, 1968, 1969; Nation, 1981), Hawaiian drosophilids (Spieth, 1974), and the cecidomyiid, *Mayetiola destructor* (McKay and Hatchett, 1984), release pheromone during "calling." Many species of Diptera have pheromone dissolved in the cuticular lipids on the surface and, therefore, have no behavioral mechanism to control pheromone release (Table I).

It is assumed, however, that it is beneficial for the female to regulate the time of mating so that it coincides with a period of peak fertility and that the male will either respond to the female or demonstrate calling behavior when mature sperm are present. When pheromones are involved the time of mating can be regulated by controlling pheromone release ("calling"), by regulating pheromone biosynthesis, or by regulating pheromone perception. These types of control (shown diagrammatically in Fig. 1) indicate that both external and internal factors can interact to influence pheromone synthesis, release, and mating behavior.

Several external factors have been shown to influence pheromone release or synthesis in Diptera. Photoperiod influences the time at which *Mayetiola destructor* (McKay and Hatchett, 1984) and *Dacus oleae* (Haniotakis, 1974) release pheromone during calling. The blood meal in *Stomoxys calcitrans* stimulates both pheromone production and oogenesis (Meola *et al.*, 1977), and liverfed female *Lucilia cuprina* are more attractive to males than sugar-fed flies (Bartell *et al.*, 1969). The mechanisms by which these external factors influence

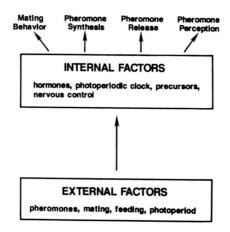

Fig. 1. Diagram of interacting factors that are responsible for mating in Diptera.

pheromone production and/or release must involve internal factors in some way, and these factors are discussed later (Section IV).

Flies that are monocoitic (mate only once) (Nelson *et al.*, 1969) or demonstrate cyclical polygamy may use mating-derived factors to decrease pheromone release, synthesis, or perception. The following flies lose their attractiveness for a period of time after mating: *Mayetiola destructor* (McKay and Hatchett, 1984), *Bradysia tritici* (Casartelli *et al.*, 1971), *Culicoides nebeculosus* (Ismail and Kremer, 1983), *Dacus oleae* (Haniotakis, 1974), and *Lucilia cuprina* (Bartell *et al.*, 1969). These mechanisms of interference with pheromone production have not been investigated in detail, but the studies of these mechanisms could result in the discovery of potential inhibitors of pheromone biosynthesis.

Other monocoitic or cyclically polygamous dipterans use different strategies to prevent further matings. Mated female *Musca domestica* (Riemann *et al.*, 1967), *Drosophila melanogaster* (Shorey and Bartell, 1970), and *Glossina* species (Huyton and Langley, 1982) will reject courting males and will not allow copulation to occur. In *Drosophila melanogaster* the male transfers *cis*-vaccenyl acetate (Z11-18 : Ac) to the female during mating which will inhibit subsequent courtship for 24 hr (Averhoff and Richardson, 1976). In addition to Z11-18 : Ac, the male also transfers esterase 6 to the female, which then hydrolyzes Z11-18 : Ac to *cis*-vaccenol (Z11-18 : OH) (Mane *et al.*, 1983). Both the alcohol and acetate ester are reported to be antiaphrodisiacs that decrease male courtship of inseminated females thereby reducing the probability of further mating (Zawistowski and Richmond, 1986). However, a recent report (Vander Meer *et al.*, 1986) has challenged the role of Z11-18 : Ac and esterase 6 in the regulation of mated female sexual attractiveness. Their chemical analysis did not support the contention that esterase 6, Z11-18 : Ac and Z11-18 : OH act in concert as an antiaphrodisiac pheromone system. Thus, the role of these male-produced chemicals has now become controversial.

When female *Anastrepha ludens* are mated they demonstrate a decreased attraction (perception?) to the male-produced pheromone which persists for 40 days (Robacker *et al.*, 1985). This decreased attraction has also been reported for *Ceratitis capitata* (Feron, 1962) and *Dacus opiliae* (Fitt, 1981a). The mating factor(s) responsible for this reduction in attraction and their site of action are unknown.

Male-produced pheromones have been reported in 17 species of Diptera belonging to the families Culicidae, Tephritidae, Drosophilidae, and Sarcophagidae (Table I). In the tephritids the females only respond to the male-produced pheromones when the female is sexually mature (Katsoyannos, 1982). This could reflect a humorally induced activating mechanism for pheromone perception, but this remains to be examined.

Male attractiveness to female *Ceratitis capitata* is reduced by precocene II treatments (Chang and Hsu, 1982; Chang *et al.*, 1984; Hsu and Chang, 1982), and JH III reversed the effect (Hsu and Chang, 1982). Thus, juvenile hormone (JH) is implicated in pheromone production in this tephritid, but no pheromone biosynthesis studies have been reported.

II. REPRODUCTIVE BIOLOGY OF THE HOUSEFLY

The remainder of this chapter will focus on the biosynthesis and endocrine regulation of the housefly sex pheromone. In order to put this discussion in context, a brief review of the reproductive biology of the housefly is presented.

Oogenesis in the housefly has been divided into a series of 10 stages (Adams, 1974) that have been used as indicators of physiological age. Flies contain stage 2 follicles at emergence and start to deposit yolk during stage 4 ($\sim$36 hr postemergence). Maximum yolk deposition in the oocyte occurs during stages 6, 7, and 8 ($\sim$48 hr postemergence). The chorion starts forming during stage 9, and the mature stage 10 follicle is found in flies at 60–70 hr postemergence. These ages apply to flies held at 27°C.

Oogenesis is both cyclical and synchronous, with only one cycle of eggs completing maturation at any given time. When developing follicles or stage 10 follicles are present in the ultimate cycle, the penultimate cycle does not develop past stage 4 (Adams, 1981a,b). All ovarioles contain the same stage sequence, and this type of synchrony has been termed interovariole synchrony (Adams, 1981a).

Vitellogenin is synthesized by the fat body, is released into the hemolymph, and cycles during oogenesis (Adams and Filipi, 1983). Maximal levels are found during midvitellogenesis. No vitellogenin is found in flies with stage 2 and 3 follicles, and low levels are found in flies with stage 10 follicles.

Female houseflies mate during stages 4–10 with the preferred stages being stages 6–10 (Adams *et al.*, 1984b) and produce attractant during stages 4–10 (Adams *et al.*, 1984b). Thus, mating, pheromone production, and vitellogenin synthesis are all initiated at stage 4, indicating the possibility of responding to the same set of internal cues.

III. HOUSEFLY SEX PHEROMONE

A. Isolation and Activity

A sex pheromone was first demonstrated in the housefly by Rogoff *et al.* (1964), identified as (Z)-9-tricosene (Z9-23 : Hy)[2] (muscalure) (Carlson *et al*, 1971), and shown to attract males in an olfactometer at doses as low as 0.07 μg (Adams *et al.*, 1984b). Subsequently, (Z)-9,10-epoxytricosane (C_{23} epoxide) and (Z)-14-tricosen-10-one (C_{23} ketone) (Uebel *et al.*, 1978a) and methylalkanes (Uebel *et al.*, 1976; Rogoff *et al.*, 1980) (Fig. 2) were shown to enhance the activity of muscalure. A detailed study by Adams and Holt (1987) showed that these pheromone components had different roles in male courtship behavior. Muscalure increased male mating strike activity toward females and other males. The nonhydrocarbon fraction, including both the epoxide and the ketone, decreased the number of homosexual mating strikes when muscalure was present. Thus, the nonhydrocarbon fraction contained sex recognition factors. Both the methylalkanes and the nonhydrocarbon fraction increased the number of copulatory attempts made by the test males (Adams and Holt, 1987). This was not observed with muscalure. Finally, the methylalkane fraction acted as an arrestant and increased the amount of time that a male spent with a treated model.

B. Correlation of Pheromone Production with Oogenesis

Newly emerged female houseflies do not have detectable amounts of any of the C_{23} sex pheromone components (alkene, epoxide, or ketone), whereas by day 4 they have large quantities of these and also show increased levels of methylalkanes. To examine the timing of sex pheromone production, both the amounts and relative rates of biosynthesis of sex pheromone components were monitored during oogenesis. The relative rates of pheromone biosynthesis were determined by assaying the incorporation of [1-^{14}C]acetate into C_{23} pheromone components after a 2 hr incubation period for each stage of oogenesis. We

---

[2]In this chapter Z9-23 : Hy denotes (Z)-9-tricosene, Z9-27 : Hy denotes (Z)-9-heptacosene, C_{23} epoxide denotes (Z)-9,10-epoxytricosane, and C_{23} ketone denotes (Z)-14-tricosen-10-one.

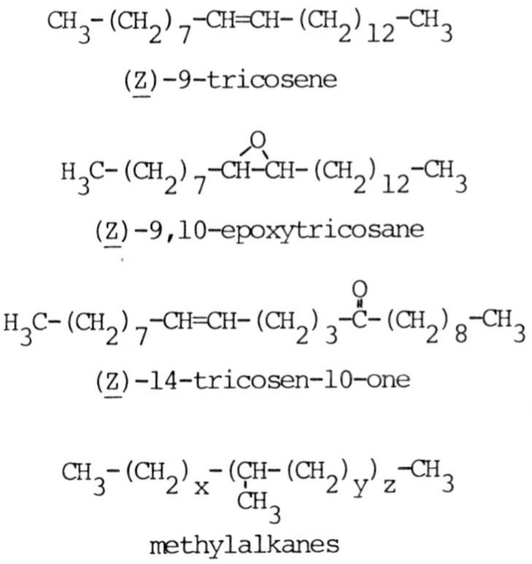

$$CH_3-(CH_2)_7-CH=CH-(CH_2)_{12}-CH_3$$

$$(\underline{Z})-9-\text{tricosene}$$

$$H_3C-(CH_2)_7-\overset{\overset{\text{O}}{\diagup\diagdown}}{CH-CH}-(CH_2)_{12}-CH_3$$

$$(\underline{Z})-9,10-\text{epoxytricosane}$$

$$H_3C-(CH_2)_7-CH=CH-(CH_2)_3-\overset{\overset{\text{O}}{\|}}{C}-(CH_2)_8-CH_3$$

$$(\underline{Z})-14-\text{tricosen-10-one}$$

$$CH_3-(CH_2)_x-\underset{\underset{CH_3}{|}}{(CH}-(CH_2)_y)_z-CH_3$$

methylalkanes

Fig. 2.   Structures of the pheromone components of the housefly, *Musca domestica.*

determined both the relative rate of pheromone biosynthesis (with radiotracers) and the total amount of pheromone.

Females with previtellogenic ovaries at stage 2 or 3 do not have detectable amounts of any of the C_{23} sex pheromone components (Dillwith *et al.,* 1983) (Table II). Z9-23 : Hy, the C_{23} epoxide, and the C_{23} ketone first appeared on females with early vitellogenic (stage 4) ovaries and increased steadily to a maximum by stage 8 (Dillwith *et al.,* 1983) (Table II). The amount of methylalkanes also increased during oogenesis from 3.9 µg/fly at stage 4 to 6.5 µg/fly at stage 8.

These data were consistent with observations correlating female attractancy in an olfactometer to the stage of oogenetic development. Females with stage 2 or 3 ovaries (previtellogenic) did not attract males, but females with ovaries at stages 4 through 10 readily attracted males (Adams *et al.,* 1984b). Thus, behavioral data complemented the chemical analyses of the timing of housefly sex pheromone production.

The pheromone components of the housefly are modified cuticular lipids. Newly emerged males and females have similar cuticular lipid profiles; the major hydrocarbon components are (Z)-9-alkenes in which the C_{27} homolog predominates (Adams *et al.,* 1984a). From stages 4 through 8, both the percentage of alkenes and the percentage of Z9-27 : Hy in the alkene fraction decrease while the percentage of Z9-23 : Hy increases. Since Z9-23 : Hy is readily converted to both C_{23} epoxide and ketone (Blomquist *et al.,* 1984b), the increase in Z9-23 : Hy is mirrored by a concomitant increase in the C_{23} epoxide and ketone.

The incorporation of radioactivity from [1-^{14}C]acetate into the C_{23} sex phe-

TABLE II

**Correlation of Ovarian Development with Sex
Pheromone Production and Ecdysteroid Titers**

	Ovarian stage	Ecdysteroid titer[a] (pg/μl hemolymph)	C_{23} Pheromone components[b] (μg/insect)
Previtellogenic	2	15	0
	3	12	0
Vitellogenic	4	26	0.8
	5	45	1.3
	6	45	1.3
	7	45	1.7
	8	21	2.0
Postvitellogenic	9	10	1.9
	10	10	2.1
−Ovaries	—	5.2[c]	0

[a]Data from Adams et al., 1985.
[b]Data from Dillwith et al., 1983.
[c]Two-day-old insects.

romone components followed a pattern consistent with that described above and emphasized the role that the maturing ovary plays in initiating sex pheromone production (Dillwith et al., 1983). Although the total incorporation of radioactivity into hydrocarbon varied little from stages 2 through 10, the percentage of hydrocarbon as alkenes decreased from 60–70% at stages 2 and 3 to 20–30% at stages 8–10. The percentages of alkenes present as Z9-23 : Hy changed even more dramatically (Fig. 3). Radioactivity in alkenes at stages 2 and 3 was primarily in the Z9-27 : Hy component and first appeared in Z9-23 : Hy during stage 4; from stages 7–10, the major labeled component was Z9-23 : Hy. Associated with the increased radioactivity in Z9-23 : Hy was a large increase in the incorporation of radioactivity into the C_{23} epoxide and ketone during egg stages 3 to 8 (Dillwith et al., 1983). In addition, there was a dramatic increase in the incorporation of [1-^{14}C]propionate into methylalkanes as the female became reproductively mature (Dillwith et al., 1981). Thus, both mass studies and radiotracer experiments documented the association of ovarian maturation with sex pheromone production.

C. Role of Ovary and CA–CC Complex

Since pheromone production was correlated with ovarian development, it was possible either that both processes were regulated by a common factor, such as occurs in some cockroaches and beetles where JH induces vitellogenesis and sex

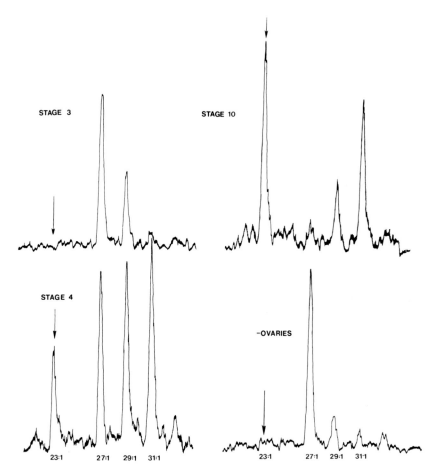

Fig. 3. Radioactivity traces from the alkene fractions of females that were injected with [1-¹⁴C]acetate. Radio-gas–liquid chromatography was performed on the alkenes from a typical previtellogenic fly with stage 3 ovaries, a vitellogenic insect with stage 4 ovaries, a postvitellogenic insect with stage 10 ovaries (6 days old), and an ovariectomized insect that was 6 days old. Each extract was prepared from 10 insects. Arrows indicate where Z9-23 : Hy elutes or would elute if present. (Reprinted from Dillwith *et al.*, 1983, Copyright © 1983, Pergamon Books Ltd.)

pheromone production, or that a product from the developing ovary was responsible for initiating pheromone production. To determine which occurs in the housefly, experiments were performed to examine the effect of removing the corpus allatum–corpus cardiacum (CA–CC) complex and of ovariectomy on sex pheromone production. Female houseflies that had the CA–CC complex removed within 6 hr of eclosion still produced Z9-23 : Hy, C_{23} epoxide, and C_{23}

ketone when assayed at 4 days postemergence (T. S. Adams, G. J. Blomquist, and J. W. Dillwith, unpublished), developed ovaries to stage 4, but did not mate (Adams and Hintz, 1969). Mating and ovarian maturation were restored in these insects by methoprene injections (Adams *et al.*, 1984b). This suggested that JH or other products from the CA–CC complex were not directly required for C_{23} pheromone production. In contrast, flies ovariectomized within 6 hr of emergence did not produce detectable amounts of Z9-23 : Hy, C_{23} epoxide, or C_{23} ketone when assayed at 4 or 6 days after emergence (Fig. 3), indicating that a product from the maturing ovary was required for sex pheromone production (Dillwith *et al.*, 1983).

Females that were ovariectomized did not attract males in the olfactometer (Adams *et al.*, 1984b) but mated normally (Adams and Hintz, 1969). Furthermore, males courted ovariectomized flies and inseminated them if they extended their ovipositor. This indicates that visual cues are important for successful courtship and mating. The female-produced attractants appear to be regulated by an ovarian factor whereas female mating behavior is regulated by a factor from the CA–CC complex.

If a product from the developing ovary were involved in inducing sex pheromone synthesis, then implantating ovaries into ovariectomized insects should restore pheromone production. Insects ovariectomized within 6 hr of emergence were implanted on day 4 with stage 2 and 3 ovaries from 12- to 24-hr-old donors and were maintained for 3–4 days. All of the implants reached the vitellogenic phases of development with stages varying from 4 to 6. Analysis of the incorporation of [1-^{14}C]acetate showed that Z9-23 : Hy was synthesized at levels similar to those found in stage 5 females (Adams *et al.*, 1984a). Thus, a product from the ovary stimulated pheromone synthesis and provided evidence for the hypothesis that housefly sex pheromone biosynthesis was humorally mediated.

IV. ENDOCRINE REGULATION OF PHEROMONE PRODUCTION

A. Early Observations

Since females of some insects have repeated reproductive cycles and mate only during specific periods within each cycle, it was suggested that pheromone production might be humorally mediated. Engelmann (1960) first suggested that products from the corpora allata mediated sex pheromone production in the female cockroach *Leucophaea maderae*. Subsequent studies with the Cuban cockroach, *Byrsotria fumigata* (Barth, 1961, 1962), showed that females required functional corpora allata to produce sex pheromone. Allatectomized females did not produce sex pheromone nor did they mate (Barth, 1961, 1962;

Barth and Bell, 1970), but the implantation of corpora allata or application of JH restored sex pheromone production (Barth, 1962; Bell and Barth, 1970). Furthermore, JH was shown to mediate sex pheromone production in other insects, such as the cockroaches *Pycnoscelus indicus* (Barth, 1965), *Periplaneta americana* (Barth, 1965), and *Blaberus discoidalis* (Barth and Lester, 1973) and the beetles *Tenebrio molitor* (Menon, 1970, 1976), *Ips paraconfusus* (Hughes and Renwick, 1977; Borden et al., 1969), and three species of *Pityokteines* (Harring, 1978). Since JH induced vitellogenesis and regulated ovarian development in many insect species, the observation that JH also regulated sex pheromone production suggested that the same hormone may be used to coordinate different reproductive events (see review by Blomquist and Dillwith, 1983).

B.   Ecdysteroids Induce Sex Pheromone Production

1.   Role in Females

In many Diptera, ecdysteroids have been shown to play a role in regulating reproductive processes, including vitellogenin synthesis (Adams et al., 1985; Hagedorn, 1985; Bownes, 1986; Huybrechts and De Loof, 1977, 1981; Jowett and Postlethwait, 1980). To determine if ecdysteroids would restore sex pheromone production in ovariectomized flies, a single large dose (10 µg/insect) of 20-hydroxyecdysone was injected into insects that had been ovariectomized within 6 hr after emergence. Flies were analyzed for [1-^{14}C]acetate incorporation into C_{23} pheromone at various postinjection times. Although no detectable incorporation of [1-^{14}C]acetate into Z9-23 : Hy was observed at 8 hr, increasing levels of incorporation were observed at 16 and 24 hr (Adams et al., 1984a). Furthermore, a single injection of 10 µg of 20-hydroxyecdysone into ovariectomized flies resulted in 18% incoporration of the label into alkenes to be in Z9-23 : Hy by 24 hr postinjection (Adams et al., 1984a). Even this amount of 20-hydroxyecdysone did not induce the pattern that was found in 4-day controls. There was also a time-dependent increase in [1-^{14}C]propionate incorporated into methylalkanes after 20-hydroxyecdysone injection.

Because of the controversy concerning the requirements for large doses of 20-hydroxyecdysone to induce vitellogenin synthesis in mosquitoes (Hagedorn, 1983, 1985; Borovsky and Van Handel, 1979; Fuchs and Kang, 1981; Lea, 1982; Bownes, 1986; Borovsky et al., 1985, 1986), the dosage of 20-hydroxyecdysone needed to induce sex pheromone production in the housefly was examined. Studies to monitor the removal of free ecdysteroid from the hemolymph were also performed, and it was shown that 20-hydroxyecdysone was metabolized very rapidly with a half-life of 16 min (Adams et al., 1985). Since it took 16 hr to detect C_{23} pheromone synthesis after the injection of 20-hydroxyecdysone, it was reasoned that high hormone doses were needed to maintain the necessary hemolymph titer over the time period required to obtain detectable amounts of C_{23} pheromone. This was examined further by injecting smaller doses of 20-hydroxyecdysone repeatedly at regular intervals into ovariectomized flies. Doses as small as 50 ng injected repeatedly at 3- to 4-hr intervals into ovariectomized flies induced Z9-23 : Hy synthesis (Adams et al., 1984a). Thus, although these doses were still many times the physiological levels, these data supported the hypothesis that an ecdysteroid produced by the ovary is the physiological inducer of sex pheromone synthesis.

2.   Ecdysteroids in Vivo

Hemolymph ecdysteroid levels cycled during oogenesis from a low of 10–15 pg/μl at stages 2 and 3 and again at stages 9 and 10 to a high of 40–50 pg/μl at stage 6 or 7 (Table II) (Adams et al., 1985). Ovariectomized flies had lower ecdysteroid levels at 2 days than controls (5 versus 27 pg/μl), but by 6 days postemergence ecdysteroid levels were 22 pg/μl and did not differ from the controls. Flies without the CA–CC complex contained about 10 pg/μl of ecdysteroid at both 2 and 6 days postemergence. Thus, a discrepancy exists; ovariectomized flies with higher ecdysteroid levels than those without the CA–CC complex do not synthesize C_{23} pheromone whereas those without the CA–CC complex do. Subsequent studies utilizing high-pressure liquid chromatography–radioimmunoassay (HPLC–RIA) showed that 20-hydroxyecdysone levels varied from 3 to 5.6 pg/μl in 4-hr, 2-day, 4-day, and ovariectomized flies. In contrast, ecdysone levels varied from 0.04 to 0.4 pg/μl in newly emerged and ovariectomized flies, reached a peak of 3.3–3.6 pg/μl in 2-day old insects, and declined to 1.1–1.6 pg/μl in 4-day-old flies (Kelly et al., 1986). Direct comparisons between the ecdysteroid levels in these studies (Adams et al., 1985; Kelly et al., 1986) cannot be made because different antisera were used and some ecdysteroid was lost during HPLC purification. The data do suggest that ecdysone production by the developing ovary is responsible for the elevated levels of total ecdysteroid that was observed during mid-vitellogenesis. The roles of ecdysone, 20-hydroxyecdysone, and their titer fluctuations in inducing C_{23} pheromone synthesis require further study.

3.   Role in Males

Vitellogenin is normally produced only by females, but the injection of 20-hydroxyecdysone into males of Drosophila melanogaster (Bownes, 1982) and Sarcophaga bullata (Huybrechts and De Loof, 1977, 1981) induced vitellogenin synthesis. Thus, experiments were performed to determine whether male houseflies, which do not produce C_{23} sex pheromone and produce only small amounts of methylalkanes, could be induced to produce female-specific pheromone after ovary implants or injections of 20-hydroxyecdysone.

Implanting ovaries or injecting 20-hydroxecdysone into male houseflies induced sex pheromone production, including production of Z9-23:Hy (muscalure), C_{23} epoxide, and C_{23} ketone, which normally occurs only in vitellogenic females (Blomquist *et al.*, 1984a). Control males did not produce detectable amounts of these compounds. Injection of 20-hydroxyecdysone (5 μg/insect per day) for 3 days resulted in the accumulation of 1.81 μg/insect of Z9-23:Hy, 0.97 μg/insect of C_{23} epoxide, and 0.12 μg/insect of C_{23} ketone. Multiple injections of 20-hydroxyecdysone at doses as low as 50 ng (1) resulted in the accumulation of Z9-23:Hy, C_{23} epoxide, and C_{23} ketone; (2) shifted the distribution of label within the alkenes from Z9-27:Hy to Z9-23:Hy; and (3) decreased the amount of label in the hydrocarbon fractions as alkenes. The chemical identity of the C_{23} alkene and epoxide produced by the males was verified by gas chromatography–mass spectrometry (Blomquist *et al.*, 1984a).

Radioactivity from [1-^{14}C]acetate was incorporated into the C_{23} alkene (Fig. 4), epoxide, and ketone in male insects after ovaries were implanted or after they were injected with 20-hydroxyecdysone. Synthesis of the C_{23} pheromone components decreased rapidly within several days after the administration of 20-hydroxyecdysone, indicating that the enzymes involved in sex pheromone production were not permanently induced by hormone treatment. Ecdysone was also effective in initiating pheromone production in males, whereas inokosterone and cholesterol were not effective. These data demonstrate that male houseflies possess the metabolic capability to produce the sex pheromone components, and this suggests that 20-hydroxyecdysone alters the production of cuticular hydrocarbons such that the C_{23} sex pheromone components become major products.

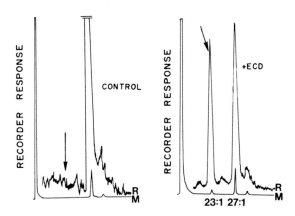

Fig. 4. Radio-gas–liquid chromatography traces of the alkenes of control and 20-hydroxyecdysone (ECD)-treated male houseflies. Arrows indicate where Z9-23:Hy elutes or would elute when present. M is the mass trace; R is the radioactivity trace. (Reprinted from Blomquist *et al.*, 1984a, Copyright © 1984, Pergamon Books Ltd.)

Work is currently being pursued in our laboratory (G.J.B.) to determine which enzymes are affected by 20-hydroxyecdysone.

C. Models for Endocrine Regulation of Pheromone Production

Barth (1965) presented a model that was designed to predict the types of insects that would have pheromone production under endocrine regulation. The females of these species would be characterized by (1) long life span, (2) multiple cycles of egg development, and (3) multiple matings interspersed with intervals when mating would not be advantageous. Insects not having pheromone production so regulated would be characterized by (1) short life span, (2) initiation of reproduction shortly after emergence, (3) monocoitic behavior, and (4) no cyclical egg production, i.e., females lay their eggs and then die. The housefly does not fit into either of these groups because (1) its life span is 2 weeks to 1 month, (2) it produces eggs in cycles, (3) it mates once (monocoitic), and (4) it mates soon after emergence (2 days) and oviposits at 3 days and then at subsequent intervals of 2–3 days.

Many but not all of the insects that regulate pheromone production by hormones (Raina and Menn, Chapter 5, this volume) have several things in common (Table III). These insects produce eggs in cycles and some cannot control phe-

TABLE III

Selected Examples of Female Insects That Regulate Pheromone Production with Hormones

Classification	Pheromone site	Hormone/ gland	Eggs develop in cycles	References
Dictyoptera				
Leucophaea maderae	—	CA	+	Engelmann, 1960
Pycnoscelus indicus	—	CA	+	Barth, 1965
Byrsotria fumigata	—	CA, JH	+	Barth, 1962; Bell and Barth, 1970
Blattella germanica	Surface	CA, JH	+	C. Shal, unpublished
Blaberus discoidalis	—	CA	+	Barth and Lester, 1973
Coleoptera				
Tenebrio molitor	Surface	CA, JH	+	Menon, 1976
Diptera				
Musca domestica	Surface	Ovary, ecdysone	+	Adams *et al.*, 1984a

romone release behaviorally because the pheromone is present on their cuticular surface. They are different from most other insect species which produce sex pheromones in glandular structures and which can control the release of pheromone behaviorally by extruding or exposing the gland during "calling behavior." Thus it appears important for the insect to regulate the release of pheromone either behaviorally or by initiating or terminating its synthesis. We suggest that many of the insects that regulate pheromone production by hormones would have the following characteristics: (1) the insects would have cycles of synchronous egg production that are regulated by cyclic hormone levels and (2) they would have no behavioral control over pheromone release.

Thus far, the hormone regulation of pheromone biosynthesis has been demonstrated in only one dipteran, *Musca domestica*. *Musca domestica* females show changes in their hydrocarbon profiles during the first gonotrophic cycle of ovarian maturation, and these changes do not occur in males (Dillwith *et al.*, 1983; Nelson *et al.*, 1981). Other Diptera demonstrating this pattern change include *Musca autumnalis* (Uebel *et al.*, 1975b), *Fannia femoralis* (Uebel *et al.*, 1978b), and *Stomoxys calcitrans* (Harris *et al.*, 1976), thus indicating that pheromone synthesis may be under humoral control.

Another situation that indicates a possible humoral involvement in sex pheromone biosynthesis includes flies which become attractive during a particular period during each gonotropic cycle, such as *Bradysia impatiens* (Alberts *et al.*, 1981), *Culicoides nubeculosus* (Ismail, 1982), *Hippelates collusor* (Adams and Mulla, 1968), and *Lucilia cuprina* (Bartell *et al.*, 1969), or show cycles in pheromone levels as in *Dacus oleae* (Mazomenos, 1984).

Thus it can be seen that much more remains to be done on the endocrine control of pheromone biosynthesis in Diptera, and there are many economically and medically important species for further study.

V. BIOSYNTHESIS OF SEX PHEROMONES IN DIPTERA

As in other insects, much more is known about the biology and chemistry of dipteran pheromones than about their biosynthesis. Extensive biosynthetic studies on pheromones have been done only with the housefly, *Musca domestica*, and the pathways in this insect are now well understood. Additional work has been performed on the biosynthesis of the pheromone of the tsetse fly, *Glossina morsitans morsitans*. In both of these insects, the sex pheromones are closely related to the hydrocarbon components of the epicuticular wax layer (Table I). The biosynthetic pathways for cuticular hydrocarbons have been studied in a number of non-dipteran species and apply directly to dipteran sex pheromone biosynthesis (Blomquist and Dillwith, 1985).

A. Site of Biosynthesis

The synthesis of insect cuticular hydrocarbons is carried out by either epidermal cells or oenocytes (Diehl, 1975; Domer, 1980). However, Schlein *et al.* (1980) reported that in both the housefly and tsetse fly the pheromone was produced by a unicellular gland on the legs of the female. In subsequent studies, using radiolabeled substrates, it was shown that C_{23} pheromone synthesis occurred in the housefly abdominal integument with the subsequent transfer of the pheromone to the legs of the insect through grooming (Dillwith and Blomquist, 1982). Thus, a large portion of the total pheromone was found on the legs of the female even though very little biosynthesis occurred on the legs. This could explain Schlein *et al.*'s (1980) bioassay data implicating a gland on the legs as the site of pheromone biosynthesis. The specific cells responsible for the production of the housefly pheromone have not yet been identified.

Using radiotracer methods, Langley and Carlson (1983) showed that pheromone synthesis in the female tsetse fly also occurred mainly in the abdominal cuticle. Using bioassay methods to measure pheromone production (Ismail and Kremer, 1983; Ismail and Zachary, 1984), it was found that the abdomen was the source of pheromone in the hematophagous Diptera, *Culicoides nubeculosus.* Thus it appears that in Diptera which use modified cuticular lipids as sex pheromones, biosynthesis occurs in cells associated with the abdominal cuticle.

A specialized pheromone gland does not exist in the housefly, as is the case for the majority of Diptera (Table I); rather, pheromone synthesis occurs through the biosynthetic pathways that produce cuticular lipids. The specificity of the enzymes involved in cuticular lipid biosynthesis are apparently modified to produce the sex pheromone components. The male housefly can also synthesize sex pheromone components when properly stimulated (see Section IV,B,3, this chapter). Thus, both male and female insects possess the basic genetic information and metabolic systems necessary for pheromone production (Blomquist *et al.*, 1984a).

B. Biosynthetic Pathways of the Housefly Sex Pheromone

1. (Z)-9-Tricosene

The synthesis of Z9-23 : Hy in female houseflies occurs by the elongation of oleoyl-CoA to a 24-carbon fatty acyl moiety which is then converted to an alkene one carbon shorter (Blomquist and Dillwith, 1985). The synthesis of this C_{23} pheromone component is humorally regulated (see Section IV,B). Through the use of radiolabels and stable isotopes it was shown that the female insect synthesized Z9-23 : Hy from acetate (Dillwith *et al.*, 1981, 1982) (Fig. 5). The pathway involves the synthesis of stearic acid which is then desaturated at the Δ^9 position to produce oleic acid (Z9-18 : Acid). This reaction involves a microsomal acyl-

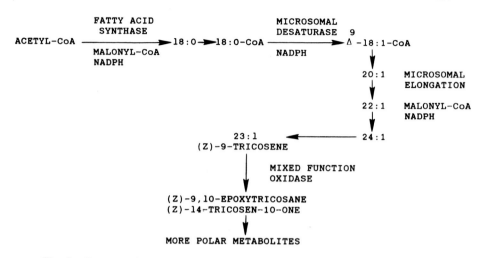

Fig. 5. Summary of the biochemical pathways involved in the metabolism of the C_{23} sex pheromones in the housefly.

CoA desaturase which can utilize NADPH or NADH as the electron donor (Wang *et al.*, 1982). Oleic acid from storage or dietary sources may enter the pathway at this point. The oleic acid is then elongated to form n9-24:1 (Z15-24:Acid) by a microsomal elongation system. The elongation of oleoyl-CoA to 20-, 22-, and 24-carbon monounsaturated acyl derivatives requires malonyl-CoA and either NADPH or NADH and has been demonstrated in microsomal preparations by both radio-gas–liquid chromatography (radio-GLC) (de Renobales *et al.*, 1986) and radio-high-pressure liquid chromatography (radio-HPLC) (Vaz *et al.*, 1987). Microsomes prepared from abdomens have higher activity than those prepared from either thorax or head tissue (Vaz *et al.*, 1987). The resulting 24-carbon acyl moiety is then apparently converted to Z9-23:Hy. *In vivo*, the enzyme systems that elongate oleoyl-CoA and then convert the acyl moiety to an alkene are apparently tightly coupled; once oleic acid enters the system, the elongation and conversion to hydrocarbon occur without release of intermediates.

In the housefly, as in most other insects, long-chain fatty acids are not found. When [15,16-³H]tetracosanoic acid was injected into female insects, it was not converted to *n*-tricosane but was metabolized to shorter chain fatty acids (16:0 and 18:0) (J. W. Dillwith and G. J. Blomquist, unpublished observations). This rapid chain shortening of long-chain fatty acids suggests that if fatty acids are released during the elongation process they are rapidly chain-shortened and thus do not show up in the fatty acid profiles. The synthesis of *n*-tricosane also occurs in the female housefly, but its desaturation to Z9-23:Hy does not occur (Dillwith *et al.*, 1981).

The hydrocarbon biosynthetic pathway in which oleic acid serves as a precursor is used to produce other cuticular alkenes (Dillwith *et al.*, 1981). The major difference is the chain length at which elongation is terminated. The specificity of the chain length is under hormonal control, and it represents a major difference between male and female houseflies (see Section IV,B). Both males and females appear to have the same biosynthetic mechanisms that can be modified to produce the appropriate chain-length alkenes to give the insects their characteristic age- and sex-dependent alkene patterns.

2. (Z)-9,10-Epoxytricosane and (Z)-Tricosen-10-one

The two pheromone components (Z)-9,10-epoxytricosane and (Z)-14-tricosen-10-one occurred only on females and appeared at the inception of Z9-23 : Hy synthesis (Blomquist *et al.*, 1984b). These findings and the structures of these two components suggested that they were derived from Z9-23 : Hy. The distribution of the epoxide and ketone on the insect body coincided with that of Z9-23 : Hy. The application of 9,10-^{3}H-labeled Z9-23 : Hy to the cuticle of female houseflies resulted in the appearance of labeled epoxide and ketone. The metabolism of Z9-23 : Hy applied to the surface of the insect apparently involves transport of the hydrocarbon through the cuticle followed by a mixed-function oxidase reaction (Ahmad *et al.*, 1987). This internalization and oxidation is apparently chain-length specific because Z9-27 : Hy is not oxidized, nor are other longer chain alkenes.

Various body parts of both male and female insects, including antennae, legs, fat body, thorax, and abdominal cuticle, converted Z9-23 : Hy to the corresponding C_{23} epoxide and C_{23} ketone. The highest rates of metabolism occurred in the antennae of male insects. More polar metabolites of 9,10-^{3}H-labeled Z9-23 : Hy have been isolated and tentatively identified as mono- and dihydroxy derivatives (Ahmad *et al.*, 1987). These data suggest that one function of the oxidation reactions in male insects is to initiate catabolism of the pheromone to prevent attenuation, perhaps functionly analogous to the esterase activity in many moths. The roles of esterases, alcohol oxidases, and dehydrogenases are discussed in Chpater 4 (Morse and Meighen, this volume). The role of mixed-function oxidases in beetle pheromone biosynthesis is examined in depth in Chapter 6 (Vanderwel and Oehlschlager). Finally, chemical studies of epoxide hydration, ω-oxidation, and other functional group transformations of pheromone catabolism in termites and in moths are described in Chapter 14 (Prestwich).

Both microsomal and mitochondrial preparations from male and female insects converted Z9-23 : Hy to the corresponding epoxide and ketone in the presence of NADPH (Ahmad *et al.*, 1987), with the microsomes having the highest activity. Piperonyl butoxide, a mixed-function oxidase inhibitor, markedly decreased the rate of metabolism by microsomal fractions but had no effect on the

mitochondrial activity. Piperonyl butoxide also affected the amounts of other more polar metabolites formed from Z9-23 : Hy. Thus it appears that mixed-function oxidase enzymes (Hodgson, 1985) play a critical role in both the synthesis of the C_{23} pheromone components in females and the catabolism of the C_{23} pheromone components in males.

3. Methylalkanes

The methylalkanes which act as "arrestants" are synthesized by a system similar to that involved in the production of the alkene components. The unique feature of this pathway is the insertion of a methylmalonyl unit in place of an malonyl unit during chain elongation which results in branching methyl groups in the final product (Blomquist and Dillwith, 1985). Our current knowledge of how methyl-branched alkanes are synthesized in the housefly is summarized in Fig. 6. Methyl-branched hydrocarbons occur in both male and female flies but are major components only in females (Nelson et al., 1981).

Radiotracer studies showed that female houseflies could synthesize methylalkanes from acetate and propionate (Dillwith et al., 1981). It was shown by radio-GLC that [1-^{14}C]propionate labeled only methyl-branched hydrocarbon. This specific labeling allowed methyl-branched hydrocarbon synthesis to be

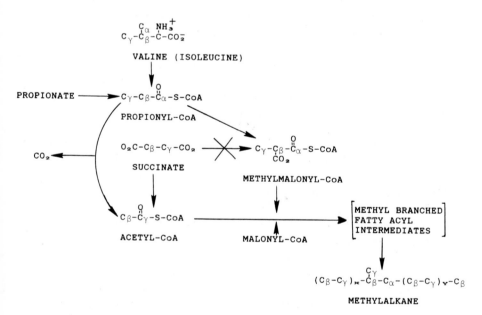

Fig. 6. Summary of the biochemical pathways involved in methylalkane synthesis in the housefly.

monitored. By using this method, it was shown that methyl-branched hydrocarbon synthesis increased dramatically at 2 days postemergence and coincided with Z9-23 : Hy production.

An important discovery regarding propionate metabolism in the housefly came from studies with propionates labeled in different positions. When [2-^{14}C]propionate or [3-^{14}C]propionate was injected into houseflies the alkenes were labeled in the same manner as that observed from labeled acetate, whereas [1-^{14}C]propionate did not label the alkenes. Studies using propionate labeled with ^{13}C in the 1, 2, or 3 position confirmed that propionate was metabolized via an acetate unit. The pathway involves the loss of the number 1 carbon of propionate with the number 3 carbon of propionate becoming the carboxyl carbon of acetate and the 2 carbon of propionate becoming the methyl carbon of acetate (Dillwith *et al.*, 1982; Halarnkar *et al.*, 1986). The pathway involves the hydroxylation of propionate in the 3 position and is entirely mitochondrial.

It is possible that the conversion of propionate to acetate in the housefly results from the absence of the methylmalonyl-CoA mutase reaction which interconverts methylmalonyl-CoA and succinate in mammals. The housefly lacks vitamin B$_{12}$ which serves as a cofactor for the mutase reaction (Wakayama *et al.*, 1984). This is supported by studies with [2,3-^{13}C]succinate which showed that succinate did not serve as a source of the methyl-branching carbon in the housefly (Dillwith *et al.*, 1982) as it did in a termite (Blomquist *et al.*, 1980). Instead, in the housefly, succinate labels hydrocarbons in the same pattern as acetate, which suggests that succinate can be metabolized to acetate via the tricarboxylic acid cycle to malate and then to pyruvate by the action of the malic enzyme and then to acetate. Recent studies have shown that [2,3-^{13}C]succinate labels saturated hydrocarbons in the housefly with labeling patterns demonstrating that carbons 2 and 3 are metabolized via acetate and that the housefly contains high levels of the malic enzyme (Halarnkar *et al.*, 1987).

Since the housefly does not appear to use succinate as a precursor of methylmalonyl-CoA for methylalkane synthesis, another source must be available. Certain amino acids can be metabolized to propionyl-CoA and methylmalonyl-CoA. In the housefly, radiolabeled valine was shown to label the methylalkanes preferentially, and incorporation increased dramatically between days 2 and 4, consistent with the initiation of pheromone synthesis (P. P. Halarnkar and G. J. Blomquist, unpublished results). Carbon-13 nuclear magnetic resonance (NMR) studies with [3,4,5-^{13}C]valine confirmed that it can efficiently serve as a precursor to methylalkanes (Dillwith *et al.*, 1982) (Fig. 7) and showed that the labeled carbons become the methyl branch, the tertiary carbon, and the carbon adjacent to the tertiary carbon. In addition, a portion of the labeled valine was converted to acetate and labeled carbons 1 and 2 of the methylalkanes. Further studies have indicated that isoleucine, but not threonine, can also serve as the methyl-branch donor (P. P. Halarnkar and G. J. Blomquist, unpublished results).

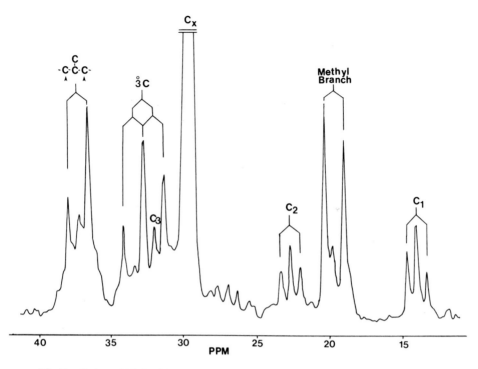

Fig. 7. Carbon-13 NMR of the methylalkanes of the housefly enriched from [3,4,5-¹³C]valine. The spectrum shows that the three labeled carbons from valine were incorporated as an intact unit to become the methyl-branch carbon, the tertiary carbon, and the carbon adjacent to the tertiary carbon. (Reprinted from Dillwith *et al.* 1982, with permission.)

The synthesis of methylalkanes involves the synthesis of a long-chain methyl-branched fatty acid which is converted to an alkane that is one carbon unit shorter (Fig. 6). As in the synthesis of the alkenes, this elongation and subsequent conversion of very long chain fatty acids to hydrocarbon must be tightly coupled since no long-chain methyl-branched fatty acids are found in the housefly. One question that arises concerning synthesis is the specificity of placement of methyl groups in the growing fatty acid chain. The housefly produces a complex mixture of methylalkanes with methyl branches in specific locations that cannot be accounted for by the random insertion of methylmalonyl-CoA during synthesis (Nelson *et al.*, 1981). Thus the specificity must either arise from the fatty acid synthase involved in the formation of the 16- and 18-carbon fatty acids or in the subsequent elongation system. It is, therefore, important to know whether the methyl branches were added early or late during synthesis. This question was answered in the housefly by feeding the female [1-¹³C]propionate which resulted in the synthesis of methylalkanes that were highly enriched with ¹³C at specific

carbons. The methylalkanes were separated and analyzed by gas chromatography coupled to a mass spectrometer. The fragmentation patterns in which the carbon-13 could be localized clearly showed that the methyl branches were added during the early part of chain synthesis (Dillwith *et al.*, 1982). Therefore, the fatty acid synthase that is involved in chain synthesis somehow determines the specific order in which methyl groups are added. The mechanism of this control is not known nor is it known if a single enzyme or multiple enzymes are involved.

4. Other Diptera

Langley and Carlson (1983) studied the biosynthesis of the sex pheromone of the tsetse fly and showed that [2,3-^{14}C]succinate labeled the cuticular hydrocarbons which contain large amounts of very long chain methyl- and dimethylalkanes. The assumption was made that succinate would specifically label methylalkanes as in the termite (Blomquist *et al.*, 1980). However, from the results with succinate in the housefly, it may be that succinate is being converted to acetate and that the radioactivity from [2,3-^{14}C]succinate is incorporated as an acetate unit. Since no data on acetate incorporation were presented in this study, direct comparisons are not possible. Succinate did label the alkene fraction, however, which suggests that at least a portion of it is probably metabolized to acetate prior to incorporation into hydrocarbon. The tsetse fly does contain vitamin B$_{12}$ (Wakayama *et al.*, 1984) suggesting the possibility that succinate could also be converted to methylmalonyl-CoA. More detailed studies are required to establish the metabolic pathways being used by this insect.

VI. SUMMARY

The number of Diptera that are reported to possess a sex pheromone is relatively small when compared to the total number of described species. Except for the tephretids, the dipteran sex pheromones are active only at close range or on contact and their release cannot be behaviorally controlled. Therefore, we hypothesize that control would be exercised at different levels, such as pheromone biosynthesis, pheromone perception, or mating behavior.

In *Musca domestica*, pheromone biosynthesis is initiated by the same hormones that induce ovarian maturation. We suggest that other dipterans demonstrating a qualitative change in cuticular lipids after the initiation of vitellogenesis should be examined for endocrine regulation of sex pheromone biosynthesis.

The ecdysteroids, ecdysone and 20-hydroxyecdysone, induced the synthesis of Z9-23 : Hy, C$_{23}$ epoxide, and C$_{23}$ ketone in ovariectomized flies and in males and also increased the amount of methylalkanes. Ecdysteroids appear to induce

the switch from Z9-27 : Hy to Z9-23 : Hy synthesis by influencing the chain elongation or chain termination process. The role of ecdysteroids in regulating the enzymes involved in this process requires examination.

Z9-23 : Hy is readily metabolized to the corresponding epoxide and ketone and to more polar products. This process involves the cytochrome P-450 enzyme system.

ACKNOWLEDGMENTS

The studies from our laboratories described here were supported in part by National Science Foundation Grants DCB-8416558 and PCM-8118305. A contribution of the Nevada Agricultural Experiment Station.

REFERENCES

Adams, T. S. (1974). The role of juvenile hormone in housefly ovarian follicle morphogenesis. *J. Insect Physiol.* **20**, 263–276.

Adams, T. S. (1981a). The role of ovarian hormones in maintaining cyclical egg production in insects. In "Advances in Invertebrate Reproduction" (W. H. Clark and T. S. Adams, eds.), pp. 109–125. Elsevier, Amsterdam.

Adams, T. S. (1981b). Activation of successive ovarian gonotrophic cycles by the corpus allatum in the housefly, *Musca domestica. Int. J. Invert. Reprod.* **3**, 41–48.

Adams, T. S., and Filipi, P. A. (1983). Vitellin and vitellogenin concentrations during oogenesis in the first gonotrophic cycle of the housefly, *Musca domestica. J. Insect Physiol.* **29**, 723–733.

Adams, T. S., and Hintz, A. M. (1969). Relationship of age, ovarian development, and the corpus allatum to mating in the housefly, *Musca domestica. J. Insect Physiol.* **15**, 201–215.

Adams, T. S., and Holt, G. G. (1987). Effect of pheromone components when applied to different models on male sexual behavior in the housefly, *Musca domestica. J. Insect Physiol.* **33**, 9–18.

Adams, T. S., and Mulla, M. S. (1968). Ovarian development, pheromone production, and mating in the eye gnat, *Hippelates collusor. J. Insect Physiol.* **14**, 627–635.

Adams, T. S., Dillwith, J. W., and Blomquist, G. J. (1984a). The role of 20-hydroxyecdysone in housefly sex pheromone biosynthesis. *J. Insect Physiol.* **30**, 287–294.

Adams, T. S., Holt, G. G., and Blomquist, G. J. (1984b). Endocrine control of pheromone biosynthesis and mating behavior in the housefly, *Musca domestica. In* "Advances in Invertebrate Reproduction 3" (W. Engels, ed.), pp. 441–456. Elsevier, Amsterdam.

Adams, T. S., Hagedorn, H. H., and Wheelock, G. D. (1985). Haemolymph ecdysteroid in the housefly, *Musca domestica,* during oogenesis and its relationship with vitellogenin levels. *J. Insect Physiol.* **31**, 91–97.

Ahmad, S., Kirkland, K. E., and Blomquist. G. J. (1987). Evidence for a sex pheromone metabolizing cytochrome P-450 monooxygenase in the housefly. *Arch. Insect Biochem. Physiol.* (in press).

Akre, R. D., Alpert, G., and Alpert, T. (1973). Life cycle and behavior of *Microdon cothurnatus* in Washington. *J. Kansas Entomol. Soc.* **46**, 327–338.

Alberts, S. A., Kennedy, M. K., and Carde, R. T. (1981). Pheromone-mediated anemotactic flight and mating behavior of the sciarid fly *Bradysia impatiens. Environ. Entomol.* **10**, 10–15.

Antony. C., and Jallon, J. (1982a). Aphrodisiaques cuticulaires de la drosophile et des dipteres. *Bull. Soc. Zool. Fr.*, 1–5.

Antony, C., and Jallon, J. (1982b). The chemical basis for sex recognition in *Drosophila melanogaster*. *J. Insect Physiol.* **28,** 873–880.

Averhoff, W. W., and Richardson, R. H. (1976). Multiple pheromone system controlling mating in *Drosophila melanogaster*. *Proc. Natl. Acad. Sci. U.S.A.* **73,** 591–593.

Baker, R., Herbert, R., Howse, P. E., Jones, O. T., Franke, W., and Reith, W. (1980). Identification and synthesis of the major sex pheromone of the olive fly, *Dacus oleae. J. Chem. Soc. Chem. Commun.* **1,** 52–54.

Bartell, R. J., Shorey, H. H., and Browne, L. B. (1969). Pheromonal stimulation of the sexual activity of males of the sheep blowfly *Lucilia cuprina* (Calliphoridae) by the female. *Anim. Behav.* **17,** 576–585.

Barth, R. H. (1961). Hormonal control of sex attractant production in the Cuban cockroach. *Science* **133,** 1598–1599.

Barth, R. H. (1962). The endocrine control of mating behavior in the cockroach *Byrsotria fumigata* (Guerin). *Gen. Comp. Endocrinol.* **2,** 53–69.

Barth, R. H. (1965). Insect mating behavior: Endocrine control of a chemical communication system. *Science* **149,** 882–883.

Barth, R. H., and Bell, W. J. (1970). Physiology of the reproductive cycle in the cockroach *Byrsotria fumigata* (Guerin). *Biol. Bull.* **139,** 447–460.

Barth, R. H., and Lester, L. J. (1973). Neuro-hormonal control of sexual behavior in insects. *Annu. Rev. Entomol.* **18,** 445–472.

Bell, W. J., and Barth, R. H. (1970). Quantitative effects of juvenile hormone on reproduction in the cockroach *Byrsotria fumigata. J. Insect Physiol.* **16,** 2303–2313.

Blomquist, G. J., and Dillwith, J. W. (1983). Pheromones: Biochemistry and physiology. *In* "Endocrinology of Insects" (R. G. H. Downer and H. Laufer, eds.), Vol. 1, pp. 527–542. Alan R. Liss, New York.

Blomquist, G. J., and Dillwith, J. W. (1985). Cuticular lipids. *In* "Comprehensive Insect Physiology Biochemistry and Pharmacology" (G. A. Kerkut and L. I. Gilbert, eds.), Vol. 3, pp. 117–154. Pergamon, Oxford.

Blomquist, G. J., Chu, A. J., Nelson, J. H., and Pomonis, J. G. (1980). Incorporation of [2,3-^{13}C]succinate into methyl branched alkanes in a termite. *Arch. Biochem. Biophys.* **204,** 648–650.

Blomquist, G. J., Adams, T. S., and Dillwith, J. W. (1984a). Induction of female sex pheromone production in male houseflies by ovarian implants or 20-hydroxyecdysone. *J. Insect Physiol.* **30,** 295–302.

Blomquist, G. J., Dillwith, J. W., and Pomonis, J. G. (1984b). Sex pheromone of the housefly: Metabolism of (Z)-9-tricosene to (Z)-9,10-epoxytricosane and (Z)-14-tricosene-10-one. *Insect Biochem.* **14,** 279–284.

Bolton, H. T., Butler, J. F., and Carlson, D. A. (1980). A mating stimulant pheromone of the horn fly, *Haematobia irritans* (L.): Demonstration of biological activity in separated cuticular components. *J. Chem. Ecol.* **6,** 951–964.

Borden, J. H., Nair, K. K., and Slater, C. E. (1969). Synthetic juvenile hormone: Induction of sex pheromone production in *Ips confusus. Science* **166,** 1626–1627.

Borovsky, D., and Van Handel, E. (1979). Does ovarian ecdysone stimulate mosquitoes to synthesize vitellogenin? *J. Insect Physiol.* **25,** 861–865.

Borovsky, D., Thomas, B. R., Carlson, D. A., Whisenton, L. R., and Fuchs, M. S. (1985). Juvenile hormone and 20-OH-ecdysone as primary and secondary stimuli of vitellogenesis in *Aedes aegypti. Arch. Insect Biochem. Physiol.* **2,** 75–90.

Borovsky, D., Whisenton, L. R., Thomas, B. R., and Fuchs, M. S. (1986). Biosynthesis and distribution of ecdysone and 20-OH-ecdysone in *Aedes aegypti. Arch. Insect Biochem. Physiol.* **3**, 19–30.

Bownes, M. (1982). The role of 20-hydroxyecdysone in yolk polypeptide synthesis by male and female fat bodies of *Drosophila melanogaster. J. Insect Physiol.* **28**, 317–328.

Bownes, M. (1986). Expression of the genes coding for vitellogenin (yolk protein). *Annu. Rev. Entomol.* **31**, 507–531.

Carlson, D. A., Mayer, M. S., Silhacek, D. L., James, J. D., Beroza, M., and Bierl, B. A. (1971). Sex attractant pheromone of the housefly: Isolation, identification and synthesis. *Science* **174**, 76–78.

Carlson, D. A., Langley, P. A., and Huyton, P. (1978). Sex pheromone of the tsetse fly: Isolation, identification, and synthesis of contact aphrodisiacs. *Science* **201**, 750–753.

Carlson, D. A., Nelson, D. R., Langley, P. A., Coates, T. W., Davis, T. L., and Leegwater-Van Der Linden, M. E. (1984). Contact sex pheromone in the tsetse fly *Glossina pallidipes* (Austen): Identification and synthesis. *J. Chem. Ecol.* **10**, 429–450.

Casartelli, C., Schrieber, L. R., Toledo, L. A., De Magalhaes, L. E., and Basilio, V. L. (1971). Sex-pheromone in *Bradysia tritici. Experientia* **27**, 1096–1097.

Chang, F., and Hsu, C. L. (1982). Effect of precocene II on sex attractancy in the Mediterranean fruitfly *Ceratitis capitata. Ann. Entomol. Soc. Am.* **75**, 38–42.

Chang, F., Hsu, C. L., Jurd, I., and Williamson, D. L. (1984). Effect of precocene and benzyl-13-benzodioxole derivatives on sex attractancy in the Mediterranean fruit fly. *Ann. Entomol. Soc. Am.* **77**, 147–151.

Chaudhury, M. F. B., Ball, H. J., and Jones, C. M. (1972). A sex pheromone of the female face fly, *Musca autumnalis,* and its role in sexual behavior. *Ann. Entomol. Soc. Am.* **65**, 607–611.

de Renobales, M., Wakayama, E. J., Halarnkar, P. P., Reitz, R. C., Pomonis, J. G., and Blomquist, G. J. (1986). Inhibition of hydrocarbon biosynthesis in the housefly by 2-octadecynoate. *Arch. Insect Biochem. Physiol.* **3**, 75–86.

Diehl, P. A. (1975). Synthesis and release of hydrocarbons by the oenocytes of the desert locust, *Schistocerca gregaria. J. Insect Physiol.* **21**, 1237–1246.

Dillwith, J. W., and Blomquist, G. J. (1982). Site of sex pheromone biosynthesis in the female housefly, *Musca domestica* L. *Experientia* **38**, 471–473.

Dillwith, J. W., Blomquist, G. J., and Nelson, D. R. (1981). Biosynthesis of the hydrocarbon components of the sex pheromone of the housefly, *Musca domestica* L. *Insect Biochem.* **11**, 247–253.

Dillwith, J. W., Nelson, J. H., Pomonis, J. G., Nelson, D. R., and Blomquist, G. J. (1982). A ^{13}C-NMR study of methyl-branched hydrocarbon biosynthesis in the housefly. *J. Biol. Chem.* **257**, 11305–11314.

Dillwith, J. W., Adams, T. S., and Blomquist, G. J. (1983). Correlation of housefly sex pheromone production with ovarian development. *J. Insect Physiol.* **29**, 377–386.

Downes, J. A. (1966). Observations on the mating behavior of the crab hole mosquito *Deinocerites cancer. Can. Entomol.* **98**, 1169–1177.

Engelmann, F. (1960). Mechanisms controlling reproduction in two viviparous cockroaches (Blattaria). *Ann. N.Y. Acad. Sci.* **89**, 516–536.

Feron, M. (1959). Attraction chimique du male de *Ceratitis capitata* pour la femelle. *Acad. Sci. Paris* **248**, 2403–2404.

Feron, M. (1962). L'instinct de reproduction chez la mouche mediteraneeane des fruits *Ceratitis capitata.* Comportement sexuel. Comportement de Poute. *Rev. Pathol. Ves. Entomol. Agric. Fr.* **41**, 1–129.

Fitt, G. P. (1981). Inter- and intraspecific responses to sex pheromones in laboratory bioassays by females of three species of tephritid fruit flies from northern Australia. *Entomol. Exp. Appl.* **30,** 40–44.

Fletcher, B. S. (1968). Storage and release of a sex pheromone by the Queensland fruit fly, *Dacus tryoni. Nature (London)* **219,** 631–632.

Fletcher, B. S. (1969). The structure and function of the sex pheromone glands of the male Queensland fruit fly, *Dacus tryoni. J. Insect Physiol.* **15,** 1309–1322.

Fletcher, B. S., and Giannakakis, A. (1973). Factors limiting the response of females of the Queensland fruit fly, *Dacus tryoni,* to the sex pheromone of the male. *J. Insect Physiol.* **19,** 1147–1155.

Fuchs, M. S., and Kang, S. H. (1981). Ecdysone and mosquito vitellogenesis: A critical appraisal. *Insect Biochem.* **11,** 627–633.

Girard, J. E., and Budris, J. P. (1975). Sex pheromone in the flesh fly, *Sarcophaga bullata. Melsheimer Entomolog. Ser.* **20,** 1–5.

Girard, J. E., Hendry, L. B., and Snetsinger, R. (1974). Sex pheromone in a mushroom infesting sciarid fly, *Lycoriella mali. Mushroom J.* **13,** 29–31.

Girard, J. E., Germino, F. J., Budris, J. P., Vita, R. A., and Garrity, M. P. (1979). Pheromone of the male flesh fly, *Sarcophaga bullata. J. Chem. Ecol.* **5,** 125–130.

Gjullin, C. M., Whitfield, T. L., and Buckley, J. F. (1967). Male pheromones of *Culex quinquefasciatus, C. tarsalis* and *C. pipiens* that attract females of these species. *Mosq. News* **27,** 382–387.

Hagedorn, H. H. (1983). The role of ecdysteroids in the adult insect. *In* "Invertebrate Endocrinology" (R. G. H. Downer and H. Laufer, eds.), Vol. 1, Endocrinology of Insects, pp. 271–304. Alan R. Liss, New York.

Hagedorn, H. H. (1985). The role of ecdysteroids in reproduction. *In* "Comprehensive Insect Physiology, Biochemistry, and Pharmacology" (G. A. Kerkut and L. I. Gilbert, eds.), Vol. 8, pp. 205–262. Pergamon, Oxford.

Halarnkar, P. P., Heisler, C. R.. and Blomquist, G. J. (1986). Propionate catabolism in the housefly *Musca domestica* and the termite *Zootermopsis nevadensis. Insect Biochem.* **16,** 455–461.

Halarnkar, P. P., Heisler, C. R., and Blomquist, G. J. (1987). Succinate metabolism in the housefly *Musca domestica:* Role of the malic enzyme. *Arch. Insect Biochem. Physiol.* (in press).

Hammack, L. (1986). Pheromone mediated copulatory response of the screwworm fly, *Cochliomyia hominivorax. J. Chem. Ecol.* **12,** 1623–1631.

Haniotakis, G. E.(1974). Sexual attraction in the olive fruit fly, *Dacus oleae. Environ. Entomol.* **3,** 82–86.

Haniotakis, G. E., Mazomenos, B. E., and Tumlinson, J. H. (1977). A sex attractant of the olive fruit fly, *Dacus oleae,* and its biological activity under laboratory and field conditions. *Entomol. Exp. Appl.* **21,** 81–87.

Harring, C. M. (1978). Aggregation pheromones of the European fir engraver beetles *Pityokteines curvidens, P. spinidens,* and *P. vorontzovi* and the role of juvenile hormone in pheromone biosynthesis. *Z. Angew. Entomol.* **85,** 281–317.

Harris, R. L., Frazar, E. D., Grossman, P. D., and Graham, O. H. (1966). Mating habits of the stable fly. *J. Econ. Entomol.* **59,** 634–636.

Harris, R. L., Oehler, D. D., and Berry, I. L. (1976). Sex pheromone of the stable fly: affect on cuticular hydrocarbon of age, sex, species and mating. *Environ. Entomol.* **5,** 973–977.

Hodgson, E. (1985). Microsomal mono-oxygenases. *In* "Comprehensive Insect Physiology, Biochemistry, and Pharmacology" (G. A. Kerkut and L. I. Gilberts, eds.), Vol. 11, pp. 225–321. Pergamon, Oxford.

Hodosh, R. J., Keough, E. M., and Ringo, J. M. (1979). The morphology of the sex pheromone gland in *Drosophila grimshawi. J. Morphol.* **161,** 177–184.

Hsu, C. L., and Chang, F. (1982). Interference with JH production as a possible cause for the effect of precocene II on sex attractancy in the Mediterranean fruit fly (Diptera: Tephritidae). *Ann. Entomol. Soc. Am.* **75**, 363–365.

Hughes, P. R., and Renwick, J. A. A. (1977). Neural and hormonal control of pheromone biosynthesis in the bark beetle *Ips confusus. Physiol. Entomol.* **2**, 117–123.

Huybrechts, R., and De Loof, A. (1977). Induction of vitellogenin synthesis in male *Sarcophaga bullata* by ecdysterone. *J. Insect Physiol.* **23**, 1359–1362.

Huybrechts, R., and De Loof, A. (1981). Effect of ecdysterone on vitellogenin concentration in haemolymph of male and female *Sarcophaga bullata. Int. J. Invert. Reprod.* **3**, 157–168.

Huyton, P. M., and Langley, P. A. (1982). Copulatory behavior of the tsetse flies *Glossina morsitans* and *G. austeni. Physiol. Entomol.* **7**, 167–174.

Huyton, P. M., Langley, P. A., Carlson, D. A., and Coates, T. W. (1980a). The role of sex pheromones in initiation of copulatory behavior by male tsetse flies, *Glossina morsitans morsitans. Physiol. Entomol.* **5**, 243–252.

Huyton, P. M., Langley, P. A., Carlson, D. A., and Schwarz, M. (1980b). Specificity of contact sex pheromones in tsetse flies *Glossina* spp. *Physiol. Entomol.* **5**, 253–264.

Ismail, M. T. (1982). Factors affecting pheromone secretion and oviposition by fertilized females of *Culicoides nubeculosus* (Diptera: Ceratopogonidae). *J. Insect Physiol.* **28**, 835–840.

Ismail, M. T., and Kremer, M. (1982). Factors associated with fertilization inducing a decrease in pheromone secretion by females of *Culicoides nubeculosus. Mosq. News* **42**, 525–526.

Ismail, M. T., and Kremer, M. (1983). Determination of the site of pheromone emission in the virgin females *Culicoides nubeculosus* Meigen (Diptera: Ceratopogonidae). *J. Insect Physiol.* **29**, 221–224.

Ismail, M. T., and Zachary, D. (1984). Sex pheromones in *Culicoides nubeculosus* (Diptera, Ceratopogonidae): Possible sites of production and emission. *J. Chem. Ecol.* **10**, 1385–1398.

Jacobson, M., Ohinata, K., Chambers, D. L., Jones, W. A., and Fujimoto, M. S. (1973). Insect sex attractants. 13. Isolation, identification, and synthesis of sex pheromones of the male Mediterranean fruit fly. *J. Med. Chem.* **16**, 248–251.

Jallon, J. M., Antony, C., and Benamar, O. (1981). Un antiaphrodisiaque produit par les males *Drosophila melanogaster* et transfere aux femelles lors de la copulation. *C. R. hebd. Seanc. Acad. Sci. Paris* **292**, 1147–1149.

Jowett, T., and Postlethwait, J. H. (1980). The regulation of yolk polypeptide synthesis in *Drosophila* ovaries and fat body by 20-hydroxyecdysone and a juvenile hormone analog. *Dev. Biol.* **80**, 225–234.

Katsoyannos, B. I. (1976). Female attraction to males in *Rhagoletis cerasi. Environ. Entomol.* **5**, 474–476.

Katsoyannos, B. I. (1982). Male sex pheromone of *Rhagoletis cerasi:* Factors affecting release and response and its role in mating behavior. *Z. Angew. Entomol.* **94**, 187–198.

Kelly, T. J., Adams, T. S., and Woods, C. W. (1986). Ecdysteroids and dipteran vitellogenesis. *In* "Symposium—Proceedings on Host-Regulated Developmental Mechanisms in Vector Arthropods" (D. Borovsky and A. Speilman, eds.), pp. 66–72. Univ. of Florida Press, Gainesville.

Kliewer, J. W., Miura, T., Husbands, R. C., and Hurst, C. H. (1966). Sex pheromones and mating behavior of *Culiseta inornata* (Diptera: Culicidae). *Ann. Entomol. Soc. Am.* **59**, 530–533.

Kostelc, J. G., Hendry, L. B., and Snetsinger, R. J. (1975). A sex pheromone complex of the mushroom-infesting sciarid fly, *Lycoriella mali* Fitch. *J. N.Y. Entomol. Soc.* **83**, 255–256.

Kostelc, J. G., Garcia, B. J., Gokel, G. W., and Hendry, L. B. (1979). Macrocyclic polyethers as probes into pheromone receptor mechanisms of a sciarid fly, *Lycoriella mali* Fitch. *J. Chem. Ecol.* **5**, 179–186.

Kostelc, J. G., Girard, J. E., and Hendry, L. B. (1980). Isolation and identification of a sex attractant of a mushroom-infesting sciarid fly. *J. Chem. Ecol.* **6**, 1–11.

Kremer, M., Ismail, M. T., and Rebholtz, C. (1979). Detection of a pheromone released by the females of *Culicoides nubeculosus* attracting the males and stimulating copulation. *Mosq. News* **39**, 627–631.

Lang, J. T. (1977). Contact sex pheromone in the mosquito *Culiseta inornata. J. Med. Entomol.* **14**, 448–454.

Lang, J. T., and Foster, W. A. (1976). Is there a female sex pheromone in the mosquito *Culiseta inornata? Environ. Entomol.* **5**, 1109–1115.

Langlev, P. A., and Carlson, D. A. (1983). Biosynthesis of contact sex pheromone in the female tsetse fly, *Glossina morsitans morsitans* Westwood. *J. Insect Physiol.* **29**, 825–831.

Langley, P. A., Pimley, R. W., and Carlson, D. A. (1975). Sex recognition pheromone in tsetse fly *Glossina morsitans. Nature (London)* **254**, 51–53.

Lea, A. O. (1982). Artifactual stimulation of vitellogenesis in *Aedes aegypti* by 20-hydroxyecdysone. *J. Insect Physiol.* **28**, 173–176.

Linley, J. R. (1983). Bodily stimulus gradients and precopulatory orientation in the midge, *Culicoides melleus. Physiol. Entomol.* **8**, 403–412.

Linley, J. R., and Carlson, D. A. (1978). A contact mating pheromone in the biting midge, *Culicoides melleus. J. Insect Physiol.* **24**, 423–427.

McKay, P. A., and Hatchett, J. H. (1984). Mating behavior and evidence of a female sex pheromone in the Hessian fly, *Mayetiola destructor* (Say) (Diptera: Cecidomyiidae). *Ann. Entomol. Soc. Am.* **77**, 616–620.

Mackley, J. W., and Broce, A. B. (1981). Evidence of a female sex recognition pheromone in the screwworm fly. *Environ. Entomol.* **10**, 405–408.

Mane, S. D., Tompkins, L., and Richmond, R. C. (1983). Male esterase 6 catalyzes the synthesis of a sex pheromone in *Drosophila melanogaster* females. *Science* **222**, 419–421.

Mazomenos, B. E. (1984). Effect of age and mating on pheromone production in the female olive fruit fly, *Dacus oleae* (Gmel.) *J. Insect Physiol.* **30**, 765–769.

Mazomenos, B. E., and Haniotakis, G. E. (1981). A multicomponent female sex pheromone of *Dacus oleae. J. Chem. Ecol.* **7**, 437–444.

Menon, M. (1970). Hormone–pheromone relationships in the beetle, *Tenebrio molitor. J. Insect Physiol.* **16**, 1123–1139.

Menon, M. (1976). Hormone–pheromone relationship of male *Tenebrio molitor. J. Insect Physiol.* **22**, 1021–1023.

Meola, R. W., Harris, R. L., Meola, S. M., and Oehler, D. D. (1977). Dietary-induced secretion of sex pheromone and development of sexual behavior in the stable fly. *Environ. Entomol.* **6**, 895–897.

Muhammed, S., Butler, J. F., and Carlson, D. A. (1975). Stable fly sex attractant and mating pheromones found in female body hydrocarbons. *J. Chem. Ecol.* **1**, 387–398.

Nation, J. L. (1972). Courtship behavior and evidence for a sex attractant in the male Caribbean fruit fly, *Anastrepha suspensa. Ann. Entomol. Soc. Am.* **65**, 1364–1367.

Nation, J. L. (1981). Sex-specific glands in tephritid fruit flies of the genera *Anastrepha, Ceratitis, Dacus* and *Rhagoletis. Int. J. Morphol. Embryol.* **10**, 121–129.

Nelson, D. R., Adams, T. S., and Pomonis, J. G. (1969). Initial studies on the extraction of the active substance inducing monocoitic behavior in houseflies, black blow flies and screw-worm flies. *J. Econ. Entomol.* **62**, 634–639.

Nelson, D. R., Dillwith, J. W., and Blomquist, G. J. (1981). Cuticular hydrocarbons of the housefly, *Musca domestica. Insect Biochem.* **11**, 186–197.

Nijhout, H. F., and Craig, G. B. (1971). Reproductive isolation in *Stegomyia* mosquitoes. III. Evidence for a sexual pheromone. *Entomol. Exp. Appl.* **14**, 399–412.

Offori, I. I., Carlson, D. A., Gadzama, N. M., and Bozimo, H. T. (1981). Sex recognition pheromone in the West African tsetse fly, *Glossina palpalis* (Robineau-Desvoidy). *Insect Sci. Appl.* **1**, 417–420.

Ohinata, K., Jacobson, M., Kobayashi, R. M., Chambers, D. L., Fujimoto, M. S., and Higa, H. H. (1982). Oriental fruit fly and melon fly: Biological and chemical studies of smoke produced by males. *J. Environ. Sci. Health* **17**, 197–216.

Pritchard, G. (1967). Laboratory observations on the mating behavior of the islands fruit fly *Rioxa pornia*. *J. Aust. Entomol. Soc.* **6**, 127–132.

Prokopy, R. J. (1982). Getting to know a fruit fly. *J. Georgia Entomol. Soc. Second Suppl.* **17**, 30–38.

Riemann, J. G., Moen, D. J., and Thorson, B. J. (1967). Female monogamy and its control in houseflies. *J. Insect Physiol.* **13**, 407–418.

Robacker, D. C., Ingle, S. J., and Hart, W. G. (1985). Mating frequency and response to male-produced pheromone by virgin and mated females of the Mexican fruit fly. *Southwest. Entomol.* **10**, 217–221.

Rogoff, W. M., Beltz, A. D., Johnsen, J. O., and Plapp, F. W. (1964). A sex pheromone in the housefly, *Musca domestica* L. *J. Insect Physiol.* **10**, 239–246.

Rogoff, W. M., Gretz, G. H., Jacobson, M., and Beroza, M. (1973). Confirmation of (Z)-9-tricosene as a sex pheromone of the housefly. *Ann. Entomol. Soc. Am.* **66**, 739–741.

Rogoff, W. M., Gretz, G. H., Sonnet, P. F., and Schwarz, M. (1980). Response of male houseflies to muscalure and to combinations of hydrocarbons with and without muscalure. *Environ. Entomol.* **9**(5), 605–606.

Romer, R. (1980). Histochemical and biochemical investigations concerning the function of larval oenocytes of *Tenebrio molitor* L. (Coleoptera, Insecta). *Histochemistry* **69**, 69–84.

Schlein, T., Galun, R., and Ben-Eliahu, M. N. (1980). The legs of *Musca domestica* and *Glossina morsitans* females as the site of sex pheromone release. *Experientia* **36**, 1174–1175.

Shorey, H. H., and Bartell, R. J. (1970). Role of a volatile female sex pheromone in stimulating male courtship behavior in *Drosophila melanogaster*. *Anim. Behav.* **18**, 159–164.

Sloane, C., and Spiess, E. B. (1971). Stimulation of male courtship behavior by female odor in *D. pseudoobscura*. *Drosophila Inform. Ser.* **46**, 53.

Sonnet, P. E., Uebel, E. C., and Miller, R. W. (1976). Sex pheromone of the face fly and compounds influencing pheromone activity. *Environ. Entomol.* **4**, 761–764.

Sonnet, P. E., Uebel, E. C., Harris, R. L., and Miller, R. W. (1977). Sex pheromone of the stable fly: Evaluation of methyl- and 1,5-dimethylalkanes as mating stimulants. *J. Chem. Ecol.* **3**, 245–249.

Spieth, H. T. (1966). Courtship behavior of endemic Hawaiian *Drosophila*. *Univ. Tex. Publ.* **6615**, 245–313.

Spieth, H. T. (1974). Courtship behavior in *Drosophila*. *Annu. Rev. Entomol.* **19**, 385–405.

Tompkins, L., and Hall, J. C. (1981). The different effects on courtship of volatile compounds from mated and virgin *Drosophila* females. *J. Insect Physiol.* **27**, 17–21.

Tychsen, P. H. (1977). Mating behavior of the Queensland fruit fly, *Dacus tryoni*, in field cages. *J. Aust. Entomol. Soc.* **16**, 459–465.

Uebel, E. C., Sonnet, P. E., Bierl, B. A., and Miller, R. W. (1975a). Sex pheromone of the stable fly: Isolation and preliminary identification of compounds that induce mating strike behavior. *J. Chem. Ecol.* **1**, 377–385.

Uebel, E. C., Sonnet, P. E., Miller, R. W., and Beroza, M. (1976b). Sex pheromone of the face fly, *Musca autumnalis* De Geer (Diptera: Muscidae). *J. Chem. Ecol.* **1**, 195–202.

Uebel, E. C., Sonnet, P. E., and Miller, R. W. (1976). Housefly sex pheromone: Enhancement of mating strike activity by combination of (Z)-9-tricosene with branched saturated hydrocarbons. *J. Econ. Entomol.* **5**, 905–908.

Uebel, E. C., Sonnet, P. E., Menzer, R. E., Miller, R. W., and Lusby, W. R. (1977). Mating stimulant pheromone and cuticular lipid constituents of the little house fly, *Fannia canicularis* (L.). *J. Chem. Ecol.* **3,** 269–278.

Uebel, E. C., Schwarz, M., Lusby, W. R., Miller, R. W., and Sonnet, P. E. (1978a). Cuticular non-hydrocarbons of the female housefly and their evaluation as mating stimulants. *Lloydia* **41,** 63–67.

Uebel, E. C., Schwarz, M., Sonnet, P. E., Miller, R. W., and Menzer, R. E. (1978b). Evaluation of the mating stimulant pheromones of *Fannia canicularis, F. pusio,* and *F. femoralis* as attractants. *Florida Entomol.* **61,** 139–144.

Vander Meer, R. K., Obin, S. M., Zawistowski, S., Sheehan, K. B., and Richmond, R. C. (1986). A reevaluation of the role of *cis*-vaccenyl acetate, *cis*-vaccenol, and esterase 6 in the regulation of mated female sexual attractiveness in *Drosophila melanogaster. J. Insect Physiol.* **32,** 681–686.

Vaz, A. H., Blomquist, G. J., Wakayama, E. J., and Reitz, R. C. (1987). Characterization of the microsomal fatty acyl elongation system in the housefly, *Musca domestica.* (In preparation.)

Wakayama. E. J., Dillwith, J. W., Howard, R. W., and Blomquist, G. J. (1984). Vitamin B_{12} levels in selected insects. *Insect Biochem.* **14,** 175–179.

Wang, D. L., Dillwith, J. W., Ryan, R. O., Blomquist, G. J., and Reitz, R. C. (1982). Characterization of the acyl-CoA desaturase in the housefly, *Musca domestica* L. *Insect Biochem.* **12,** 545–551.

Zawistowski, S., and Richmond, R. C. (1986). Inhibition of courtship and mating of *Drosophila melanogaster* by the male-produced lipid, *cis*-vaccenyl acetate. *J. Insect Physiol.* **32,** 189–192.

8

Alkaloid-Derived Pheromones and Sexual Selection in Lepidoptera

THOMAS EISNER
JERROLD MEINWALD
Section of Neurobiology and Behavior
and Department of Chemistry
Cornell University
Ithaca, New York 14853

I. INTRODUCTION

Courtship in insects may involve more than the copulatory act itself. Following the initial phases of the behavior, in which male recognition, attraction, and localization are at play, the prospective partners do not necessarily proceed at once to mate, but may first show elaborate precopulatory interactions, obviously communicative in nature. What it is that the sexes "say" to one another in that context, and why they should even "bother" to communicate once they have achieved the proximity necessary for copulation, is often a mystery.

Our primary purpose in this chapter is to describe work from our laboratories that is leading us to believe that, in certain insects at least, "foreplay" is basically a sexually selective process, involving assessment by the female of certain male traits that are a measure of an eventual benefit to the offspring. The foreplay is in the nature of a pheromone-mediated dialogue, and the insects are certain butterflies and moths. Our collaborators in these studies are former graduate students, undergraduates, and postdoctoral fellows, instrumental not only in doing much of the research but in generating and refining some of the ideas.

Pheromone Biochemistry

Much work related to these studies has been the subject of useful and in some measure highly comprehensive reviews by others (Ackery and Vane-Wright, 1984; Boppré, 1984; Edgar, 1984). Our treatment of the subject here, to the extent that it draws on work from other laboratories and shows overlap with these reviews, is different in emphasis and deliberately more speculative. We have also chosen for inclusion reference to some of our unpublished findings.

II. DANAIDONE: FIRST CHARACTERIZATION OF A HAIRPENCIL SECRETION (*Lycorea ceres*)

What kindled our interest in this area of research was the seminal paper by Brower *et al.* (1965) on the courtship of the queen butterfly, *Danaus gilippus,* and the motion picture that these investigators made of this behavior. Their data showed clearly that the two brushlike structures, or "hairpencils," that the males ordinarily keep tucked away in their abdomen are in fact everted and splayed during courtship, and brushed against the female prior to copulation. Glandular in nature, the hairpencils seemed to function as an "aphrodisiac" device that effected its action chemically. But the nature of the presumed pheromone and its precise communicative significance remained unknown.

No butterfly pheromone had previously been characterized, let alone assayed for activity, and we were intrigued by the prospects of doing so. We knew that hairpencils occurred in other danaid butterflies (family Nymphalidae; subfamily Danainae) beside the queen butterfly. Through the help of Jocelyn Crane, Lincoln Brower, and others, we were able to secure a source of *Lycorea ceres* (Fig. 1A), a beautiful tropical danaid with particularly large hairpencils (Fig. 1B). Extirpation of the brushes proved easy, and we proceeded to excise dozens of

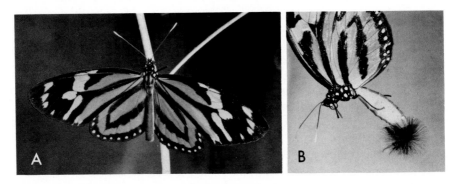

Fig. 1.   (A) *Lycorea ceres* from Trinidad. (B) Male of same, with hairpencils everted. [Photos by T. Eisner, from Meinwald *et al.,* Major components in the exocrine secretion of a male butterfly (*Lycorea*). *Science* **151**, 583–585, 1966, © AAAS.]

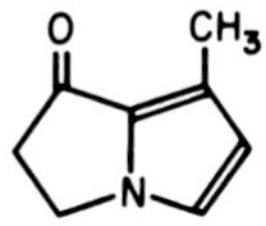

I

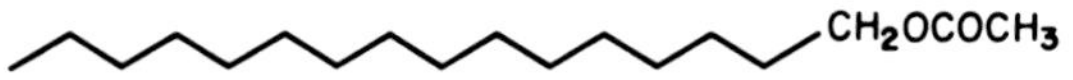

II

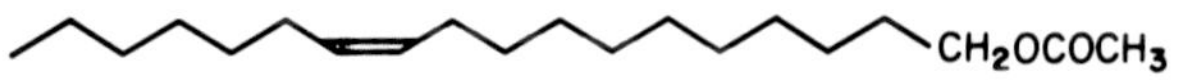

III

them for chemical extraction, partly from individuals shipped to use live from Trinidad. Three major components were characterized from these extracts, a crystalline, nitrogenous ketone, for which we could establish structure **I**, and two aliphatic esters, **II** and **III** (Meinwald *et al.*, 1966; Meinwald and Meinwald, 1966). The relative inaccessibility of *Lycorea,* plus the fact that the animal courts in dense tropical forest, made possibilities for bioassaying the compounds dim.

We were struck by one concomitant of our finding, however, and speculated at the time about its possible significance. The pyrrolizidine **I**, since named "danaidone," bore no resemblance to any previously characterized natural products except certain alkaloids, the so-called senecio or pyrrolizidine alkaloids (PAs), present not in animals but in a diversity of plants. This led us to suggest that the *Lycorea* compound might be obtained or derived from a food source (Meinwald *et al.*, 1966; Meinwald and Meinwald, 1966). We proceeded to look into the question experimentally, but were thwarted by happenstance. *Lycorea* male collection had proven relatively easy for our suppliers in Trinidad because the butterflies could be lured in numbers to senescent branches of a plant known locally as "fedegoso," a species of *Heliotropium* (Boraginaceae). We secured extracts of these plants with the intent of looking into the chemistry, but the material proved so allergenic to one of our associates that we discontinued the project. We turned instead to a study of the queen butterfly in Florida.

III. DANAIDONE: PROVEN PHEROMONAL FUNCTION
(*Danaus gilippus*)

The hairpencils of *Danaus gilippus* (Figs. 2A and 2C) turned out to be chemically similar to those of *Lycorea.* While they lacked the esters, and had instead the viscous terpenoid alcohol **IV**, they too were laden with danaidone (**I**) (Meinwald *et al.*, 1969). Structurally they were notable in that their bristles were densely beset with tiny cuticular pellets, the hairpencil "dust" (Fig. 2D). Our

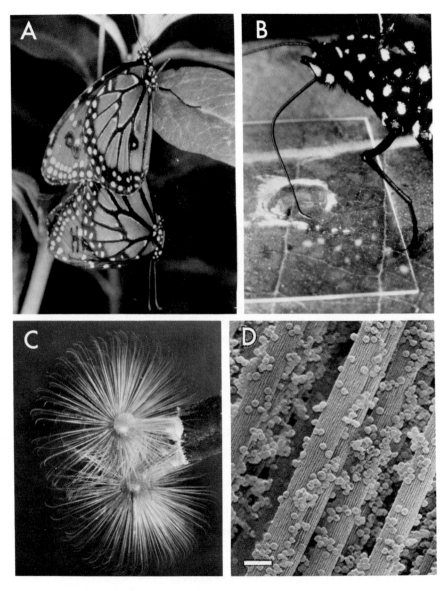

Fig. 2. *Danaus gilippus,* the queen butterfly, from Florida. (A) Mating pair; the female is hanging downward, coupled to the abdomen of the perched male. (B) Male, feeding on mono-crotaline (*N*-oxide) crystals. The animal has liquified some of the crystals with regurgitated fluid and is imbibing the solution. (C) Everted hairpencils of male. (D) Scanning electron micrograph of bristles of a hairpencil, showing the cuticular pellets that are transferred to the surface of the female during courtship and are carriers of the pheromone (danaidone, **I**). Bar = 10 μm. [(C) From Pliske and Eisner, Sex pheromones of the queen butterfly: Biology. *Science* **164,** 1170–1172, 1969, © AAAS.]

hypothesis had it that the pellets acted as a carrier for the pheromonal secretion of the hairpencils and that they were transferred to the surface of the female during precopulatory "hairpencilling." Transfer of pellets was readily demonstrated. Virgin females that were recaptured after they had been courted by males within a large experimental cage that we had built for our purposes in Florida could be shown on surface examination with powerful epi-illumination optics to bear pellets on their antennae, where principal chemoreceptors could be expected to be located.

Through an unforeseen circumstance we were able to prove that danaidone is indeed a pheromone. Male *Danaus* that we had raised indoors in cages had proven singularly unsuccessful in courtship. They pursued females normally and hairpencilled them but vis à vis wild males were only about 20% as likely to be accepted by a female. Such laboratory-raised males were found to be virtually devoid of danaidone. We did not initially know the reason for the deficiency but did find that the males were not irreversibly impotent. By subsidizing them with danaidone, added to their hairpencils either as native secretion from wild males or as synthesized material (dissolved in synthetic **IV** or in mineral oil), one could restore their potency. The danaidone, we concluded, was not only the principal communicative component of the secretion but possibly the only one. The terpene alcohol seemed to act primarily as carrier and as glue for the dust pellets (Pliske and Eisner, 1969). Independent work by Schneider and Seibt (1969) showed the antennae of *Danaus* to be electrophysiologically sensitive to danaidone but only minimally sensitive to the terpene alcohol, and Myers and Brower (1969) showed in behavioral experiments that certain antennal zones in the female are essential for chemical signal reception in courtship.

IV

Much information has been added since to our knowledge of courtship behavior in danaid butterflies. First, it is becoming clear that danaidone and closely related pyrrolizidines are very generally present in the hairpencils of these insects, having been found in a number of genera beside *Danaus* and *Lycorea* (references in Ackery and Vane-Wright, 1984). Accompanying compounds are also present, but these are variable and have been identified in only a few species (e.g., Meinwald *et al.*, 1974; Petty *et al.*, 1977).

Second and perhaps most interesting, the pyrrolizidines do indeed appear to be derived from dietary PAs (Edgar *et al.*, 1973; Edgar, 1984; Schneider *et al.*, 1975). Adult male danaids visit PA-containing plants (including species of *He-*

liotropium) and routinely feed on the fluid excrescences that ooze from senescent parts of such plants (they may even scratch the plants to induce excrescence; Boppré, 1984). Feeding on these fluids, or on PA sources that can be offered to them as laboratory alternatives (Fig. 2B), is essential if they are to produce hairpencil pyrrolizidine, hence the lack of danaidone in our laboratory-reared *Danaus* males and their consequent lack of success in courtship. Additional factors complicate the story. Subsidiary glandular structures on the wings of the males (wing pouches, scent patches), present in some (e.g., *Danaus, Amauris*) but not all danaids (e.g., *Lycorea*), which the males periodically wipe or otherwise bring into contact with the hairpencils, may contribute in important ways to the derivation of pyrrolizidine pheromone from alkaloid precursor, but the precise basis of interaction of these glandular structures remains to be clarified (Seibt *et al.,* 1972; Boppré *et al.,* 1978).

Moreover, there is one exceptional species, the monarch butterfly (*Danaus plexippus*), anomalous also by virtue of its migratory habits, which, although a visitor to PA-containing plants and a sequesterer of the PAs, fails to produce a pheromonal pyrrolizidine (Meinwald *et al.,* 1968; Pliske, 1975a; Edgar *et al.,* 1971, 1976a). These complications do not obscure the central fact: danaids as a group show male sequestration of PAs and production, by degradation of these PAs, of pheromonal pyrrolizidines. The pheromones—if generalization from the single proven case (Pliske and Eisner, 1969) of the queen butterfly is justified— serve the males as a critical key to success in mating.

Further relevant findings are being made in butterflies related to the danaines, the so-called ithomiines (family Nymphalidae; subfamily Ithomiinae). Male ithomiines have tufts of hair on the costal margins of the hindwings, which are "aired" behaviorally, as if for scent dissemination, under various conditions (aggregation, male–male interaction, female attraction), not all clearly defined or understood (Pliske, 1975b; Haber, 1978). Ithomiines also visit PA-containing plants, and chemical analyses of the wing glands showed presence of a lactone (**V**), which by virtue of its structural similarity to the acid moiety of certain PAs (such as lycopsamine, **VI**) is suspected to be a derivative of these plant products (Edgar *et al.,* 1976b).

V   V I

IV. PYRROLIZIDINE ALKALOIDS: PROVEN DEFENSIVE ROLE (*Utetheisa ornatrix*)

Pyrrolizidine alkaloids (PAs) are secondary metabolites and as such can be viewed to play defensive roles in the organisms that produce them. They are known to be toxic, certainly to vertebrates (Bull *et al.*, 1968; Mattocks, 1972), and could therefore serve in plants for protection against at least some herbivores. Sequestration of PAs by insects could thus be viewed as an adaptive strategy on their part to arm themselves with prefabricated, and hence relatively "low-cost," defenses. Since sequestration of PA is by no means restricted to adult danaids, but can potentially occur in any of the diverse insects known to feed on PA-containing plants as larvae or adults, it seemed that the strategy might be fairly widespread. Proof that PA sequestration actually conveys a defensive advantage, however, was lacking. We came upon the opportunity to provide such proof in a fortuitous way.

Work from our laboratories of some years back had shown that Lepidoptera are protected against entanglement in spiderwebs by their investiture of scales. Instead of sticking to webs as "naked" insects typically do, they simply lose scales to points of contact with an orb and flutter free (Eisner *et al.*, 1964). The site in Florida where we made these observations was the habitat of *Utetheisa ornatrix*, a well-protected aposematic arctiid moth which, like its congeners (Rothschild, 1972, 1973), feeds as a larva on PA-containing food plants (Leguminosae of the genus *Crotalaria*) (Bull *et al.*, 1968) (see Fig. 5B). *Utetheisa*, we noted, makes no effort to struggle loose in a spiderweb, but simply folds its wings and remains quiescent. The spider pounces upon it, but on contact–inspection immediately pulls it from the web or, as we observed many times with our chief experimental spider *Nephila clavipes*, frees it by severance of the entangling threads. The *Utetheisa* invariably survives uninjured.

In the laboratory we succeeded in rearing *Utetheisa* on a semisynthetic diet based on pinto beans, totally devoid of PAs (Miller *et al.*, 1976). Such moths, although visually and in every other respect indistinguishable from *Crotalaria*-fed counterparts, proved palatable to *Nephila* (Figs. 3 and 4). Further experiments provided proof that the PAs themselves are deterrent to *Nephila*. Mealworms with a topical additive of monocrotaline (**VII,** the principal PA of *Crotalaria spectabilis*, one of *Utetheisa*'s food plants) proved substantially less acceptable to the spider than untreated controls (Eisner, 1980, 1982) (Fig. 4). PA sequestration, it seemed, could be adaptive to any insect capable of withstanding systemic incoporation of the compounds, including, of course, danaid butterflies, in which the PAs could be viewed as an adult supplement of the defensive cardenolides incorporated by these insects from the milkweed plants (Asclepiadaceae) they eat as larvae (Eisner, 1980; Ackery and Vane-Wright, 1984;

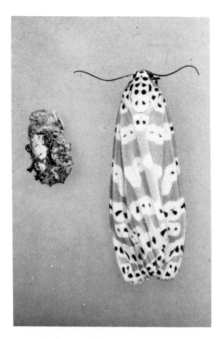

Fig. 3. *Utetheisa ornatrix* that were offered to the orb-weaving spider *Nephila clavipes*. The specimen on right, rejected intact, was raised on one of its normal, pyrrolizidine alkaloid-containing food plants (*Crotalaria mucronata*). The one on left, raised on artificial diet devoid of alkaloid, was eaten. See also Fig. 4. [From Eisner, T., *BioScience* **32**, 321, 1982, Copyright American Institute of Biological Science.]

Boppré, 1984). More recently, it has been shown that PAs may play a protective role vis à vis spiders in ithomiine butterflies as well (Brown, 1984; Vasconcellos-Neto and Lewinsohn, 1984) and may offer protection also against other predators (T. Eisner, W. Conner, and K. Hicks, unpublished results).

VII

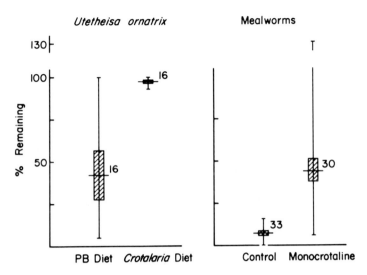

Fig. 4. Percent of prey item (*Utetheisa*, mealworms) remaining following attack by the orb-weaving spider *Nephila clavipes*. Items were placed into individual webs with forceps (mealworms) or flipped from vials (*Utetheisa*). The field-collected *Utetheisa* can be expected to have fed as larvae on normal pyrrolizidine alkaloid–containing food plants (*Crotalaria* spp.). The control *Utetheisa* were laboratory reared on alkaloid-free [pinto bean (PB)-based] diet. The experimental mealworms were treated by topical addition of 200 μg monocrotaline (free base); controls were alkaloid free. With *Utetheisa*, the percent remaining was calculated from weighings of each moth before and after the test (all field-collected *Utetheisa* survived the tests without noticeable injury; the pinto bean–fed *Utetheisa* were all killed and partly to almost totally eaten (see Fig. 3). With the mealworms, the percent remaining was calculated from final dry weight relative to mean dry weight of a sample of 10 mealworms. Sample sizes are given by numbers in parentheses. From T. Eisner, W. Conner, K. Hicks, and D. Aneshansley (unpublished).

V. HYDROXYDANAIDAL: PHEROMONAL INDICATOR OF SYSTEMIC ALKALOID LOAD (*Utetheisa ornatrix*)

A paper by Culvenor and Edgar (1972), reporting the presence of two pyr-rolizidines closely related to danaidone, danaidal (**VIII**) and hydroxydanaidal (**IX**), from the coremata (analogs of hairpencils) of Australian *Utetheisa*, set us looking into the courtship of *U. ornatrix*. The question was whether this moth also produced a corematal pyrrolizidine, and whether it used the substance for sexual communicative purposes as danaids do. The potential for parallel was striking, since these aldehydes seemed also to be derived from PAs, albeit from PAs ingested by larvae rather than adults.

CHO   OH   CHO

VIII   IX

Courtship in *Utetheisa* turned out to proceed in two stages (Conner *et al.*, 1980, 1981). The initial stage, in which the sexes are brought together, and which in danaids and other butterflies involves visual pursuit by day, is mediated by a sex attractant in *Utetheisa*. The female broadcasts the pheromone after sunset while stationary, luring males from downwind. Principal components of the attractant, which is released from a pair of tubular abdominal glands, are three C_{21} unsaturated hydrocarbons, **X, XI,** and **XII** (Conner *et al.*, 1980; Huang *et al.*, 1983; Jain *et al.*, 1983). An incidental finding—providing a first demonstration of temporal patterning in an aerial pheromonal signal—was that the secretion is released discontinuously, in short pulses, which is presumed to aid the male in pinpointing the female and to aid the female possibly in economizing on pheromonal output. Female *Utetheisa* raised on a pinto-bean diet had normal titers of attractant, indicating that production of the hydrocarbons is, as was to be expected, independent of PA intake (Conner *et al.*, 1980).

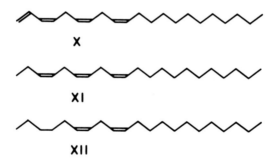

X

XI

XII

Utetheisa uses its coremata at close range during what we used to call the ''seductant'' phase of the behavior but prefer now to call the sexually selective phase. Once the male has reached the female, he flutters around her and periodically thrusts his abdomen against her, simultaneously everting the coremata. The eversions are momentary and involve direct strokings of the female (Figs. 5A and 5C). Chemical analyses showed the coremata to contain hydroxydanaidal, but only in moths reared on *Crotalaria*. Such moths proved consistently successful in courtship, unlike individuals with excised hairpencils or those raised on pinto-bean diet that were shown to be lacking in hydroxydanaidal. Further tests showed hydroxydanaidal, as its R-(−) isomer, **XIII,** to induce the

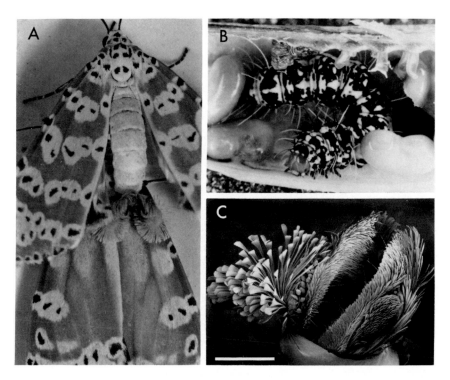

Fig. 5. *Utetheisa ornatrix.* (A) Male (above) stroking its everted coremata against female during courtship. (B) Larva, feeding on seed pod of one of its natural, pyrrolizidine alkaloid–containing food plants (*Crotalaria spectabilis*). (C) Scanning electron micrograph of abdominal tip of male, showing coremata in everted (left) and retracted condition. Bar = 1 mm. [(A) and (C) From Eisner, 1980.]

wing-raising response in females that is the usual prelude to copulation (Conner *et al.*, 1981). The pheromonal role of hydroxydanaidal seemed established, as was the apparent dependence of hydroxydanaidal production on dietary PAs.

XIII

The nagging question was whether the derivation of a sexual pheromone from phytotoxin, a phenomenon now demonstrated for two disparate phyletic lineages, was to be viewed strictly as a manifestation of metabolic expediency or whether it could be justified on entirely different adaptive grounds. What we proposed is that the pheromonal pyroolizidines could function, in both *Utetheisa* and *Danaus*, as a chemical yardstick by which the female gauges the PA load of her suitor. By exercising such assessment, and by favoring males of higher PA content, the females could be selecting for mates adept at PA sequestration, a trait that could be heritable. In *Utetheisa* the adeptness could manifest itself in improved larval competitive ability for *Crotalaria* seeds, the parts of the plant richest in PAs (Culvenor and Smith, 1957; Sawhney *et al.*, 1967), favored not only by fellow larvae but other herbivores as well (on *Crotalaria mucronata*, for example, larvae of another moth, *Etiella zinkeniella*, compete with *Utetheisa* for the seed pods). In *Danaus*, the favored male would be one with proven ability to locate and sequester PAs as an adult.

We recognized, when we advanced the hypothesis (Eisner and Conner, in Eisner, 1980), that it was contingent on a number of premises, including major uncertainties. Is sequestrative ability genetically controlled? Is the pheromonal titer a quantitative expression of PA content? While many details remain unknown, some facts are falling into place. Preliminary evidence tells us that, in *Utetheisa* at least, there is quantitative proportionality of hydroxydanaidal to body PA content. Also interesting are data from other hydroxydanaidal-producing arctiid moths (*Creatonotos* spp.) in which the *size* of the coremata is a function of systemic PA load (Schneider *et al.*, 1982; Boppré and Schneider, 1986). Whether effectiveness of the organs in courtship is also a function of size, and whether sequestrative ability finds expression through this morphogenetic effect, remains unclear. In *Creatonotos*, where the males seemingly show lek behavior, the hairpencils may also mediate aspects of female attraction and male–male interaction (Schneider, 1983). Such may be the case also in other arctiid moths (Willis and Birch, 1982).

Courtship in arctiids, as in danaids, both sizable groups, is subject to considerable adaptive variation. *Utetheisa* and *Danaus*, therefore, while illustrative of striking behavioral convergence, cannot each be taken to typify the courtship strategy of its group. We do feel, however, that the notion that close-range precopulatory interactions in insects are sexually selective in character, and that they involve assessment by the female, through indirect, measurable characters manifest by the male, of traits indicative of fitness, is worth pondering and could be broadly applicable. The courtship of that most deviant of all danaid butterflies, the monarch, might itself be interpretable in such light. Male monarchs produce no pyrrolizidine pheromone (Meinwald *et al.*, 1968) and may entirely forego use of their rudimentary hairpencils in courtship. They seize females forcibly and bring them down for mating after capture in midair (Pliske, 1975a), an approach that has been likened to rape (Rothschild, 1978). But might not the female be assessing the male for vigor when she is in his aerial grasp, and by so doing put him to the test for a trait that is eminently adaptive in the context of migration? Needless to say, such reasoning on our part, and particularly its applicability to insects other than Lepidoptera, or for that matter to animals other than insects, will itself need to be put to the test.

Most recently, evidence from our laboratories has shown that the sexually selective aspects of PA appraisal in *Utetheisa* and the queen butterfly may be fraught with yet additional complexity.

VI. PYRROLIZIDINE ALKALOIDS: PARENTAL TRANSMISSION TO EGG (*Utetheisa ornatrix* and *Danaus gilippus*)

When an *Utetheisa* female raised on a pinto-bean diet is mated with a male raised on *Crotalaria,* she lays eggs endowed with PA, indicating that she must have obtained a nuptial gift of PA from the male which she transmitted to the eggs. The experiment was not a fortuitous one but was deliberately designed to look into the possibility of seminal transfer of PA from male to female in mating (Dussourd *et al.,* 1984; J. Resch, K. Ubik, C. Harvis, and D. Dussourd, unpublished results cited in Dussourd, 1986). Within the eggs, moreover, the PA acts protectively. Coccinellid beetles, for example, which are relatively reluctant to consume eggs containing PA, find PA-free eggs (from parents both raised on a pinto-bean diet) significantly more palatable (Dussourd, 1986). The female, if herself raised on *Crotalaria,* provides a subsidy of her own PA to the eggs, complementing the amount supplied by the male. The joint contribution adds to approximately 0.5% of egg mass.

The paternal provisioning of eggs puts the sexual selective strategy of *Utetheisa* in a new light. In choosing males of high PA load, the female could be selecting not only for the genetic capacity to compete favorably in the larval race for PA but also for the immediate benefit of the PA gift that she bestows on the eggs. The two traits could be linked. Preliminary data indicate that there is in males proportionality not only of pheromonal pyrrolizidine to body PA content but of PA content to quantity of PA transmitted to the female.

It seemed obvious that there might be a comparable egg-endowment mechanism in *D. gilippus.* Males of the queen butterfly can readily be made to sequester PA in the laboratory. Crystalline monocrotaline *N*-oxide that is offered to them by the hundreds of micrograms is first liquified with regurgitated fluid and then imbibed. The males transfer the chemical largely to the reproductive accessory glands, and then at mating to the female. She in turn passes it on to the eggs (D. Dussourd, K. Ubik, and C. Harvis, unpublished results cited in Dussourd, 1986). The parallel for danaids was established and might well extend to encompass other members of the subfamily.

The story could doubtless be complicated by variation on the basic theme. In danaids, too, for example, there could be maternal contribution of PAs to the eggs, since both sexes sequester PAs as adults in some species, and in exceptional cases even as larvae from the food plants (Edgar, 1984). There are arctiids, in turn, and also species of the related family Ctenuchidae, that may sequester PAs as adults in the manner of danaids, by visitation of PA-containing plants (Pliske, 1975c; Goss, 1979) (in one species of ctenuchid, *Cisseps fulvicollis*, we have shown that PA procured by the adult male is transmitted through the female to the eggs; Dussourd *et al.*, 1984; Dussourd, 1986). And, of course, there are important questions that remain unanswered concerning the mating strategy itself. *Utetheisa* and the queen butterfly, for example, may mate with several males rather than a single one. In what sequence are the acquired PA ''gifts'' that a female obtains through multiple matings incorporated into her eggs? Does a male have paternal assurance that his gift will be allotted to eggs of his siring? And does a male ever ''lie'' about the magnitude of his potential gift? In other words, does he produce pheromone at disproportionately high levels when he is underendowed with PA? Or might deception be biochemically impossible or maladaptive for a male? Might females actually favor underendowed males under some circumstances, because such males have other, compensatory positive qualities? And can one really be certain that sequestrative ability is genetically determined?

A diversity of specifically biochemical questions also come to mind. Preliminary results suggest that *Creatonotos transiens* can produce (R)-$(-)$-hydroxy-danaidal (**XIII**) from PA esters based either on retronecine (**XIV**), which has the same absolute configuration at the corresponding asymmetric carbon atom as **XIII,** or on heliotridine (**XV**), which has the opposite configuration (Bell *et al.,* 1984; Bell and Meinwald, 1986). Does this biosynthetic plasticity reflect the ability of these insects to sequester and exploit a wide range of naturally occurring PAs for defensive purposes? What enzymatic pathways are involved in the conversion of PA to pheromone, and how are these pathways controlled? In species with male glandular wing pouches, what is the biosynthetic role of the pouch/hairpencil interaction?

XIV   **XV**

Finally, questions remain with respect to the PAs themselves. The compounds are generally regarded as defensive in plants, partly because of their toxicity (Bull *et al.,* 1968). But, vis à vis vertebrates at least, PAs are relatively innocuous as such and only become toxic after ingestion, when they are converted to pyrrolic alkylating agents by the mixed-function oxidases (MFOs) of the liver

(Mattocks, 1972). Oddly, MFOs are viewed as detoxifying agents, part of the defensive biochemical armamentarium of an organism (Brattsten, 1979). Are PAs to be regarded, in a coevolutionary sense, as an adaptive counterploy to this armamentarium, as chemicals specifically tailored by the plant to be bioactivated rather than detoxified by the MFOs of the herbivore? If so, how is one to regard an insect's ability to tolerate and sequester PAs? Do species such as *Utetheisa* and *Danaus* have a modified MFO system, or do they shield ingested PAs from exposure to MFOs? Have they, in a sense, through biochemical one-upmanship, themselves succeeded in countering the plant's defenses?

VII. POSTSCRIPT

Given the virtually explosive current interest in mating strategies and sexual selection (Blum and Blum, 1979; Rutowski, 1982; Gwynne and Morris, 1983; Thornhill and Alcock, 1983; Trivers, 1985), much is bound to be discovered about the related topic of parental investment. In insects, we feel, parental investment, and particularly parental provisioning of egg defenses, will likely be found to be widespread and to involve provisioning by either parent or both. A system currently being studied in our laboratories involves maternal endowment of eggs in *Apiomerus flaviventris,* a reduviid bug, with a surface coating of plant resin scraped by the mother from plants (e.g., the composite *Heterotheca psammophila*). The resin contains repellent terpenoids (camphor, borneol, 1,8-cineole, among others), deterrent to such egg predators as ants (T. Eisner, R. M. Silverstein, J. West, F. X. Webster, H. Hummel, M. Cazier, and G. Linsley, unpublished results). But defensive endowment by the father may be more commonplace among insects than realized. In meloid beetles, for instance, where the adult female may not produce cantharidin herself but may receive a supply of the chemical at mating (Schlatter *et al.,* 1968; Sierra *et al.,* 1976), she may transmit much of that gift to the eggs (J. Carrel and T. Eisner, unpublished results). Whether males must offer proof of their intended ''generosity'' prior to acceptance by females in such meloids remains unknown.

We feel that sexually selective strategies comparable to those of *Utetheisa* and *Danaus* are bound to be uncovered in the future (e.g., are the PAs in the eggs of the arctiid *Nyctemera annulata* partly of paternal origin? Benn *et al.,* 1979). Not nearly enough is known about the chemistry of male accessory glands, composition of spermatophores, and defensive substances in insect eggs. Nor is enough known about the numerous pheromone glands that are ''aired'' by male insects prior to mating, or even orally sampled by females, and about the chemical relationship of the products of such glands to substances that a male might transfer to the female at mating. The transferred substances, moreover, could be nutritive rather than defensive (e.g., Boggs and Gilbert, 1979; Greenfield, 1982;

Marshall, 1982; Schal and Bell, 1982), in which case the males might be assessed by females for magnitude of intended nutritive rather than defensive gift. The area of inquiry, quite clearly, is wide open, and, to the extent that it may link the field of pheromone chemistry to that of sexual selection opened by Charles Darwin over a century ago, may prove fruitful.

ACKNOWLEDGMENTS

Our studies on this general subject have been supported by the National Institutes of Health (Grants AI02908 and AI12020) and Hatch Funds. Maria Eisner was most helpful in the preparation of the illustrations and took the scanning electron micrograph in Fig. 2D. We are greatly indebted to the staff of the Archbold Biological Station, Lake Placid, Florida, where many of our studies on insect courtship were carried out.

REFERENCES

Ackery, P. R., and Vane-Wright, R. I. (1984). "Milkweed Butterflies, Their Cladistics and Biology." Cornell Univ. Press, Ithaca, New York.

Bell, T. W., and Meinwald, J. (1986). Pheromones of two arctiid moths (Creatonotos transiens and C. gangis): Chiral components from both sexes and achiral female components. J. Chem. Ecol. 12, 385–409.

Bell, T. W., Boppré, M., Schneider, D., and Meinwald, J. (1984). Stereochemical course of pheromone biosynthesis in the arctiid moth, Creatonotos transiens. Experientia 40, 713–714.

Benn, M., DeGrave, J., Gnanasunderam, C., and Hutchins, R. (1979). Host–plant pyrrolizidine alkaloids in Nyctemera annulata Boisduval: Their persistence through the life-cycle and transfer to a parasite. Experientia 35, 731–732.

Blum, M. S., and Blum, N. A. (1979). "Sexual Selection and Reproductive Competition in Insects." Academic Press, New York.

Boggs, C. L., and Gilbert, L. E. (1979). Male contribution to egg production in butterflies: Evidence for transfer of nutrient at mating. Science 206, 83–84.

Boppré, M. (1984). Chemically mediated interaction of butterflies. In "The Biology of Butterflies" (R. I. Vane-Wright and P. R. Ackery, eds.), pp. 259–275. Academic Press, New York.

Boppré, M., and Schneider, D. (1986). Pyrrolizidine alkaloids quantitatively regulate both scent organ morphogenesis and pheromone biosynthesis in male Creatonotos moths (Lepidoptera: Arctiidae). J. Comp. Physiol. A 157, 569–577.

Boppré, M., Petty, R. L., Schneider, D., and Meinwald, J. (1978). Behaviorally mediated contacts between scent organs: Another prerequisite for pheromone production in Danaus chrysippus males. J. Comp. Physiol. 126, 97–103.

Brattsten, L. B. (1979). Biochemical defense mechanisms in herbivores against plant allelochemicals. In "Herbivores, Their Interaction with Secondary Plant Metabolites" (G. A. Rosenthal and D. H. Janzen, eds.), pp. 199–270. Academic Press, New York.

Brower, L. P., Brower, J. V. Z., and Cranston, F. P. (1965). Courtship behavior of the queen butterfly, Danaus gilippus berenice. Zoologica 50, 1–39.

Brown, K. S., Jr. (1984). Adult-obtained pyrrolizidine alkaloids defend ithomiine butterflies against a spider predator. Nature (London) 309, 707–709.

Bull, L. B., Culvenor, C. C. J., and Dick, A. T. (1968). "The Pyrrolizidine Alkaloids." North Holland, New York.

Conner, W. E., Eisner, T., Vander Meer, R. K., Guerrero, A., Ghiringelli, D., and Meinwald, J. (1980). Sex attractant of an arctiid moth (*Utetheisa ornatrix*): A pulsed chemical signal. *Behav. Ecol. Sociobiol.* **7,** 55–63.

Conner, W. E., Eisner, T., Vander Meer, R. K., Guerrero, A., and Meinwald, J. (1981). Precopulatory sexual interaction in an arctiid moth (*Utetheisa ornatrix*): Role of a pheromone derived from dietary alkaloids. *Behav. Ecol. Sociobiol.* **9,** 227–235.

Culvenor, C. C. J., and Edgar, J. A. (1972). Dihydropyrrolizine secretions associated with coremata of *Utetheisa* moths (family Arctiidae). *Experientia* **28,** 627–628.

Culvenor, C. C. J., and Smith, L. W. (1957). The alkaloids of *Crotalaria spectabilis* Roth. *Aust. J. Chem.* **10,** 474–479.

Dussourd, D. (1986). Adaptations of insect herbivores to plant defenses. Ph.D. thesis, Cornell University, Ithaca, New York.

Dussourd, D., Ubik, K., Resch, J. F., Meinwald, J., and Eisner, T. (1984). Egg protection by parental investment of plant alkaloids in Lepidoptera. Abstract, *17th Intl. Congr. Entomol., Hamburg,* 840.

Edgar, J. A. (1984). Parsonsieae: Ancestral larval food plants of the Danainae and Ithomiinae. *In* "The Biology of Butterflies" (R. I. Vane-Wright and P. R. Ackery, eds.), pp. 91–93. Academic Press, New York.

Edgar, J. A., Culvenor, C. C., and Smith, L. W. (1971). Dihydropyrrolizine derivatives in hairpencil secretion of danaid butterflies. *Experientia* **27,** 761–762.

Edgar, J. A., Culvenor, C. C., and Robinson, G. S. (1973). Hairpencil dihydropyrrolizines of Danainae from the New Hebrides. *J. Aust. Entomol. Soc.* **12,** 144–150.

Edgar, J. A., Cockrum, P. A., and Frahn, J. L. (1976a). Pyrrolizidine alkaloids in *Danaus plexippus* and *Danaus chrysippus. Experientia* **32,** 1535–1537.

Edgar, J. A., Culvenor, C. C. J., and Pliske, T. E. (1976b). Isolation of a lactone, structurally related to the esterifying acids of the pyrrolizidine alkaloids, from the costal fringes of male Ithomiinae. *J. Chem. Ecol.* **2,** 263–270.

Eisner, T. (1980). Chemistry, defense, and survival: Case studies and selected topics. *In* "Insect Biology and the Future" (M. Locke and D. S. Smith, eds.), pp. 847–878. Academic Press, New York.

Eisner, T. (1982). For love of nature: Exploration and discovery at biological field stations. *BioScience* **32,** 321–326.

Eisner, T., Alsop, R., and Ettershank, G. (1964). Adhesiveness of spider silk. *Science* **146,** 1058–1061.

Goss, G. J. (1979). The interaction between moths and plants containing pyrrolizidine alkaloids. *Environ. Entomol.* **8,** 487–493.

Greenfield, M. D. (1982). The question of parental investment in Lepidoptera: male-contributed proteins in *Plodia interpunctella. Int. J. Invert. Reprod.* **5,** 323–330.

Gwynne, D. T., and Morris, G. K. (1983). "Orthopteran Mating Systems." Westview Press, Boulder, Colorado.

Haber, W. A. (1978). Evolutionary ecology of tropical mimetic butterflies. Ph.D. thesis, University of Minnesota, St. Paul.

Huang, W., Pulaski, S. P., and Meinwald, J. (1983). Synthesis of highly unsaturated insect pheromones: (Z,Z,Z)-1,3,6,9-heneicosatetraene and (Z,Z,Z)-1,3,6,9-nonadecatetraene. *J. Org. Chem.* **48,** 2270–2274.

Jain, S., Dussourd, D., Conner, W. E., Eisner, T., Guerrero, A., and Meinwald, J. (1983). Polyene pheromone components from an arctiid moth (*Utetheisa ornatrix*): Characterization and synthesis. *J. Org. Chem.* **48,** 2266–2270.

Marshall, L. D. (1982). Male nutrient investment in Lepidoptera: What nutrients should males invest? *Am. Natural.* **120**, 273–279.

Mattocks, A. R. (1972). Toxicity and metabolism of *Senecio* alkaloids. *In* "Phytochemical Ecology" (J. B. Harborne, ed.), pp. 179–200. Academic Press, New York.

Meinwald, J., and Meinwald, Y. C. (1966). Structure and synthesis of the major components in the hairpencil secretion of a male butterfly, *Lycorea ceres ceres* (Cramer). *J. Am. Chem. Soc.* **88**, 1305–1310.

Meinwald, J., Meinwald, Y. C., Wheeler, J. W., Eisner, T., and Brower, L. P. (1966). Major components in the exocrine secretion of a male butterfly (*Lycorea*). *Science* **151**, 583–585.

Meinwald, J., Chalmers, A. M., Pliske, T. E., and Eisner, T. (1968). Pheromones III. Identification of *trans,trans*-10-hydroxy-3,7-dimethyl-2,6-decadienoic acid as a major component in "hairpencil" secretion of the male monarch butterfly. *Tetrahedron Lett.* **1968**, 4893–4896.

Meinwald, J., Meinwald, Y. C., and Mazzocchi, P. H. (1969). Sex pheromone of the queen butterfly: Chemistry. *Science* **164**, 1174–1175.

Meinwald, J., Boriack, C. J., Schneider, D., Boppré, M., Wood, D. F., and Eisner, T. (1974). Volatile ketones in the hairpencil secretion of danaid butterflies (*Amauris* and *Danaus*). *Experientia* **30**, 721–722.

Miller, J. R., Baker, T. C., Cardé, R. T., and Roelofs, W. L. (1976). Reinvestigation of oak leaf roller sex pheromone components and the hypothesis that they vary with diet. *Science* **192**, 140–142.

Myers, J., and Brower, L. P. (1969). A behavioral analysis of the courtship pheromone receptors of the queen butterfly, *Danaus gilippus berenice*. *J. Insect Physiol.* **15**, 2117–2130.

Petty, R. L., Boppré, M., Schneider, D., and Meinwald, J. (1977). Identification and localization of volatile hairpencil components in male *Amauris ochlea* butterflies. *Experientia* **33**, 1324–1326.

Pliske, T. E. (1975a). Courtship behavior of the monarch butterfly, *Danaus plexippus*. *Ann. Entomol. Soc. Am.* **68**, 143–151.

Pliske, T. E. (1975b). Courtship behavior and use of chemical communication by males of certain species of ithomiine butterflies. *Ann. Entomol. Soc. Am.* **68**, 935–942.

Pliske, T. E. (1975c). Attraction of Lepidoptera to plants containing pyrrolizidine alkaloids. *Environ. Entomol.* **4**, 455–473.

Pliske, T. E., and Eisner, T. (1969). Sex pheromones of the queen butterfly: Biology. *Science* **164**, 1170–1172.

Rothschild, M. (1972). Some observations on the relationship between plants, toxic insects and birds. *In* "Phytochemical Ecology" (J. B. Harborne, ed.), pp. 2–12. Academic Press, New York.

Rothschild, M. (1973). Secondary plant substances and warning colouration in insects. *In* "Insect/Plant Relationships" (H. F. van Emden, ed.), pp. 59–83. Blackwell, London.

Rothschild, M. (1978). Hell's angels. *Antenna* **2**, 38–39.

Rutowski, R. L. (1982). Mate choice and lepidopteran mating behavior. *Florida Entomol.* **65**, 72–82.

Sawhney, R. S., Girotra, R. N., Atal, C. K., Culvenor, C. C. J., and Smith, L. W. (1967). Phytochemical studies on genus *Crotalaria:* Part VII. Major alkaloids of *C. mucronata, C. brevifolia, C. laburnifolia. Indian J. Chem.* **5**, 655–656.

Schal, C., and Bell, W. J. (1982). Ecological correlates of paternal investment of mates in a tropical cockroach. *Science* **218**, 170–173.

Schlatter, C., Waldner, E. E., and Schmid, H. (1968). Zur Biosynthese des Cantharidins. *Experientia* **24**, 994–995.

Schneider, D. (1983). Kommunikation durch chemische Signale bei Insekten: Alte und neue Beispiele von Lepidopteren. *Verhandl. Dtsch. Zool. Gesellsch.* **1983**, 5–16.

Schneider, D., and Seibt, U. (1969). Sex pheromone of the queen butterfly: Electroantennogram responses. *Science* **164**, 1173–1174.

Schneider, D., Boppré, M., Schneider, H., Thompson, W. R., Boriack, C. J., Petty, R. L., and Meinwald, J. (1975). A pheromone precursor and its uptake in male *Danaus* butterflies. *J. Comp. Physiol.* **97**, 245–256.

Schneider, D., Boppré, M., Zweig, J., Horsley, S. B., Bell, T. W., Meinwald, J., Hansen, K., and Diehl, E. W. (1982). Scent organ development in *Creatonotus* moths: Regulation by pyrrolizidine alkaloids. *Science* **215**, 1264–1265.

Seibt, U., Schneider, D., and Eisner, T. (1972). Duftpinsel, Flügeltaschen und Balz des Tagfalters *Danaus chrysippus*. *Z. Tierpsychol.* **31**, 513–530.

Sierra, J. R., Woggon, W.-D., and Schmid, H. (1976). Transfer of cantharidin during copulation from the adult male to the female *Lytta vesicatoria* (Spanish flies). *Experientia* **32**, 142–144.

Thornhill, R., and J. Alcock. (1983). "The Evolution of Insect Mating Systems." Harvard Univ. Press, Cambridge, Massachusetts.

Trivers, R. L. (1985). "Social Evolution." Benjamin/Cummings, Menlo Park, California.

Vasconcellos-Neto, J., and Lewinsohn, T. M. (1984). Discrimination and release of unpalatable butterflies by *Nephila clavipes*, a neotropical orb-weaving spider. *Ecol. Entomol.* **9**, 337–344.

Willis, M. A., and Birch, M. C. (1982). Male lek formation and female calling in a population of the arctiid moth *Estigmene acrea*. *Science* **218**, 168–170.

9

Neuroendocrine Regulation of Sex Pheromone–Mediated Behavior in Ixodid Ticks

DANIEL E. SONENSHINE
Department of Biological Sciences
Old Dominion University
Norfolk, Virginia 23508

I. INTRODUCTION

Although pheromone-mediated control of arthropod behavior and physiology is well known, the factors that regulate the production and release of these regulatory molecules have received scant attention. The immense diversity of the arthropod fauna and the incredible variety of chemical compounds that have been adapted for use as pheromones by these animals has made it difficult to identify a common basis for the control of these semiochemicals. However, some common features do exist. Most arthropods do not release sex pheromones until they are sexually competent, despite some notable exceptions, e.g., mites of the families Phytoseiidae and Tetranychidae (Cone, 1979). Typically, the timing of mating behavior is temporally determined; in insects with repeated mating cycles, pheromone is released only during periods of mating activity. In those insects that mate only during certain periods of the day or night, sex pheromone secretion release occurs only at that time (calling behavior) (Blomquist and Dillwith, 1983). Feeding is also important. In insects that convert dietary compounds into pheromone more or less directly, e.g., bark beetles, feeding greatly enhances pheromone production. In the stable fly, *Stomoxys calcitrans,* a blood meal is

Pheromone Biochemistry

required before sex pheromone synthesis can even begin (Meola *et al.*, 1977). In ticks, however, particularly metastriate ixodid ticks, sex attractant pheromone production commences soon after emergence of the imago from the nymphal molt, independent of feeding, but sex pheromone secretion is initiated only after commencement of feeding (Sonenshine *et al.*, 1982a, 1984a).

I

JUVENILE HORMONE

JH1: $R_1 = R_2 = C_2H_5$
JH2: $R_1 = C_2H_5$; $R_2 = CH_3$
JH3: $R_1 = R_2 = CH_3$
(cis-10, 11-epoxy-3,7,11-trimethyl trans,
trans-2, 6-dodecadienoic acid methyl ester)

Most of our evidence to date suggests that the hormone regulating sex pheromone production in insects is juvenile hormone (JH) (**I**). Borden *et al.* (1969) demonstrated that topical application of 25, 50, or 100 µg of 10,11-epoxyfarnesoic acid methyl ester, a synthetic juvenile hormone, induced sex pheromone production in the hindgut Malpighian tubule regions of *Ips confusus*. Twenty-four hours after treatment of male beetles with 100 µg of hormone, extracts of the hindgut malpighian tubules of these treated beetles were more attractive to females than extracts from males producing pheromone naturally in ponderosa pine logs. Similarly, Barth and Bell (1969) showed that JH in the cockroach, *Bryostria fumigata,* controls sex pheromone production as well as certain of the accessory gland secretions and oocyte maturation. In some species, age is a factor in determining when JH is most effective in stimulating sex pheromone activity. In *Tenebrio molitor,* topical application of JH onto the bodies of females induced higher pheromone activity in 3-day-old beetles, but had little or no affect on 5- or 7-day-old beetles (Menon and Nair, 1976). These data were interpreted as indicating that if the ovary was not competent to desposit yolk, the excess JH would be used for pheromone synthesis. In contrast, if the ovary was mature, exogenous JH would initiate synthesis and deposition of yolk (Menon and Nair, 1976). The role of the brain and corpora allata was also explored. Decapitation or injection of JH analogs into decapitated males had no effect on pheromone production in *T. molitor*. However, JH treatment of normal males induced pheromone production. Presumably, JH persisting from the larval stages may play a role in regulating pheromone biosynthesis in these insects (Menon. 1976).

Other evidence of the role of JH in the regulation of sex pheromone activity comes from experimental work on the corpora allata. When this organ is excised in the cockroach, pheromone production is terminated (summarized by Blomquist and Dillwith, 1983). Coating the allatectomized insects with pheromone restored their ability to mate, demonstrating that the production or secretion of the sex pheromone was interrupted. Similar findings were made by Amerasinghe (1978), who demonstrated that addition of synthetic JH restored sexual activity in allatectomized *Schistocerca gregaria.*

Clearly, juvenile hormone plays a role in stimulating sex pheromone biosynthesis in many insects. In some, such as the bark beetle, *Ips paraconfusus,* juvenile hormone acts on the corpora cardiaca to stimulate the release of an unidentified "brain hormone" that acts directly to stimulate sex pheromone biosynthesis (Blomquist and Dillwith, 1983). In others, it may act directly on the sex pheromone glands or via some other intermediary organ (e.g., the ovary).

Juvenile hormone is also believed to be present in ticks and other acarines, although direct evidence of its occurrence has not been demonstrated (Wright, 1969; Sannasi and Subramoniam, 1972; Bassal, 1974; Bassal and Roshdy, 1974; Hafez and Bassal, 1980; Ioffe and Uspenskiy, 1979; Ioffe *et al.,* 1977; McDaniel and Oliver, 1978; Mansingh and Rawlins, 1977; Solomon *et al.,* 1982). Pound and Oliver (1979) demonstrated that a JH-like compound acting as a gonadotropin was required for induction of oviposition in argasid ticks. Other workers (Leahy and Booth, 1980; Dees *et al.,* 1982; Hayes and Oliver, 1981), using the anti-allatotropin precocene II (**II**), have described evidence implicating the occurrence of a juvenile hormone and/or gonadotropin in ixodid ticks, while Oliver *et al.* (1985) demonstrated evidence of a similar role in the regulation of reproductive activity in the chicken mite, *Dermanyssus gallinae.* Nevertheless, no evidence of JH stimulation of sex pheromone activity in ticks has been reported.

II

PRECOCENE II
(6, 7-dimethoxy-2, 2-
dimethyl chromene)

Ecdysteroids also stimulate sex pheromone activity in some arthropods (Adams *et al.,* 1984, Blomquist *et al.,* 1984). Knowledge of this role for ecdysteroids is relatively recent and, undoubtedly, incomplete. Until the work of Hagedorn *et al.* (1975), who demonstrated ecdysone secretion by the ovary of adult mosquitoes, these hormones were regarded strictly as molting hormones. Following this important discovery, it soon became apparent that ecdysteroids serve several important regulatory roles in the adult animal, specifically, vitellogenesis, diapause, and, most noteworthy in relation to the present topic, sex pheromone activity. In some insects, control of sex pheromone biosynthesis is expressed via an intermediary, namely, 20-hydroxyecdysone (20-OH ecdysone), secreted by the ovary when stimulated by gonadotropic hormone (JH III) or in concert with a neuropeptide, the egg development neurotropic hormone (EDNH) (Koeppe *et al.*, 1985).

We shall first explore the evidence for hormonal regulation of sex pheromone biosynthesis and secretion in ticks, and then compare this mechanism with those operating in insects. We shall attempt to determine whether this action is direct or is expressed via other hormones in a complex series of interactions, including inhibition. Finally, we shall examine the stimulation of synthesis and regulation of pheromone secretion by different molecules.

II. SEX PHEROMONES OF IXODID TICKS

Sex pheromones of ixodid ticks have been reviewed extensively elsewhere (Sonenshine, 1984, 1985). Consequently, this discussion will highlight only the most relevant information regarding our knowledge of these pheromones.

The predominant sex attractant pheromone is 2,6-dichlorophenol (**III**) now known from at least 14 species in 5 genera of metastriate Ixodidae. The possible occurrence of other volatiles is not precluded, and the existence of other phenols, e.g., *p*-cresol, salicylaldehyde, *o*-nitrophenol, and even phenol itself, has been reported in several species of these ticks. Moreover, a blend of three phenols serves as the aggregation–attachment pheromone in *Amblyomma variegatum* (Schoeni *et al.*, 1984). Thus far, none of these other phenols have been found to serve as sex pheromones. Wood *et al.*'s (1975) designation of phenol and *p*-cresol as the sex pheromone of *Rhipicephalus appendiculatus* has since been questioned (Waladde, 1982). In addition, other unidentified volatiles have been reported to affect mating behavior. Unknown pheromones believed to be produced by the foveal glands of *Rhipicephalus evertsi evertsi* males attract unfed females to form preparasitic and precopulatory assemblages (Gothe and Neitz, 1985). In *Amblyomma limbatum, A. albolimbatum*, and *Aponomma hydrosauri*

2, 6-DICHLOROPHENOL

(all parasites of reptiles), unknown nonspecific sex attractants facilitate male orientation to the pheromone-emitting females, while species-specific volatile excitants facilitate conspecific matings (Andrews and Bull, 1982). The manner in which attached *Amblyomma* spp. males recognize and grasp females, even rotating them so that they attach venter to venter (Obenchain, 1984), or in which the females of Australian reptile parasitizing ticks recognize conspecific males implicates yet another variety of undescribed mating signals, some of which may be chemical in nature. Thus, the variety of compounds serving as sex attractant pheromones may be larger and the nature of the signals important in the mate finding processes of these ticks may be more complex than currently known.

The chlorinated phenol, 2,6-dichlorophenol (2,6-DCP), is believed to be produced in specific glands, the foveal glands located on the dorsal body surface of adult ticks. Although both male and female ticks have such glands, they are functional only in the females in most species. A notable exception occurs in the genus *Amblyomma,* specifically, *A. maculatum,* where both males and females produce 2,6-DCP in substantial quantities (Kellum and Berger, 1977). These paired glands superficially resemble dermal glands and may have evolved from them. They consist of a cluster of lobes, each lobe containing from two to five very large cells, all connected via delicate ducts to a group of tiny pores, the foveal pores. In unfed, sexually inactive females, the secretory cells in the secretory lobes contain numerous membrane-bound oil droplets. Each oil droplet is believed to contain pheromone, since X-ray microanalysis shows unusually high signals for chlorine in the oil droplets but only trace amounts anywhere else (Sonenshine *et al.,* 1981a,b). With the commencement of feeding, the vesicles containing the oil droplets break down, and the tiny droplets migrate to the foveal gland ducts. Here they coalesce and are funneled via the foveal pores through the delicate cuticle of the fovea onto the external surface. Thus, the pheromone-impregnated oily secretion reaches the exterior, allowing the pheromone to evaporate into the surrounding air. This mechanism facilitates controlled release of the pheromone from the tick body.

The formation of the sex pheromone glands and the time of production and secretion of pheromone are both rigorously controlled. The manner in which this is accomplished and the specific physiological factors that facilitate this control are discussed below.

Another type of sex pheromone, distinctly different from the volatiles produced by the foveal glands (or other organs), is the genital sex pheromone (Sonenshine *et al.,* 1982a,b). Although associated with the female reproductive organs in some unknown way, the precise site(s) of production of the genital sex pheromone is less clear. Recent evidence implicates the oviducts and, possibly, the lobular accessory gland surrounding the vestibular vagina. Also unknown is how the production of the unusual sex pheromone is regulated.

III. ROLE OF ECDYSTEROIDS IN REGULATING SEX PHEROMONE BIOSYNTHESIS IN TICKS AND INSECTS

The first report that ecdysteroids stimulate sex pheromone activity in an arthropod was by Dees *et al.* (1984a), who demonstrated this effect in the camel tick, *Hyalomma dromedarii*. These workers observed sharply elevated sex pheromone content in female ticks treated with exogenous 20-hydroxyecdysone (**IV**) by direct inoculation of engorged nymphs. Extracts of female ticks assayed (by gas chromatography) for 2,6-DCP content revealed a fourfold or greater increase in the concentration of this pheromone as compared to saline-treated controls (Table I). Females treated with 10 ng doses (as engorged nymphs) had as much as 4.6 times more 2,6-DCP than untreated or saline-treated controls. X-Ray microanalysis also revealed elevated chlorine concentrations in the pheromone glands of treated females, significantly higher than in saline-treated controls (Table II). Since almost all of the free chloride is extracted during the preparation of the specimens for X-ray microanalysis, this was interpreted as indicating increased organically bound chlorine in these tissues, i.e., more sex pheromone. Especially significant was their finding of 2,6-DCP in 20-hydroxyecdysone-treated males, since this compound is normally absent in this sex. Autoradiography of the pheromone gland tissues from [3H]ecdysone-treated females suggested the presence of specific receptors capable of binding the hormone (Fig. 1). Bioassays with sexually active males revealed that up to 25% of the exogenously treated females were attractive to males, even though these females had not fed [according to Khalil *et al.* (1981), unfed females are not believed to secrete 2,6-DCP and do not normally attract males].

IV

20-HYDROXYECDYSONE
(2β, 3β, 14α, 20, 22, 25-hexahydroxy-
5β-cholest-7-en-6-one)

Additional evidence that the foveal glands (=pheromone glands) are target organs with receptors that bind ecdysteroids is provided by recent work by

TABLE I

Sex Pheromone, 2,6-Dichlorophenol,[a] in the Ticks, *Hyalomma dromedarii* and *Dermacentor variabilis*, in Relation to Treatment with 20-Hydroxyecdysone[b]

Species and life stage	Physiological state	Number of ticks in sample	Treatment	Amount of 2,6-DCP (ng/tick)
H. dromedarii				
Nymphs	15 Days postengorgement	80	None	0.00
Females	Unfed, 2–3 weeks posteclosion	100	None	3.46
Females	Unfed, 2–3 weeks posteclosion	50	10 ng ecd*	16.00
Females	Fed 7 days	65	1% saline	5.57
Females	Fed 7 days	75	10 ng ecd*	21.30
Females	Fed 7 days	21	100 ng ecd*	4.47
Males	Unfed, 2–3 weeks posteclosion	70	None	0.00
Males	Unfed, 2–3 weeks posteclosion	106	10 ng ecd*	3.90
D. variabilis				
Females	Unfed, 2–3 weeks posteclosion	117	None	1.87
Females	Unfed, 2–3 weeks posteclosion	78	10 ng ecd*	1.68

[a]Amounts determined by gas chromatography. From Dees *et al.*, 1984a, reproduced with permission from *Acarology VI* by Griffiths & Bowman, published by Ellis Horwood Limited, Chichester, England, 1984 (please see original article for details of assay techniques).

[b]20-Hydroxyecdysone (ecd*) or 1% saline administered to engorged nymphs on the day of drop off (please see original article for details).

TABLE II

Chlorine Content of Microscopic Areas of the Foveal Glands of *Hyalomma dromedarii* as Determined by X-Ray Microanalysis[a]

	Osmium/gold (%)				
	Unfed females		Fed females, control (n = 5)	Unfed males	
	20-Hydroxyecdysone (n = 9)	Control (n = 6)		20-Hydroxyecdysone (n = 3)	Control (n = 1)
Mean	4.45	1.24	0.87	0.27	0.02
±	±	±	±	±	
S.D.	1.33	0.45	0.48	0.18	—

[a]Microanalysis by scanning electron microscopy. From Dees *et al.*, 1984a, reproduced with permission from *Acarology VI* by Griffiths & Bowman, published by Ellis Horwood Limited, Chichester, England, 1984.

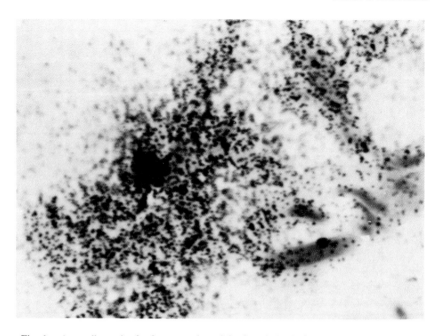

Fig. 1.   Autoradiograph of a frozen section of the foveal glands from unfed *Hyalomma dromedarii* that emerged from nymphs inoculated with [³H]ecdysone. The intense accumulation of silver grains virtually obscures the large secretory cells of the gland lobes in this frozen section. ×800. Reproduced with permission from Dees *et al.* (1984a), *Acarology VI* by Griffiths & Bowman, published by Ellis Horwood, Limited, Chichester, England, 1984.

Sonenshine *et al.* (1985a), who observed that these glands ranked second, after the synganglion, when the concentration of radioimmunoassay (RIA)-positive ecdysteroids was determined per milligram of tissue for different tissue or organ types (Table III). In view of the fact that the minute foveal gland lobes are difficult to excise without the adjacent epidermal tissues, the latter was also excised and assayed separately. When epidermis and "fat body," i.e., the diffuse fat body cells that adhere to the epidermal tissues, was assayed alone, the amount of RIA-positive activity was much lower than when the foveal glands were included. Inclusion of the foveal glands resulted in a three- to fivefold increase in immunoreactive activity as compared to that obtained with just epidermis and fat body cells. Autoradiographs (frozen sections) of the foveal glands of females treated (as nymphs) with [¹⁴C]cholesterol (a precursor of ecdysteroid biosynthesis) also revealed highly significant accumulations of silver grains over these glands, substantially greater than in the surrounding epidermis (Figs. 2 and 3). Thus the data from several different types of assays converge to suggest that the foveal glands are indeed receptive to this hormone, supporting the suggested

TABLE III

Summary of Estimates of Total Ecdysteroid Content of Selected Body Organs and Tissues of Partially Fed Virgin *Hyalomma dromedarii* and *Dermacentor variabilis*[a]

Organ/tissue	*H. dromedarii*				*D. variabilis*			
	N	mg tissue	pg/tick	pg/mg	N	mg tissue	pg/tick	pg/mg
Syneganglion	250	5.16 ± 1.31	2479 ± 1134	120,223 ± 24,361	250	5.14 ± 1.11	1901 ± 1384	92,416 ± 20,406
Hemolymph	—	1.50	1934[b] ± 85	85	—	1.50	1362[c] ± 87	86
Salivary gland	25	26.93 ± 8.55	312	290 ± 92	25	22.45 ± 2.88	957	1065 ± 120
Ovary	50	12.82 ± 2.60	115	448 ± 74	50	21.45 ± 2.22	57	133 ± 13
Muscle	25	9.58 ± 4.13	98	226 ± 46	25	4.42 ± 1.63	190	1074 ± 289
Epidermis/fat body/foveal glands	10	12.59 ± 0.91	500	397 ± 27	10	4.87 ± 0.24	1120	2300 ± 122
Epidermis/fat body	10	12.04 ± 0.90	82	68 ± 5	10	4.95 ± 0.25	360	727 ± 39
Foveal glands	49	0.67 ± 0.33	158	11,731 ± 6977	50	0.39 ± 0.07	133	17,183 ± 823
Anterior reproductive tract	100	3.99 ± 0.56	13	313	50	1.90 ± 0.19	162	4263

[a]From Sonenshine *et al.*, 1985a, reprinted by permission of the Editor, from the *Journal of Medical Entomology* 22:303–311, 1985.
[b]Average per tick = 22.7 ± 0.9 µl.
[c]Average per tick = 15.9 ± 6.9 µl.

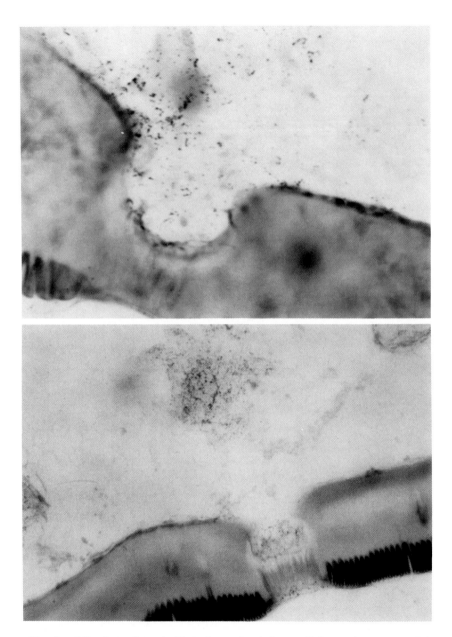

Figs. 2 and 3. Autoradiographs illustrating scattered clusters of silver grains over one of the paired foveal pores and foveal glands from a female *H. dromedarii*. Specimens inoculated as engorged nymphs with [^{14}C]cholesterol. Figure 2 (top) shows silver grains over the ducts and pore tubes, ×160. Figure 3 (bottom) shows silver grain accumulations over the secretory lobes of one of the paired foveal glands, ×80. From Sonenshine *et al.* (1985a), reprinted with permission of the Editor, from the *Journal of Medical Entomology*, 22:303–311, 1985.

role of 20-hydroxyecdysone in biosynthesis of pheromone. In contrast to these effects in *H. dromedarii*, no significant increases in 2,6-DCP content were found in *Dermancentor variabilis* females following treatment with 20-hydroxyecdysone [although Dees *et al.* (1984b) noted vesicle breakdown characteristic of feeding adults in several unfed females following treatment with 20-hydroxyecdysone].

Studies with ecdysteroid analogs suggest as great or even greater stimulation of sex pheromone production as that observed with the natural hormone. Jaffe *et al.* (1986) confirmed the increased 2,6-DCP concentration in females of *H. dromedarii* as well as its appearance in males following administration of 20-hydroxyecdysone and the ecdysteroid analog 3β,5β,14α-trihydroxy-5β-cholest-7-en-6-one (**V**) (=BSEA-28; Thompson *et al.*, 1971) by controlled-release

V

BSEA-28
(3β, 5β, 14α - trihydroxy-5β-cholest-
7-en-6-one)

methods. Implantation of the ecdysteroid analog in controlled-release plastic capsules under the skin of tick-infested rabbits led to accelerated molting and reduced feeding (reduced body weight) in the fed nymphs, especially when very large concentrations of the active ingredient were used. However, the viability and fertility of the survivors were not affected. Of special interest was the increased production of 2,6-DCP in the females and the appearance of 2,6-DCP in the males that emerged from the treated nymphs (Table IV). Although chemical analysis [high-performance liquid chromatography (HPLC)] indicated spectral shifts consistent with metabolic changes in the original analog, RIA methods specific for ecdysone demonstrated persistence of immunoreactive material in the blood of the analog-treated host rabbits for at least 95 days after implantation, from 18.5 to 72.0 ng/ml host blood.

Another ecdysteroid analog active in ticks is 2β,3β,14α-trihydroxy-5β-cholest-7-en-6-one (**VI**), also known as 22,25-dideoxyecdysone (22,25 DDE, BSEA-1). When ingested by the argasid tick, *Ornithodoros moubata*, nanogram doses (e.g., 70 ng, 100 ng) were sufficient to induce molting, supermolting, and

TABLE IV

2,6-Dichlorophenol Content in *Hyalomma dromedarii* (Unfed)
Following Treatment with Different Hormones

Treatment	Females		Males	
	Number in sample	2,6-DCP content	Number in sample	2,6-DCP content
Saline (1%)	65	5.6	75	0.0
None	100	5.7	100	0.3
20-Hydroxyecdysone (engorged nymphs)[a]	68	13.1	26	2.0
20-Hydroxyecdysone (engorged nymph + JH III)[b]	71	9.7	43	3.5
20-Hydroxyecdysone implant in host[c]	100	5.8	105	0.0
BSEA-28 implant in host[c]	49	10.1	45	5.0
22,25-DDE (BSEA-1) (implant in host)[c]	75	39.1	75	11.3
Methoprene (implant in host)	89	6.9	114	0.0

[a] A 10^{-3} M solution of 20-hydroxyecdysone in Shen's saline was inoculated into engorged nymphs.

[b] 20-Hydroxyecdysone was inoculated as described above; JH III was applied topically in acetone.

[c] 22,25-DDE, 22,25-Dideoxyecdysone. From Jaffe *et al.*, 1986. Reprinted by permission of the Editor, from the *Journal of Medical Entomology*, 23:685–691, 1986.

oviposition. Doses as low as 15–20 ng/tick induced oviposition in mated females. Treatment with higher doses resulted in considerable mortality. In contrast, ecdysone (**VII**), 20-hydroxyecdysone, and other natural ecdysteroids had no effect or provoked a response only when administered in nonphysiological (e.g., microgram) doses (Connat *et al.*, 1983). Similar findings were made by Mango *et al.* (1976) and Kitaoka (1972).

22,25-DDE was also found to be highly effective in its effects on sex phe-

22, 25-DIDEOXYECDYSONE
(2β, 3β, 14α -trihydroxy-5β-cholest-
7-en-6-one)

VII

ECDYSONE
(2β, 3β, 14α, 22, 25-pentahydroxy-5β-
cholest-7-en-6-one)

romone biosynthesis in *H. dromedarii* (Table IV). The analog was administered by the same slow-release devices implanted into the bodies of laboratory rabbits described previously (Jaffe *et al.*, 1986). Ticks fed on the treated hosts suffered high mortality; 37% died without molting. When the sex pheromone content of the mature adults that emerged from the surviving nymphs was measured, unfed females were found to have 39.1 ng of 2,6-DCP per tick, almost 8 times as much as the female controls; unfed males had 11.3 ng of 2,6-DCP, as compared to only trace amounts in the control males. These are the highest values ever recorded for this species. Unfortunately, the precise amounts of active ingredient to which the ticks were exposed was unknown, although estimates based on host body weight, probable release rates, and average blood consumption by the feeding nymphs indicated exposure to accumulated dose of approximately 6.0 ng per tick. This estimate is very similar to the effective dose range reported by Connat *et al.* (1983) for *O. moubata*, and probably explains the high mortality.

Clearly, these two different analogs proved highly effective in stimulating 2,6-DCP production in the camel tick, *H. dromedarii*. Direct inoculation of authentic hormone, 20-hydroxyecdysone, was also effective in stimulating pheromone production, as indicated by the results shown in the table. In contrast, treatment of the inoculated nymphs with the juvenoid JH III had no effect on these results.

The time when ecdysteroid stimulation of sex pheromone biosynthesis is initiated and the period of its duration are uncertain. When ixodid ticks commence the ecdysial process following the nymphal blood meal, the titer of ecdysteroids in the hemolymph rises. The peak is reached at the time of maximum mitotic activity in the epidermis, coinciding with the commencement of apolysis. In *Amblyomma hebraeum* Koch, this occurs on day 23 after commencement of feeding (at 26°C). Following this peak, estimated at about 14 ng of 20-hydroxyecdysone equivalents per tick, the titer falls, declining to about 0.5 ng per tick at the time of molting. Similar changes occur during development in *D.*

variabilis (Dees *et al.*, 1984b). Thus, the developing pheromone glands are exposed to declining hormone titers during their formative period, and relatively low titers as their development nears completion.

The site of the future pheromone gland appears in nymphal *H. dromedarii* as a simple, three-cell primordium which degenerates during feeding. This is replaced by a new structure which proliferates extensively, forming a multicellular organ 5 days postfeeding. This rapid onset of cellular activity precedes the mitotic activity of the surrounding epidermis by several days and indicates a high degree of sensitivity to hormonal stimulation. By 8 days postfeeding, or slightly less than 45% of the length of the ecdysial period in this species, the pheromone gland shows evidence of developing pore tubes and ampullae, and the separation of the large secretory cells from the duct cells. This is close to the time when maximum ecdysial titers would be expected. Further development led to the clear differentiation of the pore tubes, ampullae, and the secretory lobes, the latter with one or two large cells in pyriform lobes (Khalil *et al.*, 1983). Following ecdysis, the glands of the newly emerged ticks appeared morphologically similar to those of the mature adults, and the secretory lobes contained numerous lipid droplets (Figs. 4 and 5). However, these lipid droplets were not found to be osmiophilic. This one histochemical feature represents the only apparent distinction between these glands and those of the mature females (Fig. 6).

No 2,6-DCP was found to be present in the foveal glands of the newly emerged females, even though the structures appeared to be fully formed and ready to synthesize this pheromone (Sonenshine *et al.*, 1983). Dees *et al.* (1984a,b, 1985) compared the time of synthesis of 2,6-DCP in *D. variabilis* and *H. dromedarii* with the changing concentrations of ecdysteroids. 2,6-DCP appeared within 5 days after the nymph to adult molt in these species and increased to a maximum between 10 and 15 days postmolt (Dees *et al.*, 1984a,b, 1985). Thereafter, 2,6-DCP remained present but did not increase in concentration (Sonenshine *et al.*, 1984a). Ecdysteroid concentrations declined during this period or remained the same. When the ticks attach and begin feeding, 2,6-DCP secretion commences and is believed to be accompanied by additional 2,6-DCP production, since the concentrations of this compound in the ticks decrease only slightly or not at all. Concentrations of ecdysteroids, particularly 20-hydroxyecdysone, also increase during this period of feeding. However, whether this hormone is directly responsible for the renewed synthesis remains to be discovered.

In contrast to these findings for *H. dromedarii*, *D. variabilis* females did not appear to respond to exogenous ecdysteroids. However, ultrastructural studies demonstrated commencement of secretory activity in treated female ticks.

The generally accepted model for hormonal activation of biological function is based on vertebrate data, especially evidence from studies with steroids. In this model, the free hormone is believed to enter the cytosol by diffusion through the

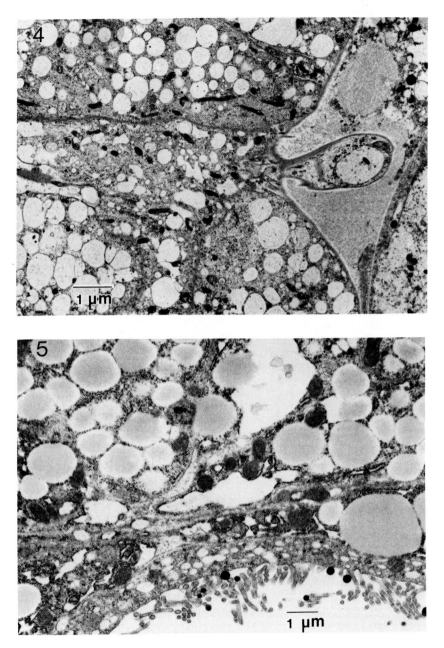

Figs. 4 and 5. Transmission electron micrographs illustrating varying states of the secretory cell contents in relation to age and feeding in *H. dromedarii* females. Figure 4 shows intact vesicles with minute granular contents but no electron-dense secretory droplets in a newly emerged female, ×10,200. Figure 5 shows intact vesicles with amorphous contents but no electron-dense secretory droplets in a newly emerged female, ×8400. From Sonenshine *et al.* (1983), reprinted with permission of the Editor, from the *Journal of Medical Entomology*, 20:424–439, 1983.

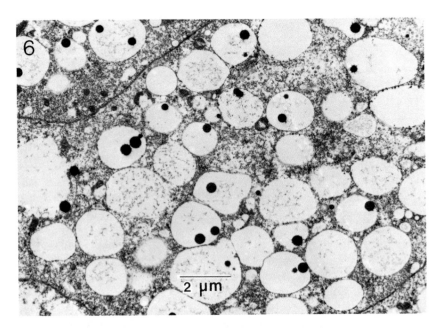

Fig. 6. Transmission electron micrograph illustrating the highly osmiophilic, electron-dense lipid droplets in the secretory lobe cells of a mature (age 2–4 weeks postmolting) *H. dromedarii* female. The droplets are compact and much smaller than the vesicles that contain them. Note the contrast with the diffuse, electron-lucent appearance in the newly emerged females. ×7200. From Sonenshine *et al.* (1983), reprinted with permission of the Editor, from the *Journal of Medical Entomology,* 20:424–439, 1983.

plasma membrane where it binds to specific receptor proteins, forming a hormone–receptor complex. The latter is then translocated to the nucleus and, after binding to specific affinity sites on the chromosomes, directs RNA transcription at these specific gene loci. In insect cells, new evidence, summarized by O'Connor (1983), suggests a more direct linkage with nuclear receptor sites, rather than via translocation of hormone–receptor complexes formed in the cytosol. These findings have almost all come from studies done *in vitro* using *Drosophila* Kc cells. *In vivo* studies did not reveal evidence of receptor binding sites, presumably because of the saturation of the relatively small number of such sites with natural hormone. JH receptor sites were also found, including a receptor binding protein of approximately 80,000 daltons, located in the cytosol (O'Connor, 1983). Nothing is known about the receptor binding sites for either 20-hydroxyecdysone or JH in ticks!

An example of how the hormone 20-hydroxyecdysone directs synthesis of new proteins is given by the study by Grzelak and Krishna Kumaran (1985) on the wax moth, *Galleria mellonella.* Addition of this hormone, in physiological concentrations, to larvae (*in vivo*) resulted in doubling of the rate of synthesis of polyadenylated [poly(A)]RNA, indicating transcription, in contrast to treatment with JH, which had no detectable effect on these tissues. This was verified by measuring uptake of ^{3}H-labeled radionucleotides. However, JH administered together with 20-hydroxyecdysone prevented ecdysteroid stimulation of RNA synthesis. When gel electrophoresis was done with an extract of larval fat body treated with 20-hydroxyecdysone *in vitro*, two new proteins, 22 and 26 kDa (kilodaltons), respectively, were found. That the proteins were new was confirmed by autoradiography of the gels from tissues incubated with hormone and ^{3}H-labeled amino acids. Controls done without hormone treatment lacked these new proteins. Clearly, 20-hydroxyecdysone stimulated synthesis of specific poly(A) RNA, as well as an increase in total RNA, which in turn directed the synthesis of two new proteins. Thus, 20-hydroxyecdysone is essential for the expression of specific genes in this insect, genes that otherwise would not be expressed!

Studies are now in progress in the author's laboratory to determine whether 20-hydroxyecdysone can induce 2,6-DCP production by female tick foveal glands maintained in culture. Preliminary evidence suggests that foveal glands removed from mature females do not respond to *in vitro* stimulation with this hormone alone but do respond to stimulation when 20-hydroxyecdysone is administered in combination with dopamine. Similarly, glands in which the neural connections with the synganglion were retained also showed elevated 2,6-DCP activity when incubated *in vitro*. Future studies will examine whether glands from very young females, young males, or from molting nymphs can be excited by this hormone and whether new enzymes are produced.

IV. ROLE OF JUVENILE HORMONE/GONADOTROPIC HORMONE IN REGULATING TICK PHEROMONE ACTIVITY

In most insects, juvenile hormone (JH) serves as the hormone inhibiting maturation of reproductive and related adult characteristics. Often, the same molecule serves as the gonadotropic hormone (GTH) in the adults. The most widespread of the various JH hormones is JH III, methyl 3,7,11-trimethyl-10,11-epoxy-2,6-dodecadienoate (**I**). In some insects, JH may antagonize ecdysteroid synthesis or inhibit ecdysteroid-dependent processes (O'Connor, 1983). Abundant evidence of a JH-like hormone in ticks has been accumulated, as noted in Section I. The synganglion, a possible site of GTH synthesis (Binnington, 1981; Marzouk *et al.*, 1985), was found to be capable of inducing oviposition when pooled homogenates from fed mated *O. moubata* females were inoculated into fed virgin females (Aeschlimann, 1968). Other evidence of synganglion involvement in regulating oogenesis, all in argasid ticks, is summarized in recent reviews (Solomon *et al.,* 1982; Diehl and Aeschlimann, 1982).

Precocene II (**II**), an anti-allatotropin associated with inhibition of JH synthesis in insects (Bowers, 1976), has been reported to inhibit oogenesis in argasid ticks (Pound and Oliver, 1979), as well as male fertility (Leahy and Booth, 1980) or embryonic develpoment (Hayes and Oliver, 1981) in ixodid ticks. Nevertheless, no evidence of a direct effect on sex pheromone activity has been reported. Dees *et al.* (1982) did not observe any alteration in mating behavior in precocene II-treated *D. variabilis,* even in partially fed females which were most severely impaired by the treatments. Similarly. tests of the effects of precocene II on *H. dromedarii* indicated toxic responses. However, no conclusive evidence of anti-hormonal activity or hormonally related disruption of mating behavior was observed.

JH was also without effect when administered to ixodid ticks. Khalil *et al.* (1984a) did not observe any alteration in *H. dromedarii* mating behavior when the hormone analog JH I was administered to nymphs or adults in various stages of development. Inadequate penetration or inability of the tick's physiological system to respond to this particular JH were offered as possible explanations for the lack of a response. More recently, Jaffe *et al.* (1986) showed that JH III, administered topically to engorged *H. dromedarii* nymphs, had no effect on sex pheromone production in the adults that emerged from the treated nymphs.

A possible explanation of the failure of exogenous JH, even when administered in relatively large doses, to affect sex pheromone activity, is the very rapid enzymatic digestion of these molecules by the tick's hemolymph. D. Sonenshine (unpublished) demonstrated the breakdown of ^{3}H-labeled JH and the production of relatively polar metabolites, tentatively identified as the free acid, diol, and the acid–diol forms. Gel electorphoresis of the tick's hemolymph revealed evidence of at least four esterases, ranging from 118 to 220 kDa. Presumably, these are the enzymes that are capable of digesting JH. Inactivation by intracellular enzymes, protein binding, or other methods are not excluded. Therefore, assuming very limited penetration through the highly resistent cuticle, it is not unlikely that little JH will remain intact to affect the tissues.

Whether JH or GTH can affect sex pheromone activity in ticks remains uncertain at present. Clearly, no evidence has been presented to indicate that it can do so directly. However, indirect effects, perhaps by regulating the timing of ecdysteroid production and/or release, are not excluded.

V. METABOLISM OF ECDYSONES IN TICKS

If we accept the premise of ecdysteroid excitation of sex pheromone biosynthesis in ticks, we must also concern ourselves with the question of the identity of the ecdysteroid metabolite(s) responsible for this regulatory activity. In addition, we must also consider how and where inactivation of the hormonally active metabolite(s) is done.

In insects, ecdysone is metabolized to 20-hydroxyecdysone, the active hormone, and a spectrum of predominantly polar ecdysteroids. Ecydsone and 20-hydroxyecdysone may then be hydroxylated further, e.g., to 20,26-hydroxyecdysone, or oxidized irreversibly to a variety of epi, dehydro, and deoxy metabolites. Conversion to highly polar 26-ecdysonoic acids is the predominant pathway for inactivation of ecdysone and 20-hydroxyecdysone in most insects that have been studied (Lafont et al., 1983; Lefont and Koolman, 1984). These metabolites, as well as the parent molecules, ecdysone and 20-hydroxyecdysone, may then be conjugated with phosphate, sulfate, or glucuronic acid, forming polar conjugates which provide convenient storage forms for latter use or for elimination. In the desert locust, *Schistocerca gregaria,* a number of polar inactivation products have been identified, e.g., 3-acetyl ecdysone-2-phosphate, ecdysone-26-oic acid, and 20-hydroxyecdysone-26-oic acid. Ecdysteroid 22-phosphates constitute the major means of storage of maternal ecdysteroids in newly laid eggs in this and several other species (Isaac et al., 1982, 1983; Isaac and Rees, 1984).

Ticks use novel means of inactivating ecdysteroids, very different from the metabolic events found in most insects. When ^{14}C-labeled cholesterol was inoculated into nymphal *H. dromedarii,* ^{14}C radioactivity was found not only coincident with 20-hydroxyecdysone and ecdysone, but with a spectrum of highly apolar compounds as well. Apolar ecdysteroids have been reported in *Ornithodoros moubata* also (Bouvier et al., 1982; Connat et al., 1984). Diehl et al. (1985) reported that most of the hormonal molecules are esterified with long-chain fatty acids, forming highly apolar molecules in this argasid tick. Similar findings were made with extracts of the cattle tick, *Boophilus microplus,* although the precise form of conjugation was not specified (Wigglesworth et al., 1985). These authors also observed that an enzyme isolated from developing tick embryos hydrolyzed the ecdysteroid esters, releasing ecdysone.

Sonenshine et al. (1986b) found that when tritiated ecdysone was administered to feeding female *H. dromedarii* and the ecdysteroid extracts analyzed by HPLC, most of the inoculated ecdysone was metabolized to highly apolar compounds that were not immunoreactive. In one experiment, only 8.1% of the ^{3}H radioactivity was coincident with 20-hydroxyecdysone and only 16.9% remained as ecdysone, while 66% of the ^{3}H was in the form of apolar compounds. When the experiment was repeated, the proportion of the ^{3}H represented by these same compounds was 7.0, 1.3, and 75.6% (Figs. 7 and 8). Moreover, the apolar fraction was found to consist of at least two major components. When [^{14}C]acetate was inoculated into the feeding females, all of the ^{14}C radioactivity in the ecdysteroid extract was coincident with these same apolar fractions. Treatment

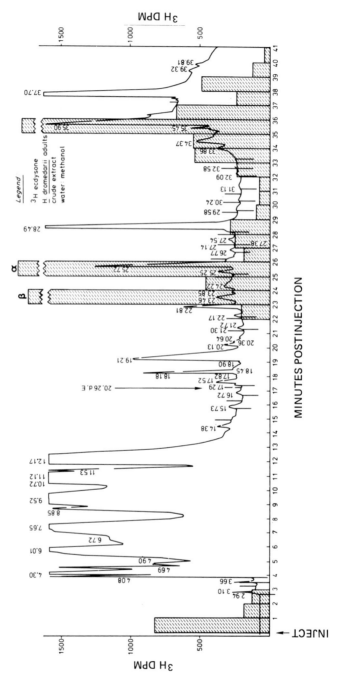

Fig. 7. Distribution of ^{3}H radioactivity in 1 min collections superimposed on an HPLC chromatogram to illustrate the distribution of ^{3}H-labeled metabolites in relation to the sample peaks. The crude extract was prepared from partially fed *H. dromedarii* females inoculated with [^{3}H]ecdysone. Chromatographic conditions comprised a gradient of different proportions of water and methanol, with the compounds retained on and eluted from a C$_{18}$ column. The retention times for 20-hydroxyecdysone (β) and ecdysone (α) are noted on the figure. From Sonenshine *et al.* (1986b), reprinted with permission of the Editor, from *Journal of Medical Entomology*, 23:630–650, 1986.

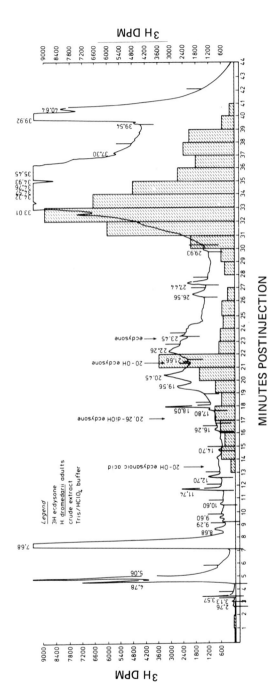

Fig. 8. Distribution of ³H radioactivity in 1 min collections superimposed on an HPLC chromatogram to illustrate the distribution of ³H-labeled metabolites when the crude extract was chromatographed using a 20 mM Tris–HClO₄ buffer, pH 6.9, using a 5-μm C₁₈ column. The retention times of ecdysone (23.45 min) and 20-hydroxyecdysone (21.66 min) as well as the more polar metabolites, 20,26-dihydroxyecdysone (17.46 min) and 20-hydroxyecdysone acid (13.35 min), are indicated by arrows. No peaks were observed that coeluted precisely with the latter compound. Chromatographic conditions were the same as in Fig. 7, except for the substitution of the buffer as the aqueous phase. From Sonenshine *et al.* (1986b), reprinted with permission of the Editor, from the *Journal of Medical Entomology,* 23:630–650, 1986.

of the female tick extract, including the apolar fractions, with *Helix* sulfatase enzymes did not release any additional immunoreactive ecdysteroids. However, treatment of these apolar ecdysteroids with porcine liver carboxylesterase released 20-hydroxyecdysone, 20,26-dihydroxyecdysone (**VIII**), and other unknown ecdysteroids (Fig. 9). In addition, four fatty acids, not previously present, were liberated, namely, palmitic, stearic, oleic, and linoletic acids, and their identification was confirmed by gas chromatography–mass spectroscopy; an unknown 9 : 0 dimethyl fatty acid was also found. Relatively small quantities of polar ecdysteroids occur (Bouvier *et al.*, 1982; Diehl *et al.*, 1985; Sonenshine *et al.*, 1986b). Radioimmunoassay and coelution with authentic radioactive standards indicated the presence of significant quantities of 20,26-dihydroxyecdysone and another unknown but highly polar ecdysteroid as well as 20-hydroxyecdysone in the tick extracts (Figs. 9 and 10).

20, 26 -DIHYDROXYECDYSONE
(2β, 3β, 14α, 20, 22, 25, 26 - heptahydroxy-
5β - cholest - 7 - en - 6 - one)

These findings demonstrate that inactivation of ecdysone is rapid. Moreover, much of this inactivation is in the form of readily hydrolyzable conjugates, suggesting their storage for later use. Studies by Diehl *et al.* (1985) support this hypothesis, indicating the presence of large quantities of the hydrolyzable conjugates in the vitellogenic ovaries. The sites of inactivation of the ecdysteroids are not known. Wigglesworth *et al.* (1985) observed that several tick tissues maintained *in vitro*, including Malpighian tubules, ovaries, midgut, and fat body, metabolized [³H]ecdysone to apolar acyl esters. Other evidence implicates the midgut as the primary organ engaged in this function (Diehl *et al.*, 1985; Sonenshine *et al.*, 1986b). Diehl *et al.* (1985) suggest that, at least in *O. moubata*, inactivation of exogenous ecdysteroids, e.g., phytoecdysteroids, may have evolved as an important adaptation to feeding on herbivorous hosts.

These findings suggest that only one or perhaps two ecdysteroids, primarily 20-hydroxyecdysone, serves as the hormone responsible for excitation of sex

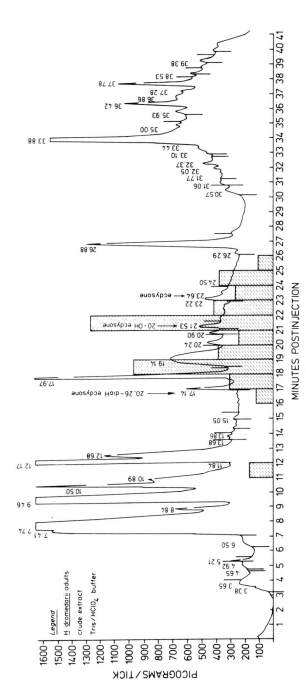

Fig. 9. Radioimmunoassay-positive fractions among the products of esterase hydrolysis of the tick extract (fraction remaining at the origin after thin-layer chromatography). The fractions were separated by HPLC, and 1 min collections were assayed by RIA using the same gradient system and column as noted in Fig. 7. The figure shows the amount detected, expressed in picograms (pg) per tick, superimposed on the HPLC chromatogram. From Sonenshine *et al.* (1986b), reprinted with permission of the Editor, from the *Journal of Medical Entomology*, 23:630–650, 1986.

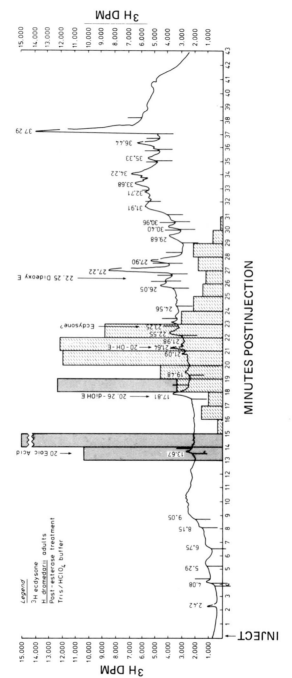

Fig. 10. Distribution of ³H radioactivity in 1 min collections. superimposed on an HPLC chromatogram of the products of esterase hydrolysis. The material hydrolyzed was the apolar ecdysteroid fraction collected from a C-18 plate, using an aliquot of a crude extract of [³H]ecdysone-inoculated ticks. HPLC conditions were the same as in Fig. 7. The dashed line shaded bars represent ³H radioactivity found in the extract. The stippled bars represent ³H radioactivity of two labeled standards, 20-ecdysonoic acid (20-Eoic Acid) and 20,26-dihydroxyecdysone (20,26-diOH E). From Sonenshine *et al.* (1986b), reprinted with permission of the Editor, from the *Journal of Medical Entomology*, 23:630–650, 1986.

pheromone activity in these ticks. Whether 20,26-dihydroxyecdysone may also excite the pheromone glands remains to be resolved. This metabolite, which is also present in substantial quantities (Sonenshine *et al*, 1986b), is very similar to 20-hydroxyecdysone. It cross-reacts readily in our radioimmunoassays. Consequently, it may also be recognized by ecdysteroid receptors, and it may also contribute to hormonally regulated functions.

VI. SITES OF ECDYSTEROID PRODUCTION IN TICKS

In insects, ecdysone is produced by the prothoracic gland in the immature stages and, in some species, by the ovary in the adult female. In mosquitoes, ovarian ecdysone acts on the fat body, initiating production of vitellogenin. Glands analogous to insect prothoracic glands have not been reported in ticks and the site, or sites, of ecdysteroid production in these parasites is unknown. Cox (1960) presented experimental evidence implicating the synganglion as a source of "moulting hormone" in *Ornithodoros turicata*. More recently, Sonenshine *et al.* (1985a) reported high RIA titers for ecdysteroids in mixed tissue extracts containing synganglion and lateral segmental organ tissues. Studies by Binnington (1981) and Marzouk *et al.* (1985) support the endocrine role of the lateral segmental organ in ixodid ticks, although they do not identify the hormones produced. In contrast to these findings, other studies implicate the "fat body" tissues as the source of ecdysteroid production in ticks. Ellis and Obenchain (1984) reported ecdysteroid production by "mixed tissues associated with the fat body" extracted from nymphal *Amblyomma variegatum* and maintained in culture. Ecdysteroid production was estimated at from 25 to 30 pg/μl of culture medium from wells containing pooled tissues from five to eight nymphal ticks. These authors suggested that the ecdysteroid-producing cell may be the basophilic fat body cell type, or nephrocyte, a cell similar to the cells that make up the molting glands of the Myriapoda.

VII. 20-HYDROXYECDYSONE AS A COMPONENT OF THE GENITAL SEX PHEROMONE OF IXODID TICKS

Certain species of ixodid ticks, e.g., *Dermacentor variabilis* and *D. andersoni*, utilize a genital sex pheromone to enable the mating male to identify and accept conspecific females (Sonenshine *et al.*, 1982b). This identification uses sensilla on the cheliceral digits (Sonenshine *et al.*, 1984b). In *D. variabilis*, 20-hydroxyecdysone appears to serve as one of the components of this still unidentified pheromone mixture. 20-Hydroxyecdysone was found to be present in the anterior reproductive tract tissues. This compound was found in methanolic extracts of the anterior reproductive organs of female *D. variabilis* analyzed by HPLC; assay of the HPLC fractions by RIA indicated 180 pg per tick in these tissues (D. Sonenshine, unpublished). Radioimmunoassays of the same tissues in *H. dromedarii* indicated only 12.5 pg per tick. To determine whether *D. variabilis* males could detect this hormone, Sonenshine and co-workers (Sonenshine *et al.*, 1986a,c) implanted glass microelectrodes filled with aqueous solutions of 20-hydroxyecdysone and other compounds over their cheliceral digits. The cheliceral digit sensillae responded with vigorous bursts of impulses when this compound was included in solutions placed in contact with these structures, as well as when the parent compound ecdysone was substituted (Fig. 11).

Ecdysteroid excitation of neuronal activity has been reported in insects (Koolman and Spindler, 1983). Bioassays of conspecific "neutered" females (vaginal connection severed) treated with 20-hydroxyecdysone also gave strong

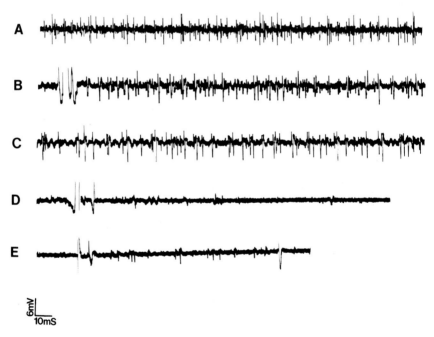

Fig. 11. Oscilloscope tracings illustrating the responses of *Dermacentor variabilis* chelicerae and palps to various chemical stimuli administered by capillary microelectrodes. (A) Response of the inner cheliceral digit sensilla to a 0.15 *M* NaCl solution. (B) Response of the inner cheliceral digit sensilla to a 1 m*M* 20-hydroxyecdysone solution. (C) Response of the inner cheliceral digit sensilla to 1 m*M* ecdysone solution. (D) Absence of a response of the palpal sensilla to 20-hydroxyecdysone (1 m*M*). (E) Absence of a response of the palpal sensilla to ecdysone (1 m*M*). From Sonenshine *et al.* (1986c), *Journal of Chemical Ecology,* with the permission of the Editor, 12:1091–1108.

TABLE V

Responses of Sexually Active Male *Dermacentor variabilis* to "Neutered" Females Treated with Authentic Known Compounds or a Known Compound Found in the ART Extract[a,b]

Treatment	Concentration (μg)	Number of trials	Summary score	Response (%)
20-Hydroxyecdysone	0.01	1	0.0	0.0
20-Hydroxyecdysone	0.1	1	7.5	83.3[c]
20-Hydroxyecdysone	2.0	2	10.8	59.8[d]
20-Hydroxyecdysone	ART II-2 (?)	1	3.5	38.9
ATP	25.0	2	3.3	18.3
Glutathione	30.0	2	0.0	0.0
"Neutered" controls	—	13	27.8	23.7

[a]Neutering was done by making an incision in the ventral body cuticle of an unfed female tick, grasping the vestibular vagina with microforceps, and severing it near its connection with the gonopore. Surviving females were allowed to feed 7 days, whereupon the ventral surface surrounding the genital pore was washed (methanol and acetone) and scraped vigorously to remove residual pheromone. Females treated in this fashion presented the same physical appearance as the untreated controls except for the wound scar located nearby. Details of the scoring system are described in the original article.

[b]From Sonenshine *et al.*, 1986a, with the permission of the editor.

[c]Significant at $p < .05$.

[d]Significant at $p < .01$.

positive responses (Table V). However, no response was obtained when conspecific neutered females were treated with ecdysone or when heterospecific females were treated with 20-hydroxyecdysone. *Dermancentor variabilis* males did not respond when the entire crude extract was implanted into heterospecific females. Based on these results, the authors suggested (1) that 20-hydroxyecdysone is a component of the genital sex pheromone in *D. variabilis*, (2) that it may be a unique component of the genital sex pheromone of that species, (3) that *D. variabilis* males can discriminate it from closely related molecules, and (4) that it is not the complete pheromone! Although unusual and certainly meriting further study, this is yet another possible role for this hormone.

VIII. ROLE OF NEUROSECRETIONS IN STIMULATING SEX PHEROMONE ACTIVITY

Adult ticks commence production of sex pheromones soon after their emergence from the juvenile stages. However, secretion, in some cases accompanied by increased synthesis, is delayed until the females attach to warm blooded hosts and commence feeding. This delayed onset of secretory activity, often 24–48 hr duration, is consistent with neurosecretory regulation of this behavior. Morphologic studies reviewed above (Sonenshine *et al.*, 1981a,b, 1983) demonstrated the occurrence of a nerve innervating the pheromone glands, the foveal nerve. The axons of this nerve have been found to contain neurosecretory vesicles, including electron-lucent vesicles characteristic of catecholamine transport vesicles, as well as electron-dense particles which may represent neuropeptides.

A recent study by Sonenshine *et al.* (1985b) provided evidence of the role of catecholamines in the excitation of sex pheromone activity. Experiments with the catecholamine-depleting agent reserpine led to highly significant reductions in sex attractant activity, reductions in foveal gland secretory droplet and chlorine content, loss of histofluorescence characteristic of monoamines, and reductions in 2,6-DCP content. These results were obtained with female ticks in which reserpine was administered prior to feeding. However, treatment of *feeding* female ticks with reserpine was ineffective, probably due to the diluting effect of the large fluid volume (blood meal) present at this stage. Treatment of female ticks with DL-α-methyl-*m*-tyrosine methyl ester hydrochloride, a compound which antagonizes the synthesis of dopamine (**IX**) from tyrosine, resulted in greatly reduced pheromone content in the treated ticks. Female ticks treated with this highly soluble antagonist were much less attractive to males than females treated with any other pharmacologically active compound. Included among those compounds that were ineffective was acetylcholine, hardly surprising in view of the widespread occurrence of acetylcholinesterase in the tick nervous system (K. A. Carson and D. Sonenshine, unpublished). Treatment of female ticks with dopamine led to elevated 2,6-DCP content in three of the five treatment groups assayed by gas chromatography, as well as to elevated chlorine content in all specimens assayed by X-ray microanalysis. The authors concluded that these findings implicated monoamines, most probably catecholamines, in the regulation of sex pheromone activity. They also noted that evidence of catecholamine stimulation of other glands, e.g., salivary gland secretion, is well known in ticks (Kaufman and Sauer, 1982) and that adrenergic regulation of foveal gland secretion may be inferred. Presumably, catecholaminergic receptor sites exist in these glands. In view of these findings and similarities with other catecholamine function in other secretory glands, it is likely that these monoamines stimulate sex pheromone secretion rather than biosynthesis.

IX

$$HO-\langle\!\bigcirc\!\rangle-CH_2-CH_2-NH_2$$
HO

DOPAMINE
(3, 4 – dihydroxyphenethylamine)

IX. PERCEPTION OF PHEROMONES

Three organs are used for detection of chemical signals in ticks: (1) the Haller's organ on the first leg tarsi, (2) the terminal segment of the palps, and (3) the cheliceral digits. Haller's organ consists of an anterior trough with six or seven setiform sensilla and a posterior capsule with both setiform and pleomorphic sensilla, exposed only by a small pore or narrow slit. The anterior trough in most ixodid species that have been studied (see Waladde and Rice, 1982, for review) has at least four types of setiform sensilla, including a large, broadly based multiporose seta (ap-1) serving as a sensillum basiconica (two such sensilla occur in *Amblyomma americanum*). In addition, a group of setae on a ridge or hump anterior to the trough contain one or more multiporose setae similar to ap-1 (=MD-3 of Waladde, 1982). This is the sensillum type that serves to detect the sex attractant pheromone, 2,6-DCP (Haggart and Davis, 1981; Wallade, 1982). These authors were unable to demonstrate any relationship between the state of feeding and sensitivity of the male tick pheromone receptors to 2,6-DCP. Unfed males, fed males, and even females were capable of detecting this compound with little apparent difference in sensitivity. Waladde (1982) observed that males of both *Amblyomma variegatum* and *Rhipicephalus appendiculatus* responded to 2,6-DCP in amounts as low as 0.4 ng/μl, with no apparent relation to species or state of feeding. This finding was all the more remarkable since neither species has been found to contain this pheromone. Clearly, this sensory modality is widespread in ixodid ticks, and it does not appear to be limited to either sex or physiological state, i.e., there does not appear to be any evidence of hormonal control of this sensory function. Haggart and Davis (1981) concluded that the behavioral responses to 2,6-DCP are based on integration of information in the central nervous system rather than at the level of peripheral neuron sensitivities.

Tick chelicerae also contain receptors that detect sex pheromones, specifically, the genital sex pheromone described by Sonenshine et al. (1982b, 1986a). Porose sensilla, including at least one innervated by chemoreceptive dendrites, occur on the inner cheliceral digits (Sonenshine et al., 1984b). In *Boophilus microplus*, electrophysiological records revealed selective responses to host blood, saline solutions, ATP, and reduced glutathione when the digit sensilla were exposed to these materials (Waladde and Rice, 1982). In *D. variabilis,* the cherliceral digit sensilla also respond to extracts of the female reproductive tract and 20-hydroxyecdysone (Sonenshine et al., 1986a). Whether the males are receptive only at certain periods of life or physiological condition is unknown.

Much less is known regarding the role of palps in sex pheromone perception. These organs were found to provide the receptors for perception of the assembly pheromone of *Ixodes ricinus* (Graf, 1975). However, they do not appear to have any role in sex pheromone perception or mating behavior in the metastriate ixodids.

At present, there is no evidence of hormonal regulation of pheromone perception in ticks, although behavioral evidence suggests that integration and interpretation of sensory information is dependent on feeding. Clearly, this is a subject that should provide fundamental insights into the nature of nervous control of behavior and the physiological or developmental factors that regulate it.

X. SUMMARY

Hormonal regulation of mate finding behavior occurs in many arthropods, including ticks. Studies with ticks suggest that biosynthesis of sex pheromone is stimulated by the ecdysteroid, 20-hydroxyecdysone, which occurs during adult life. This finding parallels similar evidence in insects and suggests that 20-hydroxyecdysone could bind to specific receptors in the pheromone-secreting cells and thereby direct the coding of specific enzymes that direct pheromone biosynthesis. The participation of other bioactive molecules, e.g., dopamine, may also be required. Other studies with ticks suggest that secretion of sex pheromone, timed to coincide with the commencement of blood sucking activity, is directed by one or more neurosecretory substances, probably including a catecholamine or even a nueropeptide.

ACKNOWLEDGMENTS

The author is most grateful to Mr. Mark Beveridge, Ms. Linda Boland, Ms. Susan Bennet, Mr. William Dees, Ms. Elizabeth Breidling, Mr. DeMar Taylor, Mr. Martin Screifer, Dr. Paul J. Homsher, and Dr. Keith A. Carson, all of whom contributed to the results described in this work. Parts of these studies were done in collaboration with Dr. R. M. Silverstein, Department of Chemistry, College of Environmental Sciences and Forestry, State University of New York, Syracuse, New York, whose incisive criticisms and encouragement are most gratefully appreciated. These studies were supported by grants, AI 10,986 and AI 10,987, from the National Institute of Allergy and Infectious Diseases, National Institutes of Health, U.S. Public Health Service, Bethesda, Maryland, and by a contract, N00014-80-C00546, with the Microbiology Program, Naval Biology Program, Office of Naval Research, Arlington, Virginia. The opinions and assertions contained herein are the private ones of the author and are not to be construed as official or as reflecting the views of the Department of the Navy or of the naval service at large.

REFERENCES

Adams, T. S., Dillwith, J. W., and Blomquist, G. J. (1984). The role of 20-hydroxyecdysone in housefly sex pheromone biosynthesis. *J. Insect Physiol.* **30**, 287–294.

Aeschlimann, A. (1968). La ponte chez *Ornithodoros moubata* Murray (Ixodoidea, Argasidae). *Rev. Suisse Zool.* **75**, 1033–1039.

Amerasinghe, F. P. (1978). Effects of JH I and JH III on yellowing, sexual activity, and pheromone production in allatectomized male *Schistocerca gregaria*. *J. Insect Physiol.* **24**, 603–612.

Andrews, R. H., and Bull, C. M. (1982). Mating behavior and reproductive isolation of three species of reptile ticks. *An. Behav.* **30**, 515–524.

Bassal, T. T. M. (1974). Biochemical and physiological studies of certain ticks (Ixodoidea). Activity of juvenile hormone analogues during embryogenesis in *Hyalaomma (H.) dromedarii* Koch (Ixodidae). *Z. Parasit.* **45**, 85–89.

Bassal, T. T. M., and Roshdy, M. A. (1974). *Argas (Persicargas) arboreus:* Juvenile hormone termination of diapause and oviposition control. *Exp. Parasitol.* **36**, 34–39.

Barth, R. H., Jr., and Bell, W. J. (1969). Effects of juvenile hormone and JH analogues on the reproductive physiology of the cockroach, *Bryostria fumigata* (Guerin). *Am. Zool.* **9**, 1085.

Binnington, K. (1981). Ultrastructural evidence for the endocrine nature of the latreal organs of the cattle tick, *Boophilus microplus. Tiss. Cell* **13**, 475–490.

Blomquist, G. J., and Dillwith, J. W. (1983). Pheromones: Biochemistry and physiology. *In* "Endocrinology of Insects" (R. G. H. Downer and H. Laufer, eds.), pp. 527–542. Alan R. Liss, New York.

Blomquist, G. J., Adams, T. S., and Dillwith, J. W. (1984). Induction of female sex pheromone production in male houseflies by ovary implants or 20-hydroxyecdysone. *J. Insect Physiol.* **30**, 295–302.

Borden, J. H., Nair, K. K., and Slater, C. E. (1969). Synthetic juvenile hormone: Induction of sex pheromone production in *Ips confusus. Science* **166**, 1626–1627.

Bouvier, J., Diehl, P. A., and Morici, M. (1982). Ecdysone metabolism in the tick, *Ornithodoros moubata* (Argasidae: Ixodoidea). *Rev. Suisse Zool.* **89**, 967–976.

Bowers, W. S. (1976). Discovery of insect anti-allatotropins. *In* "The Juvenile Hormones" (L. I. Gilbert, ed.), pp. 394–408. Plenum, New York.

Cone, W. W. (1979). *In* "Recent Advances in Acarology" (J. G. Rodriguez, ed.), Vol. 2, pp. 309–317. Academic Press, New York.

Connat, J. L., Diehl, P. A., Dumont, N., Carminati, S., and Thompson, M. J. (1983). Effects of exogenous ecdysteroids on the female tick, *Ornithodoros moubata:* Induction of supermolting and influence on oogenesis. *Z. Angst. Entomol.* **96**, 520–530.

Connat, J. L., Diehl, P. A., and Morici, M. (1984). Metabolism of ecdysteroids during vitellogenesis of the tick *Ornithodoros moubata* (Ixodoidea: Argasidae): Accumulation of apolar metabolites in the eggs. *Gen. Comp. Endocrinol.* **56**, 100–110.

Cox, B. L. (1960). Hormonal involvement in the molting process in the soft-tick, *Ornithodoros turicata* (Duges). Unpublished Ph.D. dissertation. University of Oklahoma, Norman.

Dees, W. H., Sonenshine, D. E., Breidling, E., Buford, N. P., and Khalil, G. M. (1982). Toxicity of precocene-2 for the American dog tick, *Dermancentor variabilis* (Say). *J. Med. Entomol.* **19**, 734–742.

Dees, W. H., Sonenshine, D. E., and Breidling, E. (1984a). Ecdysteroids in *Hyalomma dromedarii* and *Dermacentor variabilis* and their effects on sex pheromone activity. *In* "Acarology VI" (D. A. Griffiths and C. E. Bowman, eds.), Vol. 1, pp. 405–413, Ellis Horwood, Chichester.

Dees, W. H., Sonenshine, D. E., and Breidling, E. (1984b). Ecdysteroids in the American dog tick, *Dermacentor variabilis* (Acari: Ixodidae) during different periods of tick development. *J. Med. Entomol.* **21**, 514–523.

Dees, W. H., Sonenshine, D. E., and Breidling, E. (1985). Ecdysteroids in the camel tick, *Hyalloma dromedarii* (Acari: Ixodidae), and comparison with sex pheromone activity. *J. Med. Entomol.* **22**, 22–27.

Diehl, P. A., and Aeschlimann, A. (1982). Tick reproduction: Oogenesis and oviposition. *In* "Physiology of Ticks" (F. D. Obenchain and R. Galun, eds.), pp. 277–350. Pergamon, Oxford.

Diehl, P. A., Connat, J. L., Girault, J. P., and LaFont, R. (1985). A new class of apolar ecdysteroid conjugates: Esters of 20-hydroxyecdysone with long chain fatty acids. *Int. J. Invert. Reprod. Dev.* **8**, 1–13.

Ellis, B. J., and Obenchain, F. D. (1984). *In vivo* and *in vitro* production of ecdysteroids by nymphal *Amblyomma variegatum* ticks. *In* "Acarology VI" (D. A. Griffiths and C. E. Bowman, eds.), Vol. 1, pp. 400–404. Ellis Horwood, Chichester.

Gothe, R., and Neitz, A. W. H. (1985). Investigation into the participation of male pheromones of *Rhipicephalus evertsi evertsi* during infestation. *Onderstepoort J. Vet. Res.* **52**, 67–70.

Graf, J. F. (1975). Ecologie and ethologie D'*Ixodes ricinus* L. en Suisse (Ixodoidea: Ixodidae). Cinquieme note: Mise en evidence d'une pheromone sexuelle chez *Ixodes ricinus*. *Acarologia* **18**, 226–233.

Grzelak, K., and Krishna Kumaran, A. (1985). The effect of 20-hydroxyecdysone and juvenile hormone transcription and specific gene expression in larval fat body in *Galleria*. *J. Insect Physiol.* **31**, 315–322.

Hafez, M., and Bassal, T. T. M. (1980). Juvenilization of the brown dog tick, *Rhipicephalus sanguineus* Latr. (Ixodoidea: Acarina). *J. Egypt. Soc. Parasitol.* **10**, 301–304.

Hagedorn, H. H., O'Connor, J. D., Fuchs, M. S., Sage, B., Schlager, D. A., and Bohm, M. K. (1975). The ovary as a source of α-ecdysone in an adult mosquito. *Proc. Natl. Acad. Sci. U.S.A.* **72**, 3255–3259.

Haggart, D. A., and Davis, E. E. (1981). Neurons sensitive to 2,6-dichlorophenol on the tarsi of the tick, *Amblyomma americanum* (Acari: Ixodidae). *J. Med. Entomol.* **18**, 187–193.

Hayes, M. J., and Oliver, J. H., Jr. (1981). The immediate and latent effects induced by the anti-allatotropin precocene-2 (P2) on embryonic *Dermacentor variabilis* (Say) (Acari: Ixodidae). *J. Parasitol.* **67**, 923–927.

Ioffe, I. D., and Uspenskiy, I. V. (1979). Effect of the insect juvenile hormone analogues on ixodid tick nymphs. *Med. Parazit. Moskva* **48**, 39–46 (in Russian).

Ioffe, I. D., Uspenskiy, I. V., Bessmertnaya, I. K., and Kachanko, N. I. (1977). Effect of synthetic juvenile hormone analogue on Ixodoidea. *J. Gen. Biol.* **38**, 885–892 (in Russian; English summary).

Isaac, R. E., and Rees, H. H. (1984). Isolation and identification of ecdysteroid phosphates and acetyl ecdysteroid phosphates from developing eggs of the locust, *Schistocerca gregaria*. *Biochem. J.* **221**, 459–464.

Isaac, R. E., Rose, M. E., Rees, H. H., and Goodwin, T. W. (1982). Identification of ecdysone-22-phosphate and 2-deoxyecdysone-22-phosphate in eggs of the desert locust, *Schistocerca gregaria*, by fast atom bombardment mass spectroscopy and N.M.R. spectroscopy. *J. Chem. Soc. Chem. Commun.*, 249–251.

Isaac, R. E., Rose, M. E., Rees, H. H., and Goodwin, T. W. (1983). Identification of 22-phosphate esters of ecdysone, 2-deoxyecdysone, 20-hydroxyecdysone and 2-deoxy-20-hydroxyecdysone from newly laid eggs of the desert locust, *Schistocerca gregaria*. *Biochem. J.* **213**, 533–541.

Jaffe, H., Hayes, D. K., Sonenshine, D. E., Dees, W. H., Beveridge, M., and Thompson, M. J. (1986). Controlled release reservoir system for the delivery insect steroid analogues against ticks. *J. Med. Entomol.* **23**, 685–691.

Kaufman, W. R., and Sauer, J. R. (1982). Ion and water balance in feeding ticks: Mechanisms of tick excretion. *In* "Physiology of Ticks" (F. D. Obenchain and R. Galun, eds.), pp. 213–244. Pergamon, Oxford.

Kellum, D., and Berger, R. S. (1977). Relationship of the occurrence and function of 2,6-dichlorophenol in two species of *Amblyomma* (Acari: Ixodidae). *J. Med. Entomol.* **13**, 701–705.

Khalil, G. M., Nada, S. A., and Sonenshine, D. E. (1981). Sex pheromone regulation of mating behavior in the camel tick, *Hyalomma dromedarii* (Ixodoidea, Ixodidae). *J. Parasitol.* **67**, 70–76.

Khalil, G. M., Sonenshine, D. E., Homsher, P. J., Dees, W. H., Carson, K. A., and Wang, V. (1983). Development, ultrastructure and activity of the foveal glands and foveae dorsales of the camel tick, *Hyalomma dromedarii* (Acari: Ixodidae). 1. Primordial growth and gland formation. *J. Med. Entomol.* **20**, 414–423.

Khalil, G. M., Sonenshine, D. E., Hanafy, H. A., and Abdelmonem, A. E. (1984a). Juvenile hormone I effects on the camel tick, *Hyalomma dromedarii* (Acari: Ixodidae) *J. Med. Entomol.* **21**, 561–566.

Khalil, G. M., Shaarawy, A. A. A., Sonenshine, D. E., and Gad, S. M. (1984b). β-Ecdysone effects on the camel tick, *Hyalomma dromedarii* (Acari: Ixodidae). *J. Med. Entomol.* **21**, 188–193.

Kitaoka, S. (1972). Effects of ecdysone on ticks, especially *Ornithodoros moubata* (Acarina: Argasidae). *Abstr. 14th Int. Congr. Entomol. Canberra, Australia,* **1972.**

Koeppe, J. H., Fuchs, M., Chen, T. T., Hunt, L. M., Kovalicks, G. E., and Briers, T. (1985). The role of juvenile hormone in reproduction. *In* "Comprehensive Insect Physiology, Biochemistry and Pharmacology" (G. A. Kerkut and L. I. Gilbert, eds.), Vol. 8, pp. 165–203, Pergamon, Oxford.

Koolman, J., and Spindler, K. D. (1983). Mechanism of action of ecdysteroids. *In* "Endocrinology of Insects" (R. G. H. Downer and H. Laufer, eds.), pp. 179–201, Alan R. Liss, New York.

Lafont, R., and Koolman, J. (1984). Ecdysone metabolism. *In* "Biosynthesis, Metabolism and Mode of Action of Invertebrate Hormones" (J. Hoffman and M. Porchet, eds.), pp. 196–226. Springer-Verlag, Berlin, Heidleberg.

Lafont, R., Blais, C., Beydon, P., Modde, J. F., Enderle, U., and Koolman, J. (1983). Conversion of ecdysone and 20-hydroxyecdysone into 26-oic derivatives is a major pathway in larvae and pupae of species from three insect orders. *Arch. Insect Biochem. Physiol.* **1**, 41–58.

Leahy, M. G., and Booth, K. S. (1980). Precocene induction of tick sterility and ecdysis failure. *J. Med. Entomol.* **17**, 18–21.

McDaniel II, R. S., and Oliver, J. H., Jr. (1978). Effects of two juvenile hormone analogs and β-ecdysone on nymphal development, spermatogenesis and embryogenesis in *Dermacentor variabilis* (Say). *J. Parasitol.* **64**, 571–573.

Mango, C. K. A., Odhiambo. T. R., and Galun, R. (1976). Ecdysone and the super tick. *Nature (London)* **260**, 318–319.

Mansingh, A., and Rawlins, S. C. (1977). Anti-gonadotrophic action of insect hormone analogues on the cattle tick, *Boophilus microplus. Naturwissenschaften* **64**, 41.

Marzouk, A. S., Mohamed, F. S. A., and Khalil, G. M. (1985). Neurohemal endocrine organs in the camel tick, *Hyalomma dromedarii* (Acari: Ixodoidea: Ixodidae). *J. Med. Entomol.* **22**, 385–391.

Menon, M. D. (1976). Hormone–pheromone relationships of male *Tenebrio molitor. J. Insect Physiol.* **22**, 1021–1023.

Menon, M. D., and Nair, K. K. (1976). Age-dependent effects of synthetic juvenile hormone on pheromone synthesis in adult females of *Tenebrio molitor Ann. Entomol. Soc. Am.* **69**, 457–458.

Meola, R. W., Harris, R. L., Meola, S. M., and Oehler, D. D. (1977). Dietary induced secretion of sex pheromones and development of sexual behavior in the stable fly. *Environ. Entomol.* **6**, 895–897.

Obenchain, F. D. (1984). Behavioral interactions between the sexes, and aspects of species specificity pheromone mediated aggregation and attachment in *Amblyoma. In* "Acarology VI" (D. A. Griffiths and C. E. Bowman, eds.), Vol. 1, pp. 387–392. Ellis Horwood, Chichester.

O'Connor, J. D. (1983). Ecdysteroid and juvenile hormone receptors. *In* "Endocrinology of Insects" (R. G. H. Downer and H. Laufer, eds.), pp. 559–565. Alan R. Liss, New York.

Oliver, J. H., Jr., Pound, J. M., and Severino, G. (1985). Evidence of a juvenile hormone-like compound in the reproduction of *Dermanyssus gallinae* (Acari: Dermanyssidae). *J. Med. Entomol.* **22**, 281–286.

Pound, J. M., and Oliver, J. H., Jr. (1979). Juvenile hormone: Evidence of its role in the reproduction of ticks. *Science* **206**, 355–357.

Pound, J. M., and Oliver, J. H., Jr. (1984). Morphology of the retrocerebral organ complex in penultimate nymphal and adult female *Ornithodoros parkeri* (Cooley) (Acari: Argasidae). *In* "Acarology VI" (D. A. Griffiths and C. E. Bowman, eds.), Vol. 1, pp. 295–303. Ellis Horwood, Chichester.

Sannasi, A., and Subramoniam, T. (1972). Hormonal rupture of larval diapause in the tick, *Rhipicephalus sanguineus* (Latr.) *Experientia* **28**, 666–667.

Schoeni, R., Hess, E., Blum, W., and Ramstein, K. (1984). The aggregation-attachment pheromone of the tropical bont tick, *Amblyomma variegatum* Fabricius (Acari: Ixodidae). Isolation, identification, and action of its active components. *J. Insect Physiol.* **30**, 613–618.

Solomon, K. R., Mango, C. K. A., and Obenchain, F. D. (1982). Endocrine mechanisms in ticks. Effects of insect hormones and their mimics on development and reproduction. *In* "Physiology of Ticks" (F. D. Obenchain and R. Galun, eds.), pp. 399–438. Pergamon, Oxford.

Sonenshine, D. E. (1984). Tick pheromones. *In* "Current Topics in Vector Research" (K. F. Harris, ed.), Vol. 2, pp. 225–263. Praeger, New York.

Sonenshine, D. E. (1985). Pheromones and other semiochemicals of the Acari. *Annu. Rev. Entomol.* **30**, 1–28.

Sonenshine, D. E., Homsher, P. J., VandeBerg, J. S., and Dawson, D. (1981a). Fine structure of the foveal glands and foveae dorsales of the American dog tick, *Dermacentor variabilis* (Say). *J. Parasitol.* **67**, 627–646.

Sonenshine, D. E., Gainsburg, D. M., Rosenthal, M. D., and Silverstein, R. M. (1981b). The sex pheromone glands of *Dermacentor variabilis* (Say) and *D. andersoni* (Stiles): Sex pheromone stored in neutral lipid. *J. Chem. Ecol.* **7**, 345–357.

Sonenshine, D. E., Silverstein, R. M., and Rechav, Y. (1982a). Tick pheromone mechanisms. *In* "Physiology of Ticks" (F. D. Obenchain and R. Galun, eds.), pp. 439–468. Pergamon, Oxford.

Sonenshine, D. E., Khalil, G. M., Homsher, P. J., and Mason, S. N. (1982b). *Dermacentor variabilis* and *Dermacentor andersoni:* Genital sex pheromones. *Exp. Parasitol.* **54**, 317–330.

Sonenshine, D. E., Khalil, G. M., Homsher, P. J., Dees, W. H., Carson, K. A., and Wang, V. (1983). Development, ultrastructure, and activity of the foveal glands and foveae dorsales of the camel tick, *Hyalomma dromedarii* (Acari: Ixodidae). 2. Maturation and pheromone activity. *J. Med. Entomol.* **20**, 424–439.

Sonenshine, D. E., Silverstein, R. l., and West, J. R. (1984a). Occurrence of sex attractant pheromone, 2,6-dichlorophenol, in relation to age and feeding in American dog tick, *Dermacentor variabilis* (Say) (Acari: Ixodidae) *J. Chem. Ecol.* **10**, 95–100.

Sonenshine, D. E., Homsher, P. J., Carson, K. A., and Wang, V. G. (1984b). Evidence of the role of the cheliceral digits in the perception of genital sex pheromones during mating in the American dog tick, *Dermacentor variabilis* (Say) (Acari: Ixodidae). *J. Med. Entomol.* **21**, 296–306.

Sonenshine, D. E., Homsher, P. J., Beveridge, M., and Dees, W. H. (1985a). Occurrence of ecdysteroids in specific body organs of the camel tick, *Hyalomma dromedarii,* and the American dog tick, *Dermacentor variabilis,* with notes on their synthesis from cholesterol. *J. Med. Entomol.* **22**, 303–311.

Sonenshine, D. E., Silverstein, R. M., West, J. R., Carson, K. A., Homsher, P. J., Bennet, S., and Taylor, D. (1985b). Studies on possible role of catecholamines in regulation of sex pheromone gland activity in American dog tick, *Dermacentor variabilis* (Say). *J. Chem. Ecol.* **11**, 363–382.

Sonenshine, D. E., Silverstein, R. M., Brossut, R., Davis, E. E., Taylor, D., Carson, K. A., Homsher, P. J., and Wang, V. B. (1986a). The genital sex pheromones of ixodid ticks. 1. Morphologic, experimental and chemical evidence of their occurrence in the anterior reproductive tract of the American dog tick, *Dermacentor variabilis* (Say) (Acari: Ixodidae). *J. Chem. Ecol.* **11**, 1669–1694.

Sonenshine, D. E., Boland, L. M., Beveridge, M., and Upchurch, B. T. (1986b). Metabolism of ecdysone and 20-OH ecdysone in the camel tick, *Hyalomma dromedarii* (Acari: Ixodidae). *J. Med. Entomol.* **23,** 630–650.

Sonenshine, D. E., Taylor, D. M., and Carson, K. A. (1986c). Chemically mediated behavior in the Acari: Adaptations for finding hosts and mates. *J. Chem. Ecol.* **12,** 1091–1108.

Thompson, M. J., Robbins, W. E., Cohen, C. F., Kaplanis, J. N., Dutky, S. R., and Hutchins, R. F. N. (1971). Synthesis and biological activity of 5β-hydroxy-analogs of 2-ecdysone. *Steroids* **17,** 399–409.

Waladde, S. M. (1982). Tip-recording from ixodid tick olfactory sensilla: Responses to tick related odours. *J. Comp. Physiol.* **148,** 399–409.

Waladde, S. M., and Rice, M. (1982). The sensory basis of tick feeding behavior. *In* "Physiology of Ticks" (F. D. Obenchain and R. Galun, eds.), pp. 71–118. Pergamon, Oxford.

Wigglesworth, K. P., Lewis, D., and Rees, H. H. (1985). Ecdysteroid titre and metabolism to novel apolar derivatives in adult female *Boophilus microplus* (Ixodidae). *Arch. Insect Biochem. Physiol.* **2,** 39–54.

Wright, J. E. (1969). Hormonal termination of larval diapause in *Dermacentor albipictus. Science* **163,** 390–391.

Wood, W. F., Leahy, M. G., Galun, R., Prestwich, G. D., Meinwald, J., Purnell, R. E., and Payne, R. C. (1975). Phenols as pheromones of ixodid ticks: A general phenomenon? *J. Chem. Ecol.* **1,** 501–509.

10

Cantharidin Biosynthesis and Function in Meloid Beetles

JOHN P. McCORMICK
JAMES E. CARREL
Department of Chemistry and Division of Biological Sciences
University of Missouri
Columbia, Missouri 65211

I. INTRODUCTION

Cantharidin, a terpenoid substance found in blister beetles (Coleoptera: Meloidae), is among the most widely known insect natural products in the world. Its reputation derives principally from descriptions of its physiological activities, most notably as an aphrodisiac for humans and livestock, that are traced from oral history. Cantharidin is also the blistering agent that earned these bettles their common name. These diverse effects on humans are paralleled by activities that the beetles exploit in their reproduction and ecology. It is the latter perspective of cantharidin's role that we examine in this chapter: the pheromonal and other adaptive functions of cantharidin in blister beetles. We first discuss the chemical and biosynthetic knowledge of cantharidin in order to build a foundation for understanding its ecological roles in blister beetles.

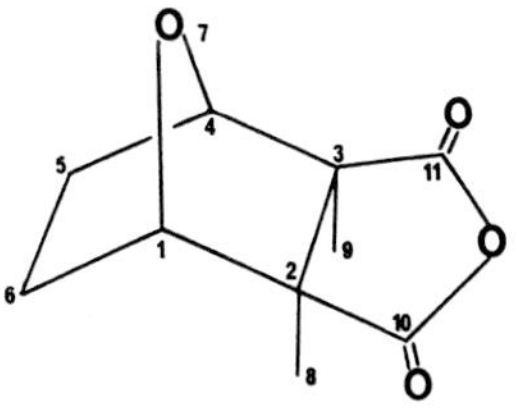

Cantharidin

307

Pheromone Biochemistry

A. Discovery and Use of Cantharidin

For more than 2,000 years, blister beetles in powdered or tincture form have been used medicinally in Europe, China, and elsewhere. In Western cultures these materials are called cantharides, derived from the Greek word for beetle (*kantharos*). They also are referred to generically as Spanish fly, the common name of the iridescent green meloid *Lytta vesicatoria* from Europe, which Kobert (1906) long ago pointed out is neither Iberian nor dipteran.

The ancient Greeks and Romans consumed cantharides as a diuretic and abortifacient as well as an aphrodisiac. To cure fevers and many other systemic maladies, they applied cantharides to the skin to induce blisters in the belief that the disease would be drawn out of the body (Keele and Armstrong, 1964). The use of cantharides grew in Western societies until the nineteenth century, at which time they were considered the most powerful drug available in medicine (Polson and Tattersall, 1959). However, in the course of the development of modern medicine, investigations produced strong evidence that cantharides have little if any therapeutic or aphrodisiac effect and that they are exceedingly toxic when taken internally (Polson and Tattersall, 1959; Nickolls and Teare, 1954; Sollman, 1948), leading to their virtual disuse in Western cultures except for removal of certain warts (Epstein and Kligman, 1959). The lethal dose of cantharidin in humans is estimated to be about 10–50 mg, but 0.5 mg lodged in the throat could cause blistering sufficient to produce death by suffocation (Nickolls and Teare, 1954; Till and Majmudar, 1981). Because the aphrodisiac properties of cantharides are legendary, they occasionally are administered illicitly to humans in an attempt to induce sexual arousal. This misguided use sometimes is lethal for the intended lover (Nickolls and Teare, 1954). In addition, poisoning of humans and livestock that accidentally consume blister beetles is reported regularly in many regions of the world (Wertelecki *et al.*, 1967; Beasley *et al.*, 1983).

An exception to the diminishing medicinal interest in cantharides is found in China, where cantharidin and various derivatives are being evaluated in laboratory and clinical trials as antitumor agents in humans (Jiang *et al.*, 1983).

B. Structural Identification of Cantharidin

The recognition that cantharidin is a white, highly crystalline substance dates from its isolation in 1810 by Robiquet (cited by Woodward and Loftfield, 1941) from Spanish blister beetles, *L. vesicatoria*. The chemical structure of this material, however, was not easily established, in spite of its relative simplicity. Piccard (1877) ascribed the correct chemical formula to this compound, but it was not until the next century that investigators made real progress in unraveling its structure. Evidence collected by Gadamer and his co-workers (Danckwortt, 1914; Gadamer, 1914a,b; Rudolph, 1916) established the correct functionality and that this substance has a highly symmetrical structure which consists of two

C_5 units joined by two carbon–carbon bonds and bonds to two oxygen atoms. Additional work by von Bruchausen and Bersch (1929) suggested that the methyl groups are attached at the ring fusion, a conclusion that was supported by additional work reported by Woodward and Loftfield (1941). This highly constrained structure accounts for the remarkable crystallinity of cantharidin.

Following establishment of the correct atomic connectivities, a more challenging question remained to be solved: the nature of the stereochemistry of ring fusion, that is, the positions of the two methyl groups relative to the oxo bridge. The exo stereochemistry of the anhydride bridge was correctly deduced by Woodward and Loftfield and supported by a total synthesis of cantharidin reported in the 1940s (Woodward and Loftfield, 1941). This stereochemistry was definitively demonstrated by a stereospecific synthesis completed by Stork et al. in 1953. Thus, a structure remarkable for its simplicity was only fully elucidated after almost 150 years of study.

It is worth noting that this long period of structural work was generated in part from the difficulty presented by the total synthesis of cantharidin. The straightforward attempts by von Bruchhausen and Bersch (1929) as well as by Diels and Alder (1929) to assemble the tricyclic system using a single Diels–Alder reaction between furan and dimethylmaleic anhydride were uniformly unsuccessful. Interestingly, the 1942 synthesis of cantharidin by Ziegler et al. (1942) utilized an alternative Diels–Alder reaction in a circuitous approach; the stereospecific synthesis in Stork's laboratory utilized two Diels–Alder reactions in ingenious applications which, however, required 12 steps to reach the cantharidin structure. In recent years, Dauben's group has reported a successful Diels–Alder approach utilizing furan and a substituted dimethylmaleic anhydride under extremely high pressures (Dauben et al., 1980). The resulting tetracycle could be reductively converted to cantharidin in a single step. Thus, the successful cantharidin syntheses that have clarified its structure and made this substance synthetically available all have employed Diels–Alder reactions, but the obvious and simplest Diels–Alder reaction has never been carried out successfully, either in the laboratory or in nature; the biosynthesis of this substance also relies on an alternative approach.

C. Apparent Relationship of Cantharidin to Terpenoids

The intriguing simplicity of the cantharidin structure belies not only the difficulties encountered establishing the details of its molecular structure but also the complexity of the metabolic process involved in its formation by blister beetles. Comparison of its structure to those of known metabolic origin readily suggests that this compound belongs to the terpenoid biosynthetic class of natural products. However, the absence of a clearly analogous structure of known biosynthetic origin left as a reasonable possibility a polyketide origin for cantharidin. In either case, the origin of the carbon atoms ultimately would be acetate and the arrangement of those acetate units would be novel. In this chapter, we discuss the methods used to establish not only the terpenoid biosynthetic origin of cantharidin but also the exact origin of each carbon atom.

D. Overview of Chapter Topics

We first describe our methodology for blister beetle collection, laboratory rearing and handling, behavioral bioassays, and administration of substrates to blister beetles. The analytical methodology related to isolation, spectroscopic characterization, and quantitative determination of cantharidin is presented. We also discuss radiolabeling procedures, the use of 6-fluoromevalonate to inhibit cantharidin biosynthesis, and the application of these methods to determine the extent and timing of cantharidin biosynthesis as well as to demonstrate its transfer from males to females during mating. We also present a summary of the evidence, obtained using radiolabeling and stable isotope labeling, regarding the origin of all the carbon, hydrogen, and oxygen atoms of cantharidin. Finally, we present experiments and results relating to the pheromonal properties and defensive properties of cantharidin in blister beetles. The chapter concludes with a summary of future research topics.

II. METHODOLOGY

A. Beetle Collection

Adult blister beetles are collected in the field using two techniques. Margined blister beetles, *Epicauta pestifera,* are located by inspection while feeding on leaves of cultivated and wild plants from July to September near Columbia, Missouri (Fig. 1A). The most common host plants are potato, *Solanum tuberosum,* tomato, *Lycopersicon esculentum,* and climbing milkweed, *Cynanchium laeve.* Beetles that are on the plants and those that have fallen to the ground are picked up, placed in containers, and transported to the laboratory.

Adults of the brassy blister beetle, *Lytta (Pomphopoea) polita,* are collected at night in ultraviolet (UV)-light traps operated from January to March at the Archbold Biological Station near Lake Placid, Florida. Our attempts to locate swarms of these beetles feeding on male flowers of native pines (Fig. 1B), their natural food source (Hedlin *et al.,* 1981), have proved unsuccessful despite hundreds of hours of searching.

B. Beetle Culture and Control of Sexual Activity

Beetles are kept either as groups by sex in screened cages or as individuals in plastic boxes. Adult *E. pestifera* are fed either freshly picked leaves of local host

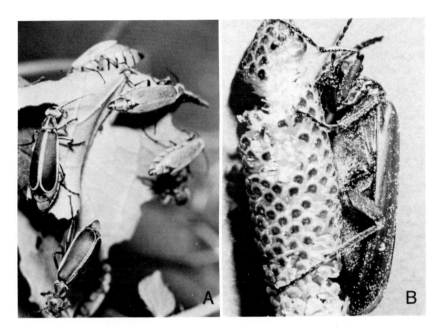

Fig. 1. (A) *Epicauta pestifera* feeding on tomato leaves; scale 2×. (B) *Lytta polita* feeding on male pine cone; scale 3×.

plants or cubes of an artificial diet developed for the southwestern cornborer (Chippendale and Cassatt, 1985). Adult *L. polita* are fed bee pollen mixed with raw honey and deionized water.

Since 1982, we have continuously reared *E. pestifera* using Selander's method (Adams and Selander, 1979). We obtain eggs deposited in moist sand by wild or laboratory-reared beetles. Triungulin larvae that emerge from these eggs are individually isolated to prevent cannibalism, and each larva is fed one egg pod of the differential grasshopper, *Melanoplus differentialis*, obtained from field-collected adults in the fall. Larvae feed for 2–3 weeks at 25°C, during which time each passes through five first grub phases; then they cease eating and shortly thereafter each molts to a diapausing coarctate larval phase. Diapause is broken by chilling coarctate larvae at 5–7°C for more than 6 months, but diapausing larvae can be maintained alive in the cold for more than 3 years until they are needed.

After warming to 25°C, postdiapause individuals develop in 4–6 weeks into adults. At 3–4 days after eclosion, adult *E. pestifera* are weighed and placed individually in plastic boxes. They then are kept at 24–26°C under continuous artificial illumination.

Virginal *E. pestifera* become sexually active approximately 1 week after eclo-

sion. However, to standardize our mating experiments, we generally use laboratory-reared adults that are about 12 days old. Because we are unable to determine
the age and previous sexual activity of *E. pestifera* and *L. polita* collected in the
field, for experimental purposes we achieve a degree of standardization in wild
beetles by isolating them for 6–8 days, during which time mated females
oviposit and once more become sexually receptive and mated males regenerate
the materials stored in their reproductive systems.

C. Behavioral Bioassays

1. Cantharidin Trapping

To evaluate the efficacy of cantharidin as a long-range attractant for blister
beetles, we conducted two series of field experiments in Boone County, Missouri, using insect traps baited with cantharidin. In the first series, 12 sticky traps
each baited with 50 µg of pure cantharidin were hung in July, 1983, on tree
branches 1–2 m above the ground, 6 in the middle of a tall grass prairie, and 6
along the interface of a deciduous forest and meadow. Randomly interspersed
with these at 10-m intervals were an equal number of unbaited traps as controls.
All traps were retrieved after 1 week and examined for blister beetles.

We conducted a second, more elaborate series of trapping experiments in
June–August, 1985. We suspended five 8-funnel Lindgren traps 1.5 m above
ground at 30-m intervals in a line along the grassy verge of a cornfield. Three
traps were baited with filter paper impregnated with 0, 200, or 2,000 µg of
cantharidin. The remaining two traps were baited with dead male or female *E.
pestifera* reared in the laboratory. All baits were wrapped once with cheesecloth
and hung off center between the middle two funnels. The order of traps was
randomly determined. The contents of the traps were checked daily for 7 weeks.

2. Sexual Selection Tests

In the last 2 years, we have tested the hypothesis that female blister beetles
may prefer to mate with males which contain relatively large amounts of cantharidin or that males may prefer low-cantharidin females (S. L. Briesacher and
J. E. Carrel, unpublished results). An overview of these experiments, all performed with laboratory-reared *E. pestifera,* is given here.

We tested whether virgin females show a short-range attraction to cantharidin
or to male beetles themselves. In the first set of tests, we assayed attractancy of
females to filter paper with and without exogenous cantharidin, located in
styrofoam cups covered with cheesecloth placed at opposite ends of a rectangular
arena. We subsequently repeated these tests using live virginal male beetles with
or without a coating of cantharidin on their elytra. These tests were performed in
the summertime in a greenhouse under environmental conditions closely match-

ing those experienced by wild beetles in the field. We used disposable materials to avoid odor contamination between different experiments.

We next tested whether virgin males show a short-range aversion to cantharidin or to mated female beetles themselves. Using the two-choice arena assays described in the previous paragraph, we recorded the movements of males relative to different baits in the cups. Baits tested were pure cantharidin, virgin females, and mated females. Controls consisted of blanks.

Finally, we tested whether female beetles prefer to mate with males containing elevated amounts of cantharidin. In these tests, we placed two male beetles of known size, age, and sexual experience simultaneously into a virginal female's cage and observed the interactions of the three beetles. As soon as the female allowed one male to mount and to initiate copulation, we isolated the two males, collected blood from each of them, and froze them for dissection and quantitative analysis of cantharidin.

3. Antifeedant Tests

In collaboration with Tom Eisner at Cornell University and Joel Maruniak and other colleagues in Columbia, Missouri, we have evaluated cantharidin as an antifeedant to many predaceous anthropods and vertebrates (Carrel and Eisner, 1974; T. Eisner, J. E. Carrel, and J. P. McCormick, unpublished results; J. E. Carrel and A. J. Slagle, unpublished results; J. E. Carrel and J. Maruniak, unpublished results). In some tests, we added known amounts of pure cantharidin either to the diet or to the water of predators. In other tests, we used whole blister beetles or their tissues as food and later determined the cantharidin content of these biological materials. The quantitative cantharidin analyses always were performed in the absence of knowledge regarding the outcome of the related biological experiments, thereby ensuring independence of biological and chemical results. The antifeedant effectiveness of cantharidin in these bioassays was determined either by its ability to reduce the quantity of food consumed by a predator or by its ability to induce cleansing in a predator.

D. Administration of Substrates to Beetles

In most biosynthetic studies, we administered metabolic substrates to blister beetles by injection into the abdomen (Fig. 2A). Injection of dosages ranging from 1 to 40 μl per beetle is easily accomplished using a micrometer syringe fitted with a 30 gauge needle. Substrates are dissolved in sterile saline, which simply consists of a 1.5% NaCl solution. To administer substrates orally to blister beetles, we mix substances of interest thoroughly into the solid diet (Fig. 2B). This method has the disadvantage that we cannot control precisely the dosage or the time course of its administration. Our attempts to force-feed blister beetles have been unsuccessful.

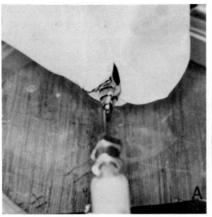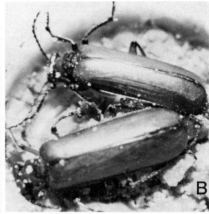

Fig. 2. (A) Injection of substrate into a male *Epicauta pestifera;* scale 1×. (B) Feeding of substrate to male *Lytta polita* in a diet of bee pollen moistened with honey and water; scale 2×.

E.   Quantitative Analysis of Cantharidin

Studies of the pharmacological and physiological activities of cantharidin as well as its ecological role in blister beetles require an effective means for cantharidin quantitation. Even the very early, relatively crude studies of its pharmacological activities relied on at least semiquantitative data obtained by biological assay methodology that was available at the time. Currently, experiments require much more accurate data regarding cantharidin content and rely on state-of-the-art detection technologies. Because these quantitative methodologies have been important in the work described and will be important in future experiments regarding the biological roles of cantharidin, we describe here the early as well as current methodology for quantitative analysis of cantharidin.

1.   Cantharidin Extraction

Quantitative analysis of materials contained in a biological matrix generally presents problems associated with the biomatrix in addition to the problem of direct quantitation of the material of interest. In the case of cantharidin, organic solvent extraction of blister beetles or desiccated tissues obtained from blister beetles provides an organic extract that contains only a small proportion of the total cantharidin in the biomatrix. The meloid tissues must be pretreated with either strong base (followed by acidification) or strong acid before organic extraction to obtain high recovery of the total cantharidin. (Although the chemical basis for the need for this pretreatment is not established, it is tempting to speculate that cantharidin is not stored as the anhydride, but rather a chemical derivative.) Some workers (Ray *et al.*, 1979; Capinera *et al.*, 1985) have reported success using treatment of the desiccated powder prepared from blister beetles with 0.2 *M* sodium hydroxide at 75–80°C. The aqueous solution thereby obtained is acidified to pH 1.0 and subsequently extracted with chloroform. This method appears to depend on initial extraction of the dicarboxylic acid disodium salt derived from cantharidin and subsequent acid-promoted reclosure of the anhydride functionality. Recovery of cantharidin in this procedure is reported to be typically 96% (Capinera *et al.*, 1985). In our experience, pretreatment of the biomatrix with concentrated HCl at 120°C followed by Soxhlet extraction using methylene chloride permits recoveries of cantharidin that are in the 95–99% range (Carrel *et al.*, 1985).

2. Blister Bioassay

The oldest method for detecting the presence of cantharidin is the blister bioassay. Through centuries of development, this technique became semiquantitative (Nickolls and Teare, 1954). Topical application of 0.05–1.0 mg of cantharidin to a person's forearm causes a complete blister to develop reliably within less than a day (Sollman, 1948). Smaller amounts of cantharidin, ranging down to 0.1 μg, produce reddening and sometimes more severe irritation of human skin (Epstein and Kligman, 1959; J. E. Carrel, unpublished results).

The blister bioassay has two major drawbacks. First, it is based on slow, somewhat variable, and often painful epidermal responses of mammalian subjects. Second, it is not sufficiently specific to exclude the presence of other vesicating agents (Fleisher and Fox, 1970). Despite these and possibly other limitations, the blister bioassay was used by forensic toxicologists to identify cantharidin until two decades ago (Simpson, 1965).

3. Colorimetry

Cantharidin determination by colorimetry has been largely unsuccessful. Bagatell (1964) used selenous acid for the microestimation of the pure compound, but he found this method did not detect cantharidin in biological fluids or in organic extracts. Yu (1957) reported that as little as 5 μg of cantharidin purified from biological materials can be detected spectrophotometrically with *p*-dimethylaminobenzaldehyde in hot sulfuric acid. We found the latter method to be unreliable (H. Eisner and J. E. Carrel, unpublished results), so we turned to chromatographic methods for quantitation of cantharidin.

4. High-Performance Liquid Chromatography (HPLC)

HPLC analysis of organic substances often offers several advantages. The analysis time for the chromatography is often short, the method is easily quantitated using common refractive index or UV–visible absorbance detectors, and the necessary equipment is found in many laboratories. HPLC analysis generally is the preferred method for materials that have low volatility or are sensitive to elevated temperatures and for compounds that have relatively highly polarity and offer a UV–visible chromophore that has relatively high absorbtivity.

Because the cantharidin chromophore is not strong at the commonly monitored 254-n wavelength, effective use of HPLC for quantitative determination of cantharidin required derivatization by a reagent that contained a more easily observed chromophore. Ray and co-workers (1979) reported derivatization of cantharidin using p-nitrobenzyloxyamine to provide a derivative that had suitable chromatographic properties and was detected with satisfactory sensitivity. HPLC analysis of this derivative could be carried out in under 10 min, with a maximal sensitivity of approximately 750 pg of cantharidin in a single injection. However, when this method was applied to typical biological materials, satisfactory sensitivities required preparative chromatography to purify cantharidin prior to derivative formation. Thus, in practical application this method suffers from the requirement of a complicated extraction, purification, derivatization procedure before the HPLC analysis can be carried out with convenience and good sensitivity.

5. Gas Chromatography (GC)

The relatively high volatility and good thermal stability that are characteristic of cantharidin make GC analysis of cantharidin the method of choice. Packed-column GC analyses have been carried out effectively both on standard solutions of cantharidin and on cantharidin derived from typical biological samples. However, the sensitivity limitations of packed-column GC present a problem. The detection limit of 120 ng per injection reported by Capinera $et\ al.$ (1985) is typical and in line with our early experience (Carrel, 1971).

Fortunately, capillary GC sensitivities are very good, and the typical high resolution achieved with capillary GC permits analyses of substances from biomatrices with minimal sample preparation. We have found that extracts prepared from HCl-treated biomaterials can be concentrated and analyzed directly by capillary GC. Using our equipment with flame ionization detection, the lower sensitivity limit for standard cantharidin solutions is approximately 30 pg; in samples from typical biological materials the detection limit is approximately 500 pg. With the aid of benzophenone as an internal standard, it is therefore possible to carry out quantitative analysis of cantharidin from blister beetle tissues rapidly and with excellent sensitivity. The method has been applied not only to biological samples derived from blister beetles but also to biological samples derived from animals that have ingested cantharidin (J. E. Carrel, T. Eisner, and J. P. McCormick, unpublished results).

F. Instrumental Characterization of Cantharidin

1. Mass Spectrometry (MS)

Characterization of cantharidin by MS provides valuable information about its structural components. Electron impact ionization (EI) and chemical ionization (CI) methods provide substantially different and complementary types of information. Figure 3 displays the mass spectra obtained using these two modes of ionization and Fig. 4 outlines key elements of the fragmentation patterns. These mass spectral data taken together provide a valuable opportunity to examine the locations of stable isotope labels incorporated into specific portions of the cantharidin molecule. Although this highly sensitive technique came too late for the earlier studies that tracked the origins of carbon and hydrogen atoms from specific precursors, it provided the essential observational tool that permitted our recent studies of the origins of the oxygen atoms from molecular oxygen and water (see Section III,E,3).

a. Electron Impact Mass Spectrometry (EI–MS).   Using EI–MS analysis of cantharidin, virtually no molecular ion is observed, and fragments above m/z 130 can be detected only at trace abundances. The base peak at m/z 128 provides useful information about the anhydride portion of the molecule, while the fragments at m/z 96 and m/z 70 provide information about the two possible tetrahydrofuranyl portions. Because these fragmentations are readily understood in terms of the loss of easily identified molecules (furan, dimethylmaleic anhydride, and ethylene plus carbon dioxide plus carbon monoxide, respectively), they provide valuable evidence for locating stable isotope labels that may be incorporated during biosynthetic precursor administration experiments. However, these EI–MS data suffer from the serious limitation of providing no evidence regarding the molecular ion and no information on ions formed by loss of single, small molecules (water, carbon monoxide, or carbon dioxide), data that would reveal specific locations of isotopically labeled atoms within the anhydride functionality.

b. Chemical Ionization Mass Spectrometry (CI–MS).   Fortunately, the CI mass spectrum permits observation of protonated cantharidin as the base peak at m/z 197. As indicated in Figure 4B, this ion undergoes loss of carbon monoxide to give m/z 169, which in turn undergoes sequential loss of water to give m/z 151 and carbon dioxide to give m/z 107. Thus, we were able to use the CI mass spectral data to differentiate the carbonyl oxygen atoms from the anhydride ether oxygen atom. Symmetry prevents any mass spectral data from revealing information that differentiates the two carbonyl groups or their constituent atoms. Importantly, the loss of carbon monoxide is the exclusive route for formation of

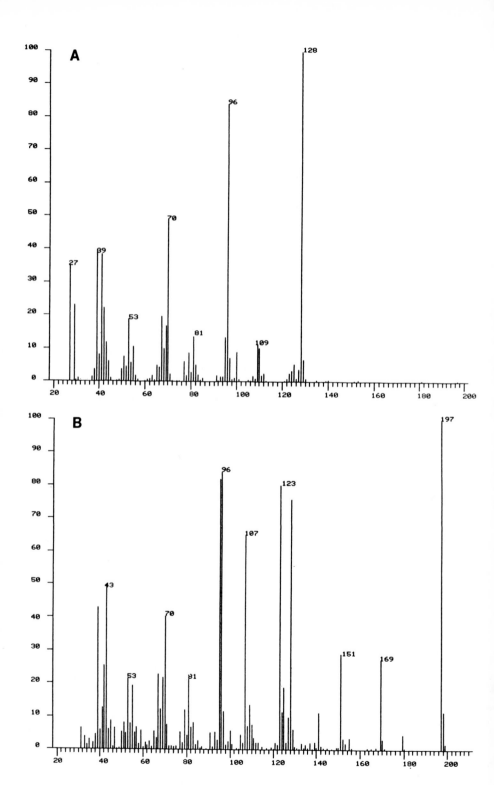

m/z 169; exact mass measurements showed that none of this ion arises from the loss of ethylene.

The CI mass spectrum also includes a fragment at m/z 128, corresponding to the base peak in the EI mass spectrum. This apparent formation of an even mass, odd electron species from an odd mass, even electron ion is interesting and seems to be unusual. Whatever the explanation of its formation may be, this m/z 128 ion (and its isotopically shifted analogs at m/z 130, 132, and 134) in the CI mass spectrum provides a useful cross-check on the composition of the m/z 128 ion (and its isotopically shifted analogs) observed as the base peak in the EI mass spectrum.

c. *Mass Spectrometry–Mass Spectrometry (MS–MS).* We were able to confirm our interpretation about the behavior of the m/z 197 ion in the CI mass spectrum by MS–MS characterization of this ion using data obtained at the Midwest Center for Mass Spectrometry in Lincoln, Nebraska. These MS–MS data confirmed that m/z 197 undergoes loss of water to give m/z 179, loss of carbon monoxide to give m/z 169, as well as subsequent loss of water to give m/z 151, and fragmentation to form m/z 128.

In addition to permitting unequivocal characterization of the m/z 197 ion fragmentation behavior, MS–MS provided an additional important capability. A general difficulty encountered with labeled-substrate administration experiments is dilution of the label in the isolated product. However, it is the maximally labeled products formed in these studies that generally provide the most information. Fortunately, MS–MS permits investigation of these maximally labeled materials without complications from materials that have less extensive isotopic incorporation. This MS–MS approach promises to offer a general method for biosynthesis studies that suffer from isotope dilution.

2. Nuclear Magnetic Resonance (NMR) Spectroscopy

NMR spectroscopic characterization of cantharidin is noteworthy for its simplicity in both spectral data and interpretation. Cantharidin possesses only four magnetically different hydrogen atoms, producing signals at 1.24 ppm (methyl), 1.78 and 1.80 ppm (methylene), and at 4.72 ppm (methine). The small difference in the chemical shifts of the exo and endo hydrogen signals does not permit assignment of these signals to specific hydrogen atoms. The geminal and vicinal coupling constants were too small to be accurately observed at 90 MHz.

The carbon spectrum also is simple but somewhat more valuable for isotope labeling studies. For our ^{18}O work (Section III,E,3), the chemical shifts of

---

Fig. 3. Mass spectra of cantharidin after (A) electron impact–induced ionization or (B) chemical ionization.

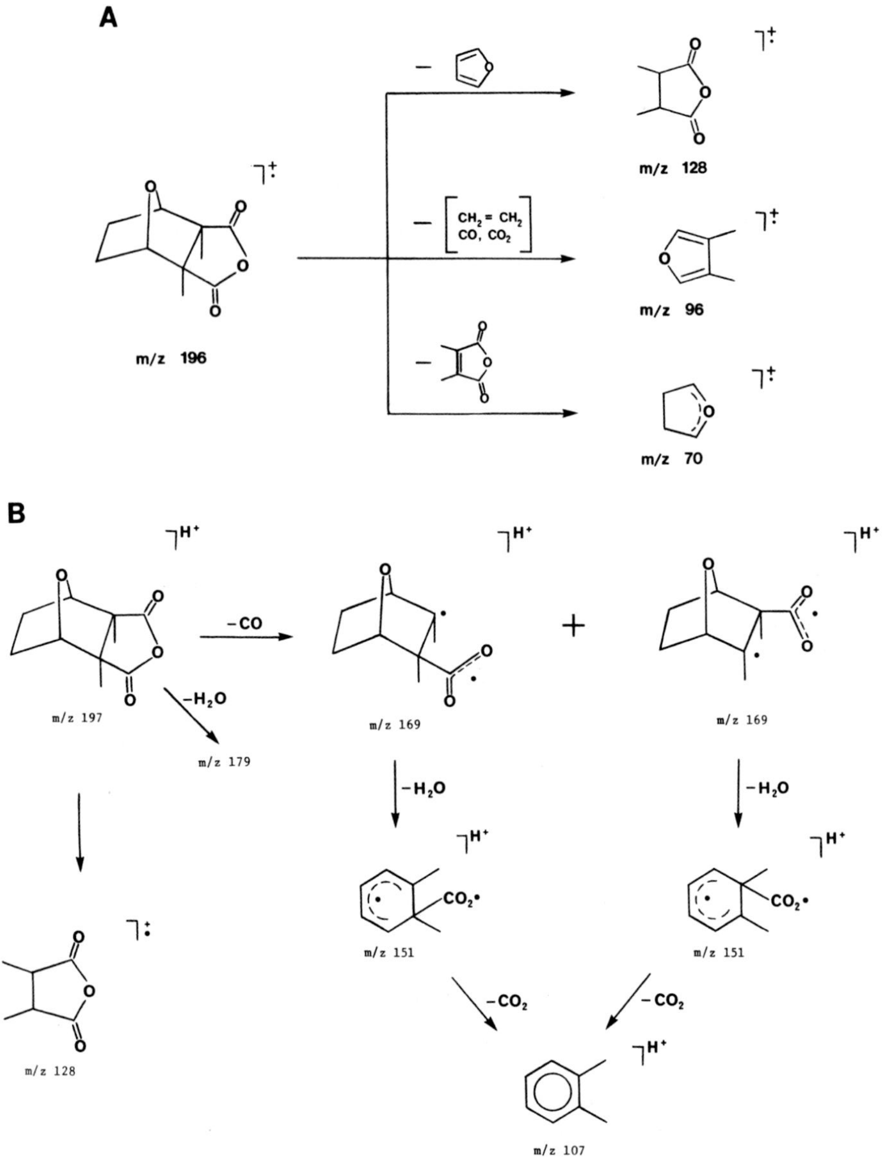

Fig. 4. Interpretations of the formation of key fragments in the mass spectra of cantharidin after (A) electron impact–induced ionization or (B) chemical ionization.

C-1/C-4 (at 84.80 ppm) and of C-10/C-11 (at 175.92 ppm) were particularly important. The excellent resolution of these carbon signals makes them ideally suited for indirect observation of isotopic changes of substituent hydrogen and oxygen atoms by detection of the resulting upfield shifts of the ^{13}C signal caused by the heavier isotopes (Hansen, 1983).

Each NMR signal in both proton and carbon spectra is derived from both halves of the cantharidin molecule, providing unusual sensitivity. Therefore, absolute amounts of cantharidin required for various NMR experiments are near typical lower limits. This was important for our ^{18}O labeling study because direct observation of the carbonyl carbons suffers from the poor sensitivity customary for this functional group owing both to the long relaxation times of these carbon atoms and to the absence of nuclear Overhauser effect (NOE) signal enhancement that requires attached hydrogen atoms.

G. Radiolabeling in Metabolism Studies

Since the pioneering days of Calvin and co-workers in the 1940s and 1950s that demonstrated the power of ^{14}C labeling studies to unravel details of metabolism, the use of radioisotope tracers has been the technique of choice for establishing metabolic precursor–product relationships. Important advantages include excellent sensitivity of detection when precursors with high levels of radioactivity are used, commercial availability of common primary metabolism precursors that are appropriately radioisotopically labeled, and general applicability to secondary metabolites comprising primarily carbon and hydrogen atoms. In particular, the high sensitivity of detection is an advantage that can be essential for studying the biosynthesis of insect metabolites that generally are formed in very small amounts. Unlike the studies of many organisms, the *in vivo* study of insect systems does not permit administration of large quantities of labeled substrates; amounts of resulting labeled products often are minute (Hammock and Quistad, 1981). Early experiments on cantharidin biosynthesis conducted when little was known about its timing and extent and when the experiments were limited by the availability of only a relatively small number of field-caught blister beetles advantageously exploited the use of [2-^{14}C]mevalonate that had a level of specific activity sufficiently high to reliably detect an incorporation rate of only 0.005% (Guenther *et al.*, 1969).

Additional technical advances made in the 1960s provided vastly improved capabilities for the use of radioisotope tracer labels in biosynthesis studies. Synthetic methodology for specifically placing hydrogen and carbon labels in desired precursors have become very powerful. As well, equipment that accurately counts both ^{3}H and ^{14}C in the same sample permitted a variety of sophisticated experiments: quantitation of substrate incorporation, quantitation of ^{3}H label retention, and experiments that quantitate relative uptake of different substrates simultaneously. Using all of these capabilities, Hans Schmid and his co-workers in Zurich conducted ingenious experiments to establish the origins of the carbon and hydrogen atoms in cantharidin.

The pioneering work of the Purdue group utilized [1-^{14}C]acetate and [2-^{14}C]mevalonate (Guenther *et al.,* 1969). These materials were coated on lettuce provided to beetles that had been starved for 4 days. The Zurich group on the other hand has consistently administered radiolabeled materials by injection. Their early studies (Schlatter *et al.,* 1968a,b; Schlatter and Duersteler-Meier, 1970) relied on [1-^{14}C]farnesol, [2-^{14}C]farnesol, [2-^{14}C]geraniol, [1-^{14}C]acetate, and [2-^{14}C]mevalonate, as well as [2-^{14}C]mevalonate administered in conjunction with mevalonate labeled with ^{3}H at either C-2, C-4, or C-5. Subsequent studies (Peter, 1973; Peter *et al.,* 1977a,b,c; Woggon *et al.,* 1977, 1983) have employed farnesol labeled with ^{14}C at C-2, C-5, C-6, and C-7 and nonstereospecifically with ^{3}H at C-11' and C-12. They used radiolabeled farnesols separately and as various mixtures to carry out double-labeling experiments. They have also utilized geraniol labeled with ^{3}H at C-7' and C-8 and other samples labeled with ^{14}C at C-2, C-7, C-7', and C-8 (Peter *et al.,* 1977b). In another study (Sierra *et al.,* 1976), the Zurich group employed methyl [2-^{14}C]farnesoate.

Experimental limitations of the radiolabeling technique, however, also have had an impact on the cantharidin biosynthesis problem. The most well recognized limitation is the requirement that radiolabels be detected by an indirect method of observation of a bulk sample. Therefore, the resulting radioactivity measurements provide data that reveal information about the entire sample but not about a particular compound in that sample, let alone particular positions in the compound of interest. Determination of exact results of precursor–product experiments is extremely labor intensive because careful product degradation studies are required to reveal the location(s) of atoms bearing radioactivity. Early studies of cantharidin biosynthesis provide classic examples. Isolated cantharidin required purification to determine the extent of radiolabeling and subsequent degradation to remove known portions of the molecule in ways that revealed the positions of radiolabeling and the extent of labeling at those positions. Each cantharidin-derived fragment was converted to a solid derivative that was rigorously purified before determination of its specific radioactivity. Such heroic efforts were well rewarded: They revealed the unprecedented biosynthetic pathway that accounts for cantharidin formation by blister beetles.

Another limitation of the radiolabeling method is less discussed but presently has an even greater impact on the cantharidin biosynthesis problem: This approach is poorly suited for detection of metabolic intermediates of unsuspected structures and low concentrations. Because the next major step in understanding this pathway clearly is the identification of metabolic intermediates that lie between farnesol and cantharidin, little additional progress has been made in recent years regarding cantharidin biosynthesis.

H. Stable Isotope Labeling in Metabolism Studies

During the decade of the 1970s, advances in several technologies made available new capabilities based on stable isotope labeling that are particularly valuable for biosynthesis investigations. The experimental advantages that led to their rapid displacement of radioactive isotopic labeling include: ready availability, applicability of synthetic techniques that already had been developed for radiolabeling but that do not involve the tedious laboratory procedures associated with handling radioactive materials, observation of ^{13}C and ^{2}H by direct spectroscopic examination using NMR, observation of ^{15}N and ^{18}O by indirect spectroscopic examination using ^{13}C NMR, and observation of all stable isotopes using MS. Unfortunately, the advantages of ^{2}H and ^{13}C labels came too late to assist the cantharidin biosynthesis studies that determined origins of its carbon and hydrogen atoms.

The vastly reduced sensitivity of the NMR and MS methods of isotope detection relative to detection of radiolabels, however, is a serious disadvantage for the use of stable isotope labeling in insect biosynthesis studies. NMR spectroscopic observation of ^{13}C generally requires amounts of materials that may exceed 1 mg. Favorable cases and good instrumentation can permit successful studies in which as little as 10–100 μg of labeled product is isolated, such as the results reported by Dillwith *et al.* (1982). In addition, because NMR detection of ^{15}N and ^{18}O relies on direct observation of ^{13}C signals, similar amounts of materials also are required for NMR observation of these stable isotope labels.

MS is substantially more sensitive, generally requiring only nanogram quantities of materials, but interpretation of the data from this technique often is very complicated. In some cases, the use of stable isotopes that shift normal ions and their fragments to higher mass units can permit simplification of data interpretation. Bjostad and Roelofs (1986) have described a particularly promising approach using stable isotopes to permit sensitive detection of labeled substrate incorporation in insect pheromone biosynthesis (see also Bjostad *et al.*, Chapter 3, this volume).

The reduced sensitivities of stable isotope detection by NMR and by MS delayed the use of the stable isotope labeling approach to study cantharidin biosynthesis. Advances in laboratory rearing techniques and understanding of the extent and timing of cantharidin biosynthesis were required before stable isotope labeling could be expected to provide sufficient quantities of labeled cantharidin for isotope analysis by MS and NMR.

The extension of the use of stable isotopes to include oxygen and nitrogen, the two heteroatoms most commonly found in secondary metabolites, opened the possibility of ready investigation of their origins and fates. In particular, the commercial availability of highly enriched ^{18}O-labeled molecular oxygen and water make it possible to investigate conveniently the utilization of these two common biological sources of oxygen.

1. NMR Analysis

^{13}C labeling coupled with the NMR observational method offers the unique advantage of uncovering the origin of carbon–carbon, carbon–hydrogen, carbon–oxygen, and carbon–nitrogen connectivities that are preserved in precursor–product relationships or, alternatively, that derive from the formation of carbon–carbon bonds during the metabolism process. This approach could be used to obtain evidence about the carbon–hydrogen connectivities in cantharidin. In particular, administration of (2R)- and (2S)-[2-^{2}H,2-^{13}C]mevalonate could usefully be employed to learn any stereoselection that occurs in the retention of one hydrogen atom on C-1 and on C-6 of cantharidin. Isotopic enrichment of those carbon atoms could more than offset the sensitivity loss resulting from signal splitting by the attached ^{2}H; as well, the differentiation of the C-5 and C-6 signals that would result from deuterium isotope effects on the ^{13}C chemical shifts would facilitate analysis of the NMR data (Hansen, 1983).

Unfortunately, the need for multimicrogram or even milligram amounts of isolated products for NMR examination has restricted the use of this technique in insect biosynthesis studies, owing to the very small amounts of materials that commonly are available. The study of defensive substances, however, can be an important exception. Because these materials commonly are built up and stored in substantially larger amounts, NMR techniques may be applicable. In the case of cantharidin, the formation and storage of multimilligram amounts of materials and the use of highly isotopically enriched $^{18}O_2$ and $H_2{}^{18}O$ have permitted the use of NMR to study the results of ^{18}O labeling experiments (Section III,E,3).

2. Mass Spectrometric Analysis

The use of stable isotope labeling permits analysis of the extent and position of label incorporation using MS. Detection sensitivities of this method are several orders of magnitude better than NMR detection capabilities and make this technique more suited to typical insect metabolism problems. Bjostad et al. (Chapter 3, this volume) and Bjostad and Roelofs (1986) have, for example, recently provided elegant examples of stable isotope labeling techniques that can be used with great sensitivity to obtain information rapidly regarding the metabolism of multiply ^{13}C-labeled substrates. Unfortunately, MS suffers from the complexity of fragmentation data that commonly are obtained, making this technique more difficult to use other than for examination of the extent of isotopic labeling in the entire molecule by observation of the molecular ion.

A particularly important potential of mass spectrometric data results from the fact that they are obtained from *sequential detection of individual ions.* This is in contrast to NMR and other spectroscopic information that is obtained only on the macroscopic level, *simultaneously* providing data resulting from all molecules, irrespective of their extent of isotopic enrichment. Data obtained exclusively from molecular species having a uniform extent of isotopic labeling can be extremely valuable. In most biosynthesis studies, for example, the dilution of isotope owing to either reduced enrichment levels in administered substrates or incomplete incorporation of labeled substrates presents problems regarding the determination of the maximal extent of label incorporation into a product of interest. Mass spectrometric examination of the product obtained can provide direct information regarding the maximal extent of labeling in a substrate incorporation experiment.

Further, MS–MS can permit examination of maximally labeled material without interference from materials labeled to a lesser extent. We have taken advantage of these capabilities to determine the maximal extent of ^{18}O labeling of cantharidin in the presence of labeled molecular oxygen and to uncover the positions of labeled oxygen in the maximally labeled material (McCormick *et al.*, 1986).

I. Metabolic Inhibition: 6-Fluoromevalonate

Fluorine, used as an abnormal substituent of a normal substrate, has been ingeniously applied in a number of biological studies to interrupt normal metabolism. Other investigators have used judicious placement of fluorine as a probe for mechanistic studies of enzymatic reactions. Walsh (1983) has reviewed some of these applications in a particularly informative and insightful manner, and Schlosser (1978) has reviewed some of the relevant synthetic methods for incorporation of fluorine into potential substrates.

Two applications that are especially relevant for cantharidin studies are related to the known 6-fluoromevalonate (Fig. 5) inhibition of cholesterol biosynthesis in mammalian systems (Singer *et al.*, 1959). Inhibition by fluoromevalonate was presumed to occur as the result of effects of the fluorine substituent on the early steps involved in cholesterol biosynthesis. Juvenile hormone biosynthesis was known to share with the cholesterol biosynthetic pathway the early steps on which fluoromevalonate was presumed to act. Therefore, Schooley and his collaborators reasoned that this substance would inhibit juvenile hormone biosynthesis (Quistad *et al.*, 1981a, 1982). Thorough studies in their laboratories demonstrated unequivocally the effective inhibition of juvenile hormone synthesis by fluoromevalonate.

Poulter and his co-workers (Poulter and Rilling, 1978; Poulter *et al.*, 1978, 1979, 1981; Muehlbacher and Poulter, 1985) employed fluorine as a mechanistic

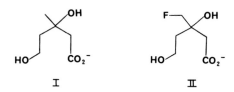

Fig. 5. Structures of mevalonate (**I**) and 6-fluoromevalonate (**II**).

probe in a series of elegant experiments designed to study the early steps of the terpenoid prenylation process, a portion of terpenoid biosynthesis that is shared by both juvenile hormone and cantharidin biosynthesis. In this series of investigations to determine mechanistic details regarding charge development in the prenylation process, this group took advantage of the destabilization of beta positive charge by the fluorine substituent. Results demonstrated that the course of the normal metabolic pathway was not altered, but that this process proceeded at a rate that was reduced by about a factor of 100 owing to the fluorine substituent. This study is important not only for its substantiation of the development of significant positive charge in the prenylation reaction mediated by porcine enzymatic preparations but also because it demonstrated that fluoro substrates could be processed in a normal manner.

For our results presented in this chapter (Section III,D), the importance of these studies is the demonstration that fluoromevalonate can substantially inhibit terpenoid biosynthesis pathways by acting on the early steps that utilize mevalonate. We have exploited this effect to obtain blister beetles that are chemically disarmed.

J. Synthesis of 6-Fluoromevalonate

It is beyond the scope of this chapter to discuss reported syntheses of mevalonate; limitation to those that could be modified to permit synthesis of 6-fluoromevalonate is still not sufficient for our focus. However, we wish to point out that this valuable mevalonate analog is reasonably available. Tschesche and Machleidt (1960) reported what to our knowledge was the first modification of a mevalonate synthesis to prepare fluoromevalonate. In our experience, this approach is useful but it suffers from difficulty associated with selective carbonyl modification.

More recently, we have found (J. P. McCormick and D. O'Bannon, unpublished results) that an improved mevalonate synthesis (Bardshiri *et al.*, 1984) works well for preparation of 6-fluoromevalonate. This synthetic route, outlined in Fig. 6, derives part of its attractiveness from use of the commercially available ethyl fluoroacetate (*Caution!* This ester is hydrolyzed under physiological conditions to form the highly toxic fluoroacetate) as the starting material, thereby

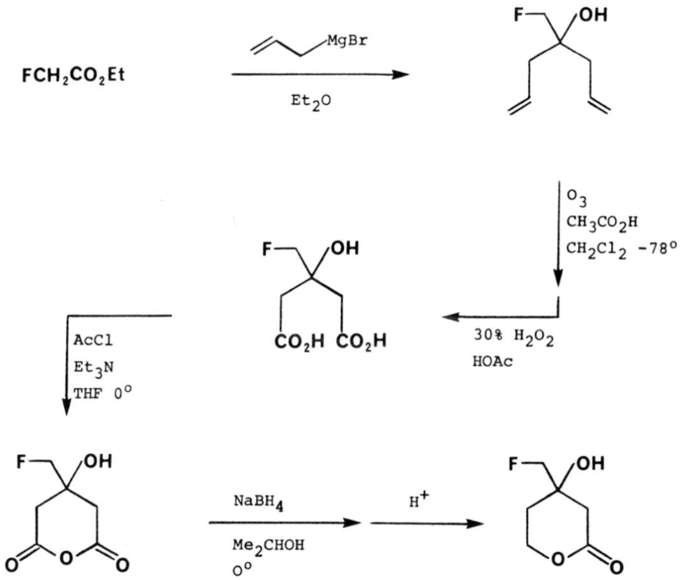

Fig. 6. Practical synthetic route for preparation of 6-fluoromevalonate.

avoiding the need to form the carbon–fluorine bond. It is important to note that this synthetic route as described contains modifications that made the procedure more reliable (Lewer and MacMillan, 1983) than the initial procedures described by Scott and Shishido (1980).

Quistad *et al.* (1981b) have reported a modification of the 6-fluoromevalonate synthesis outlined in Fig. 6. The ozonolysis of the 1,6-heptadienol intermediate is followed by reductive workup to provide a pentanetriol that can be oxidized using Jones' conditions to give the desired fluoromevalonic acid.

III. RESULTS

A. Cantharidin Biosynthesis in Isolated Beetles

Cantharidin is produced by *E. pestifera* males but apparently not by the females of this species (J. E. Carrel, J. P. McCormick, and T. Eisner, unpublished results). The amount of cantharidin accumulated by isolated males is impressive: 60–90 days after eclosion a single virginal male on average possesses 23.8 mg of the substance. This is the equivalent of 15% of his live body weight. Most (92%) of the cantharidin in these males is localized in the third pair of accessory reproductive glands. Each gland consists of a narrow, 3–4 cm long tube that becomes bloated with cantharidin-containing secretions as the males age.

In short-term studies with wild *L. polita*, we found isolated adult males definitely produce cantharidin, but they appear to make it at a relatively low rate (0.06 mg/beetle/day) in comparison to *E. pestifera* males (0.26 mg/beetle/day). Although we have little information for female *L. polita*, Schlatter and his co-workers (1968b) showed that female *L. vesicatoria*, in contrast to males of this species, do not synthesize cantharidin from radioactive acetate and mevalonate. We currently are conducting long-term studies with isolated *L. polita* adults of both sexes to determine clearly the patterns of cantharidin production in this American species.

B. Cantharidin Biosynthesis and Transfer during Mating

Observations made in early studies of cantharidin in blister beetles created a paradox (Schlatter *et al.*, 1968b). Although female meloids appear unable to biosynthesize cantharidin, nonetheless adults of both sexes collected in the field contain large amounts of the substance. The possibility that cantharidin is transferred from males to females during mating was suggested long ago by Beauregard (1890) after he detected large amounts of the blistering compound in the reproductive tract of male *L. vesicatoria*.

Transfer of cantharidin from male to female beetles has been demonstrated in several species of meloids. The Swiss (Sierra *et al.*, 1976) showed that male *L. vesicatoria* injected with radiolabeled mevalonate about 1 day prior to copulation transfer most of the newly biosynthesized cantharidin to females during mating. Using the same technique, Carrel and co-workers (1973) demonstrated transfer of radiolabeled cantharidin from male to female *Epicauta vittata* during copulation.

We have quantified the nuptial exchange of cantharidin in two additional meloid species, *E. pestifera* and *L. polita* (Fig. 7). Our data indicate that *E. pestifera* males simply transfer their reproductive reserves of cantharidin without greatly affecting their bodily reserves of the substance. In contrast, *L. polita* males actively biosynthesize cantharidin during copulation as well as draw on their bodily reserves of cantharidin to form their spermatophoral gift. *Lytta vesicatoria* males also actively synthesize cantharidin while mating (Sierra *et al.*, 1976).

Cantharidin biosynthesis patterns seem to be correlated with mating duration in meloids. *Epicauta* males produce much cantharidin before mating and then rapidly transfer this stored material into females toward the end of their copulation period, which lasts several hours (S. L. Briesacher and J. E. Carrel, unpublished results). In contrast, *Lytta* males appear to make cantharidin slowly

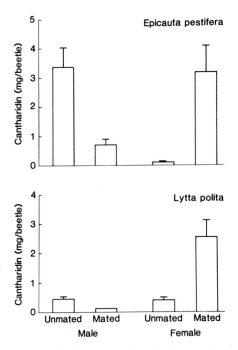

Fig. 7. Transfer of cantharidin from male to female blister beetles during mating. Bars and vertical lines, respectively, represent means and standard errors for the amount of cantharidin in adult beetles ($N = 6$ or 7 per group) belonging to two species.

before mating, but during the 20–24 hr they spend in copulation they rapidly synthesize prodigious amounts of cantharidin. A Swiss report cited above (Sierra *et al.*, 1976) provided evidence that radiolabeled cantharidin is quickly taken out of the hemolymph of copulating *L. vesicatoria* males and translocated to the females' reproductive tract.

C. Cantharidin Transfer to Meloid Eggs

Egg masses produced by meloid beetles apparently contain cantharidin or cantharidin-like substances. Beauregard (1890) first reported that meloid eggs applied to mammalian skin cause blisters to develop. Subsequently, Viehoever and Capen (1923) found eggs of *Epicauta (Macrobasis) albida* are very rich in cantharidin, as determined by sublimation and mixture melting point of extracted material.

We have determined that some, but evidently not all, *Epicauta* species deposit several hundred micrograms of cantharidin with each egg mass and that cantharidin in the egg masses comes largely from the male parent (J. E. Carrel, J. P.

McCormick, and T. Eisner, unpublished results). Our interpretation of these findings is that male meloids invest in the survivorship of their mates and ultimately of their offspring by providing them with cantharidin for defense. In the case of eggs this likely includes protection from pathogenic fungi and nematodes as well as predaceous arthropods. Paternal chemical defenses recently have been documented in two lepidopteran families. Alkaloids derived from males are present in eggs of some danaiid butterflies and arctiid moths (Eisner and Meinwald, Chapter 8, this volume).

D. Inhibition of Cantharidin Biosynthesis by Fluoromevalonate

Cantharidin biosynthesis in male blister beetles is inhibited by systemic administration of the metabolic inhibitor, 6-fluoromevalonate, which is presumed to block the utilization of mevalonate (Nave *et al.*, 1985). We have found that fluoromevalonate given either by injection or by feeding prevents cantharidin production in recently mated male *L. polita* (Carrel *et al.*, 1968b). This effect is attributable specifically to the fluorine substituent because, as illustrated in Fig. 8, beetles given doses of mevalonate matching the fluoromevalonate doses produced as much cantharidin as untreated controls. Fluoromevalonate also strongly inhibits cantharidin production in male *E. pestifera* (J. E. Carrel and J. P. McCormick, unpublished results).

Fluorolabeled substrates might possibly be used in several ways to control pest

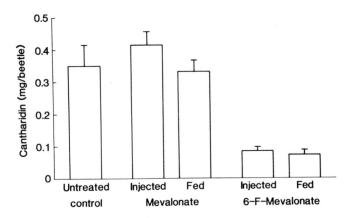

Fig. 8.   Biochemical inhibition of cantharidin production in male *Lytta polita*. Bars and vertical lines, respectively, represent means and standard errors for the amount of cantharidin in adult beetles ($N = 7$ per group). Beetles treated with the inhibitor, 6-fluoromevalonate, on average produced significantly less cantharidin than untreated or mevalonate-treated beetles. Data from Carrel *et al.* (1986b).

insects (Prestwich, 1986b). For example, as we have shown with cantharidin, fluorolabeled substrates can be employed to inhibit selectively the production of defensive substances, thereby making the host presumably more vulnerable to predation. We currently are testing this concept with fluoromevalonate-treated blister beetles. Alternatively, fluorolabeled compounds can serve as suicide substrates that kill insects by blocking essential metabolic pathways (Prestwich, 1986b). Finally, as recently reported by Prestwich (1986b), fluorolabeled sex pheromones of lepidopteran insects can be designed to be so biochemically stable that they retain their behavioral effectiveness virtually indefinitely, thereby greatly disrupting the mating systems of these insects (see also Prestwich, Chapter 14, this volume).

E. Origin of Cantharidin Constituent Atoms

1. Carbon Atoms

a. Specific Incorporation of Acetate, Mevalonate, and Farnesol. Based on recognition that cantharidin is composed of 10 carbon atoms, it was natural to speculate originally that cantharidin is derived from acetate, through either the polyketide pathway or the mevalonate pathway. The latter seemed more likely. An early study reported by Guenther *et al.* (1969) at Purdue demonstrated that $[1-^{14}C]$acetate was incorporated into cantharidin. However, degradation studies that demonstrated the extent of labeling at several positions were not readily interpretable in terms of acetate incorporation through the normal polyketide pathway or in terms of acetate incorporation through mevalonate in a normal manner.

Simultaneously, Schmid and co-workers in Zurich pursued experiments in spite of early puzzling results, following their conviction that cantharidin was of terpenoid origin. Their substrate administration studies utilized radiolabeled mevalonate, geraniol, and farnesol. Early results with $[1-^{14}C]$farnesol and $[2-^{14}C]$geraniol failed to provide incorporated radiolabel in cantharidin at meaningful levels, while an experiment in which $[2-^{14}C]$farnesol was administered provided positive incorporation results (Schlatter and Duersteler-Meier, 1970). Subsequent degradation of the radiolabeled cantharidin revealed specific incorporation of $[2-^{14}C]$farnesol and that the radiolabel was located at C-10 (or C-11) of cantharidin.

Demonstration of farnesol as a precursor provided a new puzzle: Which of the five carbon atoms are lost from farnesol in its conversion into cantharidin? From the specific incorporation of $[2-^{14}C]$farnesol it then became apparent that the failure to obtain radiolabel incorporation from $1-^{14}C$-farnesol did not result from a lack of incorporation of substrate but rather from loss of C-1 in the process. Although it is easy to presume that C-1 is lost as a one-carbon fragment, no evidence has been provided regarding this point. Since C-2 is retained, it was clear that an unparalleled process accounted for the loss of another four unidentified farnesyl carbons.

As shown in Fig. 9, the loss of two different, central C_4 fragments from farnesol could be envisioned to account for cantharidin formation without alkyl group migration. The early results reported by the Purdue group (Guenther *et al.*, 1969) using [1-^{14}C]acetate and [2-^{14}C]mevalonate indicated that it is the fragment shown as path (c) in Fig. 9 that is lost from farnesol. Subsequent experiments by the Swiss group (Schlatter and Duersteler-Meier, 1970) using (1) [2-^{14}C]- and [4-^{3}H]mevalonate and (2) [2-^{14}C]- and [5-^{3}H]mevalonate confirmed that it is the C_4 fragment shown in path (c) that is lost in the farnesol to cantharidin transformation. Thus, bond cleavages between C-1/C-2, C-4/C-5, and C-7/C-8 account for the loss of carbon fragments from farnesol, and bond formation between C-3/C-11 and C-4/C-8 tie the two farnesyl portions together to ultimately form the cantharidin skeleton.

This information brought to light an additional interesting question regarding the cantharidin carbon skeleton. Although this compound comprises two identical halves and therefore is achiral, the carbon framework contains within it a latent chirality that remained to be determined. That is, the two halves of cantharidin are distinguished from each other by their different origins from farnesol. This latent chirality that is imposed by enzymatic involvement may be schematically illustrated as shown in Fig. 10. The two indicated conformations

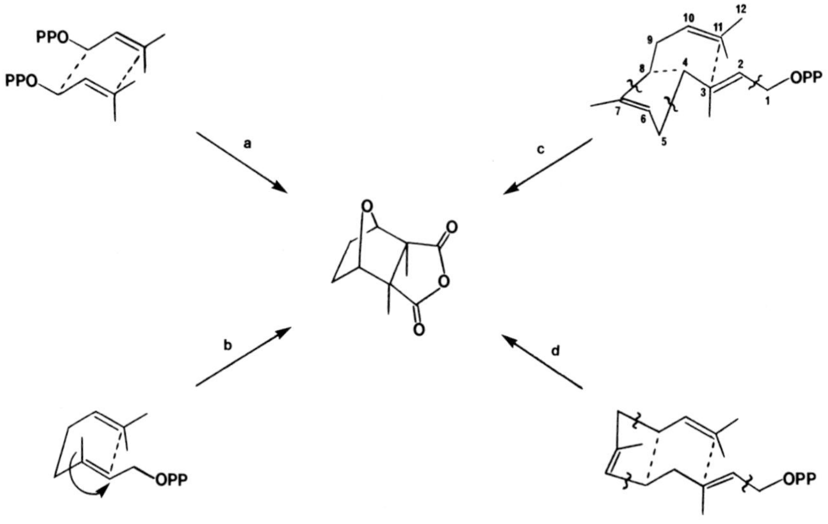

Fig. 9. Possible terpenoid pathways for the biosynthesis of cantharidin.

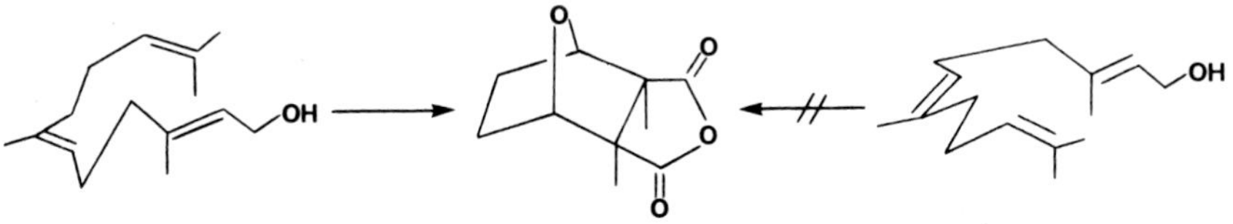

Fig. 10. Two possible chiralities for the incorporation of farnesol into cantharidin.

are not intended to convey mechanistic interpretation, but rather to show that either mirror-image half of the cantharidin skeleton could be derived from either farnesyl fragment. A sophisticated experiment reported by the Swiss group (Peter *et al.*, 1977a) demonstrated that the chirality is actually that depicted as A in Fig. 10. This determination required the production from the achiral cantharidin of a chiral derivative formed in a manner that permitted assignment of its chirality and its relationship to the two mirror-image halves of cantharidin. As shown in Fig. 11, this was accomplished (Peter *et al.*, 1974) by conversion of cantharidin into a pair of enantiomers of cantharic acid, which could be resolved by the classic brucine salt method to provide (+)-cantharic acid (**A**). That this stereoisomer has the absolute stereochemistry shown as (+)-**A** was determined by using the method of Horeau on three of its derivatives, **B–D,** providing a reasonable degree of assurance that this deductive method, which relies on structural analogies rather than definitive evidence, was applicable. With this stereochemical assignment available, degradation of cantharidin via either enantiomer of cantharic acid permits determination of which enantiomeric half originally contained biosynthetically incorporated isotopic labels.

b. Farnesol Methyl Group Scrambling. The randomization of the isopropylidene methyl groups of farnesol during their incorporation into cantharidin has been demonstrated by several of the substrate administration experiments described above. This case presents a classic example of the absolute requirement that thorough product degradation studies be used to determine the results of *radioisotopic* labeling experiments. Degradation of radiolabeled cantharidin obtained from administration of [2-^{14}C]mevalonate revealed that C-9 and C-11 carried approximately 16 and 20% of the radioactivity, respectively (Schlatter *et al.*, 1968b). Based on the normal conversion of mevalonate into farnesol (Fig. 12), label at C-2 of mevalonate resulted in labeling C-12 but not C-11′ of farnesol. Results of administration of mevalonate doubly labeled at C-2 with ^{3}H and ^{14}C similarly indicated almost complete randomization of the farnesyl methyl groups: The amount of ^{3}H labeling found at C-9 was half that expected for the amount of the labeling of C-12 of farnesol (Schlatter and Duersteler-Meier, 1970).

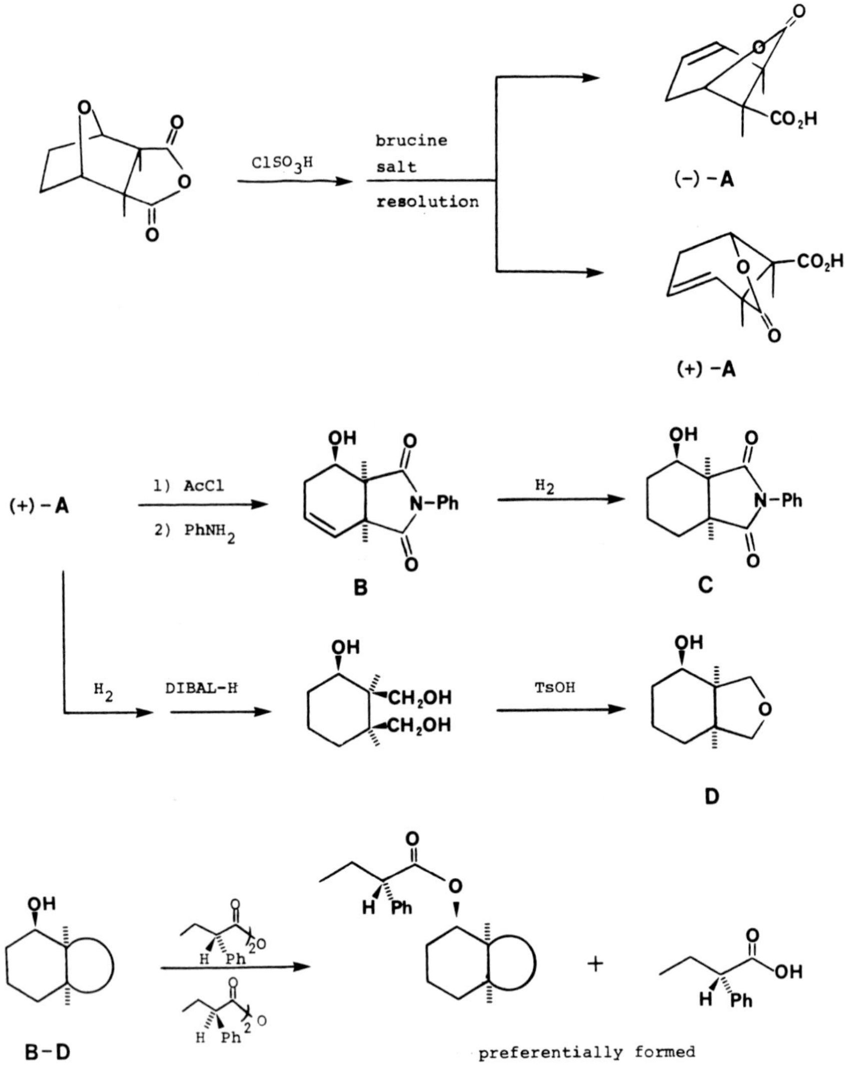

Fig. 11. Chemical transformations for differentiation and assignment of specific incorporation of farnesyl fragments into enantiomeric halves of cantharidin.

More direct evidence for terminal methyl randomization was provided by substrate administration experiments using farnesol labeled at C-11′ with ^3H and ^{14}C, with and without an additional reference ^{14}C label at C-2 (Woggon *et al.*, 1983). Determination of the $^3H/^{14}C$ ratios of the resulting cantharidin and appropriate degradation products (acetic acid and carbon dioxide) demonstrated that

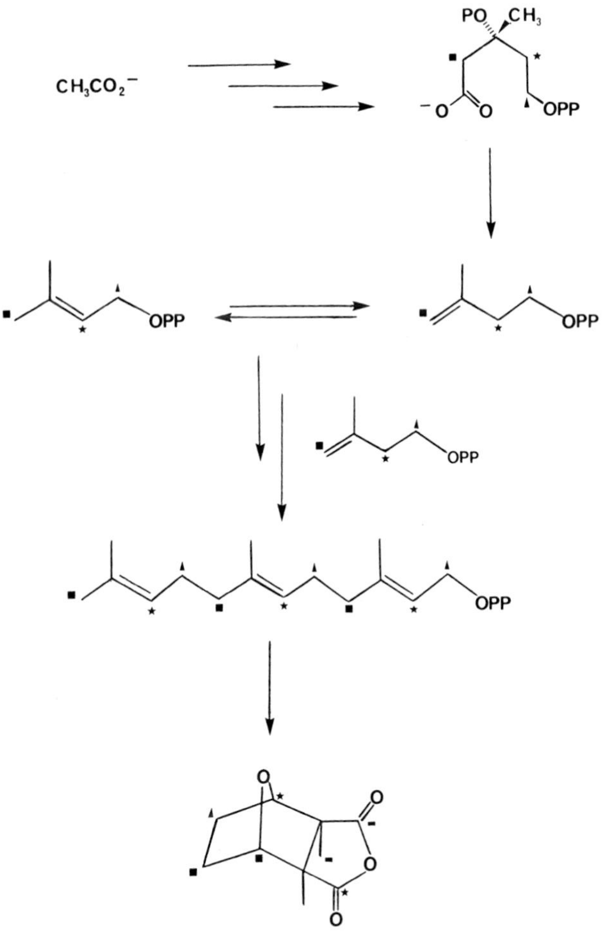

Fig. 12. Formation of mevalonate from acetate and specific incorporation of mevalonate into farnesol.

C-9 and C-11 were almost equally labeled with ^{14}C and that the C-9/(C-9 + C-11) $^3H/^{14}C$ ratio was slightly less than half that of the $^3H/^{14}C$ ratio at C-11' of the administered farnesol. These results confirmed that the farnesyl terminal methyl groups are almost completely scrambled during transformation into cantharidin, perhaps by a chemical process during which the two methyl groups become (almost) equivalent.

Although it is possible to draw an analogy between this scrambling and that documented for loganin and related terpenoid biosyntheses, which involve an intermediate in which terpenoid (geranyl) terminal methyl groups become equivalent (Escher *et al.*, 1970), the obligatory oxidation of both methyl groups in the latter processes contrast with the apparent preservation of one of the farnesyl methyl groups in cantharidin.

c. *Molecular Integrity of Farnesol Incorporation.* The loss of a *central* C_4 fragment from farnesol raises the possibility that the two separate farnesyl portions that ultimately form cantharidin arise from different molecules of farnesol. Alternatively, the excision of the C_4 piece could take place without loss of identity of these remaining portions, providing cantharidin in which all atoms are derived from the same molecule of farnesol. The question was addressed by elegant experiments (Woggon *et al.*, 1983) that utilized radiolabeled farnesol that had ^{14}C tracer labels at C-2 and C-4 together with ^3H tracer labels at C-11′ and C-12. As expected based on the nearly complete scrambling of the C-11′ and C-12 methyl groups, the resulting cantharidin possessed a $^{14}C/^3H$ ratio almost exactly twice that of the administered farnesol. Subsequent degradation experiments indicated that C-2 and C-4 of farnesol had been incorporated specifically into C-10 and C-1, respectively, of cantharidin. In a related experiment, farnesol labeled with ^{14}C at C-2 and C-11′ in a known ratio was incorporated into cantharidin that subsequent degradation showed to be labeled at C-10 and C-9 + C-11 in the same ratio.

These results provide strong evidence that the carbon atoms in any given cantharidin molecule all are derived from the same farnesol molecule. The explanation for this, however, is not yet clear. We favor interpretation of these results as evidence that some bond making precedes both C-4—C-5 and C-7—C-8 bond cleavage. An alternative possibility is that such cleavage occurs first to give two farnesyl fragments that by enzymatic direction are never allowed to mix with other such fragments before bond formation joins them.

2. Hydrogen Atoms

Information regarding the origin of the cantharidin hydrogen atoms is derived from early experiments (Schlatter and Durstetler-Meier, 1970) that were carried out with double labeling using [2-^{14}C]mevalonate for a radioactive reference and [2-^3H]-, [4-^3H]-, and [5-^3H]mevalonate to trace the fate of these hydrogen atoms. The extent of ^3H retention was determined relative to incorporation of the ^{14}C label, based on recognition that the ^{14}C label of C-2 from all three mevalonate units is incorporated into farnesol and subsequently into cantharidin. Administration of [2-^3H]mevalonate revealed that the hydrogen atoms of cantharidin on C-1 and C-9 are derived solely from farnesol and that apparently one of the hydrogen atoms on C-6 is derived from farnesol and the other from another source, presumably the aqueous medium. An experiment utilizing [4-^3H]mevalonate revealed that the hydrogen atom on C-4 of cantharidin is derived solely from farnesol, and another experiment utilizing [5-^3H]mevalonate indicated that the two hydrogen atoms on C-5 both are derived from farnesol. No information that directly addresses the origin of the hydrogen atom attached to the cantharidin C-8 methyl group is available, although it is reasonable to presume that this methyl is derived without alteration from C-3' of farnesol, which corresponds to C-6 of mevalonate. It therefore appears that, with the exception of one hydrogen at C-6 of cantharidin, all the hydrogen atoms are derived directly from farnesol and originally from mevalonate.

The radiolabeling experiments utilizing [2-^{3}H]- and [5-^{3}H]mevalonate were carried out with nonstereospecifically labeled mevalonate. Therefore, no stereochemical details are available regarding hydrogen atom incorporation into cantharidin.

3. Oxygen Atoms

Uncovering the origin of the oxygen atoms in cantharidin was a technically challenging problem that needed the development of laboratory rearing procedures for the blister beetles and appropriate detection techniques for isotopically labeled oxygen. Development of laboratory rearing techniques for *E. pestifera* was particularly important for our approach to this problem. Knowledge regarding the extent and timing of cantharidin biosynthesis and regarding the exact development of individual male blister beetles and their mating experience was critical to avoiding serious complications owing to dilution of labeled cantharidin. This information could be exploited to avoid severe dilution of labeled cantharidin by unlabeled material made prior to $^{18}O_2$ administration. Dilution by unlabeled material is an especially significant problem when determination of incorporation levels depend on a macroscopic observational technique such as NMR and also can be a complicating problem in mass spectrometric observation of label incorporation. Fortunately, mass spectrometric techniques simplified problems owing to modest amounts of product dilution by unlabeled cantharidin.

Using a slight modification of our laboratory rearing techniques, we kept five male beetles as a group during the early days of adulthood in a closed vessel. The atmospheric composition was approximately 25% O_2 and 75% N_2, with a high ^{18}O enrichment of the molecular oxygen. After 6 days of exposure, during which time the ^{18}O-enriched molecular oxygen was replenished once, the animals were bled, frozen, and dissected in the normal manner to provide four types of samples for analysis: blood, the third pair of reproductive accessory glands, the remainder of the reproductive system, and the rest of the body.

The samples from the accessory glands contained the largest amounts of cantharidin, as anticipated, but the blood-borne cantharidin contained the highest level of ^{18}O incorporation. The complementary information obtained from CI– and EI–MS data permitted location of the positions of ^{18}O in the recovered cantharidin. That the tetrahydrofuranyl oxygen was derived from molecular oxygen was clearly demonstrated by the relatively large abundances of the fragments at m/z 72 and m/z 98 in the electron impact mass spectrum. Significant dilution of the ^{18}O label during the experiment complicated analysis of the (protonated) molecular ions in the chemical ionization mass spectrum, which showed ions of significant abundance at m/z 197/199/201/203 but not at m/z 205. This information indicated that three but never four of the cantharidin oxygen atoms were derived from molecular oxygen. This conclusion was supported by analysis of the ratios of the m/z 128/130/132/134 ions in both the EI and CI mass spectra, ratios that revealed two but never three labeled oxygen atoms in the anhydride portion of cantharidin (see Fig. 4). These data did not permit determination of the distribution of ^{18}O within the anhydride portion of the molecule.

In principle, ^{13}C-NMR observation of the labeled cantharidin should reveal the distribution of ^{18}O within the anhydride functionality. However, although the presence of ^{18}O at the tetrahydrofuranyl position was clearly revealed by its upfield shift of the signals resulting from the C-1 and C-4 carbon atoms, observation of the limited amount of material available using 300 MHz (75.5 MHz for ^{13}C) did not provide data satisfactory for clear observation of the greatly reduced signals derived from the carbonyl carbons. It was possible to observe signals shifted to higher fields in a manner that suggested distribution of ^{18}O among all three anhydride oxygen atoms, but quantitation of that distribution was not possible. This difficulty arose owing not only to the limited amount of material available but also to the presence of substantial amounts of unlabeled and partially labeled cantharidin.

It was only the maximally labeled cantharidin molecules that contained unambiguous information about the distribution of atoms derived from molecular oxygen. These key, maximally labeled species could be observed without obfuscation owing to ^{16}O dilution by MS–MS CI examination of m/z 203. Observation of the loss of $C^{18}O$ and $C^{16}O$, revealed by m/z 173/175, permitted the conclusion that the carbonyl carbon atoms, which are not distinguishable by MS but need not be labeled to the same extent, bear a majority of the ^{18}O label but that the anhydride ring oxygen also was significantly labeled.

Application of MS–MS promises to provide a useful approach to dealing with the common isotope dilution problem experienced in metabolism studies that are complicated by the presence of endogenous material derived from unlabeled substrates. Typical studies of insect metabolism questions are likely to require examination of small amounts of material derived from labeled substrates and may generally benefit from the MS–MS approach to solving the isotope dilution problem.

The inference that one of the cantharidin oxygen atoms is derived from water rather than molecular oxygen was subjected to experimental verification. Although it was anticipated that labeled water would undergo substantial dilution, 95% ^{18}O-enriched water was injected abdominally into five adult male E.

pestifera. After 6 days, cantharidin was isolated from the accessory gland samples. CI–MS examination of this cantharidin revealed small but definitive enhancement of m/z 199, confirming the incorporation of one labeled oxygen atom.

F.   Cantharidin Biosynthesis: Intermediates and Chemistry

1.   Farnesol as an Intermediate

Farnesyl pyrophosphate most likely is the initial C_{15} product formed by blister beetles from the prenylation sequence, based on analogy with all other organisms in which prenylation has been studied. Nevertheless, the success observed with substrate administration experiments utilizing labeled farnesol raises the distinct possibility that this alcohol is an obligatory intermediate along the route to cantharidin. That farnesol is a genuine intermediate is demonstrated by experiments conducted in Zurich (Peter *et al.*, 1977c) in which [2-^{14}C]mevalonate and [11′,12-^{3}H]farnesol were simultaneously administered to blister beetles. Subsequent workup provided not only cantharidin that was radiolabeled with ^{3}H and ^{14}C, but also farnesol that was radiolabeled both with ^{3}H and ^{14}C. Degradation of this radiolabeled farnesol demonstrated that the ^{14}C label was specifically derived from mevalonate in the manner expected from the normal prenylation pathway (Fig. 12).

Additional experiments demonstrated that the E stereochemistry is necessary at the 6,7 double bond of farnesol for specific incorporation but that there is a reduced stereoselectivity for the stereochemistry at the 2,3 double bond (Woggon *et al.*, 1977). Using ^{14}C labeling at C-2 and ^{3}H labeling at C-11′ and C-12 of farnesol, E,E, E,Z, Z,E, and Z,Z stereoisomers were administered to adult male blister beetles. Using competition experiments, this study showed that the Z,E stereoisomer was incorporated into cantharidin at approximately half the rate of the E,E isomer. Both 6Z isomers were incorporated at greatly reduced levels that were presumed to reflect degradation of the administered farnesols to acetate and subsequent nonspecific incorporation of the labels into cantharidin. The explanation for the relatively successful incorporation of the Z,E stereoisomer is not clear. This lack of stereoselectivity may result from less demanding requirements of the enzymatic processes involved in transformation of intermediates having the 2,3 double bond, or may reflect isomerization at this double bond.

2.   Methyl Farnesoate as a Possible Intermediate

A study designed to demonstrate transfer of cantharidin during copulation from adult male to female blister beetles turned up evidence that methyl farnesoate may be a normal intermediate in cantharidin biosynthesis (Sierra *et al.*, 1976). Two experiments in this study compared the fates of (E,E)-farnesol and methyl (E,E)-farnesoate as substrates that were taken up by copulating males and incorporated into cantharidin. Isolation of cantharidin after injection of methyl [2-^{14}C]farnesoate revealed an incorporation rate into cantharidin of 1.1%. This compared to an incorporation rate of 3.6% when [11'-^{3}H]farnesol was the substrate under similar conditions and with an incorporation rate of 13.9% when [11'-^{14}C]farnesol was the injected substrate. Although methyl farnesoate was incorporated at a lower level, the incorporation rate is high enough to raise as a real possibility the involvement of methyl farnesoate as an obligatory intermediate in cantharidin biosynthesis. This possibility seems eminently reasonable in view of the known capability of insects to convert farnesol or its homologs into the corresponding methyl ester during the course of juvenile hormone biosynthesis. As well, oxidative transformation of C-1 to the carboxyl level would fit with biochemically reasonable mechanistic possibilities for the C-1—C-2 bond cleavage process. Experiments similar to those carried out to demonstrate the intermediacy of farnesol need yet to be carried out to confirm the required intermediacy of methyl farnesoate as part of the process by which farnesol is transformed into cantharidin.

3.   Summary of the Biosynthetic Events beyond Farnesol

Assuming farnesol to be an obligatory intermediate in cantharidin biosynthesis and recognizing that this molecule loses C-1 as well as C-5, C-6, C-7, and C-7', a minimum set of chemical events needed for cantharidin formation from farnesol can be identified (Fig. 13; atomic numbering refers to farnesol):

1. C-3—C-11 bond formation
2. C-4—C-8 bond formation
3. C-1—C-2 bond cleavage
4. C-4—C-5 bond cleavage
5. C-7—C-8 bond cleavage
6. Oxygen introduction at C-4
7. Oxygen introduction at C-10
8. Oxidation of C-2 to the carboxyl oxidation level
9. Oxidation of either C-11' or C-12 to the carboxyl oxidation level
10. C-2—O—C-11' (or C-2—O—C-12) bond formation
11. C-4—O—C-10 bond formation

At this point, there is little evidence to indicate the sequence in which these chemical steps occur, and we recognize that some of these events may be, even presumably are, temporally and chemically related processes that are interdependent.

Most likely there are additional, chemically distinct processes that are not *required* by present evidence. Examples include separate oxidation steps for the oxidation of the C-11' (or C-12) methyl group during its transformation to the

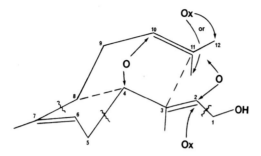

Fig. 13. Minimum set of identified chemical transformations for conversion of farnesol into cantharidin.

carboxyl level, chemical transformation(s) at C-1 prior to its loss, and chemical transformation(s) in the C-5 to C-7′ portion prior to its loss.

Within the present level of understanding, eight of the ten cantharidin carbon atoms are sites of chemical reactivity beyond farnesol; only two, C-5 and C-9, apparently remain uninvolved with the chemical transformations. Furthermore, considering the common involvement of enol/enolate functionality in biochemical bond making and bond breaking reactions, it is plausible that C-5 (C-9 of farnesol) also may be involved in the chemistry at some step of the overall process. This information has important implications regarding the choice of labeling sites as future biosynthetic experiments are designed.

G. Site of Cantharidin Biosynthesis

Discovery of the site of cantharidin biosynthesis could be valuable beyond providing interesting information relating to insect physiology. Based on experiments with the corpora allata to study the function and biosynthesis of juvenile hormone (Schooley *et al.*, 1973; Lee *et al.*, 1978; Baker and Schooley, 1978), such knowledge might present opportunities for manipulation of cantharidin biosynthesis and for tissue culture to facilitate metabolism/biosynthesis studies. Unfortunately, no direct information is available about the site of cantharidin biosynthesis, although by analogy with other insect systems it is reasonable to speculate that the site of synthesis may be in tissue associated with the site of storage, the third pair of reproductive accessory glands.

We have obtained information by analysis of the MS data from our $^{18}O_2$ incorporation studies that may relate to the site of cantharidin biosynthesis. Initial workup of incorporation experiments involved formation of four separate samples from the exposed blister beetles: (1) blood, (2) the third pair of reproductive accessory glands, (3) the rest of the reproductive system, and (4) the rest of the body. MS analysis of these samples indicated that the material in the accessory glands contained by far the largest relative amount of unlabeled material, material that was synthesized by the blister beetles prior to exposure to $^{18}O_2$. In dramatic contrast, the blood-borne cantharidin showed little unlabeled cantharidin and the highest levels of maximally labeled material. This indicates that the newly synthesized cantharidin proceeds first to the blood from which it subsequently is removed by a "cantharidin kidney" and is collected in the accessory reproductive glands. Although this observation does not preclude the synthesis of cantharidin in tissues associated with the storage glands, it is incompatible with the direct transfer of cantharidin from those tissues into the accessory glands without distribution in the hemolymph.

Correspondingly, comparison of label incorporation in the same four types of samples from the $H_2^{18}O$ administration experiments permits a similar conclusion. In this case, $H_2^{18}O$ was administered in a single injection and the insects were then allowed to develop for an additional 6 days before samples were obtained. Presumably, the availability of $H_2^{18}O$ should drop off rapidly as the experiment progressed owing to utilization and excretion. Thus, in the later days of the experiment little or no labeled cantharidin would be produced. Therefore, we anticipated that the freshest cantharidin would be minimally labeled and that ^{18}O incorporation could best be observed in cantharidin contained in the accessory glands. Our expectations were confirmed; analysis of the samples derived from the storage glands revealed the highest percentage of ^{18}O label in cantharidin. No oxygen labeling of blood-borne cantharidin was detectable.

H. Pheromonal Properties of Cantharidin

1. Releaser Effects

There is no evidence that cantharidin serves as a sex attractant or an aggregation pheromone in meloid beetles. Insect traps baited either with pure cantharidin or with blister beetles fail to capture meloids, although a number of other insects are preferentially collected in these devices (Young, 1984; J. E. Carrel, unpublished results). Female *E. pestifera* tested in arenas do not preferentially move to male beetles loaded with cantharidin or to pure cantharidin baits (S. L. Briesacher and J. E. Carrel, unpublished results).

Cantharidin does not appear to serve as a cue to male beetles for discriminating against recently mated, unreceptive females in favor of sexually receptive females. Male *E. pestifera* tested in areans do not preferentially move away from mated females toward virginal ones or away from pure cantharidin baits toward unbaited areas (S. L. Breisacher and J. E. Carrel, unpublished). In fact, male meloids often are relatively nondiscriminating in their courtship behavior and consequently some spend much time and effort attempting to mate with unreceptive females or males (Selander and Mathieu, 1969; S. L. Breisacher and J. E. Carrel, unpublished results).

Cantharidin may in some very subtle way be used by female meloids when selecting a mate at close range. If presented with two males, we found 12 of 13 *E. pestifera* females copulated with the male having the greater concentration of cantharidin in his blood. Female preference in *E. pestifera* was not significantly related to body mass, total cantharidin content, or previous mating experience of males. Careful observation of courtship interactions revealed no detectable differences involving the female beetle and the successful versus the unsuccessful male other than positioning of the tip of the abdomen by the female to control initiation of copulation (S. L. Briesacher and J. E. Carrel, unpublished results).

Other studies also indicated that precopulatory sex pheromones in blister beetles, if they exist at all, generally work at close range. Selander and his group reported that male meloids usually initiate courtship and that visual and olfactory cues may be used by males once they are within several centimeters of females (Selander and Pinto, 1967; Adams and Selander, 1979, and references therein). In many meloids, including members of the genus *Epicauta*, the presence of a female or her odor quickly stimulates conspecific males to become active and sometimes even to show part of the courtship display (Adams and Selander, 1979). Matthes (1970) observed that after courtship is begun male *Cercoma schafferi* appear to fan palpal and antennal secretions around females to induce them to copulate. Nothing apparently is known about the origin or the chemistry of olfactory cues in meloids.

2. Primer Effects of Cantharidin

Many female blister beetles generally are sexually unreceptive from copulation until oviposition (Selander and Mathieu, 1969; J. E. Carrel, unpublished results). This may in part be induced by cantharidin or its metabolites. We currently are investigating this possibility using male beetles that have been pretreated with 6-fluoromevalonate to inhibit cantharidin biosynthesis.

I. Defensive Properties of Cantharidin

1. Antifeedant against Predaceous Arthropods

Carrel (1971) and Carrel and Eisner (1974) demonstrated that cantharidin is a potent antifeedant against ants, ground beetles, and several other invertebrate predators. Pure cantharidin in submillimolar concentrations significantly reduces feeding by these animals. Blood of blister beetles, which commonly contains millimolar amounts of cantharidin, evidently is distasteful to the predators. Other investigators, such as Cuenot (1890), report that meloid blood is repugnant to insects.

Cantharidin is also very toxic to some insects. In an extensive series of pharmacological tests, Goernitz (1937) found that microgram amounts of cantharidin kill beetles, walking sticks, and caterpillars. The substance acts both as a contact as well as a systemic insecticide. Goernitz (1937) further reported that cantharides prepared from various blister beetles are effective insecticides.

2. Antifeedant against Predaceous Vertebrates

Protection of meloids from many types of vertebrates is assumed to be conferred by cantharidin present in the blood and body of the beetles. However, as pointed out by Carrel and Eisner (1974), the basis of discrimination of vertebrates against blister beetles has not been rigorously tested. Recently, J. E. Carrel and J. Maruniak (unpublished results) found that white rats rapidly learn to avoid drinking water containing minute concentrations of pure cantharidin. Because avoidance occurs within a few minutes of exposure to the substance, they conclude that rats probably discriminate against meloids on the basis of their unpalatability rather than their toxicity. Whether other vertebrates also respond in a similar fashion is under investigation in our laboratory.

IV. TOPICS FOR INVESTIGATION

A. Cantharidin Biosynthesis

1. Intermediates beyond Farnesol

Major advances in understanding how farnesol is transformed into cantharidin await isolation of intermediates derived from farnesol. Questions regarding the possible involvement of steps common to juvenile hormone biosynthesis as well as basic questions regarding the sequence of carbon–carbon bond making and carbon–carbon bond breaking steps will be answered only by the discovery of key intermediates in this pathway. As intermediates become known, it then will be possible to speculate more accurately on the timing of oxidative transformations and their relationships to carbon–carbon bond making and breaking processes.

2. Mechanism of Methyl Group Scrambling

No information is available about the chemical details that account for the nearly complete scrambling of the farnesyl terminal methyl groups, and no obvious biosynthetic analogies exist for such scrambling. Information regarding the process that accounts for this randomization will provide valuable chemical evidence regarding a portion of cantharidin biosynthesis. This process may well be linked with introduction of oxygen at C-10, oxidation of one of these methyl groups, or carbon–carbon bond formation between C-3 and C-11.

3. Fate of Farnesol Fragments Lost during Cantharidin Biosynthesis

Little information is available regarding the C_1 and C_4 portions of the farnesyl skeleton that are lost during its transformation into cantharidin. Evidence regarding the oxidation level at which the C_1 fragment is released would provide clues regarding the chemistry at C-2, possibly including C-2—C-11 bond formation. Although the Swiss group has obtained evidence that the C_4 fragment eventually produces acetate from at least a portion of this fragment, no quantitative information is available, and, more importantly, no information is available regarding the structure of the fragment as it is initially lost. Clearly, information about these fragments is essential to understanding the overall biosynthetic pathway and in particular will be crucial for unveiling the carbon–carbon bond cleavage chemistry.

4. Stereochemistry of Hydrogen Atoms Derived from Farnesol

Details regarding the stereochemical relationships of the enantiotopic hydrogen atoms of farnesol and the stereochemistries of the hydrogen atoms in cantharidin will provide chemical clues regarding the bond making and bond breaking processes that take place at C-1 and C-6 of cantharidin. What stereochemical selection, if any, is made in the removal of one of the C-4 hydrogen atoms of farnesol, and is there stereochemical selection in the removal of hydrogen from C-8 of farnesol? What is the stereochemical relationship between the retained (enantiotopic) hydrogen atom at C-4 of farnesol and the chirality at C-1 of cantharidin? Is there stereospecificity in the arrangement of hydrogen atoms at C-6 of cantharidin?

Synthetic advances over the years now permit reasonable access to precursor mevalonates stereospecifically labeled at each of the prochiral hydrogen atoms. The stereochemical fates of all of the mevalonate hydrogen atoms incorporated into farnesol are well established. Therefore, use of stereospecifically labeled $[2\text{-}^3\text{H}]$mevalonate is equivalent to utilizing farnesol stereospecifically labeled at C-4 and C-8. Use of radiolabeled mevalonate of high specific activity might permit analysis of the results by ^3H NMR, reducing the otherwise extensive amount of work required for classical stereochemical investigations carried out by ^3H labeling. Alternatively, use of stable isotope labeling and analysis of results by MS as well as NMR would permit examination of this question without the need for classical degradation studies.

5. Site of Cantharidin Biosynthesis in Adult Males

The location of the tissue(s) where cantharidin is biosynthesized in blister beetles is not known. Because cantharidin is stored in the third pair of male accessory reproductive glands, it has been suggested that the glands themselves are the site of synthesis (Blum, 1981). On the other hand, our oxygen labeling studies imply that the post-farnesyl steps in the cantharidin pathway may occur entirely in the male beetle's body outside the reproductive system and that the end product is transported and stored in the male accessory glands (McCormick *et al.*, 1986). We currently are using autoradiographic and tissue culture techniques to localize the site of cantharidin synthesis in adult male meloids.

6. Biosynthesis in Immature Meloids

Cantharidin is present in the bodies of immature meloids, but no information is available regarding whether cantharidin biosynthesis in juvenile forms is identical to that in adult males. Several questions come to mind: (1) What is the timing and extent of biosynthesis prior to adult eclosion? (2) Is the biochemical pathway the same in larval and adult instars? (3) Do adults and larvae use equivalent tissues to synthesize cantharidin?

7. Regulation

Assuming that immature meloids of both sexes generally are able to make the substance, as suggested by radiolabeling studies with larvel *L. vesicatoria* (Meyer *et al.*, 1968) and by our information regarding the cantharidin content of both sexes immediately following eclosion (Carrel *et al.*, 1986a), what are the genetic regulatory events that inhibit cantharidin production in adult females and how are these events orchestrated in them? In males, what regulatory mechanism accounts for vastly increased synthesis of cantharidin by adults, relative to immature stages? Biochemical regulation of the production of arthropod defensive substances is an important but virtually unexplored field of study (Carrel, 1984).

B. Biological Chemistry of Cantharidin

1. Protection of Blister Beetles from Cantharidin Toxicity

Cantharidin is present throughout the bodies of blister beetles (Carrel 1971; Viehoever and Capen, 1923), yet this cytotoxic substance apparently causes no cellular damage in these insects. Most of the cantharidin in meloids may be present in an inactive form; supportive evidence is provided by the requirement that beetle tissues must first be treated with strong base (Ray *et al.*, 1979) or strong acid (Carrel *et al.*, 1985) before organic solvent extraction is effective in removing most of the cantharidin. We are in the process of characterizing a cantharidin-binding protein present in abundance as a storage product in the third pair of accessory glands in male *E. pestifera*. We also are investigating the possibility that lipophorin(s) in the hemolymph of meloids simultaneously carry out roles relating to both transport and detoxification.

2. Metabolic Fate of Cantharidin Transferred to Female Meloids

Cantharidin deposited by a male meloid in a female's spermatophoral receptacle does not all simply remain there until it is voided by her. A small fraction of the male-derived cantharidin is quickly absorbed into the female's body fluids and tissues. We also found that a large part of the male's gift, approximately one-third in *E. pestifera,* is unaccountably lost by a female when kept in isolation (J. E. Carrel and J. P. McCormick, unpublished results). This observation opens the possibility that a female meloid acquires cantharidin from her mate and then transforms it biochemically into a substance or several substances useful to her, to her mate, or to their offspring. We are undertaking studies to learn more about the biochemical transformation(s) of cantharidin in female meloids.

REFERENCES

Adams, C. L., and Selander, R. B. (1979). The biology of blister beetles of the vittata group of the genus *Epicauta* (Coleoptera, Meloidae). *Bull. Am. Mus. Nat. Hist.* **162,** 137–266.

Bagatell, F. K. (1964). Studies on biological factors in acantholysis. *J. Invest. Derm.* **43,** 357–361.

Baker, F. C., and Schooley, D. A. (1978). Juvenile hormone biosynthesis: Identification of 3-hydroxy-3-ethylglutarate and 3-hydroxy-3-methylglutarate in cell-free extracts from *Manduca sexta* incubated with propionyl- and acetyl-CoA. *J. Chem. Soc. Chem. Commun.,* 292–293.

Bardshiri, E., Simpson, T. J., Scott, A. I., and Shishido, K. (1984). Studies on a synthesis of (*RS*)-mevalonic acid lactone. *J. Chem. Soc. Perkin Trans. I,* 1765–1767.

Beasley, V. R., Wolf, G. A., Fischer, D. C., Ray, A. C.. and Edwards, W. C. (1983). Cantharidin toxicosis in horses. *J. Am. Vet. Med. Assoc.* **182,** 283–284.

Beauregard, H. (1890). "Les Insectes Vesicants." Felix Alcan, Paris.

Bjostad, L. B., and Roelofs, W. L. (1986). Sex pheromone biosynthesis in the rebanded leafroller moth, studied by mass-labeling with stable isotopes and analysis with mass spectrometry. *J. Chem. Ecol.* **12,** 431–450.

Blum, M. S. (1981). "Chemical Defenses of Arthropods." Academic Press, New York.

Capinera, J. L., Gardner, D. R., and Stermitz, F. R. (1985). Cantharidin levels in blister beetles (Coleoptera: Meloidae) associated with alfalfa in Colorado. *J. Econ. Entomol.* **78,** 1052–1055.

Carrel, J. E. (1971). Arthropod chemical defenses with both immediate and delayed effects. Ph.D. thesis, Cornell University, Ithaca, New York.

Carrel, J. E. (1984). Defensive secretion of the pill millipede *Glomeris marginata.* I. Fluid production and storage. *J. Chem. Ecol.* **10,** 41–51.

Carrel, J. E., and Eisner, T. (1974). Cantharidin: Potent feeding deterrent to insects. *Science* **183,** 755–757.

Carrel, J. E., Thompson, W., and McLaughlin, M. (1973). Parental transmission of a defensive chemical (cantharidin) in blister beetles. *Am. Zool.* **13,** 1258.

Carrel, J. E., Doom, J. P., and McCormick, J. P. (1985). Quantitative determination of cantharidin in biological materials using capillary gas chromatography with flame ionization detection. *J. Chromatog. Biomed. Appl.* **342,** 411–415.

Carrel, J. E., Doom, J. P., and McCormick, J. P. (1986a). Cantharidin biosynthesis in a blister beetle: Inhibition by 6-fluoromevalonate causes chemical disarmament. *Experientia* **42,** 853–854.

Carrel, J. E., McCormick, J. P., Doom, J. P., and Smith, K. E. (1986b). Cantharidin biosynthesis: Extent, timing and inhibition. *J. Cell. Biochem. Suppl.* **10C,** 77.

Chippendale, G. M., and Cassatt, K. (1985). *Diatraea grandiosella.* In "Handbook of Insect Rearing" (P. Singh and R. F. Moore, eds.), Vol. 2, pp. 257–263. Elsevier, Amsterdam.

Cuenot, L. (1890). Le sang des *Meloe* et le role de la cantharidine dans la biologie des Coleopteres vesicants. *Bull. Zool. Fr.* **15,** 126–128.

Danckwortt, P. W. (1914). The chemical nature of cantharidin. *Arch. Pharm.* **252,** 632–636 [*Chem. Abstr.* **9,** 2083 (1915)].

Dauben, W. G., Kessel, C. R., and Takemura, K. H. (1980). Simple, efficient total synthesis of cantharidin via a high-pressure Diels–Alder reaction. *J. Am. Chem. Soc.* **102,** 6893–6894.

Diels, O., and Alder, K. (1929). Synthesen in der hydro-aromatischen Reihe, II. Mitteilung: Ueber Cantharidin. *Chem. Ber.* **62,** 554–562.

Dillwith, J. W., Nelson, J. H., Pomonis, J. G., Nelson, D. R., and Blomquist, G. J. (1982). A ^{13}C nmr study of methyl-branched hydrocarbon biosynthesis in the housefly. *J. Biol. Chem.* **257,** 11305–11314.

Epstein, W. L., and Kligman, A. M. (1959). Treatment of warts with cantharidin. *Arch. Derm.* **17,** 592–596.

Escher, S., Loew, P., and Arigoni, D. (1970). The role of hydroxygeraniol and hydroxynerol in the biosynthesis of loganin and indole alkaloids. *J. Chem. Soc. Chem. Commun.,* 823–825.

Fleisher, T. L., and Fox, I. (1970). Oedermerid beetle dermatitis. *Arch. Derm.* **101,** 601–605.

Gadamer, J. (1914a). The constitution of cantharidin. *Arch. Pharm.* **252,** 609–632 [*Chem. Abstr.* **9,** 2083 (1915)].

Gadamer, J. (1914b). The action of hydrochloric acid on cantharidin. *Arch. Pharm.* **252,** 636–663 [*Chem. Abstr.* **9,** 2084 (1915)].

Goernitz, K. (1937). Cantharidin als Gift und Anlockungsmittel fuer Insekten. *Arb. Phys. Angew. Ent. Berlin–Dahlem* **4,** 116–156.

Guenther, H., Ramstad, E., and Floss, H. G. (1969). On the biosynthesis of cantharidin. *J. Pharm. Sci.* **58,** 1274.

Hammock, B. D., and Quistad, G. B. (1981). Metabolism and mode of action of juvenile hormone, juvenoids, and insect growth regulators. *In* "Progress in Pesticide Biochemistry" (D. H. Hutson and T. R. Roberts, eds.), Vol. 1, pp. 1–83. Wiley, New York.

Hansen, P. E. (1983). Isotope effects on nuclear shielding. *In* "Annual Reports on NMR Spectroscopy" (G. A. Webb, ed.), Vol. 15, pp. 105–234. Academic Press, New York.

Hedlin, A. F., Yates, III, H. O., Tovar, D. C., Ebel, B. H., Koerber, T. W., and Merkel, E. P. (1981). "Cone and Seed Insects of North American Conifers." U.S. Forest Service, U.S. Dept. of Agriculture, Washington, D.C.

Jiang, T.-L., Salmon, S. E., and Liu, R. M. (1983). Activity of camptothecin, harringtonin, cantharidin and curcumae in the human tumor stem cell assay. *Eur. J. Cancer Clin. Oncol.* **19,** 263–270.

Keele, C. A., and Armstrong, D. (1964). "Substances Producing Pain and Itch." Edward Arnold, London.

Kobert, R. (1906). "Lehrbuch der Intoxikationen," Vol. 2, pp. 435–442. Ferdinand Enke, Stuttgart.

Lee, E., Schooley, D. A., Hall, M. S., and Judy, K. J. (1978). Juvenile hormone biosynthesis: Homomevalonate and mevalonate synthesis by insect corpus allatum enzymes. *J. Chem. Soc. Chem. Commun.,* 290–292.

Lewer, P., and MacMillan, J. (1983). Reinvestigation of a synthesis of (*RS*)-mevalonolactone. *J. Chem.Soc. Perkin Trans. I,* 1417–1420.

McCormick, J. P., Carrel, J. E., and Doom, J. P. (1986). Origin of oxygen atoms in cantharidin biosynthesized by beetles. *J. Am. Chem. Soc.* **108,** 8071–8074.

Matthes, D. (1970). Sexual stimulation by olfaction. *Umschau* **70,** 112–113.

Meyer, D., Schlatter, C., Schlatter-Lanz, I., Schmid, H., and Bovey, P. (1968). Die Zucht von *Lytta vesicatoria* im Laboratorium und Nachweis der Cantharidinsynthese in Larven. *Experientia* **24**, 995–998.

Muehlbacher, M., and Poulter, C. D. (1985). Isopentenyl diphosphate : Dimethylallyl diphosphate isomerase. Irreversible inhibition of the enzyme by active-site-directed covalent attachment. *J. Am. Chem. Soc.* **107**, 8307–8308.

Nave, J.-F., d'Orchymont, H., Ducep, J.-B., Piriou, F., and Jung, M. F. (1985). Mechanism of the inhibition of cholesterol biosynthesis by 6-fluoromevalonate. *Biochem. J.* **227**, 247–254.

Nickolls, L. C., and Teare, D. (1954). Poisoning by cantharidin. *Br. Med. J.* **2**, 1384–1386.

Peter, M. G. (1973). "Untersuchungen zur Biosynthese des Cantharidins und des Palasonins." Ph.D. thesis, Univ. of Zurich, Switzerland.

Peter, M. G., Snatzke, G., Snatzke, F., Nagarijan, K. N., and Schmid, H. (1974). Ueber die absolute Konfiguration der Cantharsaeure und des Palasonins. *Helv. Chim. Acta* **57**, 32–64.

Peter, M. G., Waespe, H.-R., Woggon, W.-D., and Schmid, H. (1977a). Einbauversuche mit (^{3}H und ^{13}C)-doppelmarkiertem Farnesol in Cantharidin. *Helv. Chim. Acta* **60**, 1262–1272.

Peter, M. G., Woggon, W.-D., Schlatter, C., and Schmid, H. (1977b). Einbauversuche mit Geraniol und Farnesol in Cantharidin. *Helv. Chim. Acta* **60**, 844–866.

Peter, M. G., Woggon, W.-D., and Schmid, H. (1977c). Identifizierung von Farnesol als Zwischenstufe in der Biosynthese des Cantharidins aus Mevalonsaeurelacton. *Helv. Chim. Acta* **60**, 2756–2762.

Piccard, J. (1877). Ueber das Cantharidin und ein in Derivat desselben. *Chem. Ber.*, 1504–1506.

Polson, C. J., and Tattersall, R. N. (1959). "Clinical Toxicology." Lippincott, Philadelphia.

Poulter, C. D., and Rilling, H. C. (1978). The prenyl transfer reaction: Enzymatic and mechanistic studies of the 1'-4 coupling reaction in the terpene biosynthetic pathway. *Acc. Chem. Res.* **11**, 307–313.

Poulter, C. D., Argyle, J. C., and Mash, E. A. (1978). Farnesyl pyrophosphate synthetase. *J. Biol. Chem.* **253**, 7227–7233.

Poulter, C. D., Mash, E. A., Argyle, J. C., Muscio, O. J., and Rilling, H. C. (1979). Farnesyl pyrophosphate synthetase. Mechanistic studies of the 1'-4 coupling reaction in the terpene biosynthetic pathway. *J. Am. Chem. Soc.* **101**, 6761–6763.

Poulter, C. D., Wiggins, P. L., and Le, A. T. (1981). Farnesylpyrophosphate synthetase. A stepwise mechanism for the 1'-4 condensation reaction. *J. Am. Chem. Soc.* **103**, 3926–3927.

Prestwich, G. D. (1986a). Chemical studies of pheromone catabolism and reception. *J. Cell. Biochem. Suppl.* **10c**, 65.

Prestwich, G. D. (1986b). Fluorinated sterols, hormones, and pheromones: Enzyme-targeted disruptants in insects. *Pest. Sci.*, **37**, 430–440.

Prestwich, G. D., Yamaoka, R., and Carvalho, J. F. (1985). Metabolism of tritiated ω-fluorofatty acids and alcohols in the termite *Reticulitermes flavipes* (Kollar) (Isoptera, Rhinotermitidae). *Insect Biochem.* **15**, 205–209.

Quistad, G. B., Cerf, D. C., Schooley, D. A., and Staal, G. B. (1981a). Fluoromevalonate acts as an inhibitor of insect juvenile hormone biosynthesis. *Nature (London)* **289**, 176–177.

Quistad, G. B., Cerf, D. C., Schooley, D. A., Staal, G. B. (1981b). Fluoromevalonate—an inhibitor of insect juvenile hormone biosynthesis. *Pr. Nauk. Inst. Chem. Org. Fiz. Politech. Wroclaw* **22**, 163–168 [*Chem. Abstr.* **96**, 176074y (1981)].

Quistad, G. B., Staiger, L. E., and Cerf, D. C. (1982). Preparation and biological activity of potential inhibitors of insect juvenile hormone biosynthesis. *J. Agric. Food Chem.* **30**, 1151–1154.

Ray, A. C., Tamulinas, S. H., and Reagor, J. C. (1979). High pressure liquid chromatographic determination of cantharidin, using a derivatization method in specimens from animals acutely poisoned by ingestion of blister beetles, *Epicauta lemniscata. Am. J. Vet. Res.* **40**, 498–504.

Rudolph, W. (1916). Cantharidin V. *Arch. Pharm.* **254**, 423–456 [*J. Chem. Soc.* **112**(I), 468–469 (1917)].

Schlatter, C., and Duersteler-Meier, A. (1970). Zur Biosynthese des kaeferinhaltsstoffes Cantharidin. *Chimia* **24**, 33.

Schlatter, C., Duersteler-Meier, A., and Schmid, H. (1968a). Zur Biosynthese des kaeferinhaltsstoffes Cantharidin. *Chimia* **22**, 498.

Schlatter, C., Waldner, E. E., and Schmid, H. (1968b). Zur Biosynthese des Cantharidins. I. *Experientia* **24**, 994–995.

Schlosser, M. (1978). Introduction of fluorine into organic molecules: Why and how. *Tetrahedron* **34**, 3–17.

Schooley, D. A., Judy, K. J., Bergot, B. J., Hall, M. S., and Siddall, J. B. (1973). Biosynthesis of the juvenile hormones of *Manduca sexta:* Labeling pattern from mevalonate, propionate, and acetate. *Proc. Natl. Acad. Sci. U.S.A.* **70**, 2921.

Scott, A. I., and Shishido, K. (1980). An easy synthesis of (*RS*)-[3′-13C]mevalonic acid lactone. *J. Chem. Soc. Chem. Commun.*, 400–401.

Selander, R. B., and Mathieu, J. M. (1969). Ecology, behavior, and adult anatomy of the albida group of the genus *Epicauta* (Coleoptera, Meloidae). *Univ. Illinois Biol. Monogr.* **41**, 1–173.

Selander, R. B., and Pinto, J. D. (1967). Sexual behavior in blister beetles (Coleoptera: Meloidae). II. *Linsleya convexa. J. Kansas Entomol. Soc.* **40**, 396–412.

Sierra, J. R., Woggon, W.-D., and Schmid. H. (1976). Transfer of cantharidin (1) during copulation from the adult male to the female *Lytta vesicatoria* ('Spanish flies'). *Experientia* **32**, 142–143.

Simpson, K. (ed.) (1965). "Taylor's Principles and Practice of Medical Jurisprudence" 12th Ed., Vol. II, pp. 575–578. Little, Brown, Boston.

Singer, F. M., Januszka, J. P., and Borman, A. (1959). New inhibitors of *in vitro* conversion of acetate and mevalonate to cholesterol. *Proc. Soc. Exp. Biol. Med.* **102**, 370–373.

Sollman, T. (1948). "A Manual of Pharmacology," 7th Ed. Saunders, Philadelphia, Pennsylvania.

Stork, G., van Tamelen, E. E., Friedman, L. J., and Burgstahler. A. W. (1953). A Stereospecific synthesis of cantharidin. *J. Am. Chem. Soc.* **75**, 384–392.

Till, J. S., and Majmudar, B. N. (1981). Cantharidin poisoning. *Southern Med. J.* **74**, 444–447.

Tschesche, R., and Machleidt, H. (1960). Synthesen von substituierten β-hydroxy-β-Methylglutarsaeuren und Mevalonsaeuren. *Justus Liebigs Ann. Chem.* **631**, 61–76.

Viehoever, A., and Capen, R. G. (1923). Domestic sources of cantharidin. I. *Macrobasis albida* Say. *J. Assoc. Off. Agric. Chem.* **6**, 489–492.

von Bruchhausen, F., and Bersch, H. W. (1929). Constitution of cantharidin. *Arch. Pharm.* **266**, 697–702 [*Chem. Abstr.* **23**, 1647 (1929)].

Walsh, C. (1983). Fluorinated substrate analogs: Routes of metabolism and selective toxicity. *In* "Advances in Enzymology" (A. Meister, ed.), Vol. 55, pp. 197–289. Wiley, New York.

Wertelecki, W., Vietti, T. J., and Kulapongs, V. (1967). Cantharidin poisoning from ingestion of a "blister beetle." *Pediatrics* **39**, 287–289.

Woggon, W.-D., Peter, W., and Schmid, H. (1977). Experimente zum kompetitiven Einbau der Stereoisomeren des Farnesols in Cantharidin. *Helv. Chim. Acta* **60**, 2288–2294.

Woggon, W.-D., Hauffe, S. A., and Schmid, H. (1983). Biosynthesis of cantharidin: Evidence for the specific incorporation of C-4 and C-11′ of farnesol. *J. Chem. Soc. Chem. Commun.*, 272–274.

Woodward, R. B., and Loftfield, R. B. (1941). The structure of cantharidine and the synthesis of desoxycantharidine. *J. Am. Chem. Soc.* **63**, 3167–3171.

Young, D. K. (1984). Cantharidin and insects: An historical review. *Great Lakes Entomol.* **17**, 187–194.

Yu Y.-H. (1957). A new micro color reaction of cantharidin. *Acta Pharm. Sinica* **5**, 168.

Ziegler, K., Schenck, G., Krockow, E. W., Siebert, A., Wenz, A., and Weber, H. (1942). Die Synthese des Cantharidins. *Justus Liebigs Ann. Chem.* **551**, 1–79.

II

Reception and Catabolism of Pheromones

11

Functional Morphology of Pheromone-Sensitive Sensilla

RUDOLF ALEXANDER STEINBRECHT

Max-Planck-Institut für Verhaltensphysiologie
D-8131 Seewiesen, Federal Republic of Germany

I. INTRODUCTION

Research on pheromone perception in insects is almost synonymous with research on insect olfaction. In particular, many fine structural and electrophysiological studies devoted to insect olfaction have been carried out with pheromone-sensitive systems. The reason is easily understood, if we remember that it was the sex attractant pheromone of the silkmoth, *Bombyx mori,* that opened the door for work on single olfactory cells in insects (for a historical retrospect, see Schneider, 1984a). Several reviews cover the morphology of arthropod olfactory receptors (Altner and Prillinger, 1980; Zacharuk, 1980, 1985; Steinbrecht, 1984; Keil and Steinbrecht, 1984). Therefore, in the context of this book, I shall primarily provide the necessary illustrations so that chemists, entomologists, and neurobiologists are quickly "put into the picture."

First, the variability of antennal and sensillar form will be demonstrated. In terms of functional morphology, antennal and sensillar shape are important for stimulus uptake. Second, we shall look into the internal structure of sensory hairs and address the question of stimulus transport: How do pheromone molecules find their way to the receptor membrane, which is isolated from the environment by the barrier of insect cuticle? If our present knowledge had allowed, the next paragraph would have been devoted to the morphology of receptor molecules and the actual recognition processes. Finally, the cellular organization of sensilla is

Pheromone Biochemistry

described in the light of what we know or should know about the functioning of the receptor organ in terms of its electrical and cell biological properties.

II. ANTENNAL SHAPE, SENSILLAR FORM AND DISTRIBUTION—UPTAKE OF PHEROMONE MOLECULES

A. Antennal Dimorphism—A Hint at Sex Pheromone Communication

Sometimes, antennal specializations for detecting pheromones are visible at the first glance: a marked sexual dimorphism of antennal size and shape is often observed in species using sex attractant pheromones. The large saturniid moths are a well-known example; the males are adorned with huge feathered antennae for perceiving the sex pheromone and locating its source, the female moths, which are themselves equipped with much feebler antennae. The size difference reflects the distribution of one sensillum type, the long sensilla trichodea, present on the male antenna in numbers over 50,000 but completely absent in the female (Boeckh *et al.*, 1960). Other examples are found in melolonthid beetles (Meinecke, 1975) and, though less spectacular, in the honeybee (Esslen and Kaissling, 1976) (Fig. 1).

In many species the overall antennal shape and size is largely the same in both sexes, with only the number of sensilla belonging to a certain type differing significantly. In *Periplaneta americana* the sensillum "swB" which contains the pheromone receptor cells is present only in the male nymph and imago (Schaller, 1978; Sass, 1983). Other examples are listed by Chapman (1982). The amount of data is small, however, since for most cases the exact sensillum type responsible for pheromone perception has not yet been identified unequivocally.

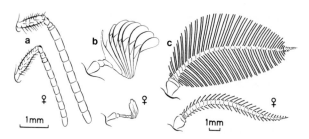

Fig. 1. Antennae of male and female (♀) insects with marked sexual dimorphism. (a) Honeybee (*Apis mellifera*); (b) scarabid beetle (genus *Rhopaea*); (c) saturniid moth (genus *Antheraea*), reduced in size as compared to a and b (see scale bars). Adapted from Kaissling (1971).

Nonchemical communication or differences in the way of living (e.g., food uptake) between the sexes, however, may also lead to antennal dimorphism. The bushy antennal flagella of male mosquitoes are well-known adaptations for acoustic communication; the blood-sucking females, on the other hand, possess a two- to fourfold larger number of olfactory sensilla than males, a feature probably connected with host location (Chapman 1982).

Sexual dimorphism can also be masked by a functional shift of the respective sensilla. In *Bombyx mori,* the antenna of the female is not much smaller than in the male. Likewise, the number of the long sensilla trichodea is not very much reduced (δ: 17,000, $\female$: 12,000; Steinbrecht, 1970a). Physiological differences are more striking. In the male, the two sensory cells associated with each sensillum respond to bombykol and bombykal, respectively (Kaissling *et al.,* 1978). In the female, neither of the cells responds to pheromone in physiological concentrations; the most effective stimuli were 2,6-dimethyl-5-hepten-2-ol and benzoic acid, respectively (Priesner, 1979a). Many noctuid moths have equal numbers of sensilla trichodea in both sexes, e.g., *Trichoplusia ni* (δ: 8,000, $\female$: 8,000; Mayer *et al.,* 1981). It would be worthwhile to look for functional changes also in these nondomesticated species. On the other hand, female *Adoxophyes orana* can detect their own pheromone with the same sensilla trichodea as the males (Den Otter *et al.,* 1978).

B. Feathered Antennae—Adaptations for Maximum Odor Uptake

The large feathered antennae of male silkmoths, often called "odor sieves," doubtless are adaptations to maximize odor uptake, thus increasing the overall sensitivity of the receiver (Fig. 2). It remains a largely open question why selection went that way instead of evolving more powerful pheromone glands. Theoretically, hundred or even thousand times higher pheromone release rates are not beyond the metabolic capacity of the female. The male on the other hand can increase its sensitivity only by increasing the number of primarily caught molecules, since the receptors themselves are already tuned to respond to single molecules (Kaissling and Priesner, 1970). We may speculate that the female "is interested" to produce offspring with "good noses" and a powerful orientation capability; thus only the fittest males in this respect are given a chance to mate, if the female reduces rather than increases its pheromone output.

In contrast to this female parsimony, the "seducing" pheromones of many male Lepidoptera are produced in microgram and even milligram quantities, even though the communication distance usually is small. Moreover, in many cases sticky particles soaked with pheromone are disseminated onto the female's antenna during courtship to make the pheromone stimulus stronger and longer lasting. The female sensilla responsible for the perception of these "aphro-

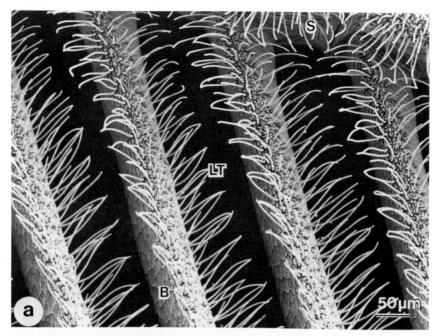

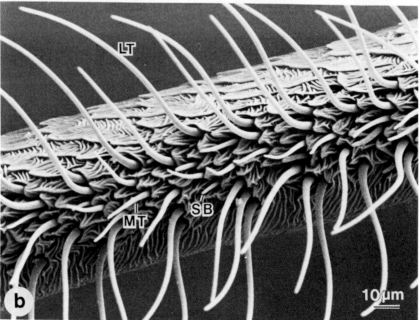

disiacs" are neither very large nor exceedingly numerous. Obviously, communication via sex pheromones evolved along highly divergent lines in female and male Lepidoptera (for review, see Schneider, 1984b).

The catchword "odor sieve" should not, however, be taken too literally. Relatively little is known about the aerodynamics of these antennae under the actual airflow situation. Vogel (1983) measured the airflow through the antenna of the saturniid *Actias luna* and found that this is much slower than the airspeed to which the antenna is exposed, e.g., 0.26 m/sec at a free airspeed of 2 m/sec. Thus, only 13% of the air directly upwind from the antenna passes through it; the rest is deflected around it and creates eddies in the wake. By contrast light transmittance is about 38%, which emphasizes the effect of viscosity. Vogel also visualized the flow situation in a water tank at equal Reynold's number and demonstrated that flow through the antenna is enough to envelope the sensory hairs in transmitted medium (water or air). Eddies of the deflected stream cannot reach the sensilla from behind. Keeping in mind that the antennae of *Actias* and *Antheraea* are flat, planar structures, it would be interesting to know whether such eddies are exploited in the basketlike antennae of *Bombyx* and *Lymantria*, where a front row of antennal branches partly covers the larger branches of the rear row.

Adsorption measurements with radioactive pheromone provide data on the fraction of molecules actually trapped on the antennal surface, which is expected to be equal to or lower than the transmissivity of an antenna. Yet surprisingly the reported values are higher: antennae of *Bombyx mori* trapped 27% of the pheromone contained in an airstream of equal cross-sectional area (airspeed 0.6 m/sec; Kaissling, 1971); with *Antheraea polyphemus* the respective adsorbance was 23–26% (airspeed 2.6 m/sec; Kanaujia and Kaissling, 1985). Since at least in the latter experiment there were no profound differences in antennal shape and airspeed to Vogel's experiments, the difference must be in the aerodynamics of the experimental setup. Vogel (1983) used a wind tunnel of 7.5 cm in diameter; Kanaujia and Kaissling (1985) blew the airstream through a glass tube with an inner diameter of 7 mm, and the antenna was placed at a distance of 5 mm to the outlet. When the distance between antenna and outlet was reduced to 1 mm, adsorbance increased to as much as 32%. It is quite conceivable, therefore, that this setup produces a higher pressure difference between front and rear side of the antenna and hence a higher transmissivity than suspending the antenna in a wind tunnel.

Fig. 2. The odor sieve of the male silkmoth, *Bombyx mori*, as seen in the scanning electron microscope. (a) The flagellar stem (S) gives rise to two rows of about 40 branches (B) each. The frame shows how the long sensilla trichodea (LT) are arranged to extend over most of the interspace between the branches. (b) Close-up view of antennal branch. In the long sensilla trichodea (LT) are found the receptors for the sex pheromone; in between some medium-sized sensilla trichodea (MT) and sensilla basiconica (SB), with olfactory receptors of largely unknown function, are visible (see also Steinbrecht, 1970a, 1973).

Kanaujia and Kaissling (1985) also checked for desorption and confirmed earlier suggestions that pheromone molecules once trapped at the antennal surface do not desorb to any measurable extent during the first few seconds after the end of stimulus. Desorption, therefore, cannot explain the rapid decline of the receptor potential (see also Kaissling, 1986a).

The next question is whether adsorption occurs equally on all antennal surfaces. Homogenous adsorption would be disadvantageous because even in the large silkmoth antennae, where the pheromone-sensitive sensilla trichodea are very long and outnumber all other sensilla, their total surface is small in relation to the remaining "insensitive surface" of the antennal stem and branches (the sensilla trichodea comprise 13% of the total antennal surface in *B. mori;* Steinbrecht, 1970a). However, as theoretically predicted by Adam and Delbrück (1968) and confirmed by measurements with radioactive pheromone, at least 80% of the initially adsorbed pheromone molecules are found on the long sensilla trichodea (*B. mori:* Steinbrecht and Kasang, 1972; *A. polyphemus:* Kanaujia and Kaissling, 1985). The thin and slender hairs (1–5 μm diameter) are arranged in such a way that the diffusion sinks created by adsorption by each single hair overlap and thus effectively clear the space inbetween the hairs from passing molecules (Adam and Delbrück, 1968). The diffusion sink toward the antennal branches is much smaller because of their larger diameter (50–100 μm).

Recently, Mankin and Mayer (1984) questioned the idea of the odor sieve. In a wind tunnel they exposed various species with feathered (*Bombyx mori* and *Lymantria dispar*) and filiform antennae (*Apis mellifera*, *Plodia interpunctella*, and *Trichoplusia ni*) to radioactive pheromone compounds. Plotting the radioactivity deposited per unit exposure time against the product of the pheromone concentration in air times the total antennal surface area, they observed a species-dependent slope, the deposition velocity. This deposition velocity was greatest in the two moths with filiform antennae and smallest in the species with feathered antennae. However, uneven deposition favoring the hairs, and even the outer half of the hairs, has been experimentally proved (Steinbrecht and Kasang, 1972; Kanaujia and Kaissling, 1985). A deposition rate averaged over the sensory hairs *and* all the insensitive antennal surfaces, therefore, is essentially meaningless for the effectivity of an antenna in terms of stimulus uptake. It certainly cannot be used to falsify the hypothesis that the dimensions of the hairs as well as their spacing is of importance for molecule catch (for a detailed treatment of how to calculate stimulus adsorption, see Kaissling, 1971, pp. 355 and 381).

C. Other Antennal and Sensillar Forms—Constraints Imposed by the Way of Living

The selective advantage of thin cylindrical surfaces for catching odor molecules as pointed out by Adam and Delbrück (1968) is of course valid for filiform antennae with hairlike olfactory sensilla as well. Feathered antennae are useful to expose a very large number of sensilla to an airstream; they have evolved convergently several times not only in Lepidoptera, but also in other insect orders with species using far-distance pheromone communication [e.g., the phengodid beetles (Tiemann, 1967) and the sawflies in Hymenoptera (Hallberg, 1979)].

Feathered antennae also have severe disadvantages, e.g., a high wind resistance, inflexibility, and sensitivity to damage and contamination. Thus, the fast flying hawk moths use filiform antennae, but these bear extraordinary long sensilla trichodea [400 μm in *Manduca sexta* (Sanes and Hildebrand, 1976a)]. Also, insects living in narrow galleries or feeding on sticky material could not possibly develop large odor sieves. Bark beetles, for example, have relatively small antennae; the only surface enlargement, the terminal club, bears the sensilla responsive for pheromone and host odor perception. Thin-walled sensilla basiconica are aligned in strands and protrude only slightly from the antennal surface, protected from damage by the stouter sensilla trichodea and chaetica (Fig. 3) (Payne *et al.*, 1973; Dickens and Payne, 1978). The whole antenna can be folded back into a groove on the head when the animal is boring into a tree.

Sensilla in lamellicorn beetles feeding on dung or nectar are found only along the inside of antennal lamellae, where they are better protected; the more delicate forms are even located in grooves (Meinecke, 1975). In hymenopterans there is the tendency to reduce the sensory hair to a pore plate flush with the antennal surface (Fig. 4), which certainly makes cleaning easier (Walther, 1981) but sacrifices molecule catch (see Kaissling, 1971, Table 5). In *Apis mellifera*, receptor cells of the pore plates respond to the female sex pheromone, queen substance, others to the pheromones of the Nassanov gland, but most are concerned with the detection of food odors (Kaissling and Renner, 1968; Vareschi, 1971). In the drone, the number of pore plates is greatly enhanced as compared to the queen or the worker bee (Esslen and Kaissling, 1976). It is intriguing that in ants the pore plates have been lifted off the hair surface to form the so-called sensilla trichodea curvata. Nevertheless, their fine structure is still very much like that of pore plates (see Figs. 11 and 12; Walther, 1979, 1981). Electrophysiological recordings revealed alarm pheromone receptors in the sensilla trichodea curvata of *Lasius fuliginosus* (Dumpert, 1972).

Finally, with respect to the sensory equipment for pheromone communication, we should bear in mind that high numbers of sensilla are not always necessary. The bedbug, *Cimex lectularius,* for example, lives in closely aggregated colonies, and the alarm pheromones (*E*)-2-hexenal and (*E*)-2-octenal which initiate dispersal on danger are released in considerable quantities; thus, the number of pheromone-receptive sensilla need not be very high. Indeed, confined to a small region on the last flagellar segment, there are not more than 29 olfactory sensilla (type E) with 58 receptor cells on each antenna. Most probably, only a fraction of these are specialists for the perception of the alarm pheromone (Fig. 5; see also Levinson *et al.*, 1974; Steinbrecht and Müller, 1976).

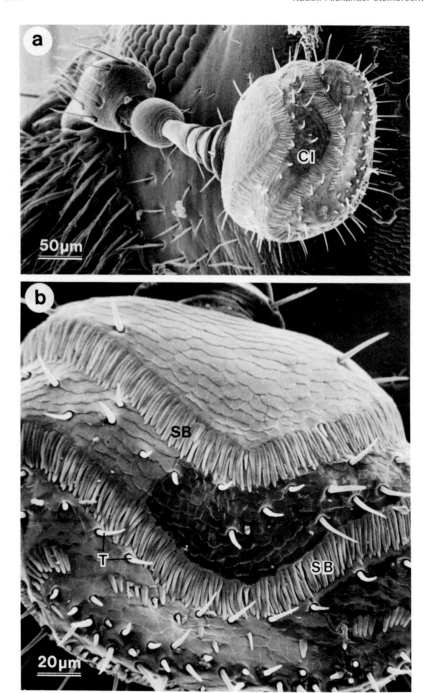

III. FINE STRUCTURE OF OLFACTORY HAIRS—STIMULUS TRANSPORT TO THE RECEPTOR SITE

However divergent the size and shape of olfactory sensilla may be (see Section II,C), their cuticular apparatus always comprises the outer dendritic segments of the olfactory cells, surrounded by an extracellular medium, the receptor lymph (sensillum lymph, sensillum liquor), confined by the cuticular wall of the sensillum (Fig. 6). In contrast to sensilla serving other modalities, e.g., gustatory, hygro-, or mechanoreceptors, the wall of olfactory sensilla is always perforated by a great number of pores (Schneider and Steinbrecht, 1968; Steinbrecht, 1984). Two fundamentally different kinds of wall pores were first distinguished by Steinbrecht (1969), the pore–tubule systems of single-walled multiporous sensilla and the spoke–channel systems of double-walled multiporous sensilla (Figs. 6b, and 6c). Both are supposed to enable the passage of odor molecules through the hair wall with minimal water loss from the dendrites and the receptor lymph.

A. Pore–Tubule Systems

1. Morphology

The pore–tubule type of wall pore has been most extensively studied in the sex pheromone sensilla of silkmoths (Steinbrecht and Müller, 1971; Steinbrecht, 1973, 1980; Keil, 1982, 1984b). The same basic components are observed in sensilla of many other species. These are an *outer pore,* widening to the outside by a pore funnel and toward inside, often leading into a wider pore kettle (Figs. 7–12). Depending on sensillum type and species, the pore diameter measures 10–40 nm. This pore structure is outlined by a very dense contour ($\sim$8.5 nm thick, sometimes trilaminar), the *L3 layer.* The pore itself looks empty but is filled with an electron-lucid material which also covers the whole cuticle of the insect with a layer of 7–10 nm thickness. This *L2 layer,* sometimes overlooked, can be observed best by the freeze-etching technique or when electron-dense material is surrounding the sensory hair, so that the contrast of the usually very faint *L1 layer* ($\sim$2.5 nm thick) is enhanced (see Fig. 10). The layers L1, L2, and L3, as defined by Steinbrecht and Kasang (1972) for sensory hairs, are not special features of insect sensilla but are observed on any kind of insect cuticle.

Fig. 3.   Pheromone-sensitive sensilla in bark beetles. (a) Antenna of a *Dendroctonus frontalis* female; the end of the flagellum forms a large club (Cl) which bears the pheromone-sensitive sensilla. (b) Detail of antennal club; long and short sensilla basiconica (SB) form sensory bands around the club. Some sensilla trichodea (T) are also seen. Both sensillum types are sensitive to bark beetle pheromones and host tree volatiles. From Payne *et al.* (1973), copyright 1973, Pergamon Press.

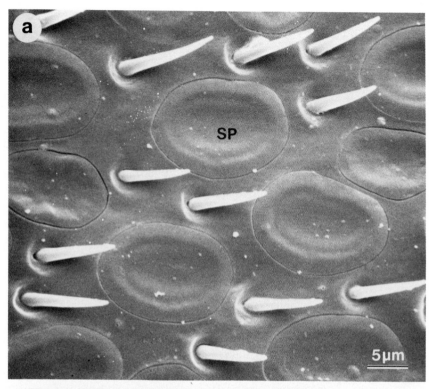

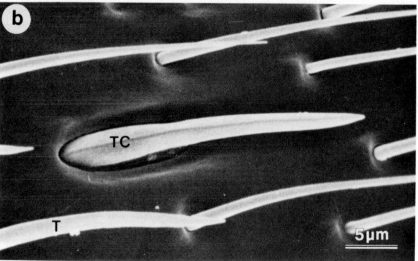

L3 is presumably the "cuticulin" layer of Locke (1966). L2 corresponds to the "outer epicuticle" as defined by Filshie (1970) and shows the same resistance to lipid solvents at room temperature; it therefore does not consist of ordinary wax. L1 may constitute the cement layer or its remnants and/or the remnants of the lipid-soluble wax layer (reviewed by Filshie, 1982).

The pore-covering L2 layer is also one of the reasons why narrow pores are usually not well demonstrated by scanning electron microscopy. Recently, however, Cuperus (1985) succeeded in obtaining very clear scanning electron micrographs of wall pores after boiling antennae of pupae in carbon tetrachloride shortly before emergence of the moth (Fig. 8). Pores of adult moths treated in the same way could not be imaged as clearly; apparently, the lipoid material inside the pores hardens in later life.

The inner end of the pore—the bottom of the pore kettle—is usually not more than 50 nm below the hair surface. This is the point where 3–30 *pore tubules* (depending on sensillum type and species) originate and traverse the rest of the hair wall. Often the thickness of the cuticle is locally reduced at the site of the pore tubules, so that they run in an extension of the hair lumen, the "liquor channel" (Figs. 9–12). The pore tubules have a dense wall and an electron-lucid core. Electron microscopy does not indicate that this core consists of material different from L2, but proof of the contrary is lacking as well. The appearance of the pore tubules depends on the preparation method, but the overall diameter is remarkably uniform (15–20 nm). The diameter of the electron-lucid core usually measures 10–15 μm. Similarities to the wax canal filaments of ordinary cuticle have been already recognized by Locke (1965). The length of the pore tubules depends mainly on the thickness of the cuticular hair, because pore tubules which protrude more than 200 nm beyond the inner surface of the hair wall are extremely rare (Steinbrecht, 1973; Keil, 1984a).

Although intermediate types were observed (Steinbrecht, 1973), two types of single-walled multiporous sensilla are usually quite distinct (Schneider and Steinbrecht, 1968): (a) the *sensilla basiconica* are fairly short, thin-walled pegs (length ~10–40 μm) with a high density of wall pores and many pore tubules per pore (20–100 pores/μm^2; 15–20 tubules/pore); the innervating dendrites divide

---

Fig. 4. Pheromone-sensitive sensilla of Hymenoptera. (a) Pore plates, sensilla placodea (SP), are especially numerous in the drone of the honeybee (*Apis mellifera*). Among general food odor receptors, they contain receptors for the female sex pheromone, queen substance, and for pheromones of the Nassanov gland. Scanning electron micrograph by courtesy of J. R. Walther. (b) A sensillum trichodeum curvatum (TC) is seen surrounded by sensilla trichodea (T) on the antenna of the ant, *Formica rufa*. The close relationship between sensilla trichodea curvata and sensilla placodea is not evident in this scanning electron micrograph, but see Figs. 11 and 12. In the ant *Lasius fuliginosus* receptors for the alarm pheromone undecane were identified in the sensilla trichodea curvata. From Walther (1981).

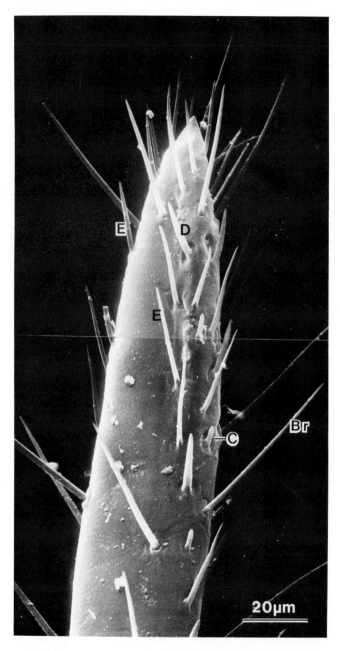

Fig. 5. Tip region of antenna of the bedbug, *Cimex lectularius*. Only in this region a very small number of presumed olfactory sensilla are found (types C, D, and E). Perception of the alarm pheromone was electrophysiologically proved for the sensilla trichodea, type E. The long bristles (Br) are mechanoreceptive. From Levinson *et al.* (1974), copyright 1974, Pergamon Press.

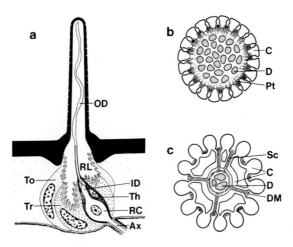

Fig. 6. General organization of insect olfactory sensilla. (a) As in sensilla serving other modalities, one or several bipolar sensory cells (RC) are surrounded by the thecogen (Th), trichogen (Tr), and tormogen cells (To). The axon (Ax) joins the antennal nerve and runs to the deutocerebrum in the brain; the dendrite is divided into an inner (ID) and outer dendritic segment (OD), which, surrounded by receptor lymph (RL), invades a cuticular hair with numerous pores. The site of stimulus transduction is the membrane of the outer dendritic segment. From Keil and Steinbrecht (1984). The two subtypes of multiporous sensilla are shown in cross section through the sensory hair; (b) single-walled sensillum basiconicum of *Necrophorus* with pore–tubule systems (Pt); (c) double-walled sensillum coeloconicum of *Locusta* with spoke–channel systems (Sc). C, Cuticle; D, dendrite; DM, dense material in spoke channels. From Steinbrecht (1969).

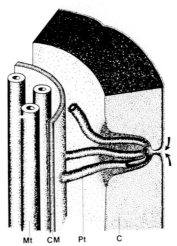

Fig. 7. Idealized drawing of pore–tubule system of a single-walled olfactory sensillum. Odor molecules are presumed to enter pores (arrows) in the cuticular wall (C), diffuse along the pore tubules (Pt), and reach the cell membrane (CM) either via direct contacts or via the receptor lymph. The electron-lucid material of L2 is drawn transparent. Mt, Microtubule. From Keil and Steinbrecht (1984).

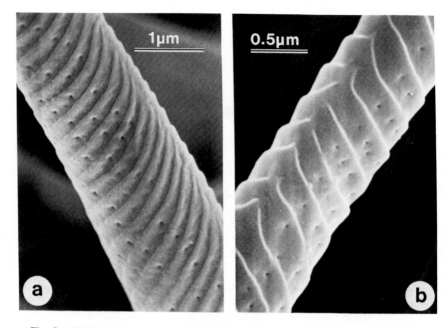

Fig. 8. High-resolution scanning electron micrographs of the wall pores in the pheromone-sensitive sensilla trichodea of male *Adoxophyes orana* (a) and *Yponomeuta vigintipunctatus* (b). Fewer pores were found in female sensilla trichodea in both species. From Cuperus (1985), copyright 1985, Pergamon Press.

into several branches. (b) In the *sensilla trichodea* (length 20–400 μm), the dendrites are essentially unbranched, and the hair wall is thicker but progressively tapers toward the tip; the density of pores and pore tubules is low (2–10 pores/μm^2; 3–6 tubules/pore). The functional significance of these differences is not yet understood. The fact that the highly sensitive sex pheromone receptors of moths have so far been found only in the sensilla trichodea is probably due to their larger size. A high density of pores and pore tubules obviously is not necessary for effective stimulus transport (Kaissling and Priesner, 1970).

The pore–tubule systems are part of the cuticle, constructed by the trichogen cell before the dendrites invade the hair lumen (Ernst, 1969, 1972). Therefore the dendrites will contact the pore tubules only secondarily. Such contacts are fairly common in basiconic sensilla, where many dendritic branches pass closely beneath the hair wall with its high density of pores and pore tubules (Myers, 1968; Steinbrecht, 1970b, 1973; for further references, see Keil, 1982). In sensilla trichodea, pore–tubule contacts were first observed by Steinbrecht and Müller (1971) after special fixation with an $OsO_4/K_2Cr_2O_7$ mixture. Keil (1982)

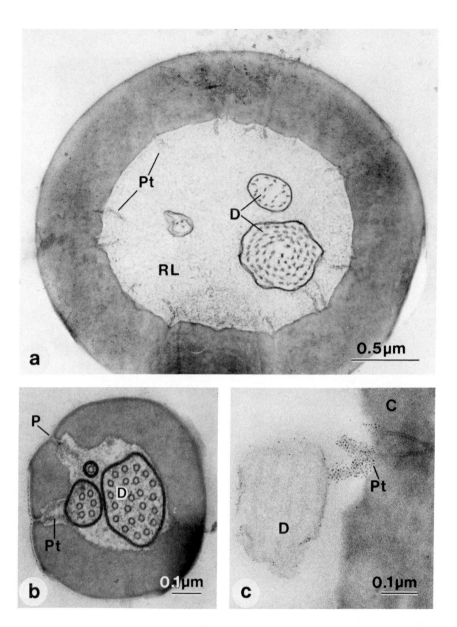

Fig. 9. Cross sections through sensory hairs of pheromone-sensitive sensilla trichodea of moths. (a) *Antheraea polyphemus*, freeze-substituted specimen. Pore tubules (Pt) penetrate the cuticular hair wall and protrude about 200 nm into the hair lumen; three of them appear to contact the largest of the three dendrites (D). RL, Receptor lymph. Micrograph courtesy of T. A. Keil. (b) *Spodoptera exempta*, tip region of freeze-substituted hair. Pore tubules (Pt) end in contact with dendrites (D); the dendrites contain microtubules in regular array. The small profile with only one microtubule is a short dendritic side branch. P, Pore. From Steinbrecht (1982). (c) *Antheraea polyphemus*, after introducing cationized ferritin (dense dots) into the hair lumen. The greatest density of ferritin is observed on the inner pore tubules (Pt); some ferritin has also bound to the membrane of the dendrite (D) but very little to the inner surface of the cuticle (C). From Keil (1984b).

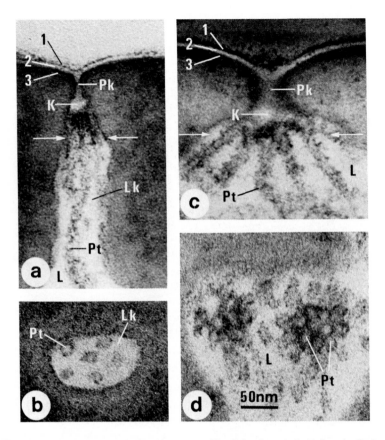

Fig. 10. Pore–tubule systems in olfactory sensilla of *Bombyx mori*. (a) Longitudinal section through pore of a long sensillum trichodeum; (b) cross section at level indicated by arrows in a; (c) longitudinal section through pore of sensillum basiconicum; (d) cross section through pore tubules of two neighboring pores at level indicated by arrows in c. The sensillar surface layers L1, L2, and L3 (1, 2, and 3) are evident in both sensillum types. Note the different diameter of the pore canal (Pk) and the different number of pore tubules (Pt) per pore in a and b and c and d, respectively. K, Pore kettle; L, receptor lymph; Lk, liquor channel. From Steinbrecht (1973).

improved the fixation by the addition of tannic acid to a glutaraldehyde fixative and by mechanically opening the hair lumen for better access of the medium. Surface coats on the pore tubules as well as on the dendrites have been demonstrated by various cationic markers and possibly play a role in establishing the contacts (see Fig. 9c) (Keil, 1984b).

Freeze-substitution, which preserves the fine structure of the dendrites better than the chemical fixatives, shows contacts between pore tubules and dendrites only in exceptional cases (Figs. 9a and 9b). In particular, the inner parts of the

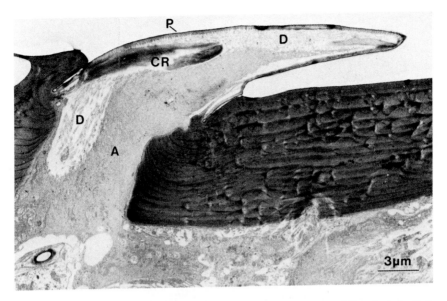

Fig. 11. Longitudinal section through sensillum trichodeum curvatum of *Formica rufa*. Only the upper cuticular wall is perforated by pores (P). This arrangement, the cuticular ridges (CR), and the location of the outermost auxiliary cell (A) underline the close relationship of this sensillum type to the pore plates of other Hymenoptera. D, Dendrites. From Walther (1981).

pore tubules are often lost; possibly they are not stable in the substitution medium (2% OsO$_4$ in acetone, Steinbrecht, 1980). In *Antheraea polyphemus*, however, after freeze-substitution in the same medium pore tubules protrude about 200 nm into the hair lumen (Keil, 1984a). Thus, the chemical nature of pore–tubules may be different in different species, as might be their outer and inner parts.

The only methods that completely avoid any chemical treatment are freeze-etching and cryosectioning. Unfortunately, with these techniques pore tubules have not yet been detected, possibly because of other preparation artifacts and a low signal to noise ratio (Steinbrecht, 1980; Steinbrecht and Zierold, 1984).

2. Stimulus Transport

Theoretically, five possible pathways of stimulus transport can be considered. These are "pore-less" transport, pore–tubule/receptor lymph transport, "pure" pore–tubule transport, and two types of multiple-hit pore finding.

a. Pore-Less Transport. In pore-less transport, the odor molecule diffuses through the cuticle of the hair wall right from the point of its impact. Once it has reached the lumen, it is conveyed to the dendritic membrane through the receptor lymph. In contrast to the following hypotheses (b)–(e), the molecule would have

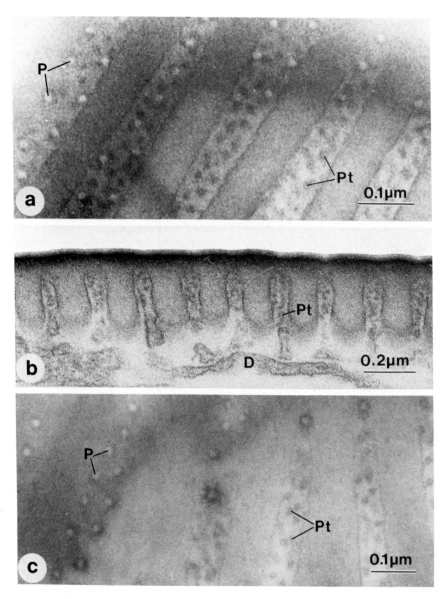

Fig. 12. The pore–tubule systems of the sensillum trichodeum curvatum of the ant *Formica rufa* [(a and b), from Walther (1981)] and of the sensillum placodeum of the honeybee, *Apis mellifera* [(c), from R. A. Steinbrecht (unpublished)], are almost identical. (a) and (c) show cross sections through pores (P) and pore tubules (Pt); (b) shows longitudinal section, with pore tubules contacting dendritic branches (D).

to traverse layer L3, the bulk of the cuticular wall, and then would have to get through the receptor lymph as discussed below in (b).

b. Pore–Tubule/Receptor Lymph Transport. Odor molecules impinging anywhere at the hair surface diffuse along the surface, e.g., in layer L2, to a pore and into a pore tubule. This could possibly take place in the same material which makes up the L2 layer. A phase shift, however, would be necessary at the end of the pore tubule unless this is in contact with the dendritic membrane. The partition coefficient between the two phases, which would be very unfavorable if the receptor lymph consisted of pure water, might be improved by the presence of proteins and proteoglycans in the receptor lymph. Moreover, proteins might bind to the stimulus molecule and function as carriers (see below).

c. Pure Pore–Tubule Transport. As in (b) transport proceeds along the surface of the hair to a pore and into a pore tubule. If this pore tubule would end blind, diffusion would carry on, back to the surface, to enter another pore tubule until eventually one is reached which contacts the dendritic membrane. Thus, the entire transport process could proceed by two- and one-dimensional diffusion, possibly even in a single phase.

d and e. Multiple-Hit Pore Finding. The multiple-hit pore finding models are essentially like (b) and (c), with the only exception that the pore is not reached by surface diffusion but by repeated impact and reflection at the hair surface. Once a pore has been encountered, transport would proceed as in (b) or (c), respectively.

Unfortunately, data which would allow selection of one of these proposals and definitely reject the others are not yet available. Not even the assumption of pore-less transport (a) can be ruled out, although it is less attractive because it disregards the morphological observation of the wall pores, which are well developed only in olfactory sensilla (Steinbrecht, 1984). Moreover, the cuticle below L3, like most arthropod exocuticles, is probably hydrophilic (Neville, 1975).

The multiple-hit models (Boeckh *et al.*, 1965; Futrelle, 1984) do not conform with the low overall desorption measured by Kanaujia and Kaissling (1985), unless the material in the pores is totally different from the rest of the hair surface and works as a molecule trap.

Direct tracing of the path of odor molecules with the required high spatial and temporal resolution and sensitivity, e.g., by autoradiographical methods, so far has not been possible. Indirect argumentation compares the latency of the first observable receptor response with the calculated transport time of a given hypothesis. Due to unknown material constants such calculations, of course, can be done only in a very crude way. Also data on the inactivation of pheromone molecules might help to give more insight into the transport process, as discussed below.

Exposing the antennae of *B. mori* to air puffs with radioactive bombykol and separating the sensory hairs from the antennal branches after different incubation times revealed a transport of radioactivity from the hairs to the branches at a rate consistent with a diffusion coefficient of $\geqq 5 \times 10^{-7}$ cm^2/sec (Steinbrecht and Kasang, 1972). Kanaujia and Kaissling (1985) repeated these experiments with *A. polyphemus* and observed the same phenomenon. Although owing to the longer sensory hairs the half-time of the transport is much longer, the diffusion coefficient is almost identical (3×10^{-7} cm^2/sec). Dried antennae showed a somewhat faster transport than fresh ones. If these diffusion constants are taken for the diffusion along the hair surface and the pore tubules (which is reasonable but not cogent), the transport time can be calculated from the morphometric data (Steinbrecht, 1973; (Keil, 1984a), according to the formulae of Adam and Delbrück (1968). In *Bombyx,* the end of a pore tubule could be reached in less than 10 msec after the impact on the hair surface (Steinbrecht, 1973). The first electrophysiological events, however, take 50–500 msec at receptor threshold (Kaissling and Priesner, 1970; Kaissling, 1974). Thus. there is ample time for a slower transport process and hardly a chance to rule out on velocity reasons any of the transport models as stated above.

Biochemical studies may give additional insight into the stimulus transport process. A pheromone-binding protein and an esterase were discovered in the receptor lymph of *A. polyphemus* (Vogt and Riddiford, 1981). Originally both were assumed to take part in the poststimulus pheromone inactivation. Later, Vogt *et al.* (1985) observed that the purified sensillar esterase *in vitro* had such a high turnover rate that the binding protein need not be involved in inactivation. Therefore, the binding protein was proposed to act as a carrier, transporting hydrophobic pheromone molecules across the aqueous receptor-lymph space from pore tubule to dendrite, at the same time protecting them from the highly active esterase (see also Vogt, Chapter 12, this volume). In intact antennae, however, the metabolism of pheromone is very slow (half-life ~3 min; Kasang and Kaissling, 1972; Kasang, 1973). Therefore, the role of the pheromone-binding protein and of the sensillar esterase *in vivo* still has to be clarified. A model of stimulus transport and inactivation which is consistent with all available data has been proposed by Kaissling (1986a,b). This model favors transport via pore tubules contacting the dendrites [possibility (c)] and ascribes to the binding protein the primary, rapid pheromone inactivation and to the esterase its subsequent enzymatic degradation.

B.   Spoke–Channel Systems

In the double-walled multiporous sensilla which have spoke–channel systems for stimulus conduction, pore tubules do not play a role in the transport pathway, but the principles of surface diffusion may apply here at least in part (Steinbrecht and Müller, 1976). It is provocative that so far no pheromone receptor has been observed which is associated with a double-walled sensillum. The number of unequivocally identified pheromone receptive sensilla with known fine structure, however, is still very small. If double-walled pheromone sensilla would be found, it would be very interesting to find out whether the stimulating pheromone molecules would be much different in their physicochemical properties from the pheromones for sensilla with pore–tubule systems.

IV. CELLULAR ORGANIZATION—IMPLICATIONS FOR ELECTROPHYSIOLOGY AND BIOCHEMISTRY

It has long been known that even sensilla serving different modalities are remarkably uniform in their cellular organization; conspicuous modality-specific specializations are restricted to the outer dendritic segments and the cuticular apparatus. However, this does not mean that the equivalent electrical network of different sensillum types necessarily is uniform too. More probably, combined fine structural and electrophysiological studies will reveal subtle but functionally important modifications also in the cellular organization of the various sensillar forms.

A. Receptor Cells

As shown schematically in Fig. 6a, the sensory process of the receptor cell is divided by a ciliary segment into an outer segment surrounded by receptor lymph and an inner segment surrounded by enveloping auxiliary cells. By experiments with local stimulation and adaptation it has been shown that the stimulus-transduction process of olfactory sensilla takes place at the membrane of the outer dendritic segment (Zack Strausfeld and Kaissling, 1986). Morphological methods, so far, are too unspecific to reveal specific features of this membrane. A high protein content is indicated by a high density of intramembrane particles in a freeze-fracture replica (Steinbrecht, 1980). Negatively stained vesicles of isolated dendritic membrane also show a particulate substructure (Klein and Keil, 1984). Various lectins bind differently to the dendritic membrane and the pore tubules, indicating differences between the cellular glycocalyx and the surface of the pore tubules (Keil, 1986).

The outer segment contains no cytoplasmic organelles except microtubules and occasionally smooth vesicles and filaments. The lack of mitochondria in the outer segment imposes the problem that a distance of up to 400 μm has to be bridged between the sites of oxidative phosphorylation and the site of the primary stimulus action. Of the possible linking mechanisms, flow of chemical energy (e.g., ATP), ions, or of a still unknown signal, Thurm (1974) favors the notion of an ionic flow, generating the action potentials in the proximal parts of the receptor. This conforms with the old electrophysiological hypothesis that action potentials are not generated in the outer segment but proximal to the ciliary region (see De Kramer and Hemberger, Chapter 13, this volume). Some more recent electrophysiological studies in mechanoreceptive and olfactory sensilla, however, argue in favor of spike generation in the outer segments (Erler and Thurm, 1981; Seyfarth *et al.*, 1982; De Kramer *et al.*, 1984; De Kramer, 1985; Oldfield and Hill, 1986; see also De Kramer and Hemberger, Chapter 13).

In the sex pheromone sensilla of *B. mori* two receptor cells are found, each responding with a characteristic spike amplitude to one of the two pheromone components, bombykol and bombykal (Kaissling *et al.*, 1978). The difference in the spike amplitude can be related to a pronounced diameter difference of the outer dendritic segments, but also the inner segments, the cell somata, and even the initial part of the axons show differences in diameter, though to a lesser degree (see Fig. 13) (Steinbrecht, 1973; Steinbrecht and Gnatzy, 1984; Gnatzy *et al.*, 1984). A similar situation prevails in *A. pernyi* and *A. polyphemus,* but here sometimes a third receptor cell is found, which has a thin dendrite like the second cell; in this case large spikes could be recorded from one unit, and small spikes from two units (electrophysiology; Kaissling, 1979; morphometry: Gnatzy *et al.*, 1984; Keil, 1984a).

Many Lepidoptera use multicomponent pheromones, and a higher number of specific receptor cells is found by single cell recording, e.g., five different receptor cells in *Choristoneura fumiferana* (Priesner, 1979b), four in *Panolis flammea* (Priesner and Schroth, 1983), and five in *Adoxophyes orana* (Priesner, 1983). In the electron microscope, however, never more than three receptor cells were found associated with a single sensillum trichodeum of these species (Den Otter *et al.*, 1978; R. A. Steinbrecht, unpublished); only the dendrites sometimes bifurcate. In these species, therefore, not all the sensilla trichodea of an antenna are functionally identical as in *Bombyx.* Hansson and co-workers (1986) report that in *Agrotis exclamationis* different pheromone components are perceived by sensillum types which differ not only in their morphology but also in their spatial localization on the antenna.

B. Auxiliary Cells

The three auxiliary cells of insect sensilla serve a well-known ontogenetic function, the construction of the cuticular apparatus. The tormogen cell forms the basal socket of the sensillum, the trichogen cell the cuticular hair, and the thecogen cell the dendrite sheath (Ernst, 1969, 1972; Sanes and Hildebrand, 1976b; for review, see Keil and Steinbrecht, 1984).

Beside their ontogenetic function, the auxiliary cells connect the receptor cells to the epidermis so that the epithelial organization is maintained. Septate junctions seal the intercellular clefts between all cells so that the transepithelial resistance is high. In pheromone-sensitive sensilla of moths, but not in mechanoreceptors of crickets and flies, septate junctions are also observed where the axon originates and the thecogen cell borders the glia cell around the axon (Keil and Steinbrecht, 1983, 1987; Steinbrecht and Gnatzy, 1984). A very close contact between the tormogen cell and the cuticle of the hair base is the morphological correlate of a high electrical resistance between neighboring sensilla (Keil, 1984c).

In sensilla trichodea of *B. mori, A. pernyi,* and *A. polyphemus* only the innermost auxiliary cell, the thecogen cell, forms a complete envelope around the inner dendritic segment and the receptor cell somata (Fig. 13). Wherever the thecogen cell contacts the receptor cell, a specialized junction of hitherto unknown function is observed in *Bombyx* after cryofixation (Steinbrecht, 1980).

Another important feature of the auxiliary cells is their apparent resemblance to the cells of ion-transporting epithelia (Fig. 14), e.g., in insect midgut and salivary glands (Harvey, 1980). Their elaborately folded apical membranes are thought to be the site of an electrogenic cation pump, which mainly pumps potassium into the receptor lymph and thereby creates a transepithelial voltage. This voltage is supposed to amplify the receptor potential (Thurm and Küppers, 1980). In *Bombyx mori* the transepithelial voltage amounts to 33 mV (Thurm and Wessel, 1979), but its influence on receptor function is still uncertain (see De Kramer and Hemberger, Chapter 13, this volume).

A characteristic feature of these electrogenic cation pumps are the so-called portasomes, particles of 9 nm diameter on the cytoplasmic face of the apical membrane which contain a K^+-ATPase (Harvey, 1980; Wieczorek, 1982). The portasomes are similar in size and arrangement to the F_1 particles of mitochondria and possibly work in an analogous way (Harvey *et al.,* 1981). Both can be observed in ultrathin sections of cryofixed silkmoth antennae (Steinbrecht, 1986). In sensilla trichodea of *B. mori,* only the trichogen cell bears portasomes (Fig. 14); it forms a deeply invaginated pouch, the surface of which is 380 times larger than a smooth and plain apical surface (Steinbrecht and Gnatzy, 1984; Gnatzy *et al.,* 1984).

A high potassium content of about 200 mM has been measured in isolated receptor lymph (Kaissling and Thorson, 1980) and also *in situ* by X-ray microanalysis of ultrathin cryosections (Steinbrecht and Zierold, 1982, 1985, 1987). The latter method allows the quantitative analysis of electrolyte elements at the resolution of the electron microscope, and preliminary data indicate that changes in the electrolyte concentrations due to stimulation of the receptors can be monitored (Kaissling and Thorson, 1980; Steinbrecht and Zierold, 1985; R. A. Steinbrecht and K. Zierold, unpublished results).

Attempts to assign electrophysiologically recorded features to defined sensillar structures have been made by a morphometric analysis in silkmoths (Gnatzy *et*

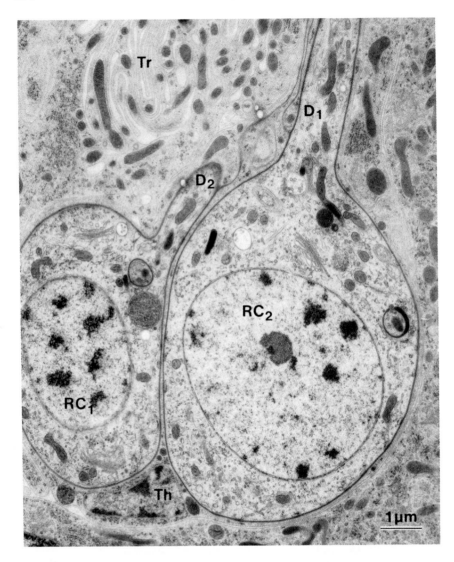

Fig. 13. *Bombyx mori,* the two receptor cells of a long sensillum trichodeum in longitudinal section (freeze-substituted specimen). The larger receptor cell (RC$_2$) responds to bombykol, the smaller one (RC$_1$) to bombykal. The dendrites (D$_1$ and D$_2$) differ in diameter too. The thecogen cell (Th) forms a very thin leaflet in between and around the receptor cells. Some lamellae of the trichogen cell (Tr) are also seen. From Steinbrecht (1980).

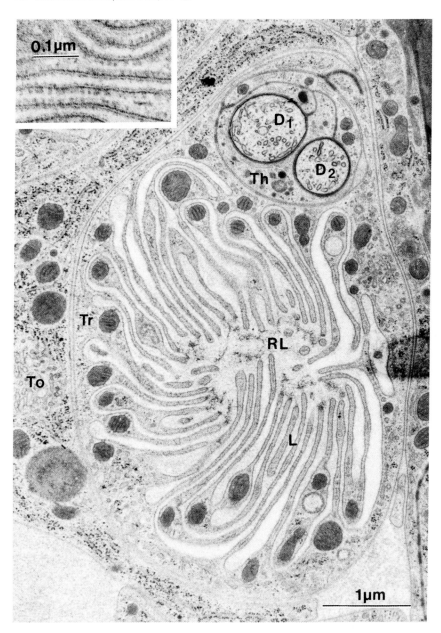

Fig. 14. *Bombyx mori,* cross section through the two inner dendritic segments (D_1 and D_2) of a sensillum trichodeum surrounded by thecogen (Th), trichogen (Tr), and, partly, by tormogen cells (To). At this level the trichogen cell forms a deeply invaginated pouch, bordered by an extensively lamellated (L) apical membrane and filled with receptor lymph (RL). The membranes of the lamellae are studded with portasomes (inset). (Freeze-substituted specimen; see also Steinbrecht and Gnatzy, 1984.)

al., 1984). Thus, the highly folded apical membrane of both the trichogen and the tormogen cell, which measures about 3000 μm^2, is the most likely candidate for the considerable capacitance of 30 pF (picofarads) observed in these sensilla (De Kramer, 1985). In addition, it was found that this membrane has the extremely high specific resistance of the order of 10^4 Ω cm^2 which is 10- to 100-fold higher than the specific resistance of the basolateral membrane of these cells (De Kramer and Hemberger, Chapter 13, this volume).

The tormogen and trichogen cells of *Bombyx* and *Antheraea* show a well-developed rough endoplasmic reticulum and numerous Golgi complexes, features indicating a high rate of protein synthesis. Coated pits are common on the apical cell membrane and to a lesser extent also on the basolateral membrane. This indicates an extensive transport of macromolecules across these cells (Steinbrecht and Gnatzy, 1984; T. A. Keil, personal communication). It is therefore tempting to speculate that there might be a continuous turnover of the proteins of the receptor lymph throughout the adult life. Autoradiographic studies are presently under way to follow this process more in detail (R. A. Steinbrecht, unpublished). A secretory role was established for the auxiliary cells of a gustatory sensillum in the blowfly, using horseradish peroxidase as a tracer (Phillips and Vande Berg, 1976).

V. SUPPLEMENTARY AND CONCLUDING REMARKS

A. Pheromone Sensilla in Other Arthropod Classes

Only few papers deal with the fine structure of sensilla in arthropod classes other than insects. Concomitant studies on their function are even more scanty (for review, see Altner and Prillinger, 1980; Steinbrecht, 1984). Pheromone-sensitive sensilla with identified function occur among the sensilla of Haller's organ on the tarsus of ticks (electron microscopy: Foelix and Axtell, 1972; Hess and Vlimant, 1982; Waladde, 1982; electrophysiology: Haggart and Davis, 1981; Waladde, 1982; see also Sonenshine, Chapter 9, this volume). In the marine crab, *Hymenocera picta,* the aesthetasc hairs on the antennules are responsible for recognition of conspecifics, their sex, sexual readiness, and even individuals, as shown by amputation experiments. The aesthetascs have a very thin, poreless wall and contain hundreds of dendrites (Wasserthal and Seibt, 1976). A complex sensory organ is the apical sensory cone of the isopod, *Hemilepistus reaumuri,* which contains mechano- and chemoreceptors, probably also for pheromones of conspecific individuals (Seelinger, 1977).

B. Central Pathway of Pheromone Messages

Most studies so far have been undertaken in the moths *Manduca sexta* and *Antheraea polyphemus,* and in the cockroach *Periplaneta americana* (for review, see Hildebrand *et al.*, 1980; Boeckh *et al.*, 1984). In these species, the sexual dimorphism of the antennae is continued at the next higher level in the brain, the deutocerebrum. Only the males possess a macroglomerular complex, where pheromone-sensitive second-order neurons are connected to the primary axons of the pheromone receptors. Possibly, the vital pheromone message is processed along a "labeled line" in a way different from general olfactory fibers which are interconnected in the numerous smaller glomeruli present in both sexes.

C. Future Prospects

Several lines of research appear promising for functional morphology of pheromone-sensitive sensilla. First, work on functionally identified pheromone receptor cells in very different insect orders and arthropod classes could provide more insight from the aspect of comparative anatomy. Second, developing and applying more sophisticated methods to the question of stimulus transport will be a challenge to the cell biologist, the electrophysiologist, and the biochemist likewise. Third, specific markers such as lectins and/or antibodies could help to find out special characteristics of the dendritic receptor membrane in relation to other nonreceptor cell membranes. Last but not least, the cell biology of the sensillum complex should be studied in more detail to find out the functional interdependence of sensillar receptor and auxiliary cells. Here, again, a joint venture of electrophysiologists and morphologists is desirable, so that the electric equivalent circuitry of sensilla can be established with greater fidelity. Cytochemical and microanalytical studies will help to accomplish this goal and provide the link between fine structural observations and biochemical data.

ACKNOWLEDGMENTS

My sincere thanks are due to Drs. P. Cuperus, T. A. Keil, T. Payne, J. R. Walther, and their publishers for the permission to use their excellent electron micrographs to illustrate this chapter. I also wish to thank Drs. J. J. De Kramer, K.-E. Kaissling, and T. A. Keil for critical reading of the manuscript, B. Müller for photographic artwork, and I. S. Rössel and G. Lamprecht for help in preparing the typescript.

REFERENCES

Adam, G., and Delbrück, M. (1968). Reduction of dimensionality in biological diffusion processes. *In* "Structural Chemistry and Molecular Biology" (A. Rich and N. Davidson, eds.), pp. 198–215. Freeman, San Francisco.

Altner, H., and Prillinger, L. (1980). Ultrastructure of invertebrate chemo-, thermo-, and hygroreceptors and its functional significance. *Int. Rev. Cytol.* **67,** 69–139.

Boeckh, J., Kaissling, K.-E., and Schneider, D. (1960). Sensillen und Bau der Antennengeissel von *Telea polyphemus*. *Zool. Jahrb. Abt. Anat. Ontog. Tiere* **78**, 559–584.

Boeckh, J., Kaissling, K.-E., and Schneider, D. (1965). Insect olfactory receptors. *Cold Spring Harbor Symp. Quant. Biol.* **30**, 263–280.

Boeckh, J., Ernst, K. D., Sass, H., and Waldow, U. (1984). Anatomical and physiological characteristics of individual neurones in the central antennal pathway of insects. *J. Insect Physiol.* **30**, 15–26.

Chapman, R. F. (1982). Chemoreception: The significance of receptor numbers. *Adv. Insect Physiol.* **16**, 247–356.

Cuperus, P. L. (1985). Inventory of pores in antennal sensilla of *Yponomeuta* spp. (Lepidoptera: Yponomeutidae) and *Adoxophyes orana* F.v.R. (Lepidoptera: Tortricidae). *Int. J. Insect Morphol. Embryol.* **14**, 347–359.

De Kramer, J. J. (1985). The electrical circuitry of an olfactory sensillum in *Antheraea polyphemus*. *J. Neurosci.* **5**, 2484–2493.

De Kramer, J. J., Kaissling, K.-E., and Keil, T. (1984). Passive electrical properties of insect olfactory sensilla may produce the biphasic shape of spikes. *Chem. Senses* **8**, 289–295.

Den Otter, C. J., Schuil, H. A., and Sander-Van Oosten, A. (1978). Reception of host-plant odours and female sex pheromone in *Adoxophyes orana* (Lepidoptera: Tortricidae): electrophysiology and morphology. *Entomol. Exp. Appl.* **24**, 370–378.

Dickens, J. C., and Payne, T. L. (1978). Structure and function of the sensilla on the antennal club of the southern pine beetle, *Dendroctonus frontalis* (Zimmermann) (Coleoptera: Scolytidae). *Int. J. Insect Morphol. Embryol.* **7**, 251–265.

Dumpert, K. (1972). Alarmstoffrezeptoren auf der Antenne von *Lasius fuliginosus* (Latr.) (Hymenoptera, Formicidae). *Z. Vergl. Physiol.* **76**, 403–425.

Esslen, J., and Kaissling, K.-E. (1976). Zahl und Verteilung antennaler Sensillen bei der Honigbiene (*Apis mellifera* L.). *Zoomorphologie* **83**, 227–251.

Erler, G., and Thurm, U. (1981). Dendritic impulse initiation in an epithelial sensory neuron. *J. Comp. Physiol.* **142**, 237–249.

Ernst, K.-D. (1969). Die Feinstruktur von Riechsensillen der Antenne des Aaskäfers *Necrophorus* (Coleoptera). *Z. Zellforsch. Mikrosk. Anat.* **94**, 72–102.

Ernst, K.-D. (1972). Die Ontogenie der basiconischen Riechsensillen auf der Antenne von *Necrophorus* (Coleoptera). *Z. Zellforsch. Mikrosk. Anat.* **129**, 217–236.

Filshie, B. K. (1970). The resistance of epicuticular components of an insect to extraction with lipid solvents. *Tiss. Cell* **2**, 181–190.

Filshie, B. K. (1982). Fine structure of the cuticle of insects and other arthropods. *In* "Insect Ultrastructure" (R. C. King and H. Akai, eds.), Vol. 1, pp. 281–312. Plenum, New York.

Foelix, R. F., and Axtell, R. C. (1972). Ultrastructure of Haller's organ in the tick *Amblyomma americanum* (L.). *Z. Zellforsch. Mikrosk. Anat.* **124**, 275–296.

Futrelle, R. P. (1984). How molecules get to their detectors. The physics of diffusion of insect pheromones. *Trends Neurosci.* **7**, 116–120.

Gnatzy, W., Mohren, W., and Steinbrecht, R. A. (1984). Pheromone receptors of *Bombyx mori* and *Antheraea pernyi*. II. Morphometric data. *Cell Tiss. Res.* **235**, 5–42.

Haggart, D. A., and Davis, E. E. (1981). Neurons sensitive to 2,6-dichlorophenol on the tarsi of the tick *Amblyomma americanum* (Acari: Ixodidae). *J. Med. Entomol.* **18**, 187–193.

Hallberg, E. (1979). The fine structure of the antennal sensilla of the pine saw fly *Neodiprion sertifer* (Insecta: Hymenoptera). *Protoplasma* **101**, 111–126.

Hansson, B. S., Hallberg, E., Löfstedt, C., and Löfqvist, J. (1986). Spatial arrangement of different types of pheromone-sensitive sensilla in a male moth. *Naturwissenschaften* **73**, 269–270.

Harvey, W. R. (1980). Water and ions in the gut. *In* "Insect Biology in the Future" (M. Locke and D. S. Smith, eds.), pp. 105–124. Academic Press, New York.

Harvey, W. R., Cioffi, M., and Wolfersberger, M. G. (1981). Portasomes as coupling factors in active ion transport and oxidative phosphorylation. *Am. Zool.* **21**, 775–791.

Hess, E., and Vlimant, M. (1982). The tarsal sensory system of *Amblyomma variegatum* Fabricius (Ixodidae, Metastriata) I. Wall pore and terminal pore sensilla. *Rev. Suisse Zool.* **89**, 713–729.

Hildebrand, J. G., Matsumoto, S. G., Camazine, S. M., Tolbert, L. P., Blank, S., Ferguson, H., and Ecker, V. (1980). Organization and physiology of antennal centres in the brain of the moth *Manduca sexta. In* "Insect Neurobiology and Pesticide Action" (F. E. Rickett, ed.), pp. 376–382. Soc. Chem. Industry, London.

Kaissling, K.-E. (1971). Insect olfaction. *In* "Handbook of Sensory Physiology" (L. M. Beidler, ed.), Vol. 4, pp. 351–431. Springer-Verlag, Berlin, Heidelberg, and New York.

Kaissling, K.-E. (1974). Sensory transduction in insect olfactory receptors. *In* "Biochemistry of Sensory Functions" (L. Jaenicke, ed.), pp. 243–273. Springer-Verlag, Berlin, Heidelberg, and New York.

Kaissling, K.-E. (1979). Recognition of pheromones by moths, especially in saturniids and *Bombyx mori. In* "Chemical Ecology: Odour Communication in Animals" (F. J. Ritter, ed.), pp. 43–56. Elsevier/North-Holland, Amsterdam.

Kaissling, K.-E. (1986a). Chemo-electrical transduction in insect olfactory receptors. *Annu. Rev. Neurosci.* **9**, 121–145.

Kaissling, K.-E. (1986b). Transduction processes in olfactory receptors of moths. *In* "Molecular Entomology" (J. Law, ed.), UCLA Symposia on Molecular and Cellular Biology, New Series, Vol. 49, pp. 1–11. Alan R. Liss, New York.

Kaissling, K.-E., and Priesner, E. (1970). Die Riechschwelle des Seidenspinners. *Naturwissenschaften* **57**, 23–28.

Kaissling, K.-E., and Renner, M. (1968). Antennale Rezeptoren für Queen Substance und Sterzelduft bei der Honigbiene. *Z. Vergl. Physiol.* **59**, 357–361.

Kaissling, K.-E., and Thorson, J. (1980). Insect olfactory sensilla: Structural, chemical and electrical aspects of the functional organization. *In* "Receptors for Neurotransmitters, Hormones and Pheromones in Insects" (D. B. Sattelle, L. M. Hall, and J. G. Hildebrand, eds.), pp. 261–282. Elsevier/North-Holland, Amsterdam.

Kaissling, K.-E., Kasang, G., Bestmann, H. J., Stransky, W., and Vostrowsky, O. (1978). A new pheromone of the silkworm moth *Bombyx mori.* Sensory pathway and behavioral effect. *Naturwissenschaften* **65**, 382–384.

Kanaujia, S., and Kaissling, K.-E. (1985). Interactions of pheromone with moth antennae: Adsorption, desorption and transport. *J. Insect Physiol.* **31**, 71–81.

Kasang, G. (1973). Physikochemische Vorgänge beim Riechen des Seidenspinners. *Naturwissenschaften* **60**, 59–101.

Kasang, G., and Kaissling, K.-E. (1972). Specificity of primary and secondary olfactory processes in *Bombyx* antennae. *In* "Olfaction and Taste IV" (D. Schneider, ed.), pp. 200–206. Wiss. Verlagsgesellschaft, Stuttgart.

Keil, T. (1982). Contacts of pore tubules and sensory dendrites in antennal chemosensilla of a silkmoth: Demonstration of a possible pathway for olfactory molecules. *Tiss. Cell* **14**, 451–462.

Keil, T. A. (1984a). Reconstruction and morphometry of silkmoth olfactory hairs: A comparative study of sensilla trichodea on the antennae of male *Antheraea polyphemus* and *Antheraea pernyi* (Insecta, Lepidoptera). *Zoomorphology* **104**, 147–156.

Keil, T. A. (1984b). Surface coats of pore tubules and olfactory sensory dendrites of a silkmoth revealed by cationic markers. *Tiss. Cell* **16**, 705–717.

Keil, T. A. (1984c). Very tight contact of tormogen cell membrane and sensillum cuticle: Ultrastructural basis for high electrical resistance between receptor-lymph and subcuticular spaces in silkmoth olfactory hairs. *Tiss. Cell* **16**, 131–135.

Keil, T. A. (1986). Lectinbindungsstudien an olfaktorischen Sensillen des Seidenspinners *Antheraea polyphemus*. *Verh. Dtsch. Zool. Ges.* **79**, 219.

Keil, T. A., and Steinbrecht, R. A. (1983). Beziehungen zwischen Sinnes-, Hüll- und Gliazellen in epidermalen Mechano- und Chemorezeptoren von Insekten. *Verh. Dtsch. Zool. Ges.* **76**, 294.

Keil, T. A., and Steinbrecht, R. A. (1984). Mechanosensitive and olfactory sensilla of insects. *In* "Insect Ultrastructure" (R. C. King and H. Akai, eds.), Vol. 2, pp. 477–516. Plenum, New York.

Keil, T. A., and Steinbrecht, R. A. (1987). Diffusion barriers in silkmoth sensory epithelia: Application of lanthanum tracer to olfactory sensilla of *Antheraea polyphemus* and *Bombyx mori*. *Tissue Cell* **19**, 119–134.

Klein, U., and Keil, T. A. (1984). Dendritic membrane from insect olfactory hairs: Isolation method and electron microscopical observations. *Cell. Mol. Neurobiol.* **4**, 385–396.

Levinson, H. Z., Levinson, A. R., Müller, B., and Steinbrecht, R. A. (1974). Structure of sensilla, olfactory perception and behaviour of the bedbug, *Cimex lectularius*, in response to its alarm pheromone. *J. Insect Physiol.* **20**, 1231–1248.

Locke, M. (1965). Permeability of insect cuticle to water and lipids. *Science* **147**, 295–298.

Locke, M. (1966). The structure and formation of the cuticulin layer in the epicuticle of an insect, *Calpodes ethlius* (Lepidoptera, Hesperiidae). *J. Morphol.* **118**, 461–494.

Mankin, R. W., and Mayer, M. S. (1984). The insect antenna is not a molecular sieve. *Experientia* **40**, 1251–1252.

Mayer, M. S., Mankin, R. W., and Carlysle, T. C. (1981). External antennal morphometry of *Trichoplusia ni* (Hübner) (Lepidoptera: Noctuidae). *Int. J. Insect Morphol. Embryol.* **10**, 185–201.

Meinecke, C.-C. (1975). Riechsensillen und Systematik der Lamellicornia (Insecta, Coleoptera). *Zoomorphologie* **82**, 1–42.

Myers, J. (1968). The structure of the antennae of the florida queen butterfly, *Danaus gilippus berenice* (Cramer). *J. Morphol.* **125**, 315–328.

Neville, A. C. (1975). "Biology of the Arthropod Cuticle." Springer-Verlag, Berlin, Heidelberg, and New York.

Oldfield, B. P., and Hill, K. G. (1986). Functional organization of insect auditory sensilla. *J. Comp. Physiol. A* **158**, 27–34.

Payne, T. L., Moeck, H. A., Willson, C. D., Coulson, R. N., and Humphreys, W. J. (1973). Bark beetle olfaction—II. Antennal morphology of sixteen species of Scolytidae (Coleoptera). *Int. J. Insect Morphol. Embryol.* **2**, 177–192.

Phillips, C. E., and Vande Berg, J. S. (1976). Mechanism for sensillum fluid flow in trichogen and tormogen cells of *Phormia regina* (Meigen) (Diptera: Calliphoridae). *Int. J. Insect Morphol. Embryol.* **5**, 423–431.

Priesner, E. (1979a). Progress in the analysis of pheromone receptor systems. *Ann. Zool. Ecol. Anim.* **11**, 533–546.

Priesner, E. (1979b). Specificity studies on pheromone receptors of noctuid and tortricid Lepidoptera. *In* "Chemical Ecology: Odour Communication in Animals" (F. J. Ritter, ed.), pp. 57–71. Elsevier/North-Holland, Amsterdam.

Priesner, E. (1983). Receptors for di-unsaturated pheromone analogues in the male summerfruit tortrix moth. *Z. Naturforsch.* **38C**, 874–877.

Priesner, E., and Schroth, M. (1983). Supplementary data on the sex attractant system of *Panolis flammea*. *Z. Naturforsch.* **38C**, 870–873.

Sanes, J. R., and Hildebrand, J. G. (1976a). Structure and development of antennae in a moth, *Manduca sexta*. *Dev. Biol.* **51**, 282–299.

Sanes, J. R., and Hildebrand, J. G. (1976b). Origin and morphogenesis of sensory neurons in an insect antenna. *Dev. Biol.* **51**, 300–319.

Sass, H. (1983). Production, release and effectiveness of two female sex pheromone components of *Periplaneta americana*. *J. Comp. Physiol.* **152**, 309–317.

Schaller, D. (1978). Antennal sensory system of *Periplaneta americana* L. *Cell Tiss. Res.* **191**, 121–139.

Schneider, D. (1984a). Insect olfaction—Our research endeavor. *In* "Foundations of Sensory Science" (W. W. Dawson and J. M. Enoch, eds.), pp. 381–418. Springer-Verlag, Berlin, Heidelberg, and New York.

Schneider, D. (1984b). Pheromone biology in the Lepidoptera: Overview, some recent findings and some generalizations. *In* "Comparative Physiology of Sensory Systems" (L. Bolis, R. D. Keynes, and S. H. P. Maddrell, eds.), pp. 301–313. Cambridge Univ. Press, Cambridge.

Schneider, D., and Steinbrecht, R. A. (1968). Checklist of insect olfactory sensilla. *Symp. Zool. Soc. London* **23**, 279–297.

Seelinger, G. (1977). Der Antennenendzapfen der tunesischen Wüstenassel *Hemilepistus reaumuri*, ein komplexes Sinnesorgan (Crustacea, Isopoda). *J. Comp. Physiol.* **113**, 95–103.

Seyfarth, E.-A., Bohnenberger, J., and Thorson, J. (1982). Electrical and mechanical stimulation of a spider slit sensillum: Outward current excites. *J. Comp. Physiol.* **147**, 423–432.

Steinbrecht, R. A. (1969). Comparative morphology of olfactory receptors. *In* "Olfaction and Taste III" (C. Pfaffmann, ed.), pp. 3–21. Rockefeller Univ. Press, New York.

Steinbrecht, R. A. (1970a). Zur Morphometrie der Antenne des Seidenspinners *Bombyx mori* L.: Zahl und Verteilung der Riechsensillen (Insecta, Lepidoptera). *Z. Morph. Tiere* **68**, 93–126.

Steinbrecht, R. A. (1970b). Stimulus transfering tubules in insect olfactory receptors. *Proc. 7th Int. Congr. Electron Microsc., Grenoble 1970*, 947–948.

Steinbrecht, R. A. (1973). Der Feinbau olfaktorischer Sensillen des Seidenspinners (Insecta, Lepidoptera): Rezeptorfortsätze und reizleitender Apparat. *Z. Zellforsch. Mikrosk. Anat.* **139**, 533–565.

Steinbrecht, R. A. (1980). Cryofixation without cryoprotectants. Freeze substitution and freeze etching of an insect olfactory receptor. *Tiss. Cell* **12**, 73–100.

Steinbrecht, R. A. (1982). Electrophysiological assay of synthetic and natural sex pheromones in the African armyworm moth, *Spodoptera exempta*. *Entomol. Exp. Appl.* **32**, 13–22.

Steinbrecht, R. A. (1984). Arthropoda: Chemo-, thermo-, and hygroreceptors. *In* "Biology of the Integument" (J. Bereiter-Hahn, A. G. Matoltsy, and K. S. Richards, eds.), Vol. 1, pp. 523–553. Springer-Verlag, Berlin, Heidelberg, and New York.

Steinbrecht, R. A. (1986). ATPase particles (portasomes) on mitochondrial cristae and the plasma membrane of an insect as demonstrated by freeze substitution. *Naturwissenschaften* **73**, 275–276.

Steinbrecht, R. A., and Gnatzy, W. (1984). Pheromone receptors of *Bombyx mori* and *Antheraea pernyi*. I. Reconstruction of the cellular organization of the sensilla trichodea. *Cell Tiss. Res.* **235**, 25–34.

Steinbrecht, R. A., and Kasang, G. (1972). Capture and conveyance of odour molecules in an insect olfactory receptor. *In* "Olfaction and Taste IV" (D. Schneider, ed.), pp. 193–199. Wiss. Verlagsgesellschaft, Stuttgart.

Steinbrecht, R. A., and Müller, B. (1971). On the stimulus conducting structures in insect olfactory receptors. *Z. Zellforsch. Mikrosk. Anat.* **117**, 570–575.

Steinbrecht, R. A., and Müller, B. (1976). Fine structure of the antennal receptors of the bedbug, *Cimex lectularius* L. *Tiss. Cell* **8**, 615–636.

Steinbrecht, R. A., and Zierold, K. (1982). Cryo-embedding of small frozen specimens for cryo-ultramicrotomy. *Proc. 10th Int. Congr. Electron Microsc., Hamburg 1982* **3**, 183–184.

Steinbrecht, R. A., and Zierold, K. (1984). A cryoembedding method for cutting ultrathin cryosections from small frozen specimens. *J. Microscopy (Oxford)* **136**, 69–75.

Steinbrecht, R. A., and Zierold, K. (1985). X-Ray microanalysis of electrolytes in cryosections of an insect olfactory sensillum. *Eur. J. Cell Biol. Suppl.* **10,** 69.

Steinbrecht, R. A., and Zierold, K. (1987). The electrolyte distribution in insect olfactory sensilla as revealed by X-ray microanalysis. *In* "Olfaction and Taste IX" (S. Roper and Y. Atema, eds.). New York Academy of Sciences, New York (in press).

Thurm, U. (1974). Mechanisms of electrical membrane responses in sensory receptors, illustrated by mechanoreceptors. *In* "Biochemistry of Sensory Functions" (L. Jaenicke, ed.), pp. 367–390. Springer-Verlag, Berlin, Heidelberg, and New York.

Thurm, U., and Küppers, J. (1980). Epithelial physiology of insect sensilla. *In* "Insect Biology in the Future" (M. Locke and D. S. Smith, eds.), pp. 735–763. Academic Press, New York.

Thurm, U. and Wessel, G. (1979). Metabolism-dependent transepithelial potential differences at epidermal receptors of Arthropods. I. Comparative data. *J. Comp. Physiol.* **134,** 119–130.

Tiemann, D. L. (1967). Observations on the natural history of the western banded glowworm *Zarhipis integripennis* (LeConte) (Coleoptera: Phengodidae). *Proc. Calif. Acad. Sci.* **35,** 235–264.

Vareschi, E. (1971). Duftunterscheidung bei der Honigbiene—Einzelzell-Ableitung und Verhaltensreaktionen. *Z. Vergl. Physiol.* **75,** 143–173.

Vogel, S. (1983). How much air passes through a silkmoth's antenna? *J. Insect Physiol.* **29,** 597–602.

Vogt, R. G., and Riddiford, L. M. (1981). Pheromone binding and inactivation by moth antennae. *Nature (London)* **293,** 161–163.

Vogt, R. G., Riddiford, L. M., and Prestwich, G. D. (1985). Kinetic properties of a pheromone degrading enzyme: The sensillar esterase of *Antheraea polyphemus. Proc. Natl. Acad. Sci. U.S.A.* **82,** 8827–8831.

Waladde, S. M. (1982). Tip-recording from ixodid tick olfactory sensilla: Responses to tick related odours. *J. Comp. Physiol.* **148,** 411–418.

Walther, J. R. (1979). Vergleichende morphologische Betrachtung der antennalen Sensillenfelder einiger ausgewählter Aculeata (Insecta, Hymenoptera). *Z. Zool. Syst. Evol.* **17,** 30–56.

Walther, J. R. (1981). Die Morphologie und Feinstruktur der Sinnesorgane auf den Antennengeisseln der Männchen, Weibchen und Arbeiterinnen der roten Waldameise *Formica rufa* Linne 1758 mit einem Vergleich der antennalen Sensillenmuster weiterer Formicoidea (Hymenoptera). Ph.D. Thesis, Free University of Berlin.

Wasserthal, L. T., and Seibt, U. (1976). Feinstruktur, Funktion und Reinigung der antennalen Sinneshaare der Garnele *Hymenocera picta* (Gnathophyllidae). *Z. Tierpsychol.* **42,** 186–199.

Wieczorek, H. (1982). A biochemical approach to the electrogenic potassium pump of insect sensilla: Potassium sensitive ATPases in the labellum of the fly. *J. Comp. Physiol.* **148,** 303–311.

Zacharuk, R. Y. (1980). Ultrastructure and function of insect chemosensilla. *Annu. Rev. Entomol.* **25,** 27–47.

Zacharuk, R. Y. (1985). Antennae and sensilla. *In* "Comprehensive Insect Physiology, Biochemistry, and Pharmacology" (G. A. Kerkut and L. I. Gilbert, eds.), Vol. 6, pp. 1–69. Pergamon, Oxford.

Zack Strausfeld, C., and Kaissling, K.-E. (1986). Localized adaptation processes in olfactory sensilla of Saturniid moths. *Chem. Senses* **11,** 499–512.

12

The Molecular Basis of Pheromone Reception: Its Influence on Behavior

RICHARD G. VOGT

Department of Chemistry
State University of New York
Stony Brook, New York 11794

I. INTRODUCTION

During a daily, species-specific window of time, usually at night, a female moth releases her sex pheromone (Rau and Rau, 1929; Haynes and Birch, 1984). This identifying mixture of volatile lipophilic molecules is carried away on air currents, the nature of which are enormously variable, being dependent on the prevailing meterological conditions. During a window of time overlapping female pheromone release, male moths fly about in a motivational state that allows them to respond behaviorally to an encounter with pheromone (Rau and Rau, 1929; Truman, 1974; Haynes and Birch, 1984).

If a male moth flies into an air space that contains an appropriate concentration of pheromone molecules, his behavior changes from an erratic flight search pattern to a highly oriented zigzag flight. He makes upwind and overground progress along the vector of the pheromone plume toward a receptive female. Meteorological conditions are quite unstable, with significant windshifts occurring every few seconds (David *et al.*, 1983). Consequently, the pheromone plume originating from a single female actually appears as a series of discontinuous packets moving in different directions, with the individual packets showing a high degree of internal discontinuity due to turbulence (David *et al.*, 1983;

Pheromone Biochemistry

Murlis, 1986; Murlis and Jones, 1981). During his precopulatory flight, it is almost certain that a male will encounter and lose numerous pheromone packets en route to a luring female. When a male loses the scent he enters a new pheromone search behavior, performing increasingly wide lateral casts, side to side, making little forward or no overground progress toward the female (Kennedy *et al.*, 1980; David *et al.*, 1983). This switch in flight behavior from overground zigzag to lateral casting is very rapid, occurring in about 0.5 sec after pheromone loss (Fig. 1) (Marsh *et al.*, 1981; Kramer, 1975; R. G. Vogt and T. C. Baker, unpublished observation).

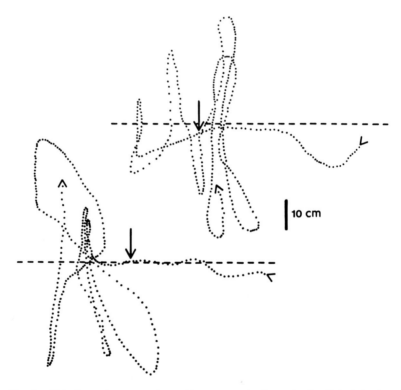

Fig. 1. This figure documents the rapid and dramatic change in the flight behavior of an *Antheraea polyphemus* male due to the abrupt loss of pheromone. Moths were videotaped during flight in a wind tunnel, and their flight paths were subsequently traced from a stop-frame video display. In these traces, the moth entered from the right, flying upwind along a pheromone plume. At the arrow, the moth encountered an abrupt loss of pheromone and rapidly changed his flight behavior from overground zigzag to lateral casting. The dots are spaced 1/30 sec apart. The latencies of this behavioral switch were approximately 0.5 sec. These experiments were conducted by T. C. Baker and the author.

Male moths use visual information to coordinate their various flight behaviors, but the manner in which they use this visual information is heavily influenced by their current and recent exposure to pheromone. In terms of the neural control of these behaviors, pheromone inputs into the brain gate the way in which visual information is used to coordinate the flight motor (Olberg, 1983; Preiss and Kramer, 1983, 1986b).

The antennae, with their complement of pheromone-sensitive sensory hairs, play an active role in these behaviors. Circuits within the male's brain rely on information about the external olfactory environment in order to make appropriate behavioral decisions. The pheromone plume has highly ephemeral temporal, spatial, and intensity characteristics, and it is the task of the antennae and particularly of the pheromone-sensitive sensory hairs and sensory neurons to translate this ever changing external chemical environment to the animal's brain. My premise is that the sensory hairs accomplish this translation by biochemically recreating the relevant external characteristics of the pheromone world. It is this biochemical recreation that is presented to the receptor proteins of the sensory dendrites and there transduced from chemical signal to electrical signal.

A male moth's sexual flight behavior is dependent on what his sensory hairs convey to his brain about the nature of the pheromone environment. Within these sensory hairs we find pheromone-binding proteins and pheromone-degrading enzymes whose tasks appear to be the rapid transport and inactivation of pheromone molecules (Vogt and Riddiford, 1981a,b, 1986a; Vogt et al., 1985; Prestwich, Chapter 14, this volume). The degradative enzymes, for example, ensure that the active life of a pheromone molecule within a sensory hair is brief, only long enough to interact with a receptor protein before being degraded (Vogt et al., 1985). These insects have evolved an extracellular biochemical network which effectively models the temporal and intensity characteristics of their external pheromone environment. The output of this biochemical network is presented to the membrane receptors and transduced.

This system is providing a detailed look at several behaviorally relevant gene-coded elements, the sensory hair proteins. Certain aspects of the male's pre-copulatory behavior appear to be encoded in the kinetic properties of these proteins. In the course of this chapter, I shall discuss experiments which have led to this view. I shall present supporting evidence that these proteins, unique to the pheromone-sensitive sensory hairs, are sexually selected elements and that they show variation in property among individuals of a species, among isolated populations of a species, and among different species. In these species, such molecular variation could provide a significant source of behavioral variation on which evolutionary selection can act. I shall close this chapter with a discussion of the significance this system has for understanding both the molecular basis of behavior and the evolution of behavior.

II. THE ANIMAL

A. Choice of Species

I have been studying proteins which appear to be involved in processing lepidopteran sex pheromone after it has been released from the pheromone gland of the female. These studies have chiefly utilized the wild silkmoth, *Antheraea polyphemus*, and more recently the gypsy moth, *Lymantria dispar*. These distantly related moths belong to the families Saturniidae and Lymantriidae, respectively.

The Saturniidae includes our most beautiful large moths: *Antheraea polyphemus, Hyalophora cecropia, Callosamia promethea, Samia cynthia* (the Ailanthus moth of New York City), and *Actias luna,* all common, nonpest species of North America. The Lymantriidae includes several common species which are serious economic pests on forest trees. In addition to *L. dispar* (gypsy moth), whose caterpillars have been feasting on oak leaves of the eastern United States since their infamous introduction at Medford, Massachusetts, in 1869 (Evans, 1985), the group includes *Orgyia pseudotsugata* (Douglas fir tussock moth), which is abundant in the Pacific Northwest and defoliates forests with some regularity. The life histories of many of these species are quite well known. The population dynamics and radiation history of species like *L. dispar* and *O. pseudotsugata* are well documented. Furthermore, species of these groups are often easy to raise and can be readily collected in the wild.

Member species of these two families, along with those of the Bombycidae (*Bombyx mori,* the commercial silkworm moth) and the Arctiidae, possess large, feathery antennae with tens of thousands of sensory hairs. The majority of these hairs are thought to be identical (Boeckh *et al.,* 1960; Keil, 1984a). This high concentration of functionally homogeneous tissue provides ideal source material for biochemical studies. Additionally, several members of these families have been extensively characterized with respect to pheromone structure, behavior, and physiology. The accessibility of these member species provides a rich opportunity for comparative studies of biochemical strategies. Through such studies it is proving possible to obtain a clearer understanding of the rules underlying both pheromone reception–transduction specifically, and the molecular basis of behavior in general.

B. Antennal and Sensory Hair Morphology, *Antheraea polyphemus*

Approximately 55,000 sensory hairs (Boeckh *et al.,* 1960) are arrayed, three abreast, in two opposing rows along the branches of the plumose antennae of male *A. polyphemus.* Until recently, we have considered these hairs to be essentially identical, each possessing two sensory dendrites. These two dendrites are specifically sensitive to, respectively, the two components of the *A. polyphemus* sex pheromone, the acetate ester (E,Z)-6,11-hexadecadienyl acetate (E6,Z11-16 : Ac) and the corresponding aldehyde E6,Z11-16 : Al (Kochansky *et al.*, 1975). Recent reports indicate that about 30% of the hairs contain a third dendrite (Keil, 1984a) and that there may be a third component to the *A. polyphemus* pheromone, the acetate ester E4,Z9-14 : Ac (K. E. Kaissling, personal communication). It may prove that the third neuron responds to this newly identified component.

The sensory hairs are hollow, cuticular structures, each about 300 μm long and 6 μm in diameter (Boeckh *et al.*, 1960), with an inner lumen volume of about 10^{-12} liter (Vogt *et al.*, 1985; Keil, 1984a). This lumen contains the sensory dendrites, whose cell bodies are buried among the epithelial cells at the base of the hair. A proteinaceous fluid, the sensory hair lymph, bathes these dendrites. Axons from the neuronal cell bodies project to the deutocerebrum of the brain via the antennal nerve. Tight-junctional complexes join the epithelial cells and neuronal cell bodies, establishing a high resistance barrier between the sensory hair lymph and the hemolymph (see De Kramer and Hemberger, Chapter 13, this volume).

The sensory hair lumen is an isolated and presumably independently modified and maintained space in the animal (see Steinbrecht, Chapter 11). The apical membrane of the base epithelial cells is highly folded, and the cytoplasmic side contains a great number of mitochondria (Steinbrecht, 1980). The presence of this energy source and the observation of membrane-bound proteins (Thurm and Küppers, 1980) suggest the presence of active transport processes across this membrane. Such transport might be used to maintain the ionic and protein compositions of the sensory hair lymph. However, it is not yet known whether active transport occurs in the adult or whether these mitochondria and membrane-bound proteins are merely remnants of antennal morphogenesis. Several studies (Steinbrecht and Zierold, 1985; Kaissling *et al.*, 1985) have indicated high concentrations of potassium and sulfur in the lymph. Our own studies have indicated that this lymph contains 30% soluble protein, the 15,000-dalton pheromone-binding protein (PBP) (Vogt and Riddiford, 1981b). The high potassium level of the lymph has supported suggestions that the initial electrical impulse of signal transduction is due to an inward potassium current (see De Kramer and Hemberger, Chapter 13). The high sulfur content may be due to methionine or cysteine residues present in the protein. The presence of both amino acids in PBP has been confirmed by recent amino acid sequence analysis (see Section VII).

C. Pheromone Entry via Pore Tubules

For pheromone molecules to be detected, they must first enter a sensory hair and arrive at presumed receptor proteins in the dendritic membrane. Pheromone molecules are assumed to enter the hair via pores through the hair cuticle. Approximately 20,000 pores penetrate each hair of *A. polyphemus* (Kaissling, 1971). As structures, these pores extend a relatively short distance into the lumen as a cluster of small diameter tubules, together called pore tubules, and are thought to be remnants of wax canals functional during antennal morphogenesis (see Steinbrecht, Chapter 11, this volume). It is generally assumed that the pore-tubule systems provide the behaviorally relevant rapid entry of pheromone mole-cules into the hair lumen.

III. SENSORY HAIR PROTEINS

The pheromone-sensitive sensory hairs of *A. polyphemus* possess at least two soluble proteins which are involved in pheromone processing: the pheromone-binding protein (PBP) and the sensillar esterase (SE) (Fig. 2) (Vogt and Rid-diford, 1981a,b). Both proteins are unique to these sensory hairs and are situated in the extracellular lymph surrounding the sensory dendrites. The PBP has a molecular weight of approximately 15,000. PBP is present at an extremely high concentration of 20 mM, indicating that the sensory hair lymph is 30% protein. The SE has a molecular weight estimated between 55,000 and 90,000 (Kaissling *et al.*, 1985) and is present at submicromolar concentrations (Vogt and Rid-diford, 1986a). The SE is very aggressive at degrading the pheromone, the pheromone having an estimated *in situ* half-life of less than 15 msec in the presence of a physiological concentration of enzyme (Vogt *et al.*, 1985). In addition to these two proteins, we presume that there are receptor proteins for the pheromone components situated in the sensory dendrite membrane, and there may be other enzymes to degrade the other components of the pheromone mixture.

A. Initial Studies

In 1970 L. M. Riddiford reported sexual dimorphism among soluble antennal proteins of the Saturniid moths *Antheraea pernyi*, *A. polyphemus*, and *Hyalo-phora cecropia* (Riddiford, 1970). In these studies, male and female antennae were dipped into saline for 30 min, and the eluted proteins were electrophoresed. A male specific protein of low mobility was observed from all three species. Riddiford suggested that such proteins unique to a functionally specific tissue such as the male antennae might be involved in the function of that tissue, i.e., the detection of sex pheromone. In support of this suggestion, sex pheromone was subsequently demonstrated to interact with the male specific protein of *A. pernyi*.

At the time of these studies, the sex pheromones of the three species were

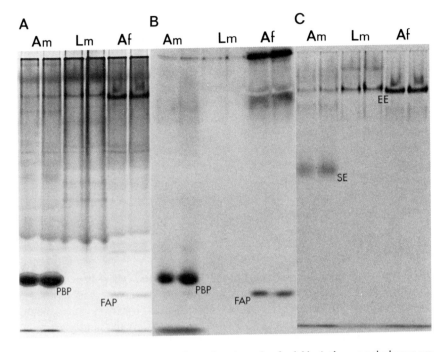

Fig. 2. This figure represents an electrophoretic study of soluble *Antheraea polyphemus* proteins, demonstrating the pheromone-binding protein (PBP) and the sensillar esterase (SE). Three tissues were compared: Am, male antenna (2 mg tissue/lane); Lm, male leg (5 mg tissue/lane); and Af, female antenna (3 mg tissue/lane). Tissue homogenates were preincubated with tritium-labeled pheromone, (E6,Z11)-[11,12-^{3}H]hexadecadienyl acetate, and electrophoresed under nondenaturing conditions. The gel was stained initially for esterase activity (C), then for total protein (A), and finally fluorographed to detect protein-associated radioactivity (B). The study revealed the male antennal-specific PBP and SE (A and C) and demonstrated the association between pheromone and PBP (B). Note the female antennal-specific protein (FAP) which also associates with pheromone. EE, Epidermal esterase referred to in Fig. 8. After Vogt and Riddiford (1981b).

structurally unknown. Riddiford relied on the ability of the female to synthesize pheromone from precursor, and injected developing female pupae of *A. pernyi,* soon to emerge as adults, with tritium-labeled sodium acetate. It was hoped that the acetate would be incorporated into the structure of the females' sex pheromone, thus producing radiolabeled pheromone. The females were allowed to release pheromone into the air, which was then passed over male antennae. The antennae were dipped in saline as before, the eluted proteins were electrophoresed, the electrophoretic gels were sliced, and the radioactivity in the slices was measured by scintillation counting. In two of eight such experiments, detectable levels of radioactivity appeared in gel slices corresponding to the position of the male specific protein, suggesting that radiolabeled sex pheromone had associated specifically with this protein. Riddiford subsequently proposed the first model for pheromone reception which was based on biochemical data (Riddiford, 1971). In this model it was presumed that these male antennal specific proteins were extracellular and soluble. Riddiford suggested that the proteins might be located within the lumen of the pore tubules, then thought to be blind-ended, and that they might function as a pheromone carrier.

These experiments illustrated two important points of strategy for the initial elucidation of the biochemical events involved in pheromone reception–transduction: (1) study proteins which show sex and tissue specificity to the antenna, and (2) utilize a highly specific radiolabeled probe which functions in a meaningful way in the context of the animal's behavior. This strategy has subsequently proved extremely successful in studies involving the silkmoth, *A. polyphemus,* as well as in more recent studies involving the gypsy moth, *L. dispar.*

B. Tritiated Probe

The identification of the structures of the *A. polyphemus* pheromone (Kochansky *et al.,* 1975) rekindled Riddiford's interest in sensory hair proteins. *Antheraea polyphemus* was not the species she had used in her previous labeling studies, but it is a sibling species and is now thought to have the same pheromone (Boeckh and Boeckh, 1979). In 1976, Simon Golec, a graduate student in Chemistry at the University of Washington who was just completing his Ph.D., was enlisted to derive a route of synthesis for an alkynyl acetate compound which would allow introduction of tritium labels at the Z-11 double bond. Golec synthesized the precursor (Prestwich *et al.,* 1984), which was then tritiated by New England Nuclear (summer of 1977) with a specific activity of 40 Ci/mmol. As a first-year graduate student at University of Washington, I was offered the opportunity to use this radiolabeled pheromone to repeat Riddiford's earlier experiments of labeling antennal proteins.

C. Pheromone-Binding Protein

My initial studies, which involved dipping antennae into saline and electrophoresing the eluate as Riddiford had done earlier, produced no clear results; no observable male-specific proteins could be extracted merely by dipping live antennae in physiological saline. I changed my approach and began examining whole tissue homogenates. Like Riddiford, I looked for proteins unique to the homogenates of male antennae and which would interact with the sex pheromone.

I prepared homogenates of both male and female antennae, as well as a variety of other tissues (wings, legs, head, trachea, brain, ventral nerve cord, fat body, epidermis, hemolymph), and compared their proteins by non–sodium dodecyl sulfate (SDS)–polyacrylamide slab gel electrophoresis. I incubated these homogenates with ^{3}H-labeled pheromone for 30 min and then electrophoresed them on 10–15% gels for about 6 hr. The gels were stained with Coomassie Blue, photographed, and then fluorographed after 1 hr treatment in 1 M salicylic acid.

These studies revealed a major protein of high mobility, unique to male antennae, which bound pheromone under the electrophoretic conditions described (Fig. 2). We named this the pheromone-binding protein (PBP) (Vogt and Riddiford, 1981a,b). The PBP has a molecular weight of 15,000 and is located extracellularly in the sensory hair lymph (Vogt and Riddiford, 1981b). The protein is very abundant: 15 μg per antenna, 3 ng per hair. This translates to a protein concentration of 20 mM, an indication that the sensory hair lymph has a 30% protein concentration. Furthermore, this type of protein appears to be a common element of pheromone-sensitive sensory hairs, present in the antennae of *Antheraea pernyi, Hyalophora cecropia, Manduca sexta,* and *Lymantria dispar* (Vogt and Riddiford, 1981a; R. G. Vogt and G. D. Prestwich, unpublished). The PBPs of *A. pernyi* and *L. dispar* have been confirmed as members of the extracellular sensory hair lymph (Kaissling and Thorson, 1980; R. G. Vogt and G. D. Prestwich, unpublished).

D. Sensillar Esterase

Throughout the 1970s a number of studies focused on pheromone degradation by antennal tissues, utilizing the species *Bombyx mori* (Kasang, 1971, 1973, 1974), *Lymantria dispar* (Kasang *et al.*, 1974), and *Trichoplusia ni* (Ferkovich *et al.*, 1973; Ferkovich, 1981). None of these studies unambiguously demonstrated a functional pheromone-degrading enzyme.

During the summer of 1979, following a suggestion of Bruce Hammock, I looked for esterases in the *A. polyphemus* antenna that might be present to degrade the pheromone. The pheromone component we had been using was an acetate ester, so an esterase was a likely candidate as a degradatory enzyme. Fortunately, esterases are easy to visualize on non-SDS gels (Shaw and Prassad, 1970). I prepared homogenates of a variety of tissues, electrophoresed these under conditions identical to those described above for the binding protein studies, stained the gels for esterase activity, and looked for the presence of esterases unique to the male antennae.

These gels demonstrated several groups of esterases, one of which was, like the binding protein, unique to the male antenna (Fig. 2). Using microgel techniques (Rüchell, 1976), I demonstrated that this esterase, also like the binding protein, was located extracellularly in the lymph of the pheromone-sensitive sensory hairs. We named this enzyme sensillar esterase (SE) (Vogt and Riddiford, 1981b). The SE has a molecular weight estimated between 55,000 and 90,000 (Kaissling *et al.*, 1985). It has the curious property of appearing as a multiband complex on gels, with different bands in this complex showing different activity (see Section VII). The SE showed a high degree of substrate specificity compared with the other, more general esterases, and it degraded sex pheromone at an impressive rate (Vogt and Riddiford, 1981a,b; Vogt et al., 1985; Prestwich et al., 1986b). The finding of this second component was very exciting to me, as it suggested dimensionality and dynamic interaction within this biochemical system.

We subsequently purified the SE by preparative gel electrophoresis, characterized its kinetic properties and its substrate specificity, and estimated its in situ activity (Vogt et al., 1985). At 25°C, pH 7.2, the enzyme displayed a K_m of 2.23 $\times 10^{-6} M$ and a V_{max} of 5.4 $\times 10^{-12}$ mol/liter-sec for the enzyme complement of one antenna. By adjusting the V_{max} to the in situ state, we estimated that pheromone in the sensory hair would have a half-life well below 15 msec.

The SE kinetic parameters closely match reported physiological and behavioral parameters. Both the enzyme and the physiological response of the sensory hair to pheromone stimulus saturate at similar pheromone concentrations, around 10^6 molecules per hair (Vogt et al., 1985; Kaissling, 1977). The physiological threshold has been reported to be well below this saturating concentration, at 1 molecule per hair (Schneider et al., 1968). Additionally, our data suggest that the enzyme can clear up to 10^6 pheromone molecules from a sensory hair in less than 0.5 sec., the time required for a male to enter a new behavioral mode on loss of pheromone (Vogt et al., 1985; Marsh et al., 1981; Kramer, 1975; R. G. Vogt and T. C. Baker, unpublished). In the absence of rapid degradation one would expect an accumulation of active pheromone molecules within the hair. Such an accumulation would not reflect external fluctuations. In the presence of degradation by SE, this accumulation of residual pheromone molecules would be prevented. This would enable the moth to detect only incoming pheromone molecules and thus to effectively monitor the external fluctuations of pheromone.

Like the pheromone-binding proteins, pheromone-degrading enzymes appear to be common features of pheromone-sensitive sensory hairs. Gypsy moth (L. dispar) antennae are the only tissue which degrade the epoxide pheromone of this species, and this enzyme activity is present in the pheromone-sensitive sensory hairs. The biochemistry of gypsy moth pheromone reception is discussed in greater detail in Section VI (see also Prestwich, Chapter 14, this volume). Heliothis virescens also appears to have antennal-specific enzyme activity directed at the aldehyde pheromone of this species (Ding and Prestwich, 1986).

Ferkovich and colleagues (Ferkovich et al., 1973; Ferkovich, 1981) reported the presence of potential pheromone-degrading esterases in the antennae of Trichoplusia ni, whose major pheromone component is (Z)-7-dodecen-1-yl acetate. This research group electrophoretically demonstrated a great many antennal esterase bands, none of which, however, could be uniquely assigned to antennae, much less sensory hairs. Consequently, it is not possible from their experiments to connect enzyme function to tissue function. Unfortunately, this group utilized tube gel electrophoresis rather than slab gel electrophoresis when comparing enzyme species between tissues. Conditions from one tube to the next are variable, and it is extremely difficult to compare one electrophoretic profile to the next. The results of their efforts would have been much clearer had they utilized slab gel electrophoresis. Nevertheless, their data were highly suggestive that there are important sensory hair enzymes present to degrade the pheromone of this species.

E. Esterase Visualization

Electrophoretic visualization of esterases is a powerful technique, as it is an easy method for analyzing enzyme systems which degrade acetate esters, common pheromone components among Lepidoptera. After electrophoresis, a gel is floated in a staining reaction mixture consisting of 0.5 mM each of 1-naphthyl acetate and 2-naphthyl acetate, and 0.1% Fast Blue in 50 mM Tris, pH 7.0. Fast Blue (0.1 g) is added to 10 ml of 0.5 M Tris, pH 6.8, and magnetically stirred for about 1 min. Distilled water (90 ml) is added and stirring is continued until most of the dye dissolves. A combined stock solution of the naphthyl acetates is prepared (0.1 M each in ethanol), and this is slowly added to the Fast Blue mixture during rapid stirring (0.5 ml/100 ml stain). The completed staining reaction mixture is immediately poured onto the gel through glass wool. In the reaction the product alcohols couple to and precipitate the dye, so that where there is an esterase which will utilize one of these substrates, a brownish band appears. 2-Naphthol yields a more reddish pigment than 1-naphthol, thus enzyme–substrate specificity can be qualitatively assessed as well.

The esterase visualization technique is extremely powerful, as it allows a rapid, one-step purification of any esterase which will utilize one of these substrates. The dye does not attach to the esterase, nor does it interfere with subsequent kinetic studies. After staining, the esterase bands can be precisely sliced from the rest of the gel, and the enzyme can be eluted. This enzyme may not be pure with respect to other proteins, but it is free from other enzymes utilizing the same substrate. As desired, detailed kinetics can then be obtained from this partially purified enzyme.

A very worthy project would be the establishment of gel staining reactions to visualize enzymes for other pheromone types, i.e., oxidoreductases for aldehydes, ketones, and alcohols and epoxide hydrolases and transferases for epoxides. With increasing identification of degradative pathways (see Prestwich, Chapter 14, this volume) this should now be feasable.

F. Analysis of Sensory Hair Contents

For the pheromone researcher, it is tempting to claim that a protein which demonstrates an ability to interact with pheromone has that function. This is not sufficient. The protein, be it enzyme, binding protein, or receptor, must also be demonstrated to reside in the sensory hair proper. Indeed, it is the challenge of these systems to demonstrate such site specificity.

We initially localized the *A. polyphemus* PBP and SE to the sensory hairs simply by cutting off these long hairs using microscissors and electrophoresing homogenates of these hairs (Vogt and Riddiford, 1981a,b). We were subsequently able to associate these proteins with the sensory hair lymph by directly collecting expressed hair lymph and analyzing this by microcapillary gel electrophoresis (Vogt and Riddiford, 1981b; Kaissling and Thorson, 1980; Rüchell, 1976). The collection technique, developed by Kaissling (Kaissling and Thorson, 1980), involved removing an antennal branch and slipping its cut end over a saline-filled glass capillary. The tips of the sensory hairs were cut using special clippers fashioned by bending and sharpening the tips of watchmaker forceps. Immediately after cutting, hydrostatic pressure was applied to the antennal branch through the saline-filled capillary. Droplets of sensory hair lymph were extruded from the cut hair tips and collected on the tip of a small glass rod ($<<1$ mm diameter). The droplets dried onto the glass surface nearly as fast as they were collected, allowing for continued collection with the same glass rod. Finally, the tip of the rod was washed in a small volume of electrophoresis sample buffer and, in our case, electrophoresed directly using microcapillary tube gels (Rüchell, 1976). The sensory hairs remain physiologically active throughout the collection process (see De Kramer and Hemberger, Chapter 13, this volume, for discussion of tip recording technique).

Ferkovich *et al.* (1980) attempted to isolate sensory hair contents by sonicating antennae to break open the sensory hairs, collecting the eluted contents, and examining esterase patterns by tube gel electrophoresis (Ferkovich *et al.*, 1980; Ferkovich, 1981). These authors argued that sonication broke the sensory hair cuticle open and dissociated the sensory dendrites, leaving the rest of the antenna untouched. This technique yielded 13 different esterase bands on electrophoresis. Though the authors suggested that these bands represented sensory hair esterases, the collection technique precluded this. One must suppose that forces powerful enough to break open the hair cuticle and dissociate the dendritic membranes could also break up the epidermal and hemolymph compartments, thus eluting their components as well. Thus the technique places no guarantee on the source location of any isolated proteins. Certainly some of the esterases could have originated from the sensory hairs, but the technique unfortunately does not assure this, nor does it suggest which esterases might be associated with sensory hairs. Our own work has demonstrated esterases of the hemolymph, epidermis, and sensory hairs present in whole antennal homogenates (Vogt and Riddiford, 1981a,b, 1986a).

An effective technique for the unambiguous isolation of sensory hairs in high yield was developed by U. Klein of the Kaissling group at Seewiesen, West Germany (Klein and Keil, 1984). Klein and I (Vogt *et al.*, 1985) both have independently used this technique with great success to collect sensory hairs from *A. polyphemus,* and I have recently used this technique with equal success for the collection of *Lymantria dispar* sensory hairs. The technique is thoroughly described for *A. polyphemus* in both of the above-cited papers. For *L. dispar,* branches of 100 male antennae were cut using a razor blade and mixed with 2 ml each 0.1- and 0.5-mm diameter glass beads in a 15-ml Corex tube covered with a rubber septum. The tube and contents were frozen in liquid nitrogen and mixed on a vortex mixer for 3–5 sec. Mixing allowed the glass beads to break the brittle sensory hairs from the antennal branches. Freezing ensured that there was no contamination of sensory hairs by epidermal or hemolymph components. (During mixing it is absolutely essential to vent the tubes by piercing the rubber septum with a large bore syringe needle. This allows venting of expanding gasses due to warming and prevents the rubber septum cap from exploding off and the tube contents from scattering across the lab bench.) The contents were than lyophilized to dryness, thus avoiding the melting of tissue and the mixing of cellular components. Hairs were separated by dumping the tube contents into specially constructed 15-cm diameter petri dishes. Glass rings were glued to disks of flat glass, to the approximate dimensions of a normal petri dish. (Normal glass petri dishes do not have flat bottoms due to their mode of manufacture, and are difficult to scrape efficiently.) The small sensory hairs stuck to the glass surface and the glass beads and antennal branches were simply shaken away. Hairs were collected by scraping using a fresh single edge razor blade, with a yield of approximately 0.5 mg hair material isolated from 100 antennae. Hairs collected in this manner can be stored at or below −70°C in sealed vials.

IV. DYNAMIC INTERACTIONS BETWEEN PHEROMONE AND SENSORY HAIR PROTEINS: MODELS OF PHEROMONE RECEPTION

It is my premise that certain aspects of a male moth's precopulatory behaviors are encoded in the kinetic properties of the sensory hair proteins. To justify this view, it is necessary to present the historical development of the models which have described our understanding of the workings of the olfactory sensory hairs. These models focus on the events surrounding the transduction of chemical into electrical information. For a thorough discussion of these transductory events, see also Chapter 13 (De Kramer and Hemberger, this volume).

A. Sensory Hair Morphology: Historical Review of Pore Tubules

In order to understand the workings of an olfactory sensory hair, it is first necessary to understand its structural anatomy. Many of these details are discussed in Section II and in Steinbrecht, Chapter 11, this volume. It is appropriate at this time to review the history of the investigations into the pore–tubule systems of these sensory hairs, as these structures have played and continue to play a significant role in discussions concerning these sensory hairs.

The ultrastructure of olfactory sensory hairs was first examined at the electron microscope level by E. Slifer and colleagues around 1960 (Slifer, 1961; Slifer *et al.*, 1957, 1959; Slifer and Sekhon, 1964). These studies examined the olfactory hairs of grasshoppers, and they showed what appeared to be finely branched dendritic fibers terminating at the many pores which penetrated the hair cuticle (Fig. 3A). Slifer's studies suggested that the sensory dendrite endings actually terminated at the surface of the hair, making direct contact with air. This idea was presented in textbook form in the sixth (1965) edition of Wigglesworth's *The Principles of Insect Physiology* (Wigglesworth, 1972).

In 1969, K.-D. Ernst, a student of Prof. D. Schneider at the Max Planck

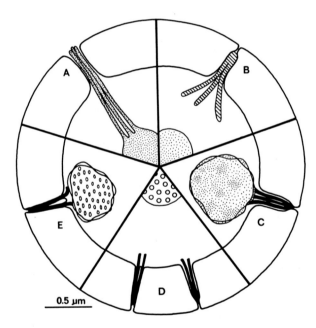

Fig. 3.   This figure represents the historical development of anatomical models of the insect olfactory hair, emphasizing the relationship between pore tubules and dendrites. Drawings are after the following sources: (A) Figs. 1 and 35 of Slifer *et al.* (1959); (B) Fig. 15 of Ernst (1969); (C) Fig. 3d of Steinbrecht and Müller (1971); (D) Figs. 28 and 29 of Steinbrecht (1980) and Fig. 3 of Keil (1984a), and (E) Fig. 8 of Keil (1982). C and E represent the result of chemical fixation; D represents the results of both freeze substitution and freeze etching. The microtubules of the dendritic cytoplasm are drawn to represent their states in the indicated micrographs. The sensory hair cross section is drawn to radial scale, after Keil (1984a). See text for discussion.

Institute at Seewiesen, demonstrated that these pore fibers were not dendritic extrusions but rather were cuticular intrusions, not at all neural in origin (Ernst, 1969). These "pore tubules," morphogenic remnants of wax canals (Steinbrecht, Chapter 11), were demonstrated to be blind-ended, making no contact with the sensory dendrites (Fig. 3B).

Ernst's studies suggested that pheromone molecules entered a sensory hair via pore tubules but then had to somehow pass through a presumed aqueous barrier, the sensory hair lymph, in order to reach the sensory dendrite. The lipophilic nature of the molecules seemed to preclude this. In 1971, R. A. Steinbrecht, also a member of the Schneider group at Seewiesen, published electron micrographs which showed pore tubules actually contacting dendritic membrane (Fig. 3C) (Steinbrecht and Müller, 1971). In the introduction to their text, these authors noted the total lack of previously observed tubule–dendrite contacts in electron micrographs, but suggested that this might be due to artifacts caused by poor fixation technique. In their text, the authors demonstrated that the appearance of tubules in electron micrographs was grossly affected by the method of tissue preparation. Steinbrecht and Müller established chemical fixation techniques which occasionally revealed tubule–dendrite contact, suggested that these contacts were the normal condition, and offered this system as a direct way that pheromone molecules could reach the dendritic membrane without ever entering the aqueous sensory hair lymph. These micrographs, however, showed badly distorted dendritic membranes. Later studies using freeze-substitution techniques which yielded well-preserved dendritic structures never showed such contacts (Fig. 3D) (Steinbrecht, 1980).

Recent publications by T. Keil, another member of the Seewiesen group, again show contacts between pore tubules and dendrites (Fig. 3E) (Keil, 1982, 1984a,b). However, these contacts are reported to have been infrequently observed, and then only when the dendrite was sitting in section very close to the inner cuticle wall of the hair. As in Steinbrecht's micrographs, Keil's micrographs demonstrated tubules contacting only badly distorted dendrites. Nevertheless, the Seewiesen group has, over the years, tended to argue that with appropriate fixation, i.e., chemical cross-linking, pore tubules can be seen in their natural state attached to the dendritic membrane.

I feel that that the importance of observed tubule–dendrite contacts has been overemphasized, invoked only as a mechanism to salve a researcher's dilemma. How does a highly lipophilic molecule cross a simple aqueous space at presumed high efficiency if not by these ephemeral structural tunnels? It is now clear that the hair lumen is not a simple aqueous fluid but rather a highly proteinaceous fluid which has the apparent property of being able to readily solubilize lipophilic molecules at high capacity. Indeed, a new picture of sensory hair function is emerging from molecular level studies. In this picture, the biochemical milieu of the sensory hair appears to be organized in a specific manner, based on the gene-coded properties of proteins, to accomplish the task of pheromone reception. That task is to translate to the brain, in a behaviorally relevant context, the temporal aspects of ambient pheromone levels.

B. Pheromone Reception: Kaissling Model

In 1974, Kaissling published a six-step model describing the events of pheromone reception (Kaissling, 1974):

1. Adsorption of the pheromone molecule to the surface of a sensory hair;
2. Diffusion down a pore tubule to the dendritic membrane;
3. Binding to a membrane-bound receptor molecule;
4. Activation of the receptor;
5. Increased membrane conductance;
6. Early inactivation of the stimulus molecule.

Two of the model's steps are of particular relevance to our work: step 2, the movement of the pheromone molecules to the receptor protein, and step 6, its subsequent "early inactivation."

Kaissling accepted the idea that pore tubules provided a direct conduit by which pheromone molecules traveled to the dendritic membrane. He also accepted that the pheromone molecule must have a short active lifetime within the sensory hair, but the mechanism for the inactivation of pheromone was unclear. Electrophysiological data strongly suggested that active stimulus molecules did not persist within the hair. Within seconds of ceasing a nonoverloading stimulus pulse, the electrical activity of a sensory cell returned to background levels. However, chemical experiments suggested that degradation of pheromone applied to the antenna was very slow, with 50% of the pheromone still in an active form after 4 min. This enormous temporal disparity between physiology and chemistry led Kaissling to suggest a nonenzymatic "early inactivation" mechanism acting within the sensory hair.

Since 1970, members of the Seewiesen group have made a series of chemical studies examining the fate of radiolabeled pheromone molecules applied to intact antennae. These studies have utilized the silkmoths, *Bombyx mori* (Kasang, 1971; Kasang and Kaissling, 1972) and *A. polyphemus* (Kanaujia and Kaissling, 1985), and the gypsy moth, *Lymantria dispar* (Kasang *et al.*, 1974). The general protocol in these experiments was to blow the tritium-labeled pheromone onto an antenna, then at time points over the course of an hour to extract radiolabeled material out of the antenna with *n*-pentane or 2 : 1 chloroform : methanol. Analysis of this eluted material indicated that pheromone degradation on whole antennae was very slow, with a half-life of 4 min for *B. mori* (Kasang and Kaissling, 1972), 3 min for *A. polyphemus* (Kanaujia and Kaissling, 1985), and 1.4 min for *L. dispar* (Kasang *et al.*, 1974). Based on the slow pheromone turnover observed in the *B. mori* experiments, Kaissling suggested that if enzymatic degradation occurred within the antenna, it did not occur at a rate which was relevant to rapid physiological and behavioral responses of the animal. These long whole antennal half-lives are in direct contrast with our estimated *in situ* pheromone half-life of 15 msec due to enzymatic degradation (Vogt *et al.,* 1985).

In trying to understand the roles of the pheromone-binding protein and the sensillar esterase of *A. polyphemus,* we initially proposed a biochemical model for pheromone reception (Fig. 4A) in which the binding protein functioned as Kaissling's "early inactivator" by binding up pheromone away from the receptors and in which the esterase functioned as a later cleanup mechanism, degrading the pheromone at a presumed slow rate (Vogt and Riddiford, 1981a,b). Soon after proposing this scheme we purified and kinetically characterized the sensillar esterase, and a very different picture emerged.

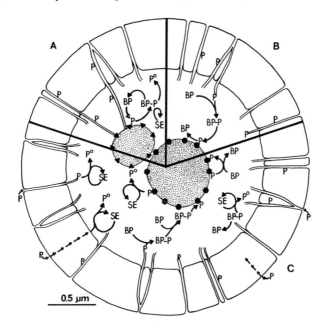

Fig. 4. This figure represents the historical development of the biochemical model of pheromone reception, proposed by Vogt and Riddiford (1986a) for *Antheraea polyphemus.* (A) After Vogt and Riddiford (1981b). (B) After Vogt *et al.* (1985). (C) Summary of the biochemical events taking place within the lumen of the sensory hair, including both the rapid entry of pheromone through the pore tubules and the slow entry of pheromone through the cuticle wall. P, Active pheromone; P°, enzymatically degraded pheromone; BP, pheromone-binding protein; BP–P, pheromone associated with binding protein; SE, sensillar esterase. The triangles and hexagons situated in the dendritic membrane represent receptor proteins. This cross section of an *A. polyphemus* sensory hair is drawn to radial scale and with a realistic number of pore–tubule structures after Keil (1984a). See text for discussion.

C. Pheromone Reception: Kinetic Equilibrium Model

It was clear from our kinetic studies that the sensillar esterase (SE) degraded pheromone fast enough to account for physiologically relevant rapid stimulus inactivation (Vogt et al., 1985). This proposed function for the enzyme allowed us to consider a carrier function for the pheromone-binding protein (PBP) (Fig. 4B). In this reevaluation of the biochemical model for pheromone reception, we suggested that pheromone molecules entered the sensory hair via pore tubules, were picked up by binding protein molecules, and transported across the lymph space to the receptor proteins. After interacting with receptors and initiating signal transduction, the pheromone molecules were degraded by the SE. This new model implied that the pheromone molecules moved along a linearly arranged biochemical pathway.

To me, this new view was still somewhat simplistic. For one thing, the proteins were not arranged in a linear fashion within the sensory hair, but rather were spatially mixed (Fig. 4C). How did pheromone molecules navigate this sea of binding protein and enzyme molecules to arrive unscathed at a receptor protein? This linear model described the result of the biochemical pheromone reception processes but did not describe the actual mechanisms which allowed this result. The new model did, however, suggest a number of testable questions, questions which address the mechanisms of the process rather than the results. (1) Does the binding protein protect pheromone from esterase enroute to the receptor? (2) Can the binding protein take pheromone from a receptor as easily as from a pore tubule? (3) What property prevents pheromone from being recycled to more receptors rather than being inactivated by enzymatic degradation? Some answers came from a series of experiments designed to examine the combined interaction between binding protein, esterase, and pheromone (Vogt and Riddiford, 1986a).

In these experiments, we examined how different concentrations of PBP influenced the rate of enzymatic degradation of pheromone (Vogt and Riddiford, 1986a). This experiment was designed to examine whether binding protein could protect the pheromone from degradation, a seeming requirement if the PBP acted as a carrier in the classic sense. In these experiments, we used a fixed concentration of purified SE throughout and compared the rate of degradation of four concentrations of pheromone (10^{-9}, 10^{-8}, 10^{-7}, and 10^{-6} M). At each pheromone concentration, we examined the rate of degradation in the presence of increasing amounts of purified PBP (6×10^{-8} to 6×10^{-5} M). We observed the following at each pheromone concentration:

1. As the PBP concentration increased to 6×10^{-6} M, there was at best only a slight decrease in the rate of degradation, reflecting an equally slight decrease in the availability of pheromone to the SE.
2. At 6×10^{-5} M protein concentration, there was a dramatic decrease in the

rate of degradation, to background rates within our assay conditions. This reflected a considerable lack of availability of pheromone to the SE, pheromone molecules now being bound to PBP.

3. Similar results were observed when a vertebrate lipid carrier, bovine serum albumin (BSA), was used instead of PBP, indicating relatively low specificity for the pheromone–protein interaction.

These results suggested the following:

1. There is a *temporally weak* association between *individual* binding protein and pheromone molecules. Even at $10^{-9}\,M$ pheromone, a 10,000-fold excess of PBP was required to reduce the availability of pheromone to another protein species, the SE.
2. There is a *temporally strong* association between the *population* of PBP molecules and individual pheromone molecules. This is seen only under conditions in which the population of PBP is at a high concentration.

The reduction in degradation rates suggests that, above critical protein concentrations ($10^{-5}\,M$), there is a strong association between binding protein population and pheromone. This effect would be profound at the *in situ* protein concentration of $2 \times 10^{-2}\,M$.

It should be noted that these experiments only indicated what was occurring between pheromone and binding protein. We were not increasing enzyme concentrations in these experiments. At the binding protein concentration where inhibition occurred, the enzyme concentration was at a 15-fold dilution from the *in situ* ratio between enzyme and binding protein. Degradation would have continued apace were the enzyme concentration increased in parallel with the binding protein concentration.

As a consequence of these experiments, we proposed a new model to describe the molecular mechanisms of pheromone reception, one consistent with shifting equilibrium states in chemical reactions (Vogt and Riddiford, 1986a). In this *kinetic equilibrium model* we proposed a multifunctional role for the binding protein and unifunctional roles for the esterase and the putative receptor proteins.

1. Pheromone molecules enter a sensory hair via pore tubules, gaining access to the internal lymph space, and encounter an extremely high concentration of PBP.
2. Pheromone is solubilized into the lymph by the high concentration of PBP.
3. Once solubilized, the pheromone moves through this proteinaceous phase of the sensory hair lymph, eventually encountering a receptor molecule, an enzyme, or some other species of binding site. These sites are, for the most part, also proteins belonging to the same phase in which the pheromone is already solubilized.
4. Pheromone molecule has a finite lifetime within a sensory hair, having an

opportunity to activate receptor molecules repeatedly until it is degraded on encounter with an enzyme molecule.

5. This finite lifetime of a pheromone molecule, and the dynamic response of the sensory hair to pheromone stimulus. is determined by the relative concentrations of the protein species involved and by their kinetic properties.

6. The pheromone-binding protein has the multifunctional properties of solubilizer, carrier, and protector of pheromone.

Figures 4C and 5 represent the chief biochemical interactions involved in this model. The rates that determine the net direction of pheromone movement depend on the concentrations of the various molecular species involved and on the mechanisms governing molecular scale diffusion around three- and two-dimensional interfaces (Berg and Purcell, 1977; Futrelle, 1984). The high concentration of PBP represents a lipophilic phase in contrast to the aqueous phase in which it is dissolved. Thus the PBP acts to solubilize pheromone molecules and provides a phase medium through which the pheromone molecules can rapidly migrate. The other proteins of import, i.e., enzymes and receptors, also belong to this proteinaceous phase through which pheromone is migrating. As a consequence of the high PBP concentration relative to SE concentration, mass action blockage insures that pheromone will have a finite lifetime within the sensory hair, albeit brief. In time the pheromone molecules will be degraded, but the high PBP concentration ensures that this time is sufficient for the bulk of pheromone to reach receptor proteins and thus initiate trandsuction. Additionally, this model suggests that individual pheromone molecules have the opportunity to interact with receptor proteins more than once prior to their degradation. This possibility

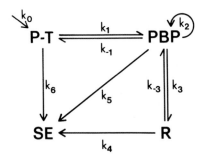

Fig. 5. This figure represents the biochemical events occurring within the sensory hair lumen during pheromone reception. A pheromone molecule enters the lumen via a pore tubule (P-T) and is removed from the system on degradation by a sensillar esterase (SE). The molecular properties of the sensory hair ensure that the majority of pheromone arrives at receptors (R), via transport by pheromone-binding proteins (PBP), prior to encountering esterase. This figure interrelates the biochemical events depicted in Fig. 4C. See text for discussion.

of repeated pheromone–receptor interaction could have a significant enhancement effect on transduction sensitivity at low pheromone concentrations.

D. Pheromone Reception: Resolving the Inconsistencies in Experimental Interpretation

Numerous experiments of a chemical or biochemical nature have been reported which concern aspects of the kinetic equilibrium model. These aspects are (1) the role of enzymatic degradation as the principal stimulus inactivator, (2) the nature of the association between binding protein and pheromone, and (3) the mechanism of pheromone transport within the sensory hair. The majority of these experiments were done prior to our biochemical studies and as such were often interpreted in a manner which is now inconsistent with new biochemical information. I shall now discuss these experiments in the light of our biochemical studies in order to reconcile these inconsistencies.

1. Pheromone Degradation

Kaissling has repeatedly proposed that primary pheromone inactivation is nonenzymatic in nature (Kaissling, 1974, 1986a,b). In contrast, we have isolated and characterized an enzyme from the sensory hairs which does appear to function as the primary pheromone inactivator (Vogt and Riddiford, 1981b; Vogt *et al.*, 1985). Kaissling based his proposal of a nonenzymatic "early inactivation" mechanism (Kaissling, 1974) on the pheromone degradation studies of G. Kasang (a chemist and member of the Seewiesen group). Although the physiological response of a sensory hair is over within seconds, these experiments were designed to examine the fate of adsorbed pheromone molecules only after they had already resided on the antenna for several seconds and up to an hour. Tritium-labeled pheromone was applied to intact antennae in an airstream. At increasing times after application, radioactivity was extracted from an intact antenna by immersion first in pentane for several minutes, followed by immersion in chloroform : methanol (2 : 1). These experiments were initially done using *Bombyx mori* (Kasang, 1971, 1973, 1974; Kasang and Kaissling, 1972) and *Lymantria dispar* (gypsy moth) (Kasang *et al.*, 1974). S. Kanaujia has recently repeated these studies using *A. polyphemus,* with similar findings (Kanaujia and Kaissling, 1985).

The solvent extractability of the tritium-labeled molecules changed with the length of time molecules were present on or in the antenna. Initially, a greater percentage of radioactivity was extractable with pentane. As time progressed, an increasing percentage of radioactivity remained on the antenna through the pentane wash but was subsequently extracted using chloroform : methanol. This movement of radioactivity from a pentane-extractable compartment to a chloroform : methanol compartment was interpreted as evidence of pheromone penetration into the antenna. Additionally, evidence for enzymatic conversion of pheromone to product was observed when the extracted material was analyzed by thin-layer chromatography.

Surprisingly, the time courses of these "fate" events were all similar, all of the order of several minutes (Fig. 6). The half-time of passage from pentane to

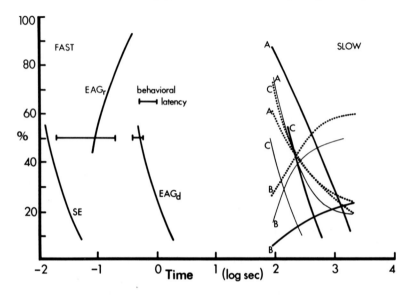

Fig. 6. This figure contrasts the experimentally determined time courses of several *fast* and *slow* pheromone-related processes. The abscissa represents time. The ordinate represents the concentration of pheromone relative to its initial concentration in each study, except in the electroantennogram (EAG) studies presented where the ordinate represents the electrical activity relative to maximal (100%). In the text discussion, it is suggested that the *fast* responses follow the rapid entry of pheromone molecules via the pore tubules, while the *slow* responses represent slow entry of phero-mone molecules via the thick cuticular hair wall.

Fast responses: SE, Estimated *in situ* rate of pheromone degradation within the sensory hair lumen by the sensillar esterase (*Antheraea polyphemus*, Vogt *et al.*, 1985). EAG_r, Rise time of the EAG response after pheromone molecules first strike a sensory hair. The horizontal bar represents the temporal range for this rate, which is negatively correlated to the stimulus concentration (*Bombyx mori*, Kaissling, 1969). EAG_d, Decline time of the EAG response. The horizontal bar represents the temporal range for this rate, which is positively correlated to the stimulus concentration (*B. mori*, Kaissling, 1969). Behavioral latency, range of the observed latency period for the behavioral switch from overground zigzag to lateral casting on loss of pheromone (*A. polyphemus*, R. G. Vogt and T. C. Baker, Fig. 1, this chapter; *B. mori*, Kramer, 1975; *Plodia interpunctella*, Marsh *et al.*, 1981). Note that the behavioral latency closely parallels the EAG decline time, EAG_d.

Slow responses: The data presented are for *A. polyphemus* (bold lines; Kanaujia and Kaissling, 1985), *Lymantria dispar* (light lines; Kasang *et al.*, 1974), and *B. mori* (dotted lines; Kasang, 1974). For each species, the falling A curve and rising B curve represent the slow movement of pheromone molecules from a pentane-extractable compartment to a chloroform : methanol-extractable compart-ment, and the C curve represents the parallel rate of degradation of these slow entering molecules.

chloroform : methanol extractability was 2 min in *B. mori* (Kasang and Kaissling, 1972), 2.5 min in *L. dispar* (Kasang *et al.*, 1974), and 6–8 min for *A. polyphemus* (Kanaujia and Kaissling, 1985). Additionally, approximately 50% of adsorbed pheromone was directly measured to have entered the sensory hair interior after 2–3 min (Kanaujia and Kaissling, 1985). Rates of degradation of applied pheromone also matched these values. The degradative half-life of applied pheromone was 4 min for *B. mori* (Kasang and Kaissling, 1972), 1.4 min for *L. dispar*, and around 3 min for *A. polyphemus*.

These researchers have demonstrated processes with half-times uniformly of several minutes, while the physiological and behavioral response times occur on a time scale of milliseconds to a second. Additionally, we have demonstrated a pheromone-degrading esterase (SE) from the sensory hair lymph that can degrade pheromone at a half-life rate of less than 15 msec (Vogt *et al.*, 1985). It seems likely that, in the Kasang and Kaissling experiments described, most of the pheromone was not entering the sensory hairs rapidly but rather was entering into the thick cuticle of the hair and either moving slowly inward through the hair wall or moving slowly laterally through surface lipids to a pore tubule and subsequently entering the hair. Once the molecules entered the hair they were rapidly degraded, as evidenced by the similar half-times for penetration and slow degradation observed in the three species described.

The likely candidate for the rapid degradation of these slow penetrating pheromone molecules is the sensillar esterase. These experiments suggest that the SE may have a dual role in noise reduction by rapidly degrading pheromone: (1) by ensuring a short residence time for behaviorally relevant pheromone molecules, and (2) by preventing slow entering background pheromone from being detected. It may yet prove the case that only pheromone molecules striking at pore openings enter the hair rapidly enough to induce a behavioral response (Futrelle, 1984).

2. The Nature of the Association between Binding Protein and Pheromone

A qualitative equilibrium binding assay was established for the *A. polyphemus* pheromone-binding protein (PBP) by J. Hemberger, at the time working with the Kaissling group at Seewiesen (Kaissling *et al.*, 1985; De Kramer and Hemberger, Chapter 13, this volume). Experimental details of this assay were never published, but the procedure utilized the fact that lipophilic pheromone molecules tend to adsorb onto the walls of a glass vessel from an aqueous solution (J. Hemberger, personal communication; see De Kramer and Hemberger, Chapter 13). Inclusion of a soluble carrier, such as soluble protein, can reduce the amount of adsorption onto glass walls. As such, the assay is really a measurement of the effectiveness of a protein to solubilize hydrophobic molecules.

Using this assay, Hemberger found that inclusion of PBP held an equimolar concentration of pheromone in solution. This suggested that the binding protein possessed a single, saturable site for association with pheromone. Hemberger compared the ability of binding protein to solubilize several other molecules (16 : Ac, E6,Z11-16 : OH, geraniol) with the pheromone (E6,Z11-16 : Ac) (De Kramer and Hemberger, Chapter 13). Both acetates showed similar increased solubility in the presence of PBP, while the two alcohols showed very little solubility in the presence of PBP, suggesting that the binding site of PBP could discriminate between alcohols and acetates. Unfortunately, these differences in solubility may be attributable to differences in glass binding-affinity among the four molecules tested, which was not controlled for in Hemberger's experiments. For example, the same results would be obtained if the alcohols have a higher affinity adsorption onto the glass walls than the acetates. Experiments of M. Tasayco (Prestwich, Chapter 14, Table I, this volume) indicate that different functional groups affect the water solubility of pheromone molecules, and that this is further influenced by the species of carrier protein present, the buffer system used, and the pretreatment conditions of the glass vessel.

Nevertheless, as the metabolic product of the *A. polyphemus* acetate pheromone is the corresponding alcohol, Hemberger's experiments suggest that the *A. polyphemus* PBP will solubilize and carry pheromone but not its degradation product. Pheromone-binding proteins thus might act to some degree as molecular filters, allowing only certain molecules entry into the hair through selective solubilization but not solubilizing degradation products. Under conditions of low solubility, these degradation products would leave the lymph, perhaps to absorb into the dendritic membrane or the hair cuticle, or be available for transport from the lymph across the apical membrane of the basal epithelial cells.

Hemberger used this glass binding assay to derive a binding constant (K_d) of 10^{-7} for the PBP–pheromone association (De Kramer and Hemberger, Chapter 13, this volume). A binding constant of this volume suggests moderate affinity between ligand and binding protein and is consistent with the ligand specificity demonstrated for this interaction. Hemberger suggested that with such an affinity the protein could act well as a carrier, delivering pheromone to a receptor which might have an expected K_d in the range of 10^{-9}. In contrast, Kaissling (Kaissling *et al.*, 1985) reported the K_d derived by Hemberger to be somewhat lower, 5×10^{-8}. Kaissling has repeatedly used this value to argue against the carrier function of PBP and in favor of pore tubules being direct conduits of pheromone from hair wall to receptor (Kaissling, 1986a,b). Kaissling argued that a binding protein of such high concentration (20 mM) and high affinity association would never release pheromone to a receptor and would greatly reduce the rate of pheromone degradation by any enzymes present. Rather, Kaissling has favored our original proposal that the PBP functions as his proposed nonenzymatic mechanism underlying "early inactivation" (Kaissling, 1986a).

In order to determine experimentally a binding constant, one must demonstrate that the receptor (PBP) can be saturated by the ligand (pheromone). The only saturation data which these researchers have published (Kaissling *et al.*, 1985) indicate that their repeated binding constants (K_d) are in error. A K_d is analogous to a K_m of an enzymatic reaction and would approximate the pheromone concentration where half the receptor population is in the bound state. In their data (Kaissling *et al.*, 1985), this half-saturation point clearly is presented as occurring around $2 \times 10^{-6} M$. Thus, their data actually suggest a considerably higher K_d than reported, in the micromolar range.

While the glass binding assay may be suited to rapid and qualitative analysis of several parameters of binding protein action, it does not seem valid for the derivation of a kinetically relevant binding constant. The lipophilic pheromone molecule will not stay in aqueous solution if a less polar surface is available. Thus the molecules adsorb onto glass surfaces. Given a soluble phase of similar affinity as the glass wall, i.e., binding protein, one would predict a distribution of pheromone between these two relatively lipophilic species of binding site. This is what Hemberger observed in his experiments. Pheromone was observed bound either to glass walls or to protein; only trace amounts were observed free in aqueous solution (Kaissling *et al.*, 1985). The nature of molecular interactions within this biochemical system preclude the validity of this method of analysis.

In our experiments with the PBP, there does not appear to be a tight association between it and pheromone, and thus we would expect a higher binding constant than those proposed by Hemberger and Kaissling. Certainly, we did not see binding protein interfere with the rate of pheromone degradation until protein concentration exceeded $10^{-5} M$ (Vogt and Riddiford, 1986a). This held even for the lowest pheromone concentrations of $10^{-9} M$. One might expect more protein interference were the K_d in the range of 5×10^{-8}, as Kaissling suggests (Kaissling *et al.*, 1985). The behavior of PBP in our experiments suggests that the K_d might be in the micromolar range. Interestingly, the K_m for sensillar esterase–pheromone interactions is also in this same range (Vogt *et al.*, 1985).

Our experiments have suggested a weak association between individual binding protein and pheromone molecules but that at the *in situ* binding protein concentrations there is a strong bulk association. Thus, we suggested that pheromone becomes solubilized into a proteinaceous phase and migrates within this phase to receptor and enzyme. Evidence for this comes from a reevaluation of previously published fluorograms of electrophoretic gels which compared antennal proteins of different species of moths and the ability of these proteins to bind *A. polyphemus* pheromone (Vogt and Riddiford, 1981a). In these studies, we observed pheromone binding to putative binding proteins of male antennae of each species. We also observed pheromone binding to most of the other proteins present in these gels. We have since suggested that, for the majority of these associations, pheromone premixed with protein samples was phase partitioned into the gel, migrating with the respective proteins, stable within these multiple and separating proteinaceous phases (Vogt and Riddiford, 1986a).

We are left with the dilemma of how to quantify the relatively weak association between pheromone and PBP. Both Hemberger's (Kaissling *et al.*, 1985) and our experiments (Vogt and Riddiford, 1986a) suggest that the K_d could be in the micromolar range. The difficulty with determining binding constants in this range is that the ligand (i.e., pheromone) does not remain associated to its receptor (i.e., binding protein) long enough to measure the existence of the association (Pace and Lancet, Chapter 15, this volume). Recently, Pevsner *et al.* (1986) reported an odorant-binding protein (OBP) from bovine olfactory mucus, and they proposed a very similar mechanism for this protein as we propose for the PBP. Pevsner utilized a modified filter binding assay which allowed the derivation of odorant–protein binding constants in this elusive micromolar range. After incubating protein with tritium-labeled odorants, the incubate was filtered through glass fiber filters modifed with polyethylenimine (Pevsner *et al.*, 1985). The protein with bound odorant adsorbs to the modified filters, and the unbound odorant passes through. This assay may prove useful for determining binding characteristics of the PBP as well.

Regardless of the actual value of the binding constant, the experiments of Hemberger (Kaissling *et al.*, 1985; De Kramer and Hemberger, Chapter 13, this volume) show that there is a single saturable site for pheromone association with the binding protein molecule. Furthermore, the site of association may discriminate between physiologically relevant molecules, i.e., pheromone and its degradative product. This finding suggests a filtering role for the binding protein, adding new depth to its multifunctional role in pheromone reception. As De Kramer and Hemberger indicate (Chapter 13), it would be very interesting to know whether the other pheromone component of this system (E6,Z11-16 : Al, associates with the PBP as well.

3.   Invoking Diffusion as a Mechanism of Pheromone Transport: A Criticism

Adam and Delbrück (1968) presented a theoretical argument that molecules, to be caught from great spatial distance by a relatively one-dimensional receptor, must first go through a reduction in dimension. Molecules must pass from three-dimensional space to two-dimensional space, and then diffuse through two-dimensional space until encountering the one-dimensional receptor. Adam and Delbrück chose pheromone reception in *Bombyx mori* as a biological example of their theory. In this example, pheromone molecules were envisioned to move through three-dimensional space from a far distant female source and to adsorb onto a two-dimensional surface of a male sensory hair. The molecules then diffused along the two-dimensional surface of the hair to a one-dimensional pore, where they entered the hair. At the time when Adam and Delbrück proposed this scheme, the nature of the pore–tubule system was unknown.

There were two major errors in the assumptions of the applicability of pheromone reception to their theory. First, pheromone molecules do not move great distances to a sensory hair. A male moth enters air which already contains a certain concentration of pheromone molecules. The pheromone concentration threshold required to induce wing fluttering in *B. mori* was estimated at 10,000 molecules/cm³ (Schneider *et al.*, 1968), which translates to an average distribution of one molecule every 0.5 mm in space. As the pheromone concentration increases from the threshold and the intramolecular spacing decreases, pheromone molecules become increasingly space filling in behaviorally relevant time, due to their random kinetic motion (Berg and Purcell, 1977; Futrelle, 1984). Thus, even on a molecular scale, pheromone molecules are not captured from great distance by sensory hairs. The second error was an assumption that sensory hair cuticle is a nonabsorbing, two-dimensional surface. It now seems highly probable that a great deal of pheromone enters and becomes temporarily trapped within the very thick hair cuticle (see Section IV,D,1; Steinbrecht, Chapter 11, this volume; Kasang, 1973; Kanaujia and Kaissling, 1985). Thus, it is quite possible that only those molecules striking directly on a pore are internalized rapidly enough to be considered behaviorally relevant (Futrelle, 1984). Such molecules would, counter to Adam and Delbrück's theory, be moving directly from three-dimensional to one-dimensional space.

Members of the Kaissling group have repeatedly invoked two-dimensional and one-dimensional diffusion to describe the processes by which pheromone moelcules move from hair surface to receptor (Kaissling, 1974, 1986a,b; Kanaujia and Kaissling, 1985; Keil, 1982). Their arguments were based in part on Adam and Delbrück's (1968) analysis, and on Steinbrecht and Müller's (1971) demonstration of contacts between pore tubules and dendrites. Thus both Kaissling (1974, 1986a,b) and Keil (1982) suggested that pheromone arrives at a receptor in the dendritic membrane after diffusing first along the hair surface to a pore (two-dimensional), then down the pore–tubule conduit (one-dimensional) directly to the receptor. Keil (1984) noted that he only rarely observed tubule–dendrite contacts. He suggested, however, that based on estimated diffusion coefficients (Kaissling, 1974), a pheromone molecule possessed ample time to locate the rare pore–tubule complex made contact with the correct dendrite. These researchers have suggested that if a pheromone molecule diffuses down a blind tubule, it will diffuse back out again, diffuse to another pore–tubule complex, and diffuse down it, searching for a dendrite, and it will do this within several milliseconds. This scheme seems dubious in light of the Seewiesen group's own experimental data. For example, Kanaujia and Kaissling (1985) found that, even after 2 min, less than half of the applied pheromone molecules had entered the sensory hair of *A. polyphemus*. The majority of applied pheromone molecules do not appear to enter the sensory hairs within a physiologically and behaviorally relevant time period.

Diffusion is not a mechanism. It is at best a mathematical description of the time course of a process. The mathematics of diffusion assume that the field through which a described element moves is homogeneous. The tissue of a sensory hair is decidedly nonhomogeneous. For example, the mathematics of diffusion might accurately describe how a tritium-labeled ethanol molecule would move through a spatial field of absolute ethanol. In such an analysis, complexities due to different states of ethanol interactions would be ignored. Kaissling (1974, 1986a,b) determined that the time from stimulus arriving at an antenna to the first appearance of an electrical impulse was greater than the time a lipid molecule, restricted to a two-dimensional lipid monolayer, might move 3 μm, the radial distance of a sensory hair. Therefore he invoked diffusion as a mechanism for stimulus migration (Kaissling, 1974).

These insects have evolved nonhomogeneous spatial fields which we call sensory hairs. These hairs include elements of cuticle, elements of pore tubules, phase boundaries, binding proteins, enzymes, dendritic membranes, and receptors, which possess properties allowing pheromone to move through rapidly and induce a behaviorally meaningful electrical impulse in the sensory neuron. As we identify the molecular elements with which pheromone interacts, simplistic concepts of diffusion become increasingly less useful. They serve no better to describe the mechanisms of pheromone reception than to simply state that the system works, therefore it is. Rather, we are challenged by these systems to address the most fundamental question. How do the properties of a complex, multidimensional array of chemical interactions favor a functional state for the organism?

V. TRANSDUCTORY MECHANISMS

We imagine that transduction involves a pheromone molecule binding to a membrane-bound receptor protein, inducing conformational changes in that protein. We further imagine that the receptor protein is directly coupled to one or more ion channels, such that pheromone binding alters (opens?) the conductance state of those channels. Alternatively, we imagine that the receptor protein might be coupled to a second messenger system, such as cyclic nucleotides or inositol, and that this second messenger system induces a transient state change in a population of ion channels through phosphorylation of the channel proteins (Pace and Lancet, Chapter 15, this volume). Consistent with the findings of De Kramer (De Kramer and Hemberger, Chapter 13), these events presumably occur within the dendritic region of the sensory neuron.

Do receptor proteins exist? Support to the affirmative comes from a variety of indirect studies, all of which can be interpreted consistently with the existence of membrane-bound receptor proteins. Structure–activity studies (Carr *et al.*, 1986; Kaissling, 1971, Kafka, 1974a,b; Kafka and Neuwirth, 1975; Kikuchi, 1975; Löfqvist, 1986; Mustaparta *et al.*, 1979; Reed and Chisholm, 1985) suggest that the receptor mechanism shows specificity that only a protein receptor could confer. Protein modifiers, such as sulfhydryl reducing agents, inhibit the responsiveness of sensory neurons, supporting the role of proteins in sensory transductions (Villet, 1974; Norris, 1981; Ma, 1981). Electron micrographs of freeze-fractured membranes of sensory dendrites show structural features referred to as "bumps" which can be interpreted as membrane proteins, possibly receptor proteins (Steinbrecht, 1980). Receptor proteins for amino acids have been isolated from aquatic vertebrates (Cagan and Zeiger, 1978; Pace and Lancet, Chapter 15, this volume).

Recently established techniques have enabled us to search for candidate receptor proteins from the sensory dendrites of *A. polyphemus*. We have isolated sensory dendrites by a modified method of U. Klein (Klein and Keil, 1984; Vogt et al., 1985). Proteins from this preparation have been labeled using a photoaffinity analog of the *A. polyphemus* pheromone (Ganjian et al., 1978; Prestwich et al., 1984, 1986a), an analog reported to possess physiological activity (Ganjian et al., 1978). In our assay, the tritium-labeled photoaffinity analog was allowed to incubate for 15–30 min with tissue, allowing for its association with protein. The preparation was then irradiated with ultraviolet light, inducing modification in the analog allowing its covalent attachment to the protein, thus radioactively labeling the protein. The reactions were then analyzed by slab gel electrophoresis followed by fluorography. In these studies, (R. G. Vogt, G. D. Prestwich, and L. M. Riddiford, unpublished), we have repeatedly observed this pheromone analog attached to a 67,000-dalton protein isolated from the sensory dendrite membrane. Coincubation with native pheromone reduced binding significantly (Prestwich et al., 1986a). Furthermore, this protein appears to be unique to sensory hairs. We interpret these experiments to indicate that we have visualized a putative membrane-bound receptor for the *A. polyphemus* pheromone.

The secondary events of signal transduction, i.e., ion channel activation following receptor activation, also remain unclear. De Kramer (1985; De Kramer and Hemberger, Chapter 13, this volume) presents convincing evidence of a dendritic spiking mechanism, which would suggest that voltage-sensitive channels are present in the dendritic membrane. In this case one might also expect receptor-sensitive channels. There might also be one or more classes of second messenger–mediated channels, as well as other membrane-bound proteins belonging to second messenger pathways. Villet (1978) demonstrated that antennal perfusion of dibutyryl cyclic AMP produced an enhanced electroantennogram response to pheromone stimulation in *Antheraea pernyi*. Wieczorek (Hansen and Wieczorek, 1981) found a similar effect in fly taste receptors exposed to dibutyryl cyclic GMP. In both situations, the cyclic nucleotides appeared to have a role of modulation, rather than of direct signal transduction.

It is clear that the sensory dendrites provide a rich source of a family of proteins involved in signal transduction. Recently, a cyclic AMP pathway was demonstrated to be involved in olfactory transduction among vertebrates (Pace and Lancet, 1986, Chapter 15, this volume). At the 1986 International Symposium on Olfaction and Taste, July 20–24, at Snowmass Village, Colorado, there were several reports of both cyclic AMP and inositol pathways operating in olfactory transduction. At the time of this meeting, it remained a question whether these pathways were inducing or modulating the output response of these sensory neurons. Needless to say, as I write this chapter, there is an enormous renewed interest in the molecular mechanisms underlying olfaction.

VI. SPECIES COMPARISONS: THE BIOCHEMISTRY OF PHEROMONE RECEPTION IN THE GYPSY MOTH

We have proposed a molecular model for pheromone reception based on our studies of *A. polyphemus*. Can we generalize this kinetic equilibrium model to other lepidopteran insects? Support to the affirmative comes from a variety of comparative studies of other moth species. These studies indicate that biochemical elements similar to those observed in *A. polyphemus* sensory hairs are associated with male antennae of other species as well. For example, we have observed putative pheromone-binding proteins in several lepidopteran antennae (Vogt and Riddiford, 1981a). Additionally, antennal pheromone-degrading capabilities have been repeatedly demonstrated for several species beside *A. polyphemus* (Vogt *et al.*, 1985), including *Bombyx mori* (Kasang and Kaissling, 1972), *Trichoplusia ni* (Ferkovich *et al.*, 1973), *Lymantria dispar* (Kasang, 1974; Prestwich, Chapter 14, this volume), and *Heliothis virescens* (Prestwich, Chapter 14).

We (R. G. Vogt and G. D. Prestwich, unpublished) have recently begun detailed comparative studies of the biochemical mechanisms underlying pheromone reception in the gypsy moth, *Lymantria dispar*. This species has proved tremendously amenable to pheromone studies at the behavioral (David *et al.*, 1983; Preiss, 1985; Preiss and Kramer. 1983, 1986a,b) and physiological levels (Hansen, 1984), and now we are finding it equally suited to pheromone studies at the molecular level. The male moth has large, plumose antennae possessing a great number of long, trichoid sensory hairs. Like those of *A. polyphemus*, these sensory hairs are nearly all identical and specifically sensitive to the female sex pheromone. Such tissue homogeneity is requisite for biochemical studies of high resolution.

The gypsy moth has long been known throughout the Eurasian Palearctic regions, from Britain to Japan (South, 1907). Since its accidental introduction into into the Boston, Massachusetts, area in 1869 (Evans, 1985), the gypsy moth has spread throughout the eastern United States. During the last few years it has made west coast appearances in the San Francisco, California, area, areas surrounding Eugene, Oregon, and in Seattle, Washington. Both its Eurasian range and the its preferred food source (oak leaves) are shared with the sibling species nun moth, *Lymantria monacha* (South, 1907). These two species also share the same sex pheromone.

The sensory hairs of the gypsy and nun moths are reported to each possess two neurons, specifically sensitive to the epoxide *cis*-7,8-epoxy-2-methyloctadecane (Hansen, 1984). This molecule can appear in two enantiomeric forms as (7*R*,8*S*)- or (7*S*,8*R*)-7,8-epoxy-2-methyloctadecane, (+)-disparlure and (−)-disparlure, respectively. The actual sex attractant for both gypsy moth and nun moth is (+)-disparlure. However, several studies (Hansen, 1984; Preiss, 1985; Preiss and Kramer, 1983, 1986a) have suggested an interesting chemical interplay between these two species. The gypsy moth pheromone gland synthesizes only (+)-disparlure; however, its sensory hairs each possess two neurons, one sensitive to (+)- and one sensitive to (−)-disparlure. The nun moth pheromone gland synthesizes both (+)- and (−)-disparlure; however, its sensory hairs each possess two neurons, one sensitive to (+)- but neither sensitive to (−)-disparlure. Presented separately in enantiomerically pure form, (+)-disparlure elicits a behavioral response in gypsy moth and (−)-disparlure does nothing. However, when presented together, (−)-disparlure inhibits certain aspects of the gypsy moth behavior induced by (+)-disparlure (Preiss and Kramer, 1983, 1986a). Apparently, the nun moth releases a pheromone blend which is perceived as monochrome and attractive among its own males [sensory neurons only for (+)] but polychrome and inhibitory to gypsy moth males [sensory hairs for (+) and (−)]. Clearly this is a candidate mechanism for species isolation. How are these enantiomers distinguished and processed within the sensory hairs?

Kasang *et al.* (1974) demonstrated that tritium-labeled disparlure could be metabolized by intact gypsy moth antennae. Metabolites were not identifed, nor was tissue specificity investigated (see Section IV,D,1). We (Prestwich *et al.*, 1987) have synthesized enantiomerically pure and tritium-labeled (+)- and (−)-disparlure, as well as racemic tritium-labeled disparlure, and have begun using these probes in metabolic studies. These studies have demonstrated that the antennae of male and female gypsy moths possess an epoxide hydrolase that rapidly degrades disparlure by hydrating the molecule to the corresponding *threo*-diol, thus opening the epoxide ring. Both enantiomeric forms are degraded at comparable rates. This enzyme system is present in no other tissue in either sex. The enzymatic activity is present in isolated pheromone-specific sensory hairs and appears to be associated with membrane material. Allowing for the relative small size of gypsy moth antennae, the rate of degradation of the disparlure by male antennae is comparable to that seen in *A. polyphemus* studies of E6,Z11-16 : Ac degradation (Vogt *et al.*, 1985). Current studies are focusing on whether there are two enzymes involved, specific for each enantiomeric form, or

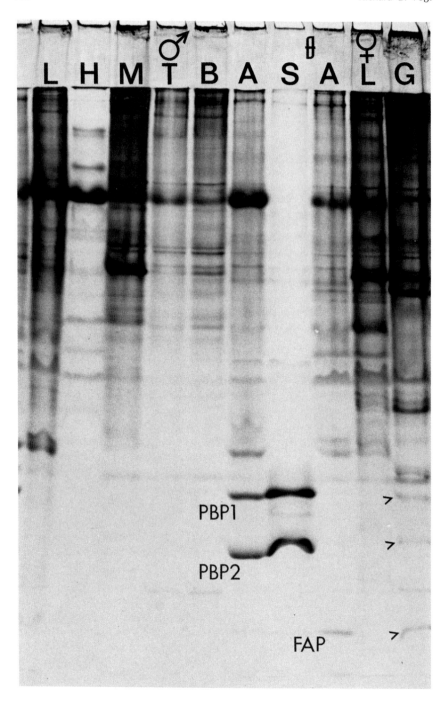

whether a single enzyme is capable of recognizing both enantiomeric forms of this pheromone.

In addition, electrophoretic analysis of homogenates of isolated sensory hairs shows two prominent soluble proteins, candidates as pheromone-binding proteins (Fig. 7). Both proteins are unique to the male antennae and are not found in blood, other neural tissue, other integumental tissue, or muscle. These proteins may be present in very low amounts in female antennae, but only at a level reflecting the equally small number of sensory hairs present on female antennae. Both proteins are associated with isolated sensory hairs in such a way to suggest that they are situated in the extracellular sensory hair lymph. Both proteins are routinely seen in preparations from individual animals, suggesting that they are not allelic forms of the same functional protein.

Though these studies are still at a preliminary stage, they clearly support the biochemical strategy demonstrated by our studies of *A. polyphemus*. That is, in pheromone-sensitive sensory hairs there are unique enzyme systems present for the rapid degradation of pheromone and high concentrations of unique proteins functioning as pheromone carriers/solubilizers. However, the gypsy moth studies may go considerably further in revealing certain basic biological principles. Consider the bizarre pheromone interplay between these two species, *L. dispar* and *L. monacha*. Clearly, the female pheromone glands and male sensory hairs have coevolved. Is it possible that the genes which code for these two organs/processes are linked? It is our hope that the proteins we are studying will give us access to the genes which code for the family of unique elements of the sensory hair and pheromone gland. Such molecular biological studies could shed light not only on (1) the connection between synthesis and reception of pheromone (see Section VII,B), but also on (2) some of the most fundamental events controlling tissue and sexual differentiation within a species and (3) the genetic

---

Fig. 7. This figure represents an electrophoretic study of soluble *Lymantria dispar* proteins, demonstrating the pheromone-binding proteins (PBP) of the sensory hairs (S). Homogenates of a variety of tissues were compared. Dissected tissues, collected on day 1 after adult eclosion, were homogenized in 10 mM Tris buffer, pH 7.0, and microcentrifuged. Supernatants were lyophilized, and fractions were electrophoresed on 15% polyacrylamide gels under nondenaturing conditions. Proteins were visualized using Coomassie blue. From left to right, tissues were as follows (with tissue amounts per lane indicated): L, male leg (6 legs); H, male hemolymph (1 μl); M, male dorsal longitudinal flight muscle (15 mg wet); T, male thoracic ganglia (2.4 mg wet); B, male brain (6 mg wet); A, male antenna (4 antennae); S, pheromone-sensitive sensory hairs isolated from male antennae (0.45 mg dry, see text for isolation procedure); A, female antenna (14 antennae); L, female leg (5 legs); and G, female abdominal tip for including sex pheromone gland (3 glands). PBP1 and PBP2 indicate the pheromone-binding proteins; FAP indicates a female antennal specific protein. Note that these three sex-specific antennal proteins appear to be associated with the sex pheromone gland (arrows, lane G). An FAP of similar mobility which associates with pheromone is also present in *Antheraea polyphemus* female antennae (see Figs. 2A and 2B).

mechanisms which underlie evolutionary changes regulating the interbreeding status between different species and subspecies (see Sections VII,A and VII,B).

VII. VARIATION IN OLFACTORY PROTEINS: EVOLVABLE ELEMENTS ENCODING INSECT BEHAVIOR

A. Pheromone Blends: Species Signatures, Behavioral Modulators

The species specificity of attractiveness of lepidopteran pheromones has long been assumed to be a powerful isolation mechanisn in mating, especially between closely related species. This specificity is certainly based on the actual chemical structures comprising a pheromone blend (Priesner, 1979, 1986; Reed and Chisholm, 1985). But specificity is also based on the precise ratio of the molecules comprising the total pheromone blend (Linn and Roelofs, 1985; Linn et al., 1986; O'Connell, 1986; O'Connell et al., 1986). For example, A. polyphemus males are trapped most effectively by a 9 : 1 ratio of acetate : aldehyde (Kochansky et al., 1975). This sibling species A. pernyi responds to the same pheromone components, but in opposite ratio (Boeckh and Boeckh, 1979).

Until recently, pheromone researchers have tended to consider the "the major component" of a pheromone blend as the attractant, chiefly because major components were often effective as trap bait (Kochansky et al., 1975). Other "minor components" were guessed to have either species-identifying roles or subtle behavioral roles. Considerable evidence now supports that the components, major and minor, can act in concert to identify the species to the male (Linn, 1986; Linn and Roelofs, 1983, 1985; Linn et al., 1986). Thus the entire pheromone blend appears to function as a species signature. The precision of this signature appears to be species specific. Miller and Roelofs (1980) observed minimal variation in the pheromone composition of individual female redbanded leafroller moths, Argyrotaenia velutinana. However, Löfstedt et al. (1985) observed quite large variation in the relative amounts of pheromone components ($\pm$32–127%) released from individual female turnip moths, Agrotis segetum. Löfstedt et al. (1985) suggested that the degree of variation in pheromone composition might be under the control of selective pressures unique to each species.

In addition to their role as species signature, the individual components of a pheromone blend also have the capacity to convey information concerning distance from a pheromone source and thereby modulate the behavior of the male. Nakamura (1981) demonstrated this phenomenon in the moth Spodoptera litura. Spodoptera litura utilizes a two-component pheromone: Z9,E11-14 : Ac and Z9,E12-14 : Ac, present in females in the ratio 10 : 1 (Tamaki et al., 1973). In this system, the minor component (Z9,E12-14 : Ac) induced a landing and walking response in the male when he was near the pheromone source in the field (Nakamura, 1981).

A similar situation was demonstrated by Howse *et al.* (1986) in the pine beauty moth, *Panolis flammea* (Noctuidae). This moth utilizes a three-component pheromone, Z9-14 : Ac, Z11-14 : Ac, and Z11-16 : Ac, present in the female in the ratio of 100 : 5 : 1 (Baker *et al.*, 1982). Howse and colleagues studied the behaviors of male moths attracted to an odor source in a wind tunnel. In these experiments, upwind flight could not be elicited by the major component, Z9-14 : Ac, alone, but required the other components as well, supporting the hypothesis that the entire blend is required to initiate male interest in pheromone (Linn, 1986). However, the studies went on to demonstrate that landing at a source and subsequent copulation were strongly influenced by Z11-14 : Ac and Z11-16 : Ac, respectively.

The Nakamura (1981) and Howse *et al.* (1986) experiments suggest that, as a male approaches a female, the concentration of the minor components increases with the resulting increase in stimulation of the neurons sensitive to these components. This increase in input stimulation leads to a modulation of the male mating behaviors.

Thus we see a situation where biosynthetic pathways within pheromone glands have been selected to produce differing levels of potential pheromone components (Van Der Pers and Löfstedt, 1986). The ratio of these components in total is recognized by the male as a species signature. The individual components can convey independent information concerning the source distance, resulting in modulation of the male's precopulatory behaviors.

B. Intraspecies Variations in Female Pheromone Production and in Male Responsiveness

The composition of a sex pheromone blend is not necessarily constant throughout a given species. For example, Klun and colleagues (Klun *et al.*, 1975; Klun and Maini, 1979) have demonstrated genetically based variation in the pheromone blend from different populations of the European corn borer, *Ostrinia nubilalis*. The pheromone of this species is a blend of the enantiomers Z11-14 : Ac and E11-14 : Ac. European and North American populations of this moth were identified to utilize $Z:E$ ratios 100 : 0, 97 : 3, 50 : 50, and 3 : 97. Males from the 97 : 3 population were unresponsive when presented with a 3 : 97 blend. Crossbreeding of 97 : 3 and 3 : 97 individuals produced hybrid females intermediate in their produced ratio (50 : 50) and hybrid males who were most attracted to this intermediate blend ratio. Thus, the control of the $Z:E$ ratio in the female and male responsiveness to this ratio were coheritable traits.

A number of studies have demonstrated similar phenomena among other insect species. Populations of the pine bark beetle, *Ips pini*, from western and eastern

United States utilize different enantiomeric ratios of ipsdienol (2-methyl-6-methylene-2,7-octadiene-4-ol) (Lanier et al., 1980; Birch et al., 1980). Eastern beetles produce and respond to a $65:35$ $(+):(-)$ ratio, while western beetles produce and respond to $(-)$-ipsdienol. Western beetles are apparently inhibited by $(+)$-ipsdienol. When these populations were crossed in breeding experiments, the hybrid females showed intermediate attractiveness to males (Piston and Lanier, 1974), and hybrid males showed intermediate numbers of enantiomeric-specific sensory neurons (Mustaparta et al., 1985).

Southern California populations of the western avocado leafroller moth, *Amorbia cuneana*, utilize the isomers (E,E)- and (E,Z)-10,12-tetradecadien-1-ol acetate for their sex pheromone. Three populations have been demonstrated based on their utilization of $E,E:E,Z$ enantiomeric ratios of $63:37$, $42:58$, and $11:89$, respectively (Bailey et al., 1986). The $42:58$ population was thought to represent a hybrid overlap of the other two populations.

Two races of larch budmoth, *Zeiraphera diniana*, coexist in a mixed habitat in the Engadine valley of Switzerland. A race with dark-colored larvae feed on larch trees, while another race with light-colored larvae feed on pine trees. The two races utilize different pheromones. The larch feeders utilize the 14-carbon acetate E11-14:Ac, while the pine feeders utilize the 12-carbon acetate E9-12:Ac (Guerin et al., 1984). Again, this specificity is observed for both pheromone synthesis and reception.

Thus we see several examples of different intraspecific populations of animals showing a high degree of evolutionary plasticity in their pheromone synthesis–reception systems. Repeatedly, pheromone synthesis and reception show co-heritability. Klun and Maini (1979) suggested that the alleles controlling the isomer composition of the female pheromone might also regulate male responsiveness, or, alternatively, that different but closely linked gene loci might be responsible for regulating the two processes. Thus, if we could gain access to the genes specifying one of the unique elements of pheromone production/reception, we might also gain access to the molecular mechanisms governing the coevolution of these two processes. We now appear to be at that stage in our studies of the molecular basis of pheromone reception.

C. Intra- and Interspecies Variation in Sensory Hair Proteins

In the course of this chapter I have presented evidence of biochemical pathways within the sensory hairs that determine critical aspects of a male moth's precopulatory flight behavior. The ability of a male to follow a pheromone plume effectively to a female seems to depend on his ability to change behavior rapidly on exit from and entry into pheromone packets (Fig. 1; David et al., 1983). But the male does not respond directly to the the external world of pheromone fluctuations. Rather, male precopulatory behaviors are modulated in response to biochemically recreated fluctuations within the sensory hairs. This poses a rather interesting question. If there were variation in the properties of the sensory hair proteins between individuals, would this be reflected in variation in the pre-copulatory behaviors of these individuals? Stated more generally, can variation in behavior between individuals be ascribed to genetic variation of the neural proteins which encode these behaviors?

I have begun assessing the type and degree of variation in the properties of the sensillar esterase (SE) and the pheromone-binding protein (PBP) in two populations of *A. polyphemus*. These populations are adults reared from wild pupae collected from Racine County, Wisconsin (fall of 1985), and wild-collected males from Long Island, New York, lured to pheromone-releasing females (summer of 1986). I have electrophoretically examined the pattern and activity of these proteins isolated from individual animals (Fig. 8). Typically, the SE appears as a quartet to octet of uniformly spaced bands. All males yield multiple esterase bands; however, the presence of a particular identifiable band varies from one individual to the next. Esterase activity varies between the different bands of one individual, as well as between identifiable bands from different individuals. At this time I have no knowledge of the nature of these differences, though they may be caused by a combination of allelic differences between individuals complicated by sequential modification (i.e., glycosylation) and polygenic expression. The PBP shows two forms, one form migrating slightly faster than the other. An individual male may yield either band singly, or a doublet of the two (Fig. 8).

It is difficult as yet to draw conclusions on differences in variation between the Wisconsin and New York populations, as insufficient numbers of animals have been analyzed ($n = 20$ for each population). However, there is strong evidence for significant genetic drift between these populations. A genetic marker distinguishing these populations is present in the form of an epidermal esterase (EE, Fig. 8) (Vogt and Riddiford, 1986b). This esterase is present in gels of Wisconsin and Indiana (source in Vogt and Riddiford, 1986b) animals, but completely absent in gels of the New York animals. This may reflect actual absence of the enzyme, or the presence of an esterase in the New York animals with very different substrate specificity in the gel staining procedure. The presence of this marker suggests that a physical barrier, such as the Appalachian Mountains, provides a basis of population isolation for this species.

We have obtained partial N-terminal amino acid sequences of 30 out of an estimated 135 amino acids for the New York and Wisconsin PBPs, combining techniques of electroblotting (Aebersold *et al.*, 1986) and gas-phase microsequencing (Applied Biosystems 470A). These sequences were

```
        5                10                15
N-Ser Pro Glu Ile Met Lys Asn Leu Ser Leu Asn Phe Gly Lys Ala Met Asp Gln Ser
20                  25                30
Lys Asp Glu Leu Asn/Ser Leu Pro Asp Ser Val Val
```

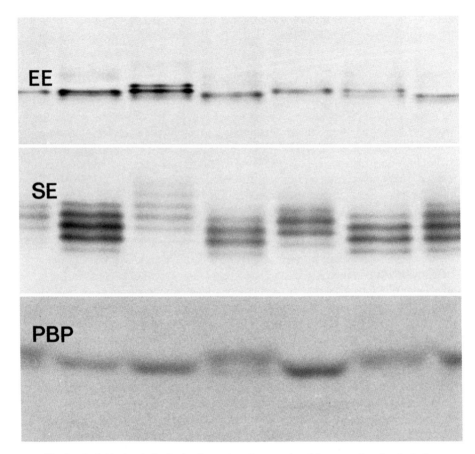

Fig. 8. Individual variation in the electrophoretic properties of three proteins of male *Antheraea polyphemus* antennae. Each lane represents two-thirds of one antenna, isolated from different animals. Adult animals were raised from pupae collected in Wisconsin during the fall of 1985. Tissue was treated as described in the legend to Fig. 7. EE, Epidermal esterase, identified in Vogt and Riddiford (1986b) (see also Fig. 2); SE, sensillar esterase; PBP, pheromone-binding protein. The EE appears to be present as a monomer of several allelic forms, with both homozygous and heterozygous individuals represented. SE is present in a multiplex of bands, with complex individual variation represented. PBP appears to be present as a monomer of two alleles, with both homozygous and heterozygous individuals represented. See text for discussion.

The Wisconsin and New York proteins differed in residue 24, asparagine from New York and serine from Wisconsin. The sequence differences and the presence/absence of the epidermal esterase presumably represent evolved population differences.

We have also obtained a partial N-terminal sequence (20 amino acids) of the higher mobility gypsy moth PBP. This sequence was:

```
         5                    10                   15
N-Ser Lys Asp Val Met His Gln Met Ala Leu Gln Phe Gly Lys Pro Ile Lys Leu Ala/Leu
20                  25                  30
Gln Gln Glu Leu Gly Ala Asp Asp Ser Val Val
```

On inspection, the gypsy moth sequence shows a relatively high degree of amino acid homology (37%) with the *A. polyphemus* proteins. This homology increases considerably (to 63%) with respect to amino acid property (neutral/hydrophobic, neutral/polar, basic, acidic). This interspecies sequence similarity suggests the possibility that, in the course of evolution, as the species diverged, their sensory hair proteins also diverged with respect to amino acid sequence. However, amino acid substitutions were only acceptable if they maintained the overall property function of these proteins. The degree of difference between gypsy moth and *A. polyphemus* PBPs presumably reflects the degree of relatedness of these two species and the differences in the chemical structures comprising their pheromones.

In order to ascribe behavioral variation to protein variation, it is necessary to establish a behavioral assay in which variation in behavior can unequivocally be correlated with variation in protein properties. As such, one might establish a wind tunnel performance test, or a electrophysiological screen, correlated with some aspect of protein property that shows individual variation. We hope to make a first attempt at addressing this issue during the summer of 1987, utilizing Wisconsin-caught *A. polyphemus*. In this study we will compare the electrophoretic variation of these proteins between individuals collected as pupae during the fall of 1986, representing the full genetic potential of the population, with individuals lured to pheromone-releasing females during the summer of 1987, representing behaviorally successful males. Consistent with the proposal favoring skewed variation, we will look for some tightness in the degree of variation in the sexually trapped animals relative to those collected as pupae.

The task of a nervous system is to temporally coordinate muscular activity into a meaningful behavioral output. A major source for temporal control in the nervous system are neural proteins, which exercise their temporal influence through kinetic properties. Thus temporal properties of a neurosynapse would be determined and regulated through the kinetic properties of channel proteins, receptor proteins, proteins involved in transmitter synthesis and release, and proteins involved in second messenger modulation, to name a few. Similarly, the temporal properties of the pheromone-sensitive sensory hairs would be determined and regulated through kinetic properties of the PBPs, pheromone receptors, and pheromone-degrading enzymes. One might well expect that individual variation in any of these elements would yield nervous systems with different temporal properties and individuals with different behavioral personalities (Fig. 9).

Our studies thus far suggest that the population genetics which determine the degree and type of behavioral variability within a population are expressed

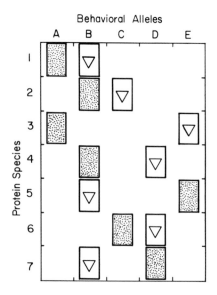

Fig. 9. This figure represents two hypothetical individuals which have inherited different alleles of a set of behaviorally relevant neural proteins. Seven protein species are depicted, each represented at the population level by five allelic forms. If these forms possess different kinetic properties, then individuals inheriting different alleles will possess neuronal components with different temporal properties. The result would be individuals with different temporal personalities with respect to behavioral expression controlled by these proteins.

through individual variability in the properties of neural proteins. It is essential to understand the rules governing this molecular variation in order to understand the behavioral genetics of a population of animals. In the context of controlling populations of insects feeding on economically important crops, such an understanding seems paramount.

VIII. THE FUTURE: THE MOLECULAR BASIS OF PHEROMONE RECEPTION, THE MOLECULAR BASIS OF BEHAVIOR

We have identified a family of proteins which are involved not merely in the functioning of pheromone-sensitive sensory hairs but in the control of an extremely important aspect of sexual behavior. In addition, we have observed individual variation with respect to the properties of these proteins. These studies have led to the assemblage of models which address the mechanisms underlying sensory hair function (kinetic equilibrium model) and mechanisms underlying the temporal aspects of behavior and the evolution of behavior.

Molecular level studies give us access to the mechanisms underlying biological events. Traditional physiological and behavioral experiments inform us of the output of a process, but they fail to describe what the actual process is. Thus we still debate the mechanism underlying sensory transduction of pheromone sensitive sensory hairs (from this volume: Steinbrecht, Chapter 11; De Kramer and Hemberger, Chapter 13; Pace and Lancet, Chapter 15; this chapter, Section V). We now have the tools to isolate and characterize the biochemical mechanism underlying the transductory process, to turn debate into knowledge.

This extends to other areas of research as well. (1) Molecular tools will allow a detailed understanding of the morphogenesis of these sensory hairs. What is the temporal sequence of the molecular construction of a sensory hair? How is this sequence regulated during adult development? How is a pheromone-sensitive sensory hair specified as distinct from other classes of sensory hair? (2) Utilizing techniques of biochemistry and molecular biology we can gain knowledge of the mechanisms underlying evolutionary plasticity. What is the basis of coheritability of the properties of pheromone production and pheromone reception/transduction? What is the basis of the species- and population-isolating properties of the pheromone system? (3) The molecular basis of pheromone reception presents a simple model system for understanding how biochemical processes interact to coordinate behavior. How do the properties of a complex, multidimensional array of chemical interactions favor a functional state for the organism? What are the kinetics governing the reaction rates for these interactions: pheromone–PBP; pheromone–receptor; receptor–channel or receptor–cyclase? How do these proteins interact in concert in the presence of pheromone? How are these rates influenced by pheromone concentrations? Are all interactions equally specific toward the pheromone of the species? Can these reactions be modulated from within the animal, either through regulation of protein turnover or by second messenger mechanisms based on cyclic AMP or inositol?

Above all else, we shall learn what pheromone reception is and how it works. Insect pheromone reception is an outstanding model system for the examination of the mechanistic basis of behavior, amenable to studies at all levels from field to gene. Among strategies for insect control, the insect pheromone system continues to offer one of the few opportunities for management methods which are nonhazardous to other species. Only with a clear knowledge of the true mechanisms underlying pheromone biology can we hope to develop specific and safe insect management strategies which successfully utilize the sex pheromone system.

ACKNOWLEDGMENTS

I am grateful for support of National Service Awards GM07270, GM07108, and N507394. Collaborative research was supported by grants from the National Science Foundation (PCM-80-11152 to L. M. Riddiford and DMB-83-16931 to G. D. Prestwich) and by the U.S. Department of Agriculture Competitive Grants Program 85 CRCR 11736 (to G. D. Prestwich).

REFERENCES

Adam, G., and Delbrück, M. (1968). Reduction of dimensionality in biological diffusion processes. *In* "Structural Chemistry and Molecular Biology" (A. Rich and N. Davidson, eds.), pp. 198–215. Freeman, San Francisco.

Aebersold, R. H., Teplow, D. B., Hood, L. E., and Kent, S. B. H. (1986). Electroblotting onto activated glass. High effeciency preparation of proteins from analytical sodium dodecyl sulfate–polyacrylamide gels for direct sequence analysis. *J. Biol. Chem.* **261**, 4229–4238.

Bailey, J. B., McDonough, L. M., and Hoffmann, M. P. (1986). Western avocado leafroller, *Amorbia cuneana* (Walsingham), (Lepidoptera: Tortricidae), discovery of populations utilizing different ratios of sex pheromone components. *J. Chem. Ecol.* **12**, 1239–1245.

Baker, R., Bradshaw, J. W. S., and Speed, W. (1982). Methoxymercuration–demercuration and mass spectrometry in the identification of the sex pheromones of *Panolis flammea,* the pine beauty moth. *Experientia* **38**, 233–234.

Berg, H. C., and Purcell, E. M. (1977). Physics of chemoreception. *Biophys. J.* **20**, 193–219.

Birch, M. C., Light, D. M., Wood, D. L., Browne, L. E., Silverstein, R. M., Bergot, B. J., Ohloff, G., West, J. R., and Young, J. C. (1980). Pheromonal attraction and allomonal interruption of *Ips pini* in California by the two enantiomers of ipsdienol. *J. Chem. Ecol.* **6**, 703–717.

Boeckh, J., and Boeckh, V. (1979). Threshold and odor specificity of pheromone-sensitive neurons in the deutocerebrum of *Antheraea pernyi* and *A. polyphemus* (Saturnidae). *J. Comp. Physiol.* **132**, 235–242.

Boeckh, J., Kaissling, K. E., and Schneider, D. (1960). Sensillen und Bau der Antennengeissel von *Telea polyphemus* (Vergleiche mit weiteren Saturniden: *Antheraea, Platysamia,* und *Philosamia*). *Zool. J. Anat.* **78**, 559–584.

Cagan, R., and Zeiger, W. N. (1978). Biochemical studies of olfaction: Binding to an isolated olfactory preparation from rainbow trout (*Salmo gardneri*). *Proc. Natl. Acad. Sci. U.S.A.* **75**, 4679–4683.

Carr, W. E. S., Gleeson, R. A., Ache, B. W., and Milstead, M. L. (1986). Olfactory receptors of the spiny lobster: ATP-sensitive cells with similarities to P2-type purinoceptors of vertebrates. *J. Comp. Physiol. A* **158**, 331–338.

David, C. T., Kennedy, J. S., and Ludlow, A. R. (1983). Finding of a sex pheromone source by gypsy moths released in the field. *Nature (London)* **303**, 804–806.

De Kramer, J. J. (1985). The electrical circuitry of an olfactory sensillum in *Antheraea polyphemus.* *J. Neurosci.* **5**, 2484–2493.

Ding, Y.-S., and Prestwich, G. D. (1986). Metabolic transformation of tritium labeled pheromone by tissues of *Heliothis virescens* moths. *J. Chem. Ecol.* **12**, 411–429.

Ernst, K.-D. (1969). Die Feinstruktur von Riechsensillen auf der Antenne des Aaskafers *Necrophorus* (Coleoptera). *Z. Zellforsch.* **94**, 72–102.

Evans, H. E. (1985). "The Pleasures of Entomology, Portraits of Insects and the People Who Study Them." Smithsonian Institution Press, Washington, D.C.

Ferkovich, S. M. (1981). Enzymatic alteration of insect pheromones. *In* "Perception of Behavioral Chemicals" (D. M. Norris, ed.), pp. 165–185. Elsevier/North Holland, Amsterdam.

Ferkovich, S. M., Mayer, M. S., and Rutter, R. R. (1973). Sex pheromone of the cabbage looper: Reactions with antennal proteins *in vitro. J. Insect Physiol.* **19**, 2231–2243.

Ferkovich, S. M., Van Essen, F., and Taylor, T. R. (1980). Hydrolysis of sex pheromone by antennal esterases of the cabbage looper, *Trichoplusia ni. Chem. Senses Flavour* **5**, 33–45.

Futrelle, R. P. (1984). How molecules get to their detectors, the physics of diffusion of insect pheromones. *Trends Neurosci.* **7**, 116–120.

Ganjian, I., Pettei, M. J., Nakanishi, K., and Kaissling, K. E. (1978). A photoaffinity-labelled insect sex pheromone for the moth *Antheraea polyphemus. Nature (London)* **271**, 157–158.

Guerin, P. M., Baltrensweiler, W., Arn, H., and Buser, H.-R. (1984). Host race pheromone polymorphism in the larch budmoth. *Experientia* **40**, 892–894.

Hansen, K. (1984). Discrimination and production of disparlure enantiomers by the gypsy moth and the nun moth. *Physiol. Entomol.* **9**, 9–18.

Hansen, K., and Wieczorek, H. (1981). Biochemical aspects of sugar reception in insects. *In* "Biochemistry of Taste and Olfaction" (R. H. Cagen and M. R. Kare, eds.), pp. 139–162. Academic Press, New York.

Haynes, K. E., and Birch, M. C. (1984). The periodicity of pheromone release and male responsiveness in the artichoke plume moth, *Platyptilia carduidactyla. Physiol. Entomol.* **9**, 287–295.

Howse, P. E., Lisk, J. C., and Bradshaw, J. W. S. (1986). The role of pheromones in the control of behavioural sequences in insects. *In* "Mechanisms in Insect Olfaction" (T. L. Payne, M. C. Birch, and C. E. J. Kennedy, eds.), pp. 157–162. Oxford Univ. Press (Clarendon), London and New York.

Kafka, W. A. (1974a). Physiochemical aspects of odor reception in insects. *Ann. N.Y. Acad. Sci.* **237**, 76–88.

Kafka, W. A. (1974b). A formalism on selective molecular interactions. *In* "Biochemistry of Sensory Functions" (L. Jaenicke, ed.), pp. 275–278. Springer-Verlag, New York.

Kafka, W. A., and Neuwirth, J. (1975). A model of pheromone molecule–acceptor interaction. *Z. Naturforsch.* **30**, 278–282.

Kaissling, K. E. (1969). Kinetics of olfactory receptor potentials. *In* "Olfaction and Taste" (C. Pfaffman, ed.), pp. 52–70. Rockefeller University Press, New York.

Kaissling, K. E. (1971). Insect olfaction. *In* "Handbook of Sensory Physiology (L. M. Beidler, ed.), Vol. 4, pp. 351–431. Springer-Verlag, Berlin.

Kaissling, K. E. (1974). Sensory transduction in insect olfactory receptors. *In* "Biochemistry of Sensory Functions" (L. Jaenicke, ed.), pp. 243–273. Springer-Verlag, Berlin.

Kaissling, K. E. (1977). Control of insect behavior via chemoreceptor organs. *In* "Chemical Control of Insect Behavior—Theory and Application" (H. H. Shorey and J. J. McKelvey, eds.), pp. 45–65. Wiley, New York.

Kaissling, K. E. (1986a). Chemo-electrical transduction in insect olfactory receptors. *Annu. Rev. Neurosci.* **9**, 121–145.

Kaissling, K. E. (1986b). Transduction processes in olfactory receptors of moths. *In* "Molecular Entomology" (J. Law, ed.). UCLA Symposia, Alan R. Liss, New York.

Kaissling, K. E. (1969). Kinetics of olfactory receptor potentials. *In* "Olfaction and Taste III" (C. M. Pfaffmann, ed.), pp. 52–70. Rockefeller University Press, New York.

Kaissling, K. E., and Thorson, J. (1980). Insect olfactory sensilla: Structural, chemical and electrical aspects of the functional organization. *In* "Receptors for Neurotransmitters, Hormones and Pheromones in Insects" (D. B. Sattelle, L. M. Hall, and J. G. Hildebrand, eds.), pp. 261–282. Elsevier/North Holland, Amsterdam.

Kaissling, K. E., Klein, U., De Kramer, J. J., Keil, T. A., Kanaujia, S., and Hemberger, J. (1985). Insect olfactory cells: Electrophysiological and biochemical studies. *In* "Molecular Basis of Nerve Activity" (Proc. Int. Symp. in Memory of D. Nachmansohn, Oct. 1984) (J. P. Changeux, F. Hucho, E. Maelicke, and E. Neumann, eds.), pp. 173–183. de Gruyter, Berlin.

Kanaujia, S., and Kaissling, K. E. (1985). Interactions of pheromone with moth antennae: Adsorption, desorption and transport. *J. Insect Physiol.* **31**, 71–81.

Kasang, G. (1971). Bombykol reception and metabolism on the antennae of the silkmoth *Bombyx mori. In* "Gustation and Olfaction" (G. Ohloff and A. F. Thomas, eds.), pp. 245–250. Academic Press, New York.

Kasang, G. (1973). Physikochemische Vorgange beim Riechen des Seidenspinners. *Naturwissenschaften* **60**, 95–101.

Kasang, G. (1974). Uptake of the sex pheromone ³H-bombykol and related compounds by male and female *Bombyx* antennae. *J. Insect Physiol.* **20**, 2407–2422.

Kasang, G., and Kaissling, K. E. (1972). Specificity of primary and secondary olfactory processes in *Bombyx* antennae. *In* "International Symposium Olfaction and Taste IV" (D. Schneider, ed.), pp. 200–206, Wiss. Verlagses, Stuttgart.

Kasang, G., Knauer, B., and Beroza, M. (1974). Uptake of the sex attractant ³H-disparlure by male gypsy moth antennae (*Lymantria dispar*). *Experientia* **30**, 147–148.

Keil, T. A. (1982). Contacts of pore tubules and sensory dendrites in antennal chemosensilla of a silkmoth: Demonstration of a possible pathway for olfactory molecules. *Tiss. Cell* **14**, 451–462.

Keil, T. A. (1984a). Reconstruction and morphometry of silkmoth olfactory hairs: A comparative study of sensilla trichodea on the antennae of male *Antheraea polyphemus* and *Antheraea pernyi* (Insecta, Lepidoptera). *Zoomorphology* **104**, 147–156.

Keil, T. A. (1984b). Surface coats of pore tubules and olfactory sensory dendrites of a silkmoth revealed by cationic markers. *Tiss. Cell* **16**, 705–717.

Kennedy, J. S., Ludlow, A. R., and Sanders, C. J. (1980). Guidance system used in moth sex attraction. *Nature (London)* **288**, 475–477.

Kikuchi, T. (1975). Correlation of moth sex pheromone activities with molecular characteristics involved in conformers of bombykol and its derivatives. *Proc. Natl. Acad. Sci. U.S.A.* **72**, 3337–3341.

Klein, U., and Keil, T. A. (1984). Dendritic membrane from insect olfactory hairs: Isolation method and electron microscopic observations. *Cell. Mol. Neurobiol.* **4**, 385–396.

Klun, J. A., *et al.* (1975). Insect sex pheromones: Intraspecific pheromoneal variability of *Ostrinia nubilalis* in North America and Europe. *Environ. Entomol.* **4**, 891–894.

Klun, J. A., and Maini, S. (1979). Genetic basis of an insect chemical communication system: The European corn borer. *Environ. Entomol.* **8**, 423–426.

Kochansky, J., Tette, J., Taschenberg, E. F., Cardé, R. T., Kaissling, K. E., and Roelofs, W. L. (1975). Sex pheromone of the moth *Antheraea polyphemus. J. Insect Physiol.* **21**, 1977–1983.

Kramer, E. (1975). Orientation of the male silkmoth to the sex attractant bombykol. *In* "Olfaction and Taste V" (D. A. Denton and J. P. Coghlan, eds.), pp. 329–335. Academic Press, New York.

Lanier, G. N., Classon, A., Stewart, T., Piston, J. J., Silverstein, R. M. (1980). *Ips pini:* The basis for interpopulational differences in pheromone biology. *J. Chem. Ecol.* **6**, 677–687.

Linn, C. E., Jr. (1986). Book review: "Insect Communication" (edited by Trevor Lewis), Academic Press, New York, 1984 (with explanatory comments by Linn of his own work). *J. Chem. Ecol.* **12**, 1311–1317.

Linn, C. E., Jr., and Roelofs, W. L. (1983). Effect of varying proportions of the alcohol component on sex pheromone blend discrimination in male oriental fruit moths. *Physiol. Entomol.* **8**, 291–306.

Linn, C. E., Jr., and Roelofs, W. L. (1985). Response specificity of male pink bollworm moths to different blends and dosages of sex pheromone. *J. Chem. Ecol.* **11**, 1583–1590.

Linn, C. E., Jr., Campbell, M. G., and Roelofs, W. L. (1986). Male moth sensitivity to multicomponent pheromones: Critical role of female-released blend in determining the functional role of components and active space of the pheromone. *J. Chem. Ecol.* **12**, 659–668.

Löfqvist, J. (1986). Species specificity in response to pheromone substances in diprionid sawflies. *In* "Mechanisms in Insect Olfaction" (T. L. Payne, M. C. Birch, and C. E. J. Kennedy, eds.), pp. 123–129. Oxford Univ. Press (Clarendon), London and New York.

Löfstedt, C., Lanne, B. S., Löfqvist, J., Appergren, M., and Bergstrom, G. (1985). Individual variation in the pheromone of the turnip moth, *Agrotis segetum. J. Chem. Ecol.* **11,** 1181–1196.

Ma, W. C. (1981). Receptor membrane function in olfaction and gustation: Implications from modification by reagents and drugs. *In* "Perception of Behavioral Chemicals" (D. M. Norris, ed.), pp. 267–287. Elsevier/North-Holland, Amsterdam.

Marsh, D., Kennedy, J. S., and Ludlow, A. R. (1981). Analysis of zigzagging flight in moths: A correction. *Physiol. Entomol.* **6,** 225.

Miller, J. R., and Roelofs, W. L. (1980). Individual variation in sex pheromone component ratios in two populations of the redbanded leafroller moth *Argyrotaenia velutinana. Environ. Entomol.* **9,** 359–363.

Murlis, J. (1986). The structure of odour plumes. *In* "Mechanisms in Insect Olfaction" (T. L. Payne, M. C. Birch, and C. E. J. Kennedy, eds.), pp. 27–38. Oxford Univ. Press (Clarendon), London and New York.

Murlis, J., and Jones, C. D. (1981). Fine-scale structure of odour plumes in relation to insect orientation to distant pheromone and other attractant sources. *Physiol. Entomol.* **6,** 71–86.

Mustaparta, H., Angst, M. E., and Lanier, G. N. (1979). Specialization of olfactory cells to insect- and host-produced volatiles in the bark beetle *Ips pini* (Say). *J. Chem. Ecol.* **5,** 109–123.

Mustaparta, H., Tommeras, B. A., and Lanier, G. N. (1985). Pheromone receptor cell specificity in interpopulational hybrids of *Ips pini* (Coleoptera: Scolytidae). *J. Chem. Ecol.* **11,** 999–1007.

Nakamura, K. (1981). The mate searching behavior of *Spodoptera litura. In* "Regulation of Insect Development and Behaviour" (F. Sehnal, A. Zabza, J. J. Menn, and B. Cymborowski, eds.), pp. 941–954. Polytech. Univ. of Wroclaw Press, Wroclaw, Poland.

Norris, D. M. (1981). Possible unifying principles in energy transduction in the chemical senses. *In* "Perception of Behavioral Chemicals" (D. M. Norris, ed.), pp. 289–306. Elsevier/North-Holland, Amsterdam.

O'Connell, R. J. (1986). Electrophysiological responses to pheromone blends in single olfactory receptor neurones. *In* "Mechanisms in Insect Olfaction" (T. L. Payne, M. C. Birch, and C. E. J. Kennedy, eds.), pp. 217–224. Oxford Univ. Press (Clarendon), London and New York.

O'Connell, R. J., Beauchamp, J. T., and Grant, A. J. (1986). Insect olfactory receptor responses to components of pheromone blends. *J. Chem. Ecol.* **12,** 451–467.

Olberg, R. M. (1983). Pheromone-triggered flip-flopping interneurons in the ventral nerve cord of the silkworm moth. *Bombyx mori. J. Comp. Physiol.* **152,** 297–307.

Pace, U., and Lancet, D. (1986). Olfactory GTP-binding protein: Signal-tranducing polypeptide of vertebrate chemosensory neurons. *Proc. Natl. Acad. Sci. U.S.A.* **83,** 4947–4951.

Pevsner, J., Trifiletti, R. R., Strittmatter, S. M., and Snyder, S. H. (1985). Isolation and characterization of an olfactory receptor protein for odorant pyrazines. *Proc. Natl. Acad. Sci. U.S.A.* **82,** 3050–3054.

Pevsner, J., Sklar, P. B., and Synder, S. H. (1986). Odorant-binding protein: Localization to nasal glands and secretions. *Proc. Natl. Acad. Sci. U.S.A.* **83,** 4942–4936.

Piston, J. J., and Lanier, G. N. (1974). Pheromones of *Ips pini* (Coleoptera: Scolytidae). Response to interpopulational hybrids and relative attractiveness of males boring in two host species. *Can. Entomol.* **106,** 247–251.

Preiss, R. (1985). Lack of effect of (−)-disparlure on orientation towards (+)-disparlure source in walking and flying gypsy moth males. *J. Chem. Ecol.* **11,** 885–894.

Preiss, R., and Kramer, E. (1983). Stabilization of altitude and speed in tethered flying gypsy moth males: Influence of (+)- and (−)-disparlure. *Physiol. Entomol.* **8,** 55–68.

Preiss, R., and Kramer, E. (1986a). Anemotactic orientation of gypsy moth males and its modification by the attractant pheromone (+)-disparlure during walking. *Physiol. Entomol.* **11**, 185–198.

Preiss, R., and Kramer, E. (1986b). *In* "Mechanisms in Insect Olfaction" (T. L. Payne, M. C. Birch, and C. E. J. Kennedy, eds.), pp. 69–79. Oxford Univ. Press (Clarendon), London and New York.

Prestwich, G. D., Golec, R. G., and Andersen, N. H. (1984). Synthesis of a highly tritiated photoaffinity labeled pheromone analog for the moth *Antheraea polyphemus*. *J. Labelled Cmpd. Radiopharm.* **21**, 593–601.

Prestwich, D. G., Vogt, R. G., and Ding, Y.-S. (1986a). Chemical studies of pheromone catabolism and reception. *In* "Molecular Entomology" (J. Law, ed.). UCLA Symposia, Alan R. Liss, New York.

Prestwich, G. D., Vogt, R. G., and Riddiford, L. M. (1986b). Binding and hydrolysis of radiolabeled pheromone and several analogs by male-specific antennal proteins of the moth *Antheraea polyphemus*. *J. Chem. Ecol.* **12**, 323–333.

Prestwich, G. D., Graham, S., Kuo, J. W., and Vogt, R. G. (1987). Tritium labeled enantiomers of disparlure. Synthesis and *in vitro* metabolism. *J. Org. Chem.* (submitted).

Priesner, E. (1979). Progress in the analysis of pheromone receptor systems. *Ann. Zool. Ecol. Anim.* **11**, 533–546.

Rau, P., and Rau, N. (1929). The sex attraction and rhythmic periodicity in giant saturniid moths. *Trans. Acad. Sci. St. Louis* **26**, 83–221.

Reed, D. W., and Chisholm, M. D. (1985). Attraction of moth species of Tortricidae, Gelechiidae, Geometridae, Drepanidae, Pyralidae, and Gracillariidae families to field traps baited with conjugated dienes. *J. Chem. Ecol.* **11**, 1645–1657.

Riddiford, L. M. (1970). Antennal proteins of saturniid moths—Their possible role in olfaction. *J. Insect Physiol.* **16**, 653–660.

Riddiford, L. M. (1971). The insect antenna as a model olfactory system. *In* "Gustation and Olfaction" (G. Ohloff and A. F. Thomas, eds.), pp. 251–259. Academic Press, New York.

Rüchell, R. (1976). Sequential protein analysis from single identified neurons of *Aplysia californica*. A microelectrophoretic technique involving polyacrylamide gradient gels and isoelectric focusing. *J. Histochem. Cytochem.* **24**, 773–791.

Schneider, D., Kasang, G., and Kaissling, K. E. (1968). Bestimmung der Reichschwelle von *Bombyx mori* mit Tritium-markiertem Bombykol. *Naturwissenschaften* **55**, 395.

Shaw, C. R., and Prassad, R. (1970). Starch gel electrophoresis of enzymes—A compilation of recipes. *Biochem. Genet.* **4**, 297–320.

Slifer, E. H. (1961). The fine structure of insect sense organs. *Int. Rev. Cytol.* **11**, 125–159.

Slifer, E. H., and Sekhon, S. S. (1964). The dendrites of the thin-walled sensory pegs of the grasshopper (Orthoptera, Acrididae). *J. Morphol.* **114**, 393–410.

Slifer, E. H., Prestage, J. J., and Beams, H. W. (1957). The fine structure of the long basiconic sensory pegs of the grasshopper (Orthoptera, Acrididae) with special reference to those on the antenna. *J. Morphol.* **101**, 359–397.

Slifer, E. H., Prestage, J. J., and Beams, H. W. (1959). The chemoreceptors and other sense organs on the antennal flagellum of the grasshopper (Orthoptera, Acrididae). *J. Morphol.* **105**, 145–191.

South, R. (1907). "The Moths of the British Isles," Fourth Ed., 1961. Frederick Warne, London.

Steinbrecht, R. A. (1980). Cryofixation without cryoprotectants. Freeze substitution and freeze etching of an insect olfactory receptor. *Tiss. Cell* **12**, 73–100.

Steinbrecht, R. A, and Müller, B. (1971). On the stimulus conducting structures in insect olfactory receptors. *Z. Zellforsch.* **117**, 570–575.

Steinbrecht, R. A., and Zierold, K. (1985). X-Ray microanalysis of electrolytes of an insect olfactory sensillum. *Eur. J. Cell. Biol. Suppl.* **10**, 69.

Tamaki, Y., Noguchi, H., and Yushima, Y. (1973). Sex pheromone of *Spodoptera litura* (F.): Isolation, identification and synthesis. *Appl. Entomol. Zool.* **8**, 200–201.

Thurm, U., and Küppers, J. (1980). Epithelial physiology of insect sensilla. *In* "Insect Biology in the Future" (M. Locke and D. S. Smith, eds.), pp. 735–763. Academic Press, New York.

Truman, J. W. (1974). Physiology of insect rhythms. IV. Role of the brain in the regulation of the flight rhythm of the giant silkmoths. *J. Comp. Physiol.* **95**, 281–296.

Van Der Pers, J. N. C., and Löfstedt, C. (1986). Signal–esponse relationship in sex pheromone communication. *In* "Mechanisms in Insect Olfaction" (T. L. Payne, M. C. Birch, and C. E. J. Kennedy, eds.), pp. 235–241. Oxford Univ. Press (Clarendon), London and New York.

Villet, R. H. (1974). Involvement of amino and sulphydryl groups in olfactory transduction in silk moths. *Nature (London)* **248**, 707–709.

Villet, R. H. (1978). Mechanism of insect sex-pheromone sensory transduction: Role of adenyl cyclase. *Comp. Biochem. Physiol.* **61C**, 389–394.

Vogt, R. G., and Riddiford, L. M. (1981a). Pheromone deactivation by antennal proteins of Lepidoptera. *In* "Regulation of Insect Development and Behaviour" (F. Sehnal, A. Zabza, J. J. Menn, and B. Cymborowski, eds.), pp. 955–967. Polytech. Univ. of Wroclaw Press, Wroclaw, Poland.

Vogt, R. G., and Riddiford, L. M. (1981b). Pheromone binding and inactivation by moth antennae. *Nature (London)* **293**, 161–163.

Vogt, R. G., and Riddiford, L. M. (1986a). Pheromone reception: A kinetic equilibrium. *In* "Mechanisms in Insect Olfaction" (T. L. Payne, M. C. Birch, and C. E. J. Kennedy, eds.), pp. 201–208. Oxford Univ. Press (Clarendon), London and New York.

Vogt, R. G., and Riddiford, L. M. (1986b). Scale esterase: A pheromone degrading enzyme from scales of silk moth *Antheraea polyphemus. J. Chem. Ecol.* **12**, 469–482.

Vogt, R. G., Riddiford, L. M., and Prestwich, G. P. (1985). Kinetic properties of a sex pheromone–degrading enzyme: The sensillar esterse of *Antheraea polyphemus. Proc. Natl. Acad. Sci. U.S.A.* **82**, 8827–8831.

Wigglesworth, V. B. (1972). "The Principles of Insect Physiology," Seventh Ed. Chapman and Hall, London.

13

The Neurobiology
of Pheromone Reception

JACOBUS JAN DE KRAMER[1]

Abteilung für Vergleichende Neurobiologie
der Universität
D-7900 Ulm, Federal Republic of Germany

JÜRGEN HEMBERGER[2]

Max-Planck-Institut für Verhaltensphysiologie
D-8131 Seewiesen, Federal Republic of
Germany

I. GENERAL INTRODUCTION

Insects perceive the presence of pheromone through specialized receptor organs, called sensilla. These sensilla are small, multicellular organs (for morphological details, see Steinbrecht, Chapter 11, this volume) and can be found in insects and other arthropods. There are also other, sometimes less specialized types of sensilla, e.g., odor, taste, hygro-, thermo-, or mechanoreceptors, which may be distributed on various parts of an insect. Sensilla often produce cuticular protrusions, called hairs, an expression also used for entire sensilla. In many species, dense arrays of pheromone-sensitive hairs (with other types of sensilla among them) can be found on the antennae.

Pheromone-receptive sensilla are usually extremely sensitive; Kaissling and Priesner (1970) showed that, at low concentrations, every single pheromone molecule which is absorbed onto the surface of an antennal hair of a male silkmoth may elicit an action potential in one of the receptor neurons of this sensillum. Absorption of about 300 pheromone molecules per second on the entire antenna may elicit a behavioral response. Not just their sensitivity but also

[1]Present address: Landwirtschaftliche Versuchsstation BASF A.G., D-6703 Limburgerhof, Federal Republic of Germany.
[2]Present address: ENKA A.G., D-8753 Obernburg, Federal Republic of Germany.

433

their extraordinary selectivity makes pheromone receptors such interesting objects; even slight modifications in the molecular structure of a pheromone, for instance in the simple hydrocarbon n-undecane, an alarm pheromone to the worker ant, *Lasius fuliginosus,* results in an at least 100-fold loss in activity (Dumpert, 1972). Beside the sensitivity and selectivity, also the bandwidth, i.e., the ability of the pheromone-receptive system to perceive fast changes in pheromone concentration (Kramer, 1986; Kaissling, 1986a), is very astonishing.

II. TYPES OF NEUROPHYSIOLOGICAL RESEARCH AND METHODS

Research on pheromone reception is carried out at various levels of integration, ranging from molecular biology to population dynamics and evolution biology. Neurophysiological research may be subdivided into three main streams of interest: (1) determinations of which animals, or which sensilla, are sensitive to which substances (pheromones or their analogs); (2) questions on the physiology, the functioning of these receptors; and (3) mechanisms by which the central nervous system integrates pheromone-derived information. This chapter will primarily discuss the methodology and interpretation of electrophysiological experiments on single sensilla. In the aforementioned types of research electrophysiological methods are used that allow one, in contrast to many biochemical and radiochemical techniques, to work *in vivo,* near physiologically relevant concentration levels, and with a very good time resolution (down to fractions of a millisecond). Several different types of electrophysiological techniques have been employed to study pheromone receptive systems, as described below.

A.   Electrophysiological Techniques

1.   Integrated Responses

Early experiments were performed by Boistel and Coraboeuf (1953), Roys (1954), Schneider (1955), and Schneider and Hecker (1956), who used various combinations of insect antennae, odorants, electrodes, amplifiers, and oscilloscopes. In the most primitive arrangements of these components, the presentation of an olfactory stimulus increased the amount of noise in a recording; after further experiments responses of single olfactory units and slow potentials could be distinguished. In the following years, single (insect olfactory) units were no longer investigated; instead, the research was focused on the slow potentials which were given the name electroantennogram or EAG (e.g., Schneider, 1957; Schneider et al., 1967). The EAG is, like the electroolfactogram (EOG) and the electroretinogram (ERG), a recording of the response of many receptor neurons to the presentation of a stimulus. This technique is at present mainly used to screen the sensitivity of particular insects to a broad spectrum of substances (e.g., Schneider et al., 1967; Priesner, 1979; Arn et al., 1975; Light, 1983; Roelofs, 1984) or to study receptors which are too small to allow use of other techniques (e.g., Levinson et al., 1978).

2. Single Sensilla

Second, techniques were developed to make extracellular recordings of single, identified sensilla. Boeckh (1962) introduced this technique using sharpened tungsten electrodes; later nonpolarizing electrodes were also employed (Schneider and Boeckh, 1962). Both of these techniques allow the monitoring of the responses of individual receptor neurons to pheromonal stimuli. The tungsten electrode technique is very useful in investigating the responses of either very densely packed or very small sensilla (Mustaparta, 1975; Hansen, 1983; Vareschi, 1971); another advantage of this technique is that the sensilla from which recordings are made may remain normally sensitive for a very long period of time (O'Connell, 1985).

Recordings with nonpolarizing electrodes generally require some major injury to a sensillum (e.g., cutting off the tip; Kaissling, 1974) and also cause modifications with unknown effects in the composition of the receptor lymph of sensilla, which may seriously affect the responsiveness of these hairs (Van Der Pers and Den Otter, 1978). Refinements in the tip-cutting technique and in the composition of the saline in the recording electrode (Van Der Pers and Den Otter, 1978; Kaissling and Thorson, 1980; J. J. De Kramer, unpublished results) may partly cancel these disadvantages. The main advantage of this technique is that very low impedance contacts with the receptor lymph cavity of the hair can be made, thus allowing low noise, DC-coupled potential or current and impedance recordings, which are important in transduction research (Kaissling and Thorson, 1980; De Kramer, 1985; De Kramer et al., 1984). The main limitation of these single sensillum recording techniques is that contributions of the response of individual membrane areas to the overall signal cannot be easily extracted since all sensillar elements in some way contribute to the response of a sensillum.

3. Intracellular Recordings

The application of a third technique, making intracellular recordings from responses to pheromone application, has so far been successful only at the level of the central nervous system (Matsumoto and Hildebrand, 1981; Burrows et al., 1982). The integration of olfactory information in insects is not further discussed in this chapter. Oldfield and Hill (1986) were successful in making intracellular recordings of insect auditory sensilla; they stated that the dendrites of these organs were electrically active.

B. Techniques of Stimulus Presentation

Quantitative interpretations of responses to pheromone applications are hampered by the low levels of pheromone which are presented to the animals. One of the first observations of one who becomes newly involved in pheromone research may be that pheromones are basically nonvolatile substances. Many techniques have been developed and even more calibrations have been carried out in attempt to try to overcome these problems. However, physiologically relevant airborne concentrations of pheromone are still several orders of magnitude below the detection level of any analytical instrumentation.

1. Cartridge Stimulators

Many investigators make use of "cartridges" made out of glass tubing and a piece of filter paper or glass which may be loaded with a precisely known amount of pheromone. Stimuli are made by passing air (or nitrogen) over the filter paper or glass in each cartridge. The air coming from this cartridge is either directly blown onto the preparation or injected into a main airstream. Where this technique has been used, stimulus strengths are usually expressed in terms of how much pheromone was loaded onto the filter paper or glass (e.g., Kaissling and Renner, 1968; Kaissling, 1979; O'Connell, 1975, 1985). Using relatively high loads of radioactively labeled pheromone, the release of these cartridge stimulators can be measured (Kaissling and Priesner, 1970; Kanaujia and Kaissling, 1985; Mayer *et al.*, 1984); the release of cartridges with lower loads must be extrapolated, often over many orders of magnitude.

This method of stimulus presentation is very simple and cheap; however, pheromone analogs may have considerably different evaporation rates, and only little is known about the behavior of these sources as a function of time. For many components, a single cartridge (when stored overnight at $-30°C$) may, without apparent loss of effectiveness, be used for years; for others, rapid degradation of material may occur. Kaissling and Priesner (1970) investigated the temporal release from these pheromone sources. They found a peak of some 100 msec at the onset of pheromone presentation which contained up to two or more times the pheromone concentration of the steady-state level.

2. Syringe Stimulators

Another odor presentation apparatus, the so-called syringe stimulator, was introduced by Kafka (1970). In this method calibrated dilutions of pheromone in oil (in small glass vials) are inserted in plastic syringes and left to stand for some time in order to reach a steady-state distribution between pheromone in air, oil, glass, and plastic. Pheromone stimuli are here performed by pressing a distinct amount of volume per time through a hypodermic needle out of this syringe either directly onto the preparation or into a main "carrier" airstream. At high loads, the concentration of stimulus inside the syringe can be easily calibrated using a gas chromatograph. Stimulus strength here is usually expressed in molecules per liter.

3. Other

Pheromone presentations to small parts of olfactory hairs have been made by Zack (1979), Kaissling (1986a), and Zack-Straussfeld and Kaissling (1987). Local stimuli were delivered from pheromone-soaked nylon threads in a (blunt) micropipette. Absolute calibrations of these types of stimulators have not yet been made.

In numerical analyses to the dynamic response of pheromone receptors, the temporal patterns of airborne pheromone concentrations coming off the sources are interpreted as square pulses.

III. INTERPRETATION OF RESPONSES TO PHEROMONE

In research on the responses of antennae (EAG) or of single sensilla, a number of different parameters are used to describe the response. In EAG recordings these include the amplitude, rise time, and decline rate; in single sensillum recordings, the amplitude, rise time, decline rate of the extracellular receptor potential, or spike rates may be determined. Different authors tend to attribute different importances to these response parameters, which is not only related to the level of integration investigated but also depends on transduction hypotheses. Kaissling (1979), for instance, analyzes primarily extracellular receptor potentials as this parameter might be very closely related to receptor–ligand interactions; Boeckh (1962, 1967), Kafka (1970), Rumbo (1981), and O'Connell (1975, 1985) mainly analyze spike rates, as spikes may be attributed to the influence of the stimulus on particular, physiologically identified cells. Using this advantage of the single sensillum recording technique in *Trichoplusia ni*, O'Connell and co-workers (O'Connell, 1985; O'Connell *et al.*, 1986) were able to demonstrate that some mixtures of substances (pheromone blends) may evoke larger responses in some receptor neurons than could be predicted from the responses of these neurons to the individual substances. Before going further into discussion on the relationship between the neurophysiological responses and pheromone presentations, the components which may qualitatively contribute to the transduction hypotheses should therefore be analyzed in detail.

A. Transduction Hypotheses

A discussion on transduction mechanisms and functional specializations of pheromone-receptive sensilla is only significant with reference to the morphology of these organs. Figure 1 shows the proximal part of a typical olfactory hair and at its base a cellular apparatus which is, except for some modifications, representative for many types of sensilla. Olfactory hairs usually have one lumen and are filled with receptor lymph and one (or more) sensory dendrites (D). The cuticular wall and the receptor lymph of olfactory hairs contain numerous pore tubules (PT) which may be pathways for odor molecules toward the sensory dendrites. The cellular apparatus of most sensilla is composed of one or more receptor neurons (RN) and, generally, three accessory cells: the thecogen cell (TH), which tightly envelops the receptor neuron(s), and the trichogen (TR) and tormogen (TO) cells, with highly folded apical membranes bordering a proximal extension of the receptor lymph space, also called the receptor lymph cavity (RLC). For more detailed morphological information see Steinbrecht (Chapter 11, this volume; 1973), Keil and Steinbrecht (1984), Keil (1984a,b), Steinbrecht and Gnatzy (1984), and Gnatzy *et al.* (1984).

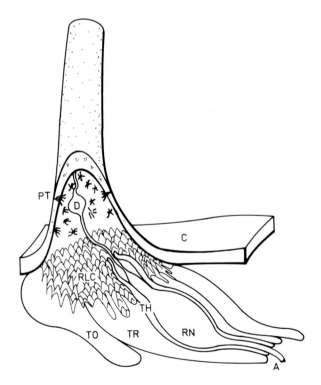

Fig. 1. Schematic diagram of a pheromone-sensitive sensillum. A, Axon; C, cuticle; D, dendrite; PT, pore tubules; RLC, receptor lymph cavity; RN, receptor neuron; TH, thecogen cell; TO, tormogen cell; TR, trichogen cell. Modified after Keil (1984a) and Steinbrecht and Gnatzy (1984).

One of the very basic questions in transduction research concerns the localization of functional properties: How do we know that certain functions are carried out by certain structures? Primary pheromone-receptive functions are presumably located in the hairs—this may seem self-evident, but apart from experiments made by Zack (1979) and Zack-Straussfeld and Kaissling (1987), who performed pheromone stimulations of various small parts of hairs and found that adaptation to pheromone presentations occurred independently at different parts of a sensory hair, there is little experimental evidence to support this.

Several structural elements of olfactory sensilla, such as the cuticle, the receptor lymph, and the sensory dendrites, may have a qualitative influence on the response to pheromone.

1. Cuticle

The cuticle of olfactory hairs has a hydrophobic surface, the epicuticle (only 10–30 nm thick), which efficiently adsorbs lipidlike pheromone molecules from the air (Steinbrecht and Kasang, 1972; Kasang, 1973; Kanaujia and Kaissling, 1985) and forms a barrier to hydrophilic substances which might interfere with pheromone reception. Recently, a discussion on the specificity with which pheromone molecules are adsorbed to the cuticle started because Mankin and Mayer (1984) found lower adsorption coefficients for (Z)-10-dodecen-1-yl acetate on a *Bombyx* antenna than the adsorption coefficients described for bombykol by Steinbrecht and Kasang (1972). According to Kaissling (1986b) this discrepancy may show a reduced adsorptivity of the *Bombyx* antenna for other pheromones. This hypothesis would have considerable implications for the interpretation of responses of antennae to a wide variety of pheromone analogs (e.g., in research as described by Boeckh, 1967, or Kafka and Neuwirth, 1975) and should therefore be carefully tested. In one of these tests, by Kasang and Kaissling (1972), it was found that a *Bombyx* antenna adsorbs two very similar substances, hexadecanol (16 : OH) and bombykol (E10,Z12-16 : OH) equally well.

Futrelle (1984) proposed that only specialized areas near the end of pore tubules in the epicuticle would adsorb pheromone. However, research on the ultrastructure of the epicuticle has not revealed differences between various epicuticular areas in pheromone-sensitive sensilla. The main layer of the sensillar cuticle (the exocuticule) is very likely hydrophilic (Scheie and Smyth, 1976; Locke, 1964; J. J. De Kramer, unpublished) and might be a barrier to pheromone molecules. They probably pass this layer through pore tubules, wax channel–like structures which contact the epicuticle and transverse the exocuticle in large numbers (Steinbrecht, 1973; Keil, 1984b). In *Bombyx* and *Antheraea* the pore density is about 10–35 per square micrometer (Keil and Steinbrecht, 1984); this value may vary considerably between different species or sensillum types. Pheromones may migrate by diffusion through the epicuticle until they reach a pore tubule (Adam and Delbrück, 1968).

2. Receptor Lymph

The receptor lymph between the cuticle and the sensory dendrites provides a hydrophilic barrier between pheromone molecules caught on the cuticle and their hypothetical receptors in the dendritic membrane. According to ultrastructural investigations by Keil (1984b), only very few of the pore tubules which extend into the receptor lymph are in contact with the dendritic membrane. Assuming that these pore tubules are sufficient to provide a pathway for pheromone molecules up to the dendritic membrane, the function of the receptor lymph—beside establishing the correct (ionic) milieu for the dendrites—could be restricted to the inactivation of pheromone molecules. Still, it is also possible that the receptor lymph plays a more substantial role in the entire transduction process (Vogt and Riddiford, 1981; Vogt et al., 1985; Kaissling, 1986b; Vogt, Chapter 12, this volume).

From a biochemical point of view, the receptor lymph (especially of *Antheraea polyphemus*) is the best known compartment of olfactory hairs. Receptor lymph can easily be collected by cutting off the tip of the hairs and extruding a droplet by applying pressure to the hemolymph space (Kaissling and Thorson, 1980). Nevertheless, only two proteins have so far been positively identifed in the receptor lymph of *Antheraea polyphemus*. The "pheromone-binding protein" (Vogt and Riddiford, 1981) dominates in quantity and is able to bind radioactive pheromone during polyacrylamide gel electrophoresis. The concentration of this protein in the receptor lymph may be as high as 20 mM.

The second known protein is an esterase and was also identified by its enzymatic activity in polyacrylamide gels (Vogt and Riddiford, 1981). Kinetic properties of this enzyme have been investigated *in vitro* in some detail (Vogt et al., 1985; Prestwich et al., 1986). This esterase could serve as an inactivator to the pheromone component (E6,Z11)-hexadecadienyl acetate (E6,Z11-16 : Ac) by converting the pheromone to the corresponding alcohol which is much less active in an electrophysiological experiment (K. E. Kaissling, personal communication).

Although this protein repertoire with binding and inactivation components might fulfill essential tasks of the receptor lymph, many questions remain unanswered. For instance,

1. How are the other, more polar degradation products which appear in the receptor lymph formed (G. Kasang, personal communication) after presentation of E6,Z11-16 : Ac?

2. What is the transport pathway for the second pheromone component, E6,Z11-16 : Al? Is it bound to the same binding protein?

3. What is the inactivation mechanism for this second pheromone component?

On the basis of the limited information on properties of the proteins in the receptor lymph outlined above, several models of the role of these proteins in the pheromone transduction process have been proposed (Vogt, Chapter 12, this volume; Kaissling, 1986b). The binding protein might act as a carrier protein responsible for the transport of pheromone to receptor sites (Vogt et al., 1985), or it might act as a pheromone inactivator or sequestering device which, by mere binding, would reduce the active pheromone concentration in the sensillum (Vogt and Riddiford, 1981; Kaissling, 1986b).

Incubation of tritiated E6,Z11-16:Ac with purified binding protein shows saturable binding (Kaissling et al., 1985) which is linearly related to the protein concentration (J. Hemberger, unpublished). Saturation occurs at a molar ratio of about 1:1. The apparent binding constant (K_D) of about 10^{-7} M indicates an interaction strong enough for capturing incoming pheromone molecules, but is still well above the dissociation constants generally observed for specific receptors $(K_D = 10^{-9}$–10^{-10} $M)$, thus allowing delivery of the ligand from the binding protein to a receptor.

Of particular interest is the specificity of the binding with modified pheromone analogs, as outlined in Fig. 2, where an inhibition of tritiated E6,Z11-16:Ac binding by certain derivatives appears. As expected, the unlabeled original acetate displaces tritiated E6,Z11-16:Ac from the binding sites most effectively. About a 10-fold higher concentration is needed for a 50% displacement by saturated 16:Ac, and an about 100-fold excess to reach only 80% competition with E6,Z11-16:OH. Geraniol, at high concentrations an inhibitor of the electrophysiological response to pheromone (Schneider et al., 1964), shows no inhibition at all. These data suggest that the functional group (acetate) contributes most to the interaction of ligand and binding protein (alcohol versus acetate); the double bonds in the pheromone, however, also play some role in specific binding as can be deduced from the decreased inhibition by 16:Ac and the modest inhibition by E6,Z11-16:OH, which lacks the acetate group.

The observed specificity of the binding protein suggests that it acts as a carrier rather than as a passive inactivator, where a specific binding is neither necessary nor useful. Inactivation of similar pheromone molecules from other species that could reach the receptor lymph as well as the natural pheromone could be achieved much better by less specific inactivators.

Another function of the receptor lymph is to provide a proper environment, i.e., a suitable ionic and osmolar milieu, to the sensory dendrites. Steinbrecht and Zierold (1985; Steinbrecht, Chapter 11, this volume), using X-ray microanalysis, found a high potassium level in the receptor lymph of male Bombyx sensilla. Earlier, Kaissling and Thorson (1980) described flame photometric and X-ray levels of 200 mM K$^+$ and 25 mM Na$^+$ and mentioned a K$^+$ activity of 145 mM and an osmolarity of 450 mOsmol for Antheraea hairs. The high

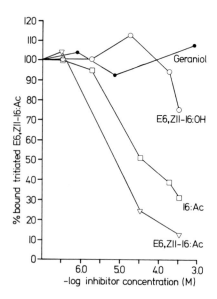

Fig. 2. Competitive displacement of the binding of tritiated E6,Z11-16:Ac to the binding protein by various pheromone analogs. The tritiated E6,Z11-16:Ac (specific activity 2.7 Ci/mmol), together with the indicated amounts of inhibitor, was freed of the solvent in a glass test tube under N_2. After incubation with 1.7 µg purified binding protein at room temperature, the protein-bound radioactivity was determined.

potassium content of the receptor lymph puts some constraints on hypotheses of the dendritic contributions to the resting potential or Nernst potential sources of the sensory dendrites, but it does not prevent the dendritic membrane from being electrically active, i.e., being able to generate action potentials (Oldfield and Hill, 1986; De Kramer, 1985). Some of the buffering properties of the receptor lymph are demonstrated in the following electrophysiological experiment.

The impedance of cut-tip olfactory sensilla in extracellular recordings can be roughly subdivided into two electrical components, R_1 and a parallel R_2-C_2 combination (see below), which may be largely attributed to the resistance of the column of receptor lymph in the hair and the cellular parts of a sensillum, respectively. If the saline solution in the recording electrode has a conductivity which is lower or higher than the resistivity of the receptor lymph, the rate with which R_1 changes is a measure for the exchange rate between recording electrode and receptor lymph. In recordings of R_1 it is very striking that the first exchange of receptor lymph takes much more time than subsequent ones (Fig. 3); some reticular mesh apparently buffers the ion activity and prevents a fast ion exchange in undamaged hairs. After disruption of the reticular structure, most ions

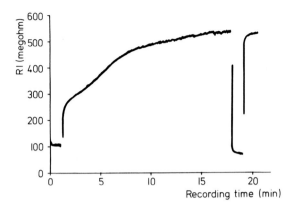

Fig. 3. Changes in R_1 caused by solutions of different conductivity in the recording electrode. During the time until the 18th minute and from the 20th minute onward, the recording electrode contained standard "receptor lymph Ringer" (Kaissling and Thorson, 1980); during the 1st and 18th minute a 10-fold less conductive saline solution was used.

in the receptor lymph can move freely. The most proximal part of the receptor lymph space, however, the receptor lymph cavity, seems to be even better protected. In cut-tip sensilla which have been chemically fixed for electron microscopic investigation, the lumen of the hair looks empty, whereas the receptor lymph cavity at the base of the hair still displays some fuzzy structure. Between the empty shaft of the hair and the receptor lymph cavity, some septum is clearly visible in cut-tip, chemically fixated material (Fig. 4). The presence of this septum, the reticular structure of the receptor lymph cavity, and its apparent buffering capacity (compare total and free K^+ concentrations mentioned above) may help explain why ion-exchange experiments investigating the effects of a change in the ionic composition of the fluid around the dendrites on the response of these hairs (Adamek et al., 1984a) have so far not led to the identification of particular ions responsible for the functioning of pheromone receptors.

3. Sensory Dendrites

It is generally expected that the actual pheromone receptor sites are located at the receptor lymph side of integral membrane proteins in the outer segments of the sensory dendrites. On one hand there is, so far, little or no experimental evidence to support this (see also Vogt, Chapter 12, this volume). On the other hand, analogies might exist with vertebrate olfactory cells whose function has been demonstrated by Adamek et al. (1984b). In some chemosensory systems intracellular receptors have also been proposed (DeSimone et al., 1984), a possibility which has not been excluded for pheromone receptors. In principle,

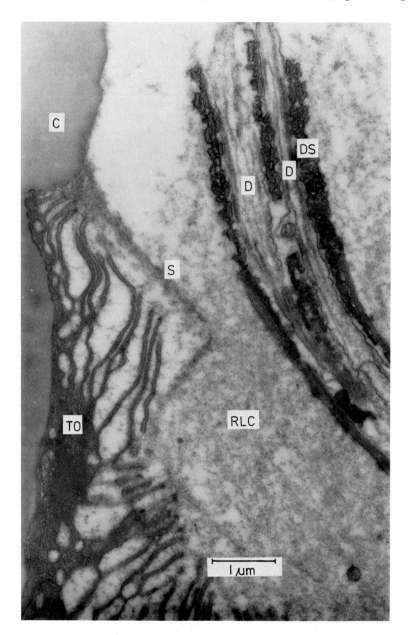

Fig. 4. The ultrastructure of the proximal end of a pheromone-receptive hair in *Antheraea polyphemus*. S, Septum between the receptor lymph space and the receptor lymph cavity; C, cuticle; TO, tormogen cell; D, dendrite, which is, in the proximal part of the hair, surrounded by a dendritic sheath (DS). Courtesy of T. A. Keil.

receptor sites for pheromone molecules may also be located within the dendritic membrane; in this case pheromones should dissolve into the dendritic membrane before they exert their influence.

Not only the location of receptor sites but also fundamentals about receptor–ligand interactions and about the complex of processes which are involved in the translation of these interactions into action potentials remain unknown. Many hypotheses on these processes are based on the dynamics of electrophysiologically recorded signals. How electrophysiologically measured parameters are related to acceptor–ligand interactions, however, is not clear; different parameters lead to different interpretations. An example of this phenomenon is the interpretation of EAGs and the extracellular receptor potentials recorded from single sensilla. Both of these signals have been proposed to be directly related to the occupancy of pheromone receptor molecules (Kaissling, 1969, 1974, 1979). However, as shown in Fig. 5, EAGs and extracellular receptor potentials may have a completely different response pattern (Kaissling, 1979; Van Der Pers *et al.*, 1980; Nagai, 1983), thus leading to significantly different affinity and inactivation constants. In order to shed some light on this complex field of transduction and

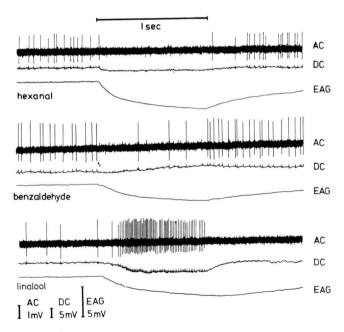

Fig. 5. Simultaneous recordings of single sensilla and EAGs in *Yponomeuta rorellus*. Note the differences in shape and even polarity between the DC traces and the EAGs in all recordings. Courtesy of Van Der Pers *et al.* (1980).

structure–function relationships, a detailed analysis of the electrical circuitry of olfactory hairs has been made, and some of the results are summarized below.

B. The Electrical Equivalent Network of Olfactory Sensilla: A Morphological–Electrophysiological Interpretation of the Preparation

Hypotheses on the distribution of functional properties over the various membrane areas in olfactory and other types of sensilla have been derived from the signals recorded by extracellular electrodes (Morita, 1959, 1963; Morita and Yamashita, 1959; Wolbarsht, 1960; Wolbarsht and Hanson, 1965; Rees, 1968; Kaissling, 1979; Kaissling and Thorson, 1980; Thurm and Küppers, 1980; Fujishiro et al., 1984). Thus, because the leading phase of (tip-recorded) spikes is positive with reference to the hemolymph space, it was concluded that action potentials would be initiated in or near the perikaryon of the sensory neuron; the negative undershoot of spikes was interpreted to be due to a retrograde propagation of action potentials into the dendrite. Simultaneous tip and sidewall measurements of spikes in contact chemoreceptive sensilla where spike peaks appeared earlier in the signal picked up by the sidewall electrode than in the tip recording supported this hypothesis (Morita and Yamashita, 1959; Wolbarsht and Hanson, 1965). The negative "receptor potential" which can be recorded from the tip of olfactory sensilla was thought to be due to an inward current at the (dendritic) site of stimulus action. Intracellularly, this receptor current was supposed to be conducted electrotonically toward a somatic spike initiator zone (Rees, 1968; Kaissling and Thorson, 1980). A few simple experiments provided reasons to start a reinvestigation of the organization of pheromone-receptive sensilla:

1. Significant phase shifts or amplitude differences between spikes recorded simultaneously from the base (sidewall electrode) and the tip of olfactory hairs could not be demonstrated (Fig. 6; De Kramer et al., 1984).

2. The potential across a sensillum ought to have a large influence on the amplitude (and polarity) of the receptor current. Using a trans-sensillar voltage clamp technique, a good correlation between receptor current and holding potential has been demonstrated in mechanoreceptive sensilla (Vohwinkel, cited in Thurm and Küppers, 1980). In pheromone-receptive sensilla, however, a noteworthy relationship between holding potential and receptor current does not exist, as can be seen in Fig. 7. Also experiments with cyanide, where (among others) the ion pumps responsible for the standing potential across a sensillum were inhibited (Levinson et al., 1973), demonstrate that in pheromone receptors the amplitude of the extracellular receptor potential is relatively insensitive to changes in the standing potential across the sensillum.

3. It is possible to perforate (or electrically short-circuit) the epithelium below

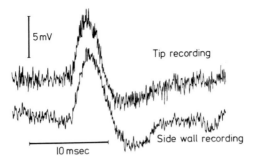

Fig. 6. Simultaneous recordings from the sidewall (near the hair base; lower trace) and the tip (upper trace) of a pheromone-receptive hair of *Antheraea polyphemus*. The recording was made upon stimulation with E6,Z11-16 : Ac at 0°C. Note that the spike recorded from the base does not lead the spike recorded from the tip.

the hair by the application of suction via the reference electrode in the hemolymph space. This treatment leads to a sudden irreversible breakdown of the epithelial resistance (R_2, see below) and the standing potential; the ability of the receptor neurons to produce spontaneous spikes or their ability to respond to pheromone, however, remains unimpaired (Kaissling, in De Kramer, 1985).

Investigations into the electrical (equivalent) network of sensilla may form the basis for electromorphological interpretations which in turn may be used in transduction hypotheses. Electrical equivalent networks, or models of the electrical circuitry of a (biological) structure, are usually reconstructed from mea-

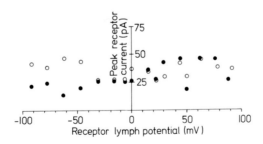

Fig. 7. The relationship between the potential across the sensillum (receptor lymph potential) and the peak receptor current. The experiments were carried out on two different hairs on the antenna of *Antheraea polyphemus* (open and filled circles) to 1 sec pheromone stimuli (E6,Z11-16 : Ac) which evoke under current clamp conditions a receptor potential of about 10 mV. In contrast to the peak receptor current, the spike rate was highly dependent on the receptor lymph potential (not shown). Individual pheromone presentations were 10 min apart, holding potentials in random sequence.

surements to the electrical impedance of this structure. The history of the branch of electrophysiology where impedance techniques have been applied represents, as Schanne and Ceretti (1978) remarked, both "unique contributions" and "great effort, greater hopes and deep frustrations." Indeed, it is very difficult to interpret voltage-to-current relationships of (pheromone) sensilla; the rather complex structure seems in no way to be represented in the complex impedance of these organs. Still, an equivalent network derived from as many measurements to the impedance of sensilla as possible will add to our knowledge on transduction; complex "best guess" models (Kaissling and Thorson, 1980; Kaissling, 1986b) are mainly of heuristic value.

One simple technique to analyze the basics of electrical connections in a structure is to analyze the voltage response to current transients (Schanne and Ceretti, 1978). The dynamic response of a pheromone-receptive sensillum in *Antheraea polyphemus* to square current pulses can be divided in two phases (De Kramer, 1985; De Kramer *et al.*, 1984) (see Fig. 8): (i) a fast component (*F*) with a time constant smaller than 50 μsec and (ii) a slow component (*S*) with a time constant of the order of 10 msec and an approximately single exponential behavior. This response to current pulses below ±50 pA is symmetric and linear and demonstrates that the passive electrical network of a sensillum is not just a resistive network but also contains capacitive elements.

The simplest equivalent scheme with a behavior like the sensillum is that of Fig. 9. Here the fast component (*F*) represents the current-induced voltage drop over R_1 according to Ohm's law, whereas the slow component (*S*) represents the steady-state (current-induced) voltage drop over R_2. From the time constant of the slow phase and R_2, the size of C_2 can be calculated:

$$R_1 = \frac{F}{I} \, , \quad R_2 = \frac{S}{I} \, , \quad C_2 = \frac{\tau}{R_2} \, .$$

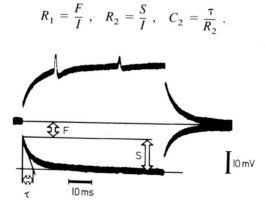

Fig. 8. Typical two-phase response of a sensillum to successive ±100-pA current pulses at 20°C. Note the different amplitude of the spikes elicited in two different cells by the +100-pA stimulus. From De Kramer *et al.* (1984).

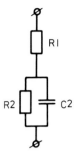

Fig. 9. Simple electrical equivalent circuit of a pheromone-receptive sensillum. The electrical response of this circuit closely mimics the response of a sensillum to current transients as shown in Fig. 8.

From the influence of lesions on the slow and fast phases, some information on the location of these elements in the equivalent network may be derived. Both the good correlation between R_1 and the length of the hair and the relationship between the conductivity of the saline in the recording electrode and R_1 (Fig. 10) indicate that R_1 will largely represent the resistance of the extracellular fluid in the sensillar hair; a small fraction of the resistance of R_1 must be attributed to electrodes and the hemolymph space. Indeed, the values found for R_1 correspond to computed resistances of morphometrically analyzed hair lumina (Keil, 1984a) when filled with an electrolyte of a specific resistance of 50 ohm · cm. The parallel elements R_2 and C_2 show no significant correlation with the length of the

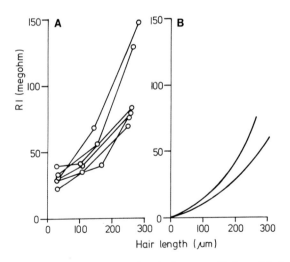

Fig. 10. (A) The relationship between the length of amputated hairs and the fast phase, or R_1, in Figs. 8 and 9. From De Kramer *et al.* (1984). (B) The resistance of the hair calculated for two morphometrically analyzed hairs (Keil, 1984b) at a conductivity of the receptor lymph of 50 ohm · cm. The offset in A is largely due to the resistivity of the branch and the electrodes.

hair (Fig. 11) and must therefore be located mainly in the epithelial cells of one sensillum (De Kramer, 1985). Between the receptor lymph space and the hemolymph space, two layers of membranes are possible locations for the R_2–C_2 combination: the apical and, not mutually exclusive, the basal and lateral membranes of the sensillar cells. Thus, from the morphology (Steinbrecht and Gnatzy, 1984), one should expect a decay of the slow component according to (see Fig. 12):

$$V(t) = I(R_a e^{-t/R_a C_a} + R_b e^{-t/R_b C_b})$$

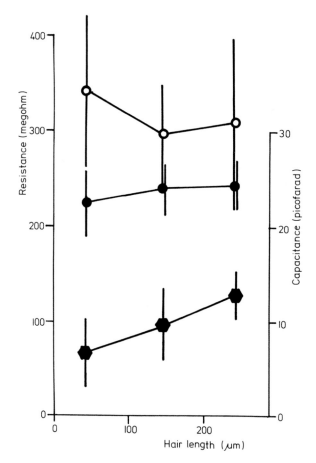

Fig. 11. The relationship between R_1 (●), R_2 (○), and C_2 (●) and the length of amputated hairs. In contrast to R_1, neither R_2 nor C_2 show a significant correlation with the length of the remaining hair stumps. Redrawn from De Kramer (1985).

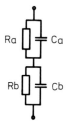

Fig. 12. The relative contributions of the apical and basolateral membranes of the supporting cells were estimated using an electrical equivalent network. R_a and C_a mimic the impedance of the apical and R_b and C_b the impedance of the basolateral membrane.

Noise, inherent in measurements, prohibits the calculation of the unknown parameters in this equation from the experimentally acquired waveform and amplitude of the slow phase alone, but by using some morphometric data and the biophysical membrane constant of 1 μF(microfarads)/cm^2 (Cole, 1972) this difficulty can be overcome. The summated area of the cells in one sensillum is about 3000 μm^2, and the summated basolateral membrane area is about 1800 μm^2 (values from *Antheraea pernyi* by Gnatzy *et al.*, 1984); values of 30 and 18 pF can therefore be assigned to C_a and C_b, respectively. As R_2 represents the DC resistance of the epithelial part of one sensillum, this value can be taken for the sum of R_a and R_b. In a computer simulation the overall time constant of the network of Fig. 13 was estimated after various partitions of R_2 between R_a and R_b; the experimentally derived time constant of the preparation is reached when the resistance ratio R_a/R_b is greater than or equal to 10, from which it can be

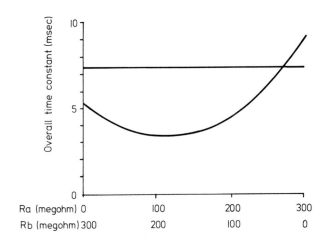

Fig. 13. Computer simulation of the response of the circuit shown in Fig. 12. The "overall" time constant of the circuit with C_a and C_b fixed at values of 30 and 18 pF at various partitions of R_2 (300 megohms) over R_a and R_b. Note that the response of the circuit (bent curve) intersects with the time constant found in experiments (straight line) when R_a is about 10 times R_b. Redrawn from De Kramer (1985).

deduced that the apical membranes of the sensillar cells contribute most to the transepithelial resistance of a sensillum.

One of the most frustrating results in the study of the relationship between passive electrical characteristics of a sensillum and the length of the remaining hair stump was that no significant relationship between R_2 and C_2 and length could be established (Fig. 11), thereby prohibiting the calculation of dendritic membrane contributions to the overall characteristics of the sensillum. Both interindividual variation between hairs and a temporal instability of the preparation are responsible for this finding. Other strategies, e.g., measurements to the amplitude of extracellularly recorded spikes, might also provide some information on the electrical properties of the sensory dendrite.

C. The Equivalent Network and Action Potentials

Two observations suggest that the shape of spikes depends on the passive network characteristics of the preparation. First, the time constant of the "tail" of spikes depends on temperature exactly as the R_2C_2 time constant does (Fig. 14). Second, when spikes are recorded from short hairs in extracellular voltage clamp configuration, their duration is considerably shorter than that of spikes which are recorded under current clamp conditions (Fig. 15). These observations

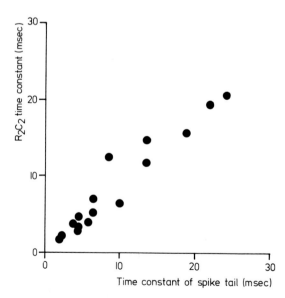

Fig. 14.   Time constants of "tails" of spikes (the repolarization following the negative under-shoot) versus time constants (R_2C_2, in milliseconds) of responses to 1-msec current pulses at temperatures between 0 and 25°C. Redrawn from De Kramer (1985).

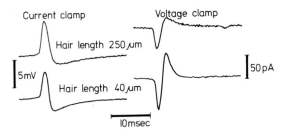

Fig. 15. Spontaneous spikes recorded under current and voltage clamp conditions from hairs that were cut to different lengths. Averages of 11 sensilla at each hair length (10 impulses/hair) are shown. Redrawn from De Kramer (1985).

may be explained if some "spike generator" (with nonideal voltage source characteristics) is inserted in parallel to the R_2-C_2 elements (see Fig. 16). This spike generator, with an (AC) potential source E_s and an inner impedance Z_s then represents electrical properties of the receptor neuron; the network of Fig. 16 is qualitatively similar to those described by Rees (1968), Thurm and Küppers (1980), and Kaissling and Thorson (1980).

Electron microscopical investigations (Keil and Steinbrecht, 1983; Steinbrecht and Gnatzy, 1984) revealed that apically and basally arranged septate junctions isolate the intercellular spaces between the receptor neurons and the thecogen cell from both the receptor and the hemolymph spaces. These findings indicate that Z_s (and possibly also E_s) must consist of some combination of neuron and thecogen elements and that the two remaining (trichogen and tormogen) accessory cells account for the $R_a C_a$ combination. An analysis of hair (dendrite) amputation might, in this configuration, provide some information about the relative contribution of the dendrite to Z_s.

Based on the hypothesis that a spatial separation between the receptor and spike initiator regions exists (Morita and Yamashita, 1959; Wolbarsht and Han-

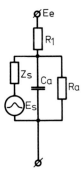

Fig. 16. An alternative equivalent network of the preparations which display a current transient response similar to that of Fig. 8 and in which "spikes" show an influence of voltage or current clamp configurations similar to those of spikes from the sensillum (Fig. 15). E_s stands for the action potential generator complex; the parallel combination Z_s, C_a, and R_a represents the previous R_2-C_2 combination.

son, 1965; Rees, 1968) and because of the high efficacy of receptor current propagation as determined by the stimulation of different parts of the dendrite (Zack, 1979; Zack-Straussfeld and Kaissling, 1987), the length constant and resistivity of the dendrite was thought to be relatively high (larger than 10,000 ohm · cm^2; Kaissling, 1980, 1986b; Rees, 1968). This high resistivity of the dendritic membrane should, in extracellular spike recordings of sensilla, become visible as a decrease in spike amplitude when sensillar hairs (and dendrites) are amputated, a phenomenon described by Wolbarsht and Hanson (1965) in taste sensilla. As shown in Fig. 17, this inverse relationship between the length of the

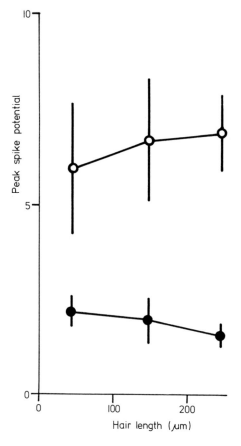

Fig. 17. The relationship between the length of amputated hairs and spike amplitude. Positive (○) and negative (●) peak spike amplitudes in current clamp configuration are shown. Only the negative phases from large and small hairs are significantly different ($p < .0005$). Redrawn from De Kramer (1985).

hair (surface area of the dendritic membrane) and the peak amplitude of spikes recorded under current clamp conditions cannot be demonstrated in the pheromone-receptive sensilla of *Antheraea*. When using voltage clamping techniques (Fig. 18) even contrary effects are observed: here the peak-to-peak spike current is inversely related to the surface area, or resistance, of the dendrite. It is just because inappropriate parameters are compared that in these voltage clamp measurements to the peak spike amplitude the sensillum seems to behave opposite to Ohm's law; in effect, this amplitude depends to a large extent on R_1, the resistance of the lumen of the hair which is directly related to the length of the hair (De Kramer, 1985).

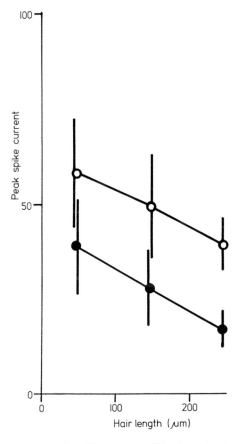

Fig. 18. Peak spike currents of first (○) and second (●) spike phases in voltage clamp configuration. Both spike phases are significantly different when long and short hairs are compared ($p < .0002$). Redrawn from De Kramer (1985).

The most significant conclusion from these spike measurements is that, in disagreement with Wolbarsht and Hanson (1965), a noteworthy contribution of the dendritic membrane to Z_s cannot be demonstrated. There are two different explanations for this lack of influence of the impedance of the dendritic membrane to the amplitude of spikes: either (1) the relative contribution is, compared to the contribution of the soma region, always very low; or (2) this low impedance of the dendrite is restricted to those moments at which spikes occur. A consequence of the first explanation would be that the transduction hypotheses which assume a high length constant of the dendrite (e.g., Kaissling and Thorson, 1980) should be rejected. In the second explanation, the length constant of the sensory dendrites might be large during interspike intervals but would decrease considerably while spikes occur. This would imply that the dendritic membrane is also electrically active during the first phase of spikes. Such an activity implies that the hypothesis about a spatial separation between receptor and spike initiator region would lose its significance, a conclusion already drawn from the simultaneous tip and sidewall recordings mentioned above (Fig. 6; De Kramer et al., 1984). The conclusion that the dendritic membrane might be electrically active during spikes does not imply that the dendritic membrane contributes much to E_s, the voltage source causing the extracellular spikes; E_s might be largely located near the soma region.

The observations on the relationship between spike amplitude and dendritic membrane area as well as the observations on the absence of demonstrable retrograde propagation of action potentials into the sensory dendrites (Fig. 6) must lead to a reinterpretation of the physiology of pheromone receptors. Many experimental building blocks for a new concept on the functioning of these receptors are available, but still many more need to be found and fitted in before we may pretend to have a true understanding of the electrophysiology of these organs. The significance of this statement for our further discussion is to emphasize that there is not enough knowledge on the electrophysiology of sensilla to make straightforward interpretations of the influence of pheromone or other stimuli on electrically measured parameters.

IV.   WHAT DO SINGLE SENSILLUM RESPONSES TELL US ABOUT PRIMARY CHEMORECEPTOR PROCESSES?

The above discussion on the meaning and interpretation of electrophysiological data might lead to the impression that this type of research is inappropriate for the investigation of pheromone receptors. This impression, however, is false; electrical recordings give considerable information on decisive aspects of pheromone perception, for instance, in view of the specificity of the sensory apparatus of an animal. Behavioral data, for example, do not inform us whether bombykol (E10,Z12-16 : OH) and bombykal (E10,Z12-16 : Al), two pheromone components of *Bombyx mori,* exert their influence through one receptor, primarily sensitive to bombykol and with a side spectrum for bombykal, or whether there are different receptors for the two substances. From electrophysiological research, however, it is very clear that there are two types of receptors, one for bombykol and one for bombykal (Kaissling *et al.,* 1978). On the other hand, electrophysiological data on the specificity of a receptor for a given key compound do not inform us about the effects of key compounds on the behavior of an animal. Some compounds may initiate anemotaxis, others may inhibit this response (e.g., Borden, 1977; Preiss and Kramer, 1983; Hansen, 1984). The question of what single sensillum responses tell us about primary chemoreceptor processes can be answered in two ways, as there are two, not yet congenial types of quantitative models on chemoreceptive transduction processes. The first focuses on the kinetics while the second tries to describe the selectivity of the interaction between stimulus molecules and hypothetical receptors.

A. Pheromone–Receptor Interactions

Pheromone molecule–receptor interactions have been investigated systematically by analyzing the response of identified receptor neurons to homologous series of compounds (Boeckh, 1967; Kafka, 1970, 1974; Vareschi, 1971; Dumpert, 1972; Kafka and Neuwirth, 1975). In these investigations it appeared that the entire molecular structure seems to be important for the excitation of a receptor. The physiology of biological chemoreceptors for hormones and drugs and their interaction with stimuli, usually called ligands, have been reviewed by Wand (1968), Cuatrecasas and Hollenberg (1976), and O'Brien (1979). Activation of a receptor evidently requires some conformational change, and pheromone receptors having a one ligand to one receptor interaction should exist in only two functional stages: (a) fully active or (b) inactive. The transition of an inactive receptor to an active one requires energy which originates from the binding of an appropriate ligand to the receptor. As summarized by Van Haastert (1980), binding of a ligand may occur in two steps.

1. The ligand approaches the receptor by diffusion, and a subsequent collision of the ligand and the receptor site causes the liberation of kinetic energy.

2. Electrical interactions, such as ionic forces, hydrogen bonds, and van der Waals forces, between atoms and atom groups of the ligand and the receptor take place, which also results in the liberation of energy. This increased energy content of the ligand–receptor complex (L–R) either causes a fast dissociation into the original components or results in a fast conformational change by which the energy content is reduced (L–R'). The magnitude of the energy content of the

ligand–receptor complex (L–R) determines whether it will dissociate or change its conformation; for a conformational change, a minimal amount of energy should be liberated at the receptor site. Since the energy of interaction will be constant for a given ligand, the liberation of kinetic energy should be larger than a minimal level of activation energy.

One difficulty in the application of these more general receptor–ligand interaction models is that many pheromone molecules are, in contrast to, for instance, hormone molecules, very simple substances where many long-range electrostatic forces cannot play an important role. Often, as in the alarm pheromone undecane (Dumpert, 1972), only weak interactions can possibly explain the efficacy of a substance. In a quantitative model on pheromone–receptor interaction, Kafka and Neuwirth (1975) stated that the discrimination between two types of stimulus molecules can be explained only if the distance between receptor and pheromone molecule is 0.15 nm or less. At this distance the total binding energy between pheromone molecule and receptor would be only 10^{-23} kcal, which in turn implies that, owing to thermal movements, receptor–ligand interactions take place only during fractions of a picosecond (provided that the conformational change of the receptor does not change the pheromone molecule). Given these numbers, it is all the more astonishing that single pheromone molecules find their way in a pheromone-receptive hair and may elicit an action potential (Kaissling and Priesner, 1970).

In the hypothesis of Wright (1961, 1974), the action of a compound is determined by the Raman (far infrared) spectrum of substances. On basis of Raman spectra, it even appeared to be possible to predict the attractiveness of specific compounds to insects. The "death of three thousand wasps" (Wright, 1974) in a behavioral experiment, however, is no validation of this intriguing vibrational theory of olfactory specificity (see above); systematic investigations of the response of single receptor neurons should be performed.

B. Kinetics of Extracellular Receptor Potentials

The study of the kinetics of the electrophysiological response of a sensillum is very complex because this response is not just determined by pheromone–receptor interactions. It is also influenced by such parameters as stimulus release by the pheromone source, stimulus uptake and transport, pheromone degradation, diffusion, and many other processes (Vogt, Chapter 12, this volume). As many of the ideas on the dynamic responses of sensilla are based on electrophysiological recordings, however, some discussion on this theme should also occur here.

The complex of processes that play a role in stimulus uptake and transport have been analyzed in some detail (Adam and Delbrück, 1968; Kasang and Kaissling, 1972; Steinbrecht and Kasang, 1972; Kasang, 1973, 1974; Kanaujia and Kaissling, 1985). In many of these studies it appears that pheromone is well adsorbed on the hairs of the antennae and later "penetrates" into the antennal tissue as expressed in the ability to elute the pheromone in different solvents (Kasang, 1973, 1974; Kanaujia and Kaissling, 1985). In these elution experiments, a kind of compartmentalization appeared. Initially, all pheromone could be eluted in pentane; the fraction eluted in pentane decreased as incubation time increased. Part of the pentane noneluable fraction could be eluted in chloroform–methanol; after 30 min a fraction of 20%, the so-called residual activity, could not be eluted any more. From these experiments it was concluded that the pheromone on the antenna passes through a number of compartments with different physicochemical properties (Kasang, 1973). Efforts have been made to try to interpret morphologically these elution compartments. Apparently, pentane extracts primarily radioactivity from the hairs, both as pheromone or degradation products. The chloroform–methanol fraction seems to originate primarily from the main stem and the antennal side branches of the antenna (Kanaujia and Kaissling, 1985).

These fractional elution experiments give a rough picture of the complexity of the antenna. The real antenna, however, will have many more subcompartments as indicated in Fig. 19, which is based on a figure by Kasang (1973) and also incorporates findings by Vogt and Riddiford (1981) and Vogt et al. (1985). Three compartments in this scheme might, in theory, be the one that provides the pheromone receptors with stimulus molecules: (1) the binding protein, (2) the pore tubule, and (3) the lipid of the dendritic membrane. Which of these compartments is sensed by the receptors, however, remains unknown.

Analysis of the dynamics of receptor potentials upon stimulus delivery (Kaissling, 1969, 1974, 1979) are based on the premise that there is a fixed relationship between amplitude of the extracellular receptor potential and concentration of pheromone available to receptor proteins on a sensory dendrite. On stimulation, the receptor potential decreases to some steady level (see Fig. 5), which is hard to interpret when one realizes that the amount of pheromone on the hair is steadily increasing during stimulus delivery. The transport of pheromone molecules out of the hairs and the *in vivo* degradation of pheromone on the antenna (Steinbrecht and Kasang, 1972; Kasang and Kaissling, 1972; Kasang, 1971; Kanaujia and Kaissling, 1985), however, occurs with a half-life of approximately 3 min (Kasang, 1973), too slow to explain why the receptor potential does not steadily decrease during stimulation. The following types of explanations could account for these effects:

1. Kaissling (1969, 1971, 1974, 1979) proposed that some (concentration-dependent) "early inactivation mechanism" might explain the dynamics of the receptor potentials; he did not explicitly mention the location of this mechanism. Kasang (1973) proposed that diffusion of pheromone into several distinct com-

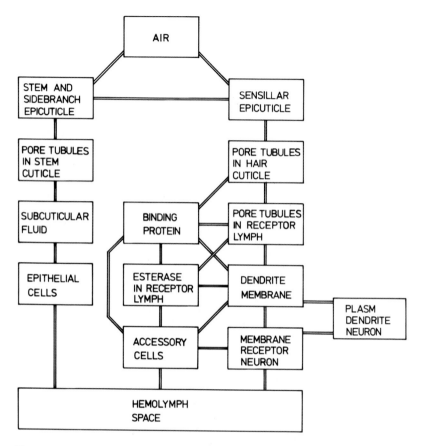

Fig. 19. Penetration and inactivation of pheromone in olfactory hairs may happen at a number of different locations (compartments) of the pheromone-sensitive apparatus, of which binding protein and sensillar esterase are only two examples. Which of the compartments is truly in connection with the receptors in the dendrite membrane is not known.

partments of the antenna (see also Fig. 19) might be the location of an inactivating mechanism.

2. Vogt and Riddiford (1981) proposed that binding of pheromone to the antennal "binding protein" might be a stimulus sink.

3. Vogt et al. (1985) concluded from in vitro experiments with purified esterase from the receptor lymph that degradation of pheromone by the esterase would be fast enough to account for the rapid inactivation.

4. Using mass-action paradigms, Kaissling (1986b) attempted to bring some coherence to in vitro and in vivo data on pheromone degradation. Using a K_D of 6 $\times$ 10^{-8} M for the binding of pheromone to the binding protein (from J. Hem-

berger, unpublished) and a K_m of 10^{-6} M for the esterase activity (Vogt et al., 1985), he proposed an in vivo half-life for the pheromone of about 5 min.

5. Another type of explanation for the dynamics of the receptor potential response would be that the pheromone receptor is not an occupancy receptor, but a rate receptor (Heck and Erickson, 1973). Under these circumstances even the receptor protein itself might be a pheromone-sequestering device. Various experimental methods to test this hypothesis have been indicated by Van Haastert (1980); these methods have not yet been used in the analysis of insect pheromone receptors.

6. The premise that the amplitude of the receptor potential represents the concentration of pheromone which is available to the receptors might be wrong. Stimulus-dependent decrease of receptor responsiveness (adaptation) might contribute to the dynamics of the receptor potential; short-term adaptation has, in contrast to long-term adaptation (Zack-Straussfeld and Kaissling, 1987), not been studied in olfactory sensilla.

C. Kinetics of Spike Responses and Receptor Potentials

Another interesting aspect of the dynamic response of pheromone receptors which has had only little attention is the change in spike rate upon stimulation. Often, the spike response of a receptor neuron has been expressed in terms of a one-dimensional number (Kafka, 1970; Boeckh, 1967; O'Connell, 1975, 1985). The modulation of spike rate, however. may also contain biologically relevant information (Van der Molen et al., 1978; Maes and Vedder, 1978; Rumbo, 1981; O'Connell et al., 1986). It has been observed (Kaissling, 1979; Kaissling and Thorson, 1980) that the poststimulus spike rate may be higher after stimulation with a key compound than after stimulation with some pheromone derivatives. As can be seen in Fig. 20, the initial responses to a low concentration of key compound and a high concentration of a pheromone analog are very similar, but the aftereffects are different.

Kaissling and Thorson (1980) proposed a mechanism for this spike modulation which is based on a direct influence of pheromone–receptor interactions on individual ion channels in the dendritic membrane. In their interpretation this influence can be observed in the behavior of what they call "elementary receptor potentials" (here miniature receptor potentials, see below). Miniature receptor potentials were defined as electrical events preceding action potentials. They can be readily observed in recordings when very low concentrations of pheromone are applied and appear as negative deflections of 0.5 mV or more in the potential across a sensillum starting some 10–40 msec before a nerve impulse. When the odor stimulus is stronger, miniature receptor potentials seem to be superimposed, thus forming a fluctuating receptor potential. Stimulation with higher concentrations of some pheromone analogs may lead to less noisy fluctuations of the

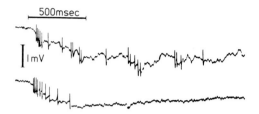

Fig. 20.   Two responses of a receptor neuron of the silkmoth *Antheraea pernyi*. The upper trace shows the response to a pheromone of this species, E6,Z11-16:Ac. The lower trace shows the response of the same cell to an approximately 1,000 times higher concentration of a partially saturated analog, Z11-16:Ac. Courtesy of Kaissling and Thorson (1980).

resulting receptor potential. This is interpreted as an indication that the amplitude or duration of miniature receptor potentials induced by pheromone analogs is reduced. As negative deflections in the receptor potential might trigger action potentials, the noisiness of the receptor potential would determine the spike rate even after termination of stimulus presentation. The supposed divisibility of the miniature potentials is one reason not to call them elementary potentials. Kaissling (1979; Kaissling and Thorson, 1980) interpreted the miniature receptor potentials to be the result of the opening of a single ion channel with a conductance of about 30 pS (picosiemens), "given appropriate parameters in the equivalent network." Since the distribution of impedances seems to be considerably different from what they proposed (see above and De Kramer *et al.*, 1984; J. J. De Kramer, unpublished), this interpretation of the miniature receptor potentials becomes very unlikely, which is another reason not to call them elementary potentials.

Quantal responses of a neuron to a stimulus are not necessarily caused by the opening of single ion channels. For instance, postsynaptic potentials display a quantal amplitude distribution (Boyd and Martin, 1956). Another example are quantal miniature potentials or "bumps" in invertebrate photoreceptors, where absorption of a photon may lead, through a row of second messenger systems (Brown *et al.*, 1984; Fein *et al.*, 1984), to the opening of 1000–10,000 ion channels. The amplitudes of these photoreceptor bumps depend on the adaptation level of the neuron (Yeandle and Fuortes, 1964; Yeandle, 1985; Stieve, 1985). Quantal responses are apparently possible when a cell responds to a quantal stimulus like the release of a single vesicle of neurotransmitter, the absorption of a single photon, or, here, the action of a single pheromone molecule. One very interesting, but also puzzling, property of the bumps with pheromone receptors is that their amplitude or duration seems to be related to the "adequacy" of the stimulus which can only be explained when more than one bit of information is transferred between receptor and receptor potential source.

How this information is transferred and amplified is a question of the second

messenger systems in chemosensory sensilla. This complex problem has been studied in gustatory sensilla especially (Felt and Vande Berg, 1977; Dailey and Vande Berg, 1976; Wieczorek and Schweikl, 1985), where some enhancement of receptor activity related to cGMP has been found. Villet (1978) describes an enhancement of the EAG amplitude after application of dibutyryl cAMP or phosphodiesterase inhibitors. In future research the role of second messengers in the pheromone-receptive system will certainly need more attention (Pace and Lancet, Chapter 15, this volume).

V. INTERPRETATION OF ELECTROANTENNOGRAMS

The electroantennogram (EAG) is usually used in screening tests for the identification of pheromones; little is known about its physiological basis. The EAG measures some slow change in the potential elicited upon presentation of a stimulus and can be recorded between two electrodes stuck into or onto an antenna. The amplitude of an EAG is well correlated with the concentration of the stimulus compound (e.g., Schneider et al., 1967; Roelofs and Comeau, 1971; Payne et al., 1970; Mayer et al., 1984) and has been called a "summated receptor potential" (Schneider, 1962). For both of these assertions, summated and receptor potential, however, there are not experimental validations. The EAG is generally much *smaller* in amplitude than the receptor potential of one single sensillum, and, as shown in Fig. 5, the shape of extracellular receptor potentials recorded from single sensilla may differ considerably from the shape of the simultaneously measured EAG (Kaissling, 1979; Van Der Pers et al., 1980; Nagai, 1983). We shall again first try to interpret the electrical circuitry of the antenna before further biological interpretations of the antennogram will be made.

The Electrical Equivalent Network of Antennae

The electrical equivalent network of antennae has been investigated using multiple electrode recordings between various different parts of the antenna (Nagai, 1983; Payne et al., 1970) and using localized olfactory stimulations. Nagai (1983) proposed that the sensory epithelium of an antenna may be considered as a core conductor, i.e., a cylinder of conducting fluid (hemolymph) surrounded by a layer of conducting medium (receptor lymph) and separated from each other by a layer of high electrical resistance (epithelial cell layer with septate junctions). Investigations of the electrical circuitry of sensilla (De Kramer, 1985) have shown that this picture needs some refinement as the receptor lymph spaces of neighboring hairs appear to be well isolated from each other; a large potential induced across one sensillum had only little influence on the

potential in a neighboring hair (Fig. 21). From these measurements and morphological observations (Keil, 1984b) it was concluded that the receptor lymph cavities of individual hairs are well isolated; current from one hair lumen to another has to pass twice through narrow clefts between the tormogen cell and the cuticle and through the subcuticular fluid, as indicated in Fig. 22. The epithelial length constant that exists in this arrangement is primarily determined by the conductance of the subcuticular fluid and the transepithelial resistance; both of these factors remain unknown. Different authors use different experimen-

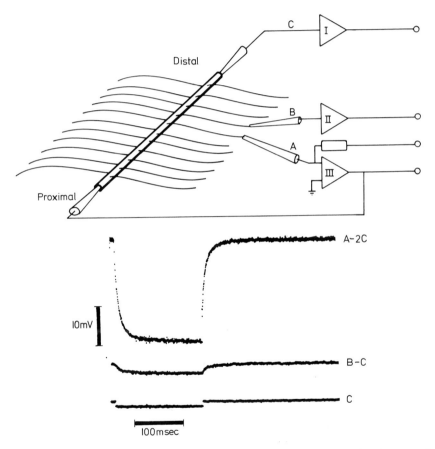

Fig. 21. Apparatus for investigation to the connections between receptor lymph spaces of neighboring sensilla. I and II, Kootsley and Johnson (1972) buffer amplifier. III, Current clamping amplifier. The oscilloscope traces show one result of such an experiment; upon stimulation of sensillum A with a current pulse of -100 pA in B only a small fraction of the potential across A is fed through. The subtraction with the signal from C is to compensate for electrode and hemolymph resistances. From De Kramer (1985).

tal arrangements in EAG measurements, which may be, next to differences due to biological variation, a reason for divergent interpretations.

1. EAG Electrode Arrangements

Most authors connect reference and recording electrodes in some way or another to proximal parts of the hemolymph space of the antenna, thereby causing artificial short circuits between the subcuticular fluid and the hemolymph space. Payne *et al.* (1970) and Nagai (1981, 1983) sometimes used extracuticular reference or recording electrodes. These extracuticular electrodes presumably measure primarily the potential of the subcuticular fluid, possibly through rather conductive intersegmental cuticular "membranes." Electrodes inside or in good contact with the hemolymph space, like those used by Schneider (1962), Roelofs and Comeau (1971), Kaissling (1979), and Mayer *et al.* (1984) might record primarily potential differences which are induced along the hemolymph core of the antenna.

2. Possible Locations for Pheromone-Dependent Potential Sources in an Antenna

The potential induced along the hemolymph core of the antenna may, as proposed by Kaissling (1971), be induced because the cellular apparatuses of sensilla are arranged in an array with the basolateral membranes directed proximally and the receptor lymph cavities directed distally. In this configuration every sensillum would be a local dipole which influences the potential of the hemolymph core, as indicated by the pluses and minuses in Fig. 22. Also field potentials introduced by the greater abundance of axons in the proximal than in the distal part of antennae may contribute to the potential gradient in the hemolymph core. The potential of the subcuticular fluid will be additionally altered by the changes in receptor lymph potential (extracellular receptor potentials) of sensilla in the neighborhood of the electrodes; the influence of sensilla farther away depends on the length constant of the epithelium.

From this brief analysis of the electrical structure of an insect antenna it may be concluded that not only the receptor potentials of single sensilla but also many other (unknown) parameters, such as the epithelial length constant or the distribution of specialized sensilla, determine the shape and amplitude of an EAG response. The inability to fully explain the EAG, however, does not make it a useless tool; it is a very relevant bioassay in olfactory research and may give first indications for the presence of receptors for a given substance. An extremely practical application of antennograms was introduced by Arn *et al.* (1975; see also Struble and Arn, 1984; Wadhams, 1984), who inserted the antenna or a single sensillum of an insect as a biological detector in parallel to the flame ionization detector at the end of the column of a gas chromatograph, a technique

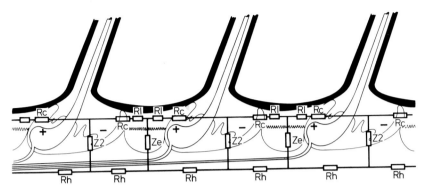

Fig. 22. Epithelial structure of the antenna. Z_2, Impedance across a sensillum (about the descriptive R_2–C_2 combination); R_c, resistance between the receptor lymph space and the subcuticular fluid; R_1, resistance of the subcuticular fluid which, together with the impedance across the nonsensillar cells in the epithelium (Z_e) and the resistance of the hemolymph core of the antenna or antennal side branch, determine the epithelial length or space constant. Note the polarized arrangement of the receptor neurons in the epithelium.

which provides the possibility of identifying biologically important substances from crude extracts.

ACKNOWLEDGMENTS

We thank all our former colleagues in Seewiesen, especially Drs. K. E. Kaissling, T. A. Keil, S. Kanaujia, G. A. Adamek, and R. A. Steinbrecht, for the many hours of constructive discussions and for supplying some figures, and R. A. Steinbrecht and G. E. Kahn for their critical reading of the manuscript. We also thank I. J. De Kramer for preparing the figures.

REFERENCES

Adam, G., and Delbrück, M. (1968). Reduction of dimensionality in biological diffusion processes. *In* "Structural Chemistry and Molecular Biology" (A. Rich and N. Davidson, eds.), pp. 198–215. Freeman, San Francisco.

Adamek, G. A., Hemberger, J., and Kaissling, K. E. (1984a). Exchange of receptor lymph in insect olfactory hairs: A method to study the role of ions and proteins in transduction. *In* "Abstracts of the ECRO VI Congress," p. 3. Lyon-Ecully, France.

Adamek, G. A., Gesteland, R. C., Mair, R. G., and Oakley, B. (1984b). Transduction physiology of olfactory receptor cilia. *Brain Res.* **310,** 87–97.

Arn, H., Städler, E., and Rauscher, S. (1975). The electroantennographic detector—a selective and sensitive tool in the gas chromatographic analysis of insect pheromones. *Z. Naturforsch.* **30C,** 722–725.

Boeckh, J. (1962). Elektrophysiologische Untersuchungen an einzelnen Geruchsrezeptoren auf Antennen des Totengräbers (*Necrophorus,* Coleoptera). *Z. Vergl. Physiol.* **41,** 212–248.

Boeckh, J. (1967). Reaktionsschwelle, Arbeitsbereich und Spezifität eines Geruchsrezeptors auf der Heuschreckenantenne. *Z. Vergl. Physiol.* **55,** 378–406.

Boistel, J., and Coraboeuf, E. (1953). L'activité électrique dans l'antenne isolée de Lépidoptere au cours de l'étude de l'olfaction. *C. R. Soc. Biol. Paris* **147,** 1172–1175.

Borden, J. H. (1977). Behavioral responses of Coleoptera to pheromones, allomones, and kairomones. *In* "Chemical Control of Insect Behaviour" (H. H. Shorey, and J. J. McKelvey, eds.), pp. 169–198. Wiley, New York.

Boyd, I. A., and Martin, A. R. (1956). The end-plate potential in mamalian muscle. *J. Physiol. (London)* **132,** 74–91.

Brown, J. E., Rubin, L. J., Ghalayini, A. J., Tarver, A. P., Irvine, R. F., Berridge, M. J., and Anderon, R. E. (1984). Myoinositol polyphosphate may be a messenger for visual excitation in *Limulus* photoreceptors. *Nature (London)* **311,** 160–163.

Burrows, M., Boeckh, J., and Esslen, J. (1982). Physiological and morphological properties of interneurons in the deutocerebrum of male cockroaches which respond to female pheromone. *J. Comp. Physiol.* **145,** 447–457.

Cole, K. S. (1972). "Membranes, Ions, and Impulses." Univ. of California Press, Berkeley, Los Angeles.

Cuatrecasas, P., and Hollenberg, M. D. (1976). Membrane receptors and hormone action. *Adv. Protein Chem.* **30,** 251–451.

Dailey, D. L., and Vande Berg, J. S. (1976). Apparent opposing effects of cyclic AMP and dibutyryl-cyclic GMP on the neuronal firing of the blowfly chemoreceptors. *Biochem. Biophys. Acta* **437,** 211–220.

De Kramer, J. J. (1985). The electrical circuitry of an olfactory sensillum in *Antheraea polyphemus. J. Neurosci.* **5,** 2484–2493.

De Kramer, J. J., Kaissling, K. E., and Keil, T. A. (1984). Passive electrical properties of insect olfactory sensilla may produce the biphasic shape of spikes. *Chem. Senses* **8,** 289–295.

DeSimone, J. A., Heck, G. L., Mierson, S., and DeSimone, S. K. (1984). The active ion transport properties of canine lingual epithelia in vivo: Implications for gustatory transduction. *J. Gen. Physiol.* **83,** 633–656.

Dumpert, K. (1972). Alarmstoffrezeptoren auf der Antenne von *Lasius fuliginosus* (Latr.) (Hymenoptera, Formicidae). *Z. Vergl. Physiol.* **76,** 403–425.

Fein, A., Payne, R., Corson, D. W., Berridge, M. J., and Irvine, R. F. (1984). Photoreceptor excitation and adaptation by inositol 1,4,5-triphosphate. *Nature (London)* **311,** 157–160.

Felt, B. T., and Vande Berg, J. S. (1977). Localization of adenylate cyclase in the blowfly labellar chemoreceptors. *J. Insect Physiol.* **23,** 543–548.

Fujishiro, N., Kijama, H., and Morita, H. (1984). Impulse frequency and action potential amplitude in labellar chemosensory neurons of *Drosophila melanogaster. J. Insect Physiol.* **30(4),** 317–325.

Futrelle, R. P. (1984). How molecules get to their detectors. The physics of diffusion of insect pheromones. *Trends Neurosci.* **7,** 116–120.

Gnatzy, W., Mohren, W., and Steinbrecht, R. A. (1984). Pheromone receptors in *Bombyx mori* and *Antheraea pernyi* II. Morphometric analysis. *Cell Tiss. Res.* **235,** 35–42.

Hansen, K. (1983). Reception of bark beetle pheromone in predaceous clerid beetle, *Thanasius formicarius* (Coleoptera: Cleridae). *J. Comp. Physiol.* **150,** 371–378.

Hansen, K. (1984). Discrimination and production of disparlure enantiomers by the gypsy moth and the nun moth. *Physiol. Entomol.* **9,** 9–18.

Heck, G. L., and Erickson, R. P. (1973). A rate theory of gustatory stimulation. *Behav. Biol.* **8,** 687–712.

Kafka, W. A. (1970). Molekulare Wechselwirkungen bei der Erregung einzelner Riechzellen. Z. *Vergl. Physiol.* **70**, 105–143.

Kafka, W. A. (1974). Physicochemical aspects of odour reception in insects. *Ann. N.Y. Acad. Sci.* **237**, 115–127.

Kafka, W. A., and Neuwirth, J. (1975). A model of pheromone molecule–acceptor interaction. Z. *Naturforsch.* **30C**, 278–282.

Kaissling, K. E. (1969). Kinetics of olfactory receptor potentials. In "Proceedings of the Third International Symposium on Olfaction and Taste" (Pfaffmann, ed.), pp. 52–70. Rockefeller Univ. Press, New York.

Kaissling, K. E. (1971). Kinetic studies of transduction in olfactory receptors of *Bombyx mori*. In "Olfaction and Taste IV" (D. Schneider, ed.), pp. 207–213. Wiss. Verlagsges, Stuttgart.

Kaissling, K. E. (1974). Sensory transduction in insect olfactory receptors. In "Biochemistry of Sensory Functions" (L. Jaenicke, ed.), pp. 243–273. Springer-Verlag, Berlin.

Kaissling, K. E. (1979). Recognition of pheromones by moths, especially in saturniids and *Bombyx mori*. In "Chemical Ecology: Odour Communication in Animals" (F. J. Ritter, ed.), pp. 43–56. Elsevier, Amsterdam.

Kaissling, K. E. (1980). Studies on the functional organization of insect olfactory sensilla (*Antheraea polyphemus* and *Antheraea pernyi*). In "Olfaction and Taste VII" (H. Van Der Starre, ed.), pp. 81. Information Retrieval, New York.

Kaissling, K. E. (1986a). Temporal characteristics of pheromone receptor cell responses in relation to orientation behaviour of moths. In "Mechanisms in Insect Olfaction" (T. Payne, ed.), pp. 193–200. Oxford Univ. Press, London and New York.

Kaissling, K. E. (1986b). Chemo-electrical transduction in insect olfactory receptors. *Annu. Rev. Neurosci.*, 121–145.

Kaissling, K. E., and Priesner, E. (1970). Die Riechschwelle des Seidenspinners. *Naturwissenschaften* **57**, 23–28.

Kaissling, K. E., and Renner, M. (1968). Antennale Rezeptoren für Queen-substance und Sterzelduft bei der Honigbiene. Z. *Vergl. Physiol.* **59**, 357–361.

Kaissling, K. E., and Thorson, J. (1980). Insect olfactory sensilla: Structural, chemical and electrical aspects of the functional organisation. In "Receptors for Neurotransmitters, Hormones and Pheromones in Insects" (D. B. Satelle, L. M. Hall, and J. G. Hildebrand, eds.), pp. 261–282. Elsevier/North Holland, Amsterdam.

Kaissling, K. E., Kasang, G., Bestmann, H. J., Stransky, W., and Vostrovksy, O. (1978). A new pheromone of the silkmoth *Bombyx mori*. Sensory pathway and behavioural effect. *Naturwissenschaften* **56**, 382–384.

Kaissling, K. E., Klein, U., De Kramer, J. J., Keil, T. A., and Hemberger, J. (1985). Insect olfactory cells: Electrophysiological and biochemical studies. In "Molecular Basis of Nerve Activity" (Proc. Int. Symp. in Memory of D. Nachmanson) (Changeux, Hucho, Maelicke, Neumann, eds.), pp. 173–183. de Gruyter, Berlin and New York.

Kanaujia, S., and Kaissling, K. E. (1985). Interactions of pheromone with moth antennae: Adsorption, desorption and transport. *J. Insect Physiol.* **31**, 71–81.

Kasang, G. (1971). Bombykol reception and metabolism on the antennae of the silkmoth *Bombyx mori*. In "Gustation and Olfaction" (Ohloff, ed.), pp. 245–250. Academic Press, New York.

Kasang, G. (1973). Physikochemische Vorgänge beim Riechen des Seidenspinners. *Naturwissenschaften* **60**, 95–101.

Kasang, G. (1974). Uptake of the sex pheromone ^{3}H-bombykol and related compounds by male and female *Bombyx* antennae. *J. Insect Physiol.* **20**, 2407–2422.

Kasang, G., and Kaissling, K. E. (1972). Specificity of primary and secondary olfactory processes in *Bombyx* antennae. In "Olfaction and Taste IV" (D. Schneider, ed.), pp. 200–206. Wiss. Verlagsges, Stuttgart.

Keil, T. A. (1984a). Very tight contact of tormogen cell membrane and sensillum cuticle: Ultrastructural basis for high electrical resistance between receptor lymph and subcuticular spaces in silkmoth olfactory hairs. *Tiss. Cell* **16**, 131–135.

Keil, T. A. (1984b). Reconstruction and morphometry of silkmoth olfactory hairs: A comparative study of sensilla trichodea on the antennae of male *Antheraea polyphemus* and *Antheraea pernyi* (Insecta, Lepidoptera). *Zoomorphology* **104**, 147–156.

Keil, T. A., and Steinbrecht, R. A. (1983). Interrelations of sensory, enveloping and glial cells in epidermal mechano- and chemoreceptors of insects. *Verh. Dtsch. Zool. Ges.* **76**, 249.

Keil, T. A., and Steinbrecht, R. A. (1984). Mechanosensitive and olfactory sensilla of insects. *In* "Insect Ultrastructure: (R. C. King, and H. Akai, eds.), pp. 477–516. Plenum, New York.

Kootsley, J. M., and Johnson, E. A. (1972). Buffer amplifier with femtofarad input capacity using operational amplifier. *I.E.E.E.* trans BME **19**, 389–391.

Kramer, E. (1986). Turbulent diffusion and pheromone triggered anemotaxis. *In* "Mechanisms in Insect Olfaction" (T. Payne, ed.), Oxford Univ. Press, London and New York.

Levinson, H. Z., Kaissling, K. E., and Levinson, A. R. (1973). Olfaction and cyanide sensitivity in the six-spot burnet moth *Zygaena filipendulae* and the silkmoth *Bombyx mori*. *J. Comp. Physiol.* **86**, 209–214.

Levinson, H. Z., Levinson, A. R., Jen, T.-L., Williams, J. L. D., Kahn, G. E., and Francke, W. (1978). Production site, partial composition and olfactory perception of a pheromone in the male hide beetle. *Naturwissenschaften* **65**, 543–544.

Light, D. M. (1983). Sensitivity of antennae of male and female *Ips paraconfusus* (Coleoptera: Scolytidae) to its pheromone and other behavior-modifying chemicals. *J. Chem. Ecol.* **9**, 585–606.

Locke, M. (1964). Permeability of insect cuticle to water and lipids. *Science* **147**, 295–298.

Maes, F. W., and Vedder, C. G. (1978). A morphological and electrophysiological inventory of labellar taste hairs of the blowfly *Calliphora vicina*. *J. Insect Physiol.* **24**, 667–672.

Mankin, R. W., and Mayer, M. S. (1984). The insect antenna is not a molecular sieve. *Experientia* **40**, 1251–1252.

Matsumoto, S. G., and Hildebrand, J. G. (1981). Olfactory mechanisms in the moth *Manduca sexta:* Response characteristics and morphology of central neurons in the antennal lobes. *Proc. R. Soc. London Ser. B* **213**, 249–277.

Mayer, M. S., Mankin, R. W., and Lemire, G. F. (1984). Quantitation of the insect electroantennogram: Measurement of sensillar contributions, elimination of background potentials, and relationship to olfactory sensation. *J. Insect Physiol.* **30**, 757–763.

Morita, H. (1959). Initiation of spike potentials in contact chemosensory hairs of insects. III. D. C. stimulation and generator potential of labellar chemoreceptor of *Calliphora*. *J. Cell. Comp. Physiol.* **54**, 189–204.

Morita, H. (1963). Generator potential of insect chemoreceptors. *Proc. Int. Congr. Zool.* **3**, 105–106.

Morita, H., and Yamashita, S. (1959). The back-firing of impulses in a labellar chemosensory hair of the fly. *Mem. Fac. Kyushu Univ. Ser. E* **3**, 81–87.

Mustaparta, H. (1975). Responses of single olfactory cells to insect- and host-produced volatiles in the bark beetle *Ips pini* (Say). *J. Comp. Physiol.* **79**, 271–290.

Nagai, T. (1981). Electroantennogram response gradient on the antenna of the European corn borer, *Ostrinia nubilalis*. *J. Insect Physiol.* **27**, 889–894.

Nagai, T. (1983). On the relationship between the electroantennogram and simultaneously recorded single sensillum response of the European cornborer. *Ostrinia nubilalis*. *Arch. Insect Bioch. Physiol.* **1**, 85–91.

O'Brien, R. D. (ed.) (1979). "The Receptors," Vol. 1. Plenum, New York.

O'Connell, R. J. (1975). Olfactory receptor responses to sex pheromone components in the red-banded leafroller moth. *J. Gen. Physiol.* **65**, 179–205.

O'Connell, R. J. (1985). Responses to pheromone blends in insect olfactory receptor neurons. *J. Comp. Physiol.* **156**, 747–761.

O'Connell, R. J., Beauchamp, J. T., and Grant, A. J. (1986). Insect olfactory receptor responses to components of pheromone blends. *J. Chem. Ecol.* **12**, 451–467.

Oldfield, B. P., and Hill, K. G. (1986). Functional organization of insect auditory sensilla. *J. Comp. Physiol.* **158**, 27–34.

Payne, T. L., Shorley, H. H., and Gaston, L. K. (1970). Sex pheromones of noctuid moths: Factors influencing antennal responsiveness in males of *Trichoplusia ni*. *J. Insect Physiol.* **16**, 1043–1055.

Preiss, R., and Kramer, E. (1983). Stabilization of altitude and speed in tethered flying gypsy moth males: Influence of (+) and (−)-disparlure. *Physiol. Entomol.* **8**, 55–68.

Prestwich, G. D., Vogt, R. G., and Riddiford, L. M. (1986). Binding and hydrolysis of radiolabelled pheromone and several analogs by male-specific antennal proteins of the moth *Antheraea polyphemus*. *J. Chem. Ecol.* **12**, 232–333.

Priesner, E. (1979). Progress in the analysis of pheromone receptor systems. *Ann. Zool. Ecol. Anim.* **11**, 533–546.

Rees, C. J. C. (1968). The effects of aqueous solutions of some 1 : 1 electrolytes on the electrical response of the type 1 ('salt') chemoreceptor cell in the labella of *Phormia*. *J. Insect Physiol.* **14**, 1331–1364.

Roelofs, W. L. (1984). Electroantennogram assays: Rapid and convenient screening procedures for pheromones. *In* "Techniques in Pheromone Research" (H. E. Hummel and T. A. Miller, eds.), pp. 131–159. Springer-Verlag, New York, Berlin, and Heidelberg.

Roelofs, W. L., and Comeau, A. (1971). Sex pheromone perception: Electroantennogram responses of the red-banded leaf roller moth. *J. Insect Physiol.* **17**, 1969–1982.

Roys, C. (1954). Olfactory nerve potentials a direct measure of chemoreception in insects. *Ann. N.Y. Acad. Sci.* **58**, 250–255.

Rumbo, E. R. (1981). Study of single sensillum responses to pheromone in the light-brown apple moth, *Epiphyas postvittana*, using an averaging technique. *Physiol. Entomol.* **6**, 87–98.

Schanne, O. F., and Ceretti, E. R. P. (1978). "Impedance Measurements in Biological Cells." Wiley, New York.

Scheie, P. O., and Smyth, T. (1976). Electrical measurements on cuticles excised from adult male *Periplaneta americana* (L.). *Comp. Biochem. Physiol.* **21**, 547–571.

Schneider, D. (1955). Mikroelektroden registrieren die elektrischen Impulse einzelner Sinnesnervenzellen der Schmetterlingsantenne. *Industrieelektronik (Hamburg)* **3**, 3–7.

Schneider, D. (1957). Elektrophysiologische Untersuchungen von Chemo- und Mechanorezeptoren der Antenne des Seidenspinners *Bombyx mori* L. *Z. Vergl. Physiol.* **40**, 8–41.

Schneider, D. (1962). Electrophysiological investigation on the olfactory specificity of sexual attracting substances in different species of moths. *J. Insect Physiol.* **8**, 15–30.

Schneider, D., and Boeckh, J. (1962). Rezeptorpotential und Nervenimpulse einzelner olfaktorischer Sensillen der Insektenantenne. *Z. Vergl. Physiol.* **45**, 405–412.

Schneider, D., and Hecker, E. (1956). Zur Elektrophysiologie der Antenne des Seidenspinners *Bombyx mori* bei Reizung mit angereicherten Extrakten des Sexuallockstoffes. *Z. Naturforsch.* **11B**, 121–124.

Schneider, D., Lacher, V., and Kaissling, K. E. (1964). Die Reaktionsweise und das Reaktionsspectrum von Riechzellen bei *Antheraea pernyi* (Lepidoptera, Saturniidae). *Z. Vergl. Physiol.* **48**, 632–662.

Schneider, D., Block, B. C., Boeckh, J., and Priesner, E. (1967). Die Reaktion der männlichen Seidenspinner auf Bombykol und seine Isomeren: Elektroantennogramm und Verhalten. *Z. Vergl. Physiol.* **54**, 192–209.

Steinbrecht, R. A. (1973). Der Feinbau olfaktorischer Sensillen des Seidenspinners (Insecta, Lepidoptera). *Z. Zellforsch.* **139**, 533–565.

Steinbrecht, R. A., and Gnatzy, W. (1984). Pheromone receptors of *Bombyx mori* and *Antheraea pernyi:* 1. Reconstruction of the cellular organization of the sensilla trichodea. *Cell Tiss. Res.* **235**, 25–34.

Steinbrecht, R. A., and Kasang, G. (1972). Capture and conveyance of odour molecules in an insect olfactory receptor. *In* "Olfaction and Taste IV" (D. Schneider, ed.), pp. 193–199. Wiss. Verlagsges, Stuttgart.

Steinbrecht, R. A., and Zierold, K. (1985). X-Ray microanalysis of electrolytes in cryosections of an insect olfactory sensillum. *Eur. J. Cell Biol. Suppl.* **10**, 69.

Struble, D. L., and Arn, H. (1984). Combined gas chromatography and electroantennogram recording of insect olfactory responses. *n* "Techniques in Pheromone Research" (H. E. Hummel and T. A. Miller, eds.), pp. 161–178. Springer-Verlag, New York, Berlin, and Heidelberg.

Stieve, H. (1985). Phototransduction in invertebrate visual cells. The present state of research—exemplified and discussed through the *Limulus* photoreceptor cell. *In* "Neurobiology" (R. Gilles and J. Balthazart, eds.), pp. 346–362.

Thurm, U., and Küppers, J. (1980). Epithelial physiology of insect sensilla. *In* "Insect Biology in the Future" (M. Locke and D. Smith, eds.), pp. 735–763. Academic Press, New York.

Van der Molen, J. N., Van der Meulen, J. W., De Kramer, J. J. and Pasveer, F. J. (1978). Computerized classification of taste cell responses. *J. Comp. Physiol.* **128**, 1–11.

Van Der Pers, J. N. C., and Den Otter, C. J. (1978). Single cell responses from olfactory receptors of small ermine moths to sex attractants. *J. Insect Physiol.* **42**, 337–343.

Van Der Pers, J. N. C., Thomas, G., and Den Otter, C. J. (1980). Interactions between plant odours and pheromone reception in small ermine moths (Lepidoptera: Yponomeutidae). *Chem. Senses,* **5**, 367–371.

Van Haastert, P. J. M. (1980). Distinction between the rate theory and the occupation theory of signal transduction by receptor activation. *Neth. J. Zool.* **30**, 473–493.

Vareschi, E. (1971). Duftunterscheidung bei der Honigbiene—Einzelzell-Ableitung und Verhaltensreaktionen. *Z. Vergl. Physiol.* **75**, 143–173.

Villet, R. H. (1978). Mechanism of insect sex-pheromone sensory transduction: Role of adenyl cyclase. *Comp. Biochem. Physiol.* **61C**, 389–394.

Vogt, R. G., and Riddiford, L. M. (1981). Pheromone binding and inactivation by moth antennae. *Nature (London)* **393**, 161–163.

Vogt, R. G., Riddiford, L. M., and Prestwich, G. D. (1985). Kinetic properties of a sex pheromone–degrading enzyme: The sensillar esterase of *Antheraea polyphemus*. *Proc. Natl. Acad. Sci. U.S.A.* **82**, 8827–8831.

Wadhams, L. J. (1984). The coupled gas chromotography–single cell recording technique. *In* "Techniques in Pheromone Research" (H. E. Hummel and T. A. Miller, eds.), pp. 179–189. Springer-Verlag, New York, Berlin, and Heidelberg.

Wand, D. R. (1968). Pharmacological receptors. *Pharmacol. Rev.* **20**, 49–88.

Wieczorek, H., and Schweikl, H. (1985). Concentrations of cyclic nucleotides and activities of cyclases and phosphodiesterases in an insect chemosensory organ. *Insect Biochem.* **6**, 723–728.

Wolbarsht, M. L. (1960). Electrical characteristics of insect mechanoreceptors. *J. Gen. Physiol.* **44**, 105–122.

Wolbarsht, M. L., and Hanson, F. E. (1965). Electrical activity in the chemoreceptors of the blowfly. III. Dendritic action potentials. *J. Gen. Physiol.* **48**, 673–683.

Wright, R. H. (1961). Odour and molecular vibration. *Nature (London)* **190**, 1101–1102.

Wright, R. H. (1974). Predicting olfactory quality from far infrared spectra. *Ann. N.Y. Acad. Sci.* **237**. 129–136.

Yeandle, S. (1985). Statistics and quantum bumps in arthropod photoreceptors. *Fed. Proc., Fed. Am. Soc. Exp. Biol.* **44,** 2947–2949.

Yeandle, S., and Fuortes, M. F. G. (1964). Probability of occurrence of discrete potential waves in the eye of *Limulus. J. Gen. Physiol.* **47,** 443–467.

Zack, C. (1979). "Sensory adaptation in the sex pheromone receptor cells of saturniid moths" Dissertation from the Faculty of Biology, Ludwig Maximilians Universität, Munich.

Zack-Straussfeld, C., and Kaissling, K. E. (1987). Localized adaptation processes in olfactory sensilla of saturniid moths (submitted).

14

Chemical Studies of Pheromone Reception and Catabolism

GLENN D. PRESTWICH

Department of Chemistry
State University of New York
Stony Brook, New York 11794-3400

I. INTRODUCTION

An understanding of the molecular basis of pheromone perception requires detailed knowledge of the sensilla-specific macromolecules which bind and degrade pheromone molecules. One approach to this problem is the use of radiolabeled pheromones and pheromone analogs to isolate and characterize both the macromolecules and the pheromone metabolites. The small amounts of tissue and the high specificity assumed for this biochemical system dictate the use of very high specific activity ligands which are both stereochemically and electronically indistinguishable from the natural pheromone components.

In this chapter, I shall first describe the methodology employed in using radiochemicals to study pheromone catabolism and pheromone reception. Second, I shall review the literature by presenting case studies for seven insect species for which detailed chemical studies have been undertaken. These examples will include previously unpublished results from my laboratories at Stony Brook.

Pheromone Biochemistry

II. METHODOLOGY

At this early stage in the chemical study of pheromone biochemistry, it is important to describe techniques for analysis of small molecule–large molecule interactions. In the 15 years since the first reported example of pheromone degradation, the analytical techniques available in chemistry and biochemistry have changed dramatically. To maximize the value of current efforts for future studies, it is important that we document how we obtained proteins, how we prepared radioligands, and how we analyzed our results.

A. Catabolic Proteins

The enzymes which degrade pheromones fall into four categories: (a) tissue- and substrate-specific, (b) tissue-specific but nonspecific for pheromone components, (c) generally distributed but pheromone-specific, and (d) generally distributed and nonspecific enzymes. Only those enzymes which are localized in pheromone-receiving tissues and those which show specificity for pheromonal molecules (regardless of tissue location) will be discussed in this chapter.

1. Tissues

a. Source.   Most pheromones are lipophilic and can adsorb to virtually any cuticular surface of an insect. For example, we can assume *a priori* that all tissues have some intrinsic ability to chemically degrade volatile fatty alcohol derivatives to prevent the receiving insect from becoming its own pheromone source. In collecting tissues for enzyme assays, therefore, it is prudent to examine legs, wing scales, body segments, hemolymph, and glandular structures as well as the antennae. Examination of tissues of both sexes will further aid in identifying the pheromone-specific processing proteins.

b. Preparation.   In obtaining cell-free protein samples, one must examine soluble and membrane-bound proteins. The best tissue preparations will minimize contamination of specific tissues, e.g., glandular epidermis or sensilla lymph, with general proteins from the hemolymph or cuticle. For example, sensory hairs can be harvested by mechanical fracturing at cryogenic temperatures (Klein and Keil, 1984) or by ultrasonic shearing (Ferkovich, 1982). Although the sonication method is quicker, especially for filiform antennae with short sensilla, it probably results in contamination by hemolymph proteins from the broken antennal base. The freeze-fracture method provides the cleanest preparation of sensillar lymph, sensillar cuticle, and dendritic membrane, but at the expense of speed and overall yield. In addition, some proteins may suffer loss of activity after freezing or lyophilization.

Similarly, the abdominal tips can be clipped to provide glandular (pheromone gland or hair pencil) materials for biogenetic studies. Contamination by general hemolymph proteins and cuticular enzymes can easily confuse the interpretation of these data; there is no substitute for a careful but expeditious dissection of glandular tissue and rinsing to remove hemolymph. After tissue specificity and protein location have been established, yield becomes paramount and the trade-off favors purification from total tissue homogenates.

c. In Vivo or In Vitro? The central dilemma in all studies is whether to examine the fate of the pheromone at very low concentrations on whole antennae, preferably attached to a moth, or to employ a binding protein or enzyme preparation with saturating ligand concentrations. The first is biologically relevant, the second biochemically informative. As a chemist, I feel that one must first determine what proteins are involved, what metabolites are produced, and what concentrations are best to measure binding and rates accurately. Subsequently, it is crucial that one reintegrates these parameters back into the intact system; this shows whether the proteins do indeed play the roles one infers for them from the in vitro assays. It is never adequate to extrapolate in the other direction, however, as has been attempted with pheromone metabolism. Without knowing cuticle composition, the nature of macromolecular processing in the sensory hair, or the net chemical conversions, it is insufficient to measure pheromone molecules impinging on and then disappearing from an antenna. Unfortunately, much of the conventional wisdom concerning pheromone processing is based on such "black box" experiments on whole antennae with inadequate chemical and biochemical follow-up. This is now changing as will be discussed in detail in this chapter.

2. Substrates

a. Radiosynthesis. In order to probe pheromone processing at realistic concentrations, particularly given the low water solubility of most aliphatic pheromones, isotopically-labeled molecules are required which are essentially carrier-free. Exciting results have been obtained in pheromone biosynthesis using stable-isotope ^{13}C-, ^{18}O-, ^{19}F-, and ^{2}H-labeled precursors in conjunction with plasma ionization or mass spectral detection of metabolites (Bjostad and Roelofs, 1986; Bjostad et al., Chapter 3, this volume; McCormick and Carrel, Chapter 10). Nonetheless, radioisotopic labels are the best choice for researchers investigating pheromone binding or catabolism, since the number of molecules involved in the olfactory process is intrinsically very small. Also, the low tolerance of the insect chemoreception system to minor alterations in chemical structure or heteroatomic substitution limits the options further. Thus, substitution of radioactive isotopes of atoms already in the pheromone offers both minimal perturbation and maximal sensitivity.

The extremely short half-lives ($<$120 min) of the positron emitters ^{18}F, ^{11}C, and ^{15}O make them unsuitable for work with antennal proteins, despite the high specific activities possible ($>$10,000 Ci/mmol). The substitution of ^{125}I ($t_{1/2}$ = 60 days, $>$2000 Ci/mmol) into the terminal methyl of fatty acid chains has been used in the study of acylglycerol metabolism in vertebrates, but the use of radioiodinated pheromones as substrates for insect olfactory receptors or catabolic enzymes has not yet been attempted. We expect to pursue this in the future. The use of the strong β emitter ^{35}S ($t_{1/2}$ = 30 days) is discouraged by the difficulty of obtaining this nuclide in a suitable chemical form, e.g., the sulfide oxidation level in the no-carrier-added state.

Carbon-14 labels can be employed, but they require additional C—C bond forming steps for introduction. The maximum specific activity per ^{14}C atom is 58 mCi/mmol. General synthetic methods for ^{14}C incorporation have been compiled by Muccino (1983), and specific methods for pheromone precursors are summarized by Bjostad *et al.* (Chapter 3, this volume). Nonetheless, the high β particle energy relative to ^{3}H and the nonlability from acidic positions makes ^{14}C a desirable level for metabolite identification. It is always the label of choice when alterations of the carbon skeleton are involved or when long incubations are required. The main limitation is that the quantity of enzymes obtained from the tissues of interest needs to be sufficient to catalyze turnover at the micromole level.

The optimal compromise for high specific activity, ease of monitoring, and ease of synthesis is tritium. The maximum specific activity is 29 Ci/mg-atom of ^{3}H for this 12-year half-life, low energy β emitter. A review of ^{3}H labeling methods, with examples, is available in a treatise on tritium nuclear magnetic resonance (^{3}H NMR) (Evans *et al.*, 1985); the major routes of interest are summarized below.

1. Tritium can be introduced in no-carrier-added form by reductive tritiation with ^{3}H$_2$ gas and an appropriate catalyst. This is the least expensive per curie and the most versatile method for obtaining products with high specific activity. Alternatively, the Evans modification of the Wilzbach method allows nonreductive exchange of tritons into amino acids, carbohydrates, lipids, steroids, and nucleosides at moderately high specific activity using tritium gas and a palladium catalyst. The exchange procedure is a poor choice for preparing ligands for pheromone catabolism studies. Many side reactions can occur, often resulting in low yields of the desired product and usually requiring extensive purification of the final products.

2. A hydride-type reduction of an aldehyde or ketone with $>$60 Ci/mmol sodium borotritide provides a direct and selective triton introduction. It is diffi-

cult to exceed 15 Ci/mmol for the specific activity of the product unless multiple hydride reductions are possible.

3. Quenching of an organometallic with tritium oxide or use of labeled water to exchange enolizable hydrogens is common. This method is generally the least suitable for two reasons. Tritiated water, particularly of high specific activity, is the most insidiously dangerous form for the laboratory worker. It is readily incorporated into the body and exchanges into OH, SH, and NH positions, which results in a prolonged biological half-life in the body. Moreover, any triton exchanged in by enolization can just as easily be exchanged back out again *in vivo* (or in subsequent chemistry). Nonetheless, a large number of generally labeled compounds are prepared by heating a target molecule with a tritiated water and a metal catalyst at >120°C in a sealed tube. Again, this gives low specific activities and nonspecific labeling and is not recommended for pheromone research.

4. Labeled borane (or its derivatives) can be prepared for hydroboration using boron trifluoride and sodium borotritide. This route has not been used extensively because it is technically more difficult and does not afford specific activities as high as in the tritium gas reductions.

5. Replacement of halogen or tosylate with tritide ($LiAlT_4$, $NaBT_4$, or $NaBT_3$ CN; T = H or ^3H depending on specific activity) under S_N2 conditions can be employed. Unfortunately, sodium cyanoborotritide is not commercially available; lithium aluminum tritide is both moisture sensitive and radiochemically unstable and should be avoided as a reagent whenever possible. The development of lithium triethylborotritide ("super-tritide") as a stereoselective and more nucleophilic single tritide labeling reagent is described by Coates *et al.* (1982), but it requires a convenient commercial source of high specific activity lithium tritide.

6. For many aromatic compounds, tritiodestannylation or catalytic substitution of iodine by tritium is possible. Although this route is important in making radiopharmaceuticals, there are few aromatic compounds in insect pheromone chemistry.

In each case, the location of the label can be confirmed indirectly by degradation (e.g., oxidation) or directly by observing the ^3H-NMR signal. With a 300-MHz spectrometer, as little as 1 mCi can be readily observed in under 1 hr acquisition. The triton is the most sensitive NMR-active nucleus and has the advantage in this case of zero natural abundance; moreover, its couplings and chemical shifts are essentially identical to those of protons. Perusal of the Evans *et al.* (1985) treatise makes it quite clear that ^3H NMR is truly the method of choice for determining triton content and location.

The choice of label location is dictated by the synthetic procedures in combination with the expected sites of metabolism. Generally, the tritons should be in a well-defined location distant from the expected sites of catabolism if simple transformations are being monitored. A triton at the site of metabolism may become labile and wash out during metabolism. Tritons on carbons undergoing oxidation or substitution may cause isotope effects on reaction rates such that the labeled material is metabolized differently from unlabeled material. In a positive sense, tritons at reactive sites can provide useful handles for verification of the structures of metabolites, as will be illustrated below.

Our radiopheromone syntheses often involve alkene reduction or alkyne semi-hydrogenation at atmospheric pressure using tritium gas. This is accomplished at the National Tritium Labeling Facility (NTLF) (Aune *et al.*, 1982), located at the Lawrence Berkeley Laboratory in Berkeley, California, where maximal safety and absolute confidence in the chemical integrity of the product are possible at a moderate cost. Tritium gas is thermally desorbed from a uranium tritritide source; the minimum volume of the gas line requires about 140 Ci at atmospheric pressure. For maximum safety, tritium gas line work is best carried out at or below atmospheric pressure; this may require redesign of synthetic procedures as in the catalytic tritiation of an alkenyl oxirane precursor to disparlure. In addition, the choice of catalyst and choice of solvent can greatly influence the ultimate number of tritons incorporated, their location, and thus the regiochemistry and stereochemistry of the labeling. Homogeneous catalysts such as Wilkinson's catalyst $[(Ph_3P)_3RhCl]$ can be presaturated with tritium gas and used as stoichiometric reagents where allylic exchange or the Lewis acidity of the catalyst is a problem (Prestwich and Wawrzeńczyk, 1985). We have used the homogeneous tritiation of an alkenyl oxirane to prepare the enantiomers of disparlure at 58 Ci/mmol (Prestwich *et al.*, 1987). Heterogeneous catalysts often cause extensive $^1H/^3H$ exchange in allylic and vinyl positions (Guilford *et al.*, 1982), particularly in protic solvents. For example, in making alkenyl pheromones by alkyne semitritiation using a quinoline-poisoned palladium on barium sulfate catalyst, we find that specific activities of 50–58 Ci/mmol can be achieved in dry tetrahydrofuran, while only 20–40 Ci/mmol products result with methanol as solvent. Additional examples of the role of ^3H NMR in elucidating these exchange reactions and in establishing selectivity of other processes can be found in Evans *et al.* (1985).

Sodium borotritide reductions and all further chemical manipulations of high specific activity compounds are performed in a specially designed Radioligand Facility at Stony Brook. ^3H NMR is now available at both locations.

b. Purification and Storage. The handling of tritiated compounds has been described in detail by Evans (1974). Caveats for the purification and storage of high specific activity fatty acid derivatives in the C_{12} to C_{20} range are summarized below.

Following the primary reaction in which tritium is introduced, secondary reactions (reductions, oxidations, esterifications, hydrolyses) are frequently required to obtain the desired radiosubstrate. After semitritiation of only 20 mg of an alkynyl acetate, up to 6 Ci of product ditritioalkene is obtained. After removal of the catalyst by filtration, exchangeable tritium must be removed by lyophilization in properly equipped facilities by trained personnel. The product can then be purified by flash chromatography (Still *et al.*, 1978) on silica gel or on silver nitrate-impregnated adsorbents to give thin-layer chromatographically (TLC) homogeneous materials. In some cases, high-performance liquid chromatographic (HPLC) purification may be required; this can also be performed routinely at the NTLF on a curie scale if necessary.

The eluting solvent is replaced with hexane–toluene mixtures which are free of water, oxygen, and acidic impurities. The samples should contain 1–1000 mCi per milliliter of solvent and should be stored as cold as possible without freezing the solvent. At higher concentrations, autoradiolysis causes more rapid degradation of the labeled material (Evans, 1975). Aromatic cosolvents are important in absorbing β particles and in trapping carbocations resulting from radioactive decay of a triton in a C—H linkage. Benzene (mp 4°C) is a poor choice relative to toluene (mp −94°C), although both can be azeotropically dried and freed from oxygen in a single process. Autoradiolysis occurs in frozen samples where labeled molecules have condensed in solvent-free aggregations. Finally, prolonged storage in very dilute solution leads to air oxidation or unpredictable effects from the glass vessel. Silanization of the glass surface (clean with methanol, then acetone, then toluene; incubate with 5% dichlorodimethylsilane in toluene; rinse and wash with reverse solvent sequence) minimizes the latter effect and is strongly advised for stock solutions of labeled pheromones.

Techniques of radiopurification and radiochromatography are discussed by Roberts (1978), by Wieland *et al.* (1985), and in a pamphlet distributed by the Amersham Corporation (Sheppard, 1975). While most techniques do not discriminate between labeled and unlabeled compounds, high resolution HPLC and capillary gas chromatography (GC) will separate the heavier, more lipophilic tritium-labeled materials from the lighter, more polar protium isotopomers. Detection of radiochemicals is generally accomplished by liquid scintillation spectrometry ("counting," or LSC) of aliquots of collected fractions or by scraping and LSC of TLC plate zones. Fluorescent autoradiography of fluor-sprayed TLC plates requires more patience, a darkroom, and a cryogenic freezer. The visualization of the data on radiochemical purity and distribution of label is satisfying, but the quantification and replicability are poorer. Older methods of scanning TLC plates (efficiency <0.1% for tritium β emissions) have been supplanted by the use of multichannel linear analyzers (efficiencies up to 2–3% for ^3H and >30% for ^{14}C) interfaced to computers for rapid visualization of the radioactivity profile on a TLC plate or an electrophoretic gel (Filthuth, 1982; Wieland *et al.*, 1985). Commercial instruments are available from Berthold or from Bioscan (Shulman and Kobayashi, 1986).

Radio-gas–liquid chromatography (radio-GLC) can be performed by the collection of peaks followed by LSC (difficult with the sharp peaks in capillary GC), or by using a gas proportional counter (Wieland *et al.*, 1985) (also difficult with capillary GC). Radio-HPLC is possible with 1% efficiency using a solid scintillator in a flow-through cell, or at higher efficiency (up to 30%) using a pumped scintillant in the flow cell (this requires splitting the sample for preparative work). Time and equipment are the most precious commodities. There is much to be said in redesigning a radiosynthesis to have several purifications which can be performed in disposable pipette silica gel columns. It is best to save the high resolution methods for analysis of metabolic products, where resolution, quantification, sample throughput, and replicability are most important.

3. Metabolic Experiments

a. Standard Procedures and Pitfalls.   Unlabeled and labeled pheromones are prepared as standard solutions in heptane, and working solutions in a water-miscible solvent such as ethanol, acetone, dimethylformamide (DMF), or dimethyl sulfoxide (DMSO) are prepared from these heptane stock solutions. Concentrations are chosen such that 0.1–1% of the organic solvent is present in the final aqueous incubation. We have used two modes of addition, depending on the sensitivity of the enzyme preparation to organic cosolvents. In the first, we prepare pheromone buffer solutions directly from the heptane stock by removal of heptane and resuspension in a phosphate or Tris buffer. Equal portions of labeled pheromone buffer, inhibitor buffer, and enzyme solution are mixed to initiate the reaction. In the second method, we add the pheromone and the inhibitor in organic solvent directly to the enzyme solution.

Neither is ideal. In both methods, adsorption to glass limits the maximum concentration usable and the stability of the concentration over time. For 16-carbon acids and acetates, we find that over 70% of the suspended pheromone at $10^{-7} M$ has been adsorbed out of solution after less than 30 min (Table I). Thus, reproducibility of the assays suffers; over a range from 10^{-5} to $10^{-9} M$, solutions used may possess concentrations which vary with time during the course of the assay. We find that the presence of a small amount of a nonspecific binding protein such as bovine serum albumin (ovalbumin is not as good) stabilizes the pheromone against adsorption to glass. Also, Pyrex is less adsorptive than the cheaper borosilicate, and siliconized surfaces are in general less adsorptive than untreated surfaces (Table I) (M. Tasayco, unpublished results). For the labeled compounds, we routinely count an aqueous aliquot of the solution and then calculate the concentration from the known specific activity. We determine the

TABLE I

**Adsorptive Loss of Carrier-Free ³H-Labeled
Z11-16 : Ac and Z11-16 : Acid from Buffer Solutions
to Glass Surfaces**[a]

| Solvent[b] | Glass treatment[c] | Percent radiolabel recovered in aqueous layer[d] | |
		Z11-16 : Ac	Z11-16 : Acid
Phosphate buffer	None	14 ± 4	13 ± 6
Phosphate buffer	$10^{-5} M$ 18 : OH	20 ± 4	20 ± 5
Phosphate buffer	DMDCS	22 ± 9	18 ± 7
Phosphate buffer	Glass Clad 6C	15 ± 5	20 ± 9
Phosphate buffer	Glass Clad 18C	17 ± 4	15 ± 9
1% DMSO	None	31 ± 10	15 ± 6
0.5% C_2H_5OH	None	25 ± 11	9 ± 3
100 μg/ml OA	None	37 ± 9	29 ± 7
100 μg/ml OA	DMDCS	10 ± 5	8 ± 1
100 μg/ml OA	Glass Clad 6C	13 ± 6	10 ± 1
100 μg/ml OA	Glass Clad 18C	11 ± 4	6.4 ± 0.1
100 μg/ml BSA	None	67 ± 11	59 ± 20
100 μg/ml BSA	DMDCS	41 ± 8	26 ± 2
100 μg/ml BSA	Glass Clad 6C	49 ± 0.5	21 ± 2
100 μg/ml BSA	Glass Clad 18C	45 ± 0.5	24 ± 2
Ethyl acetate	None	92	85

[a]M. L. Tasayco, unpublished results. Solutions were prepared by evaporation of a $1.0 \times 10^{-7} M$ hexane solution of substrate to treated or untreated glass surfaces under N_2 followed by addition of the buffer solutions indicated and vigorous vortex mixing.

[b]A 76 mM sodium phosphate buffer, pH 7.4, containing 1 mM of NAD$^+$ was modified by addition of (1) 1% (v/v) dimethyl sulfoxide (DMSO), (2) 0.5% (v/v) ethanol, (3) 0.10 mg/ml of ovalbumin (OA, M_r 43,000) or bovine serum albumin (BSA, M_r 69,000).

[c]Disposable borosilicate 10 × 75 mm tubes were used as supplied or treated with (1) 100 μM solution of octadecanol in hexane, (2) 10% solution of dichlorodimethylsilane (DCDMS) in toluene after cleaning the glass surface with methanol and toluene, (3) 10% solution Glass Clad 6C, a Pierce Co. siliconizing agent, in methylene chloride, or (4) a 1% aqueous solution Glass Clad 18C, a Pierce Co. C_{18} silanizing agent.

[d]Triplicate 10 μl aliquots were removed and counted at 1 min and 30 min. Only the 30 min values are shown; within experimental error, they somewhat exceeded or equaled the 1 min values.

time course of surface adsorption for each concentration of each pheromone molecule for each type of glass (vial, borosilicate tube, Corex tube) employed. We frequently reuse "pheromone-conditioned" vials following thorough rinsing with buffer but not an organic solvent.

In the second method, the local effect of the solvent probably denatures protein in the few seconds prior to mixing. Moreover, even at 1% organic solvent (e.g., DMSO, DMF, ethanol), many oxidases, dehydrogenases, and esterases suffer reduced activity. Often, the organic cosolvent does not solve the adsorption problem; it does allow easier introduction of precise amounts of inhibitors or substrates to an enzyme solution. Thus, although we can more accurately control the concentration of substrate or inhibitor, we may sacrifice enzyme activity.

Decomposition of pheromones and analogs in buffer solutions is difficult to control. It is crucial to use freeze-degassed buffers to eliminate oxygen when assaying aldehyde dehydrogenase or alcohol oxidase activity in order to avoid high levels of oxidation in the blanks. Ester hydrolysis occurs slowly in aqueous pheromone buffers stored overnight; similarly, ester exchange occurs at a measurable rate in alcoholic stock solutions.

The use of radiotracer techniques for measurement of enzyme assays has been critically evaluated and reviewed by Oldham (1977). He maintains that radiolabeled substrates should be stored and employed at the lowest specific activity possible consistent with needed sensitivity, and that assays will give the best results when the substrate concentration is near the enzyme K_m. For assay of the lipophilic pheromones known to be present in sub-K_m concentrations in the sensory hairs, we prefer to keep the specific activity as high as possible and the concentrations 10-fold below K_m to obtain biologically realistic data. After all, one can always dilute a high specific activity material by *adding* a radioinert material, but it is exceedingly difficult to *remove* the radioinert material from a low specific activity material. Therefore, to achieve maximal sensitivity and low blank values, assays must be conducted in minimum volumes with both high enzyme and high substrate concentrations.

b. Biological Parameters.   Biological variation must be controlled in order to obtain meaningful results in catabolism. Tissues should be collected from moths of the same age and status of sexual experience. Tissues should be collected in synchrony with photoperiod, preferrably when the female calling and male responsiveness are known to be maximal. A careful examination of individual variation of protein patterns and substrate selectivities should be undertaken. Tissues should be stored, homogenized, purified, and used following standardized protocols.

The assay of substrates for which cofactors or cosubstrates are necessary must be approached cautiously. Addition of cofactor to a protein–pheromone incubation is not the true zero time unless the homogenate has been rigorously freed of cofactor. Dehydrogenases and oxidases demand attention to these caveats. Similarly, enzyme inhibitors should be added with controlled preincubation times.

c. *Methods of Analysis.* Analysis of the results requires a rapid, quantitative, reproducible, and accurate procedure for radiopurification and scintillation counting. It is worth developing a streamlined assay when many column fractions or inhibitors are to be tested for activity. For crude homogenates at low concentrations, radio-TLC or radio-HPLC will give throughputs of 4–10 duplicate samples per hour. A partition assay or spectrophotometric assay can generate 40–100 data points in the same time period; however, to the chemist these assays can be unsatisfying since one is looking at a correlate to the conversion of substrate to product rather than the molecule-to-molecule transformation itself. Enzymatic assays can occasionally be employed, as in the luciferase assay for picomolar levels of C_{14} fatty aldehydes (Meighen *et al.*, 1981; Meighen and Grant, 1985).

4. Inhibitors

a. *Target Enzymes.* We choose as our initial target enzymes those which most rapidly catalyze the degradation of pheromone in sensory hairs of male moths. Of secondary interest but of lower priority are general hemolymph or cuticular proteins which are also able to use pheromone as substrate but for which sex and tissue specificity is lacking. Examination of pheromone-specific catabolic proteins in other tissues, such as the wing scale esterase of *Antheraea polyphemus* (Vogt and Riddiford, 1986a) will provide an abundant resource for future efforts to sort out interspecific pheromone processing by sympatric but reproductively isolated moths.

Although it may be preferable to work with purified enzymes, preliminary work is often performed with sensory hair lymph or crude antennal homogenates. For the purpose of investigating chemical agents with some hope for field use, we are comfortable in screening new compounds in the presence of all antennal proteins. In particular, some propheromones have been prepared which require enzymatic activation or even photochemical activation (Liu *et al.*, 1984).

b. *Design of Inhibitor.* Chemical inhibition of insect olfaction may be approached in two ways: hyperagonism, i.e., irreversible activation of a receptor cell, or antagonism, i.e., blockage of pheromone recognition by a receptor cell. Note that these modes are based on disruption of biochemical events in the sensilla by limited quantities of a chemical which produces in effect a selective anosmia. This approach to mating disruption is different in principle from the use of saturating quantities of pheromone or pheromone analogs for confusing males attempting to locate pheromone-producing females (see Mitchell, 1981; Wall,

1984). It is also different in principle from the use of behavioral antagonists, such as the enantiomer of a pheromone or the alcohol corresponding to an acetate pheromone; such materials are chemically unreactive but they may stimulate separate sensory cells which inhibit certain precopulatory behaviors (Beevor and Campion, 1979).

Therefore, we seek to prepare tight-binding or irreversibly binding pheromone analogs. Simple competitive inhibition is not sufficient; we require transition-state analogs or suicide substrates as mechanism-based modifiers of enzyme active sites. Similarly, reversible association with receptor proteins is insufficient; we require chemical affinity labels, preferably those which produce the chemically reactive group following processing within the antenna.

c. *Synthesis.* Inhibitors which mimic pheromone structures must be prepared with good regiochemical and stereochemical control. Specific examples will show how this can be accomplished. Frequently, new methods of preparation will be required when the functionality of the inhibitory moiety and the functionality of the lipid side chain have different chemical sensitivities.

d. *Choice of Assay.* Three assays are possible in order to assess the biological or biochemical activity of a new pheromone analog: (1) tissue homogenate or purified protein, (2) intact antenna, or (3) whole body response. A negative result in any one need not be discouraging, since each measures a different effect of the analog. The first tests for the conversion of a substrate (the pheromone) to a product (the deactivated pheromone). An inhibitor of this conversion will provide biochemical data on the enzyme mechanism, but it may not affect neuronal activity or behavior. The trifluoromethyl ketones tested on *Trichoplusia ni* (see Section III,A) were nanomolar inhibitors of the antennal esterase but failed to produce an equally dramatic behavioral effect (B. D. Hammock, personal communication). The dilemma of working with inhibition of a purified protein in contrast to the "natural mixture" of enzyme activities is resolved by performing both types of experiments.

Antennal recordings assess whether a potential inhibitor possesses any intrinsic stimulatory activity toward sensory neurons. Many compounds are undetected, while others can block or delay recovery of the electrical responsiveness of the antenna to pheromone. Again, whether or not a compound is an effective enzyme inhibitor does not simply predict its ability to affect antennal recordings. A potent inhibitor of an esterase may be totally inert as a pheromone analog. For example, O-ethyl S-phenyl phosphoramidothiolate (EPPAT) is a potent inhibitor of the *Antheraea polyphemus* sensillar esterase (Vogt *et al.*, 1985), but it has no pheromonal activity. On the other hand, both recognition by the olfactory neurons and their associated enzymes can be achieved, as in the antipheromone carbamates (Albans *et al.*, 1984) described below for *Heliothis* species.

Third, analogs may affect behavior without showing unusual electroantennogram (EAG) activity or potent biochemical activity. Such compounds are likely acting at a level different from the pheromone processing system and are discussed below. Conversely, even compounds which are potent inhibitors of pheromone catabolism and show EAG responses may prove unexpectedly inert when tested in flight tests.

B. Binding Proteins

There is now reasonable evidence in support of the existence of at least two types of proteins which reversibly bind pheromones: an abundant, soluble sensillum lymph protein of low molecular weight and low binding affinity, and a limited number of membrane-associated macromolecules with higher affinity for the pheromone (Vogt, Chapter 12, this volume). However, the ratio of experiments to speculations is still very small, and only a few insects are presently being examined. Three problems plague these studies: (1) lack of a credible binding assay by which to measure equilibrium constants and competitive displacement by analogs; (2) lack of high specific activity pheromones with which to conduct the binding assays; and (3) inability to study the putative ligand–receptor complex under denaturing conditions. We have solved the second problem for most insects, and many high specific activity pheromones are now available for use through our laboratories. The third problem has been addressed by chemical affinity labeling experiments in *Heliothis* and by photoaffinity labeling experiments in *Antheraea*, as described in Sections III,D and III,E. The first problem remains unsolved, although competitive binding to glass surfaces has been used to estimate a dissociation constant for the *A. polyphemus* binding protein (Kaissling *et al.*, 1985; Kaissling, 1986; De Kramer and Hemberger, Chapter 13, this volume).

Using our labeled pheromones and pheromone analogs, we plan to develop some generally applicable assays for pheromone-binding proteins. Some approaches to olfactory receptor proteins and transductory proteins have been described by Pace and Lancet (Chapter 15, this volume), by Dodd and Persaud (1981), by Price (1981), and by Snyder's group (Pevsner *et al.*, 1986; Sklar *et al.*, 1986). In general, the last 5 years has elevated the biochemical analysis of olfaction from a primitive state (Cagan and Kare, 1981) to a highly sophisticated problem in molecular recognition and signal transduction.

1. Antennal Tissues

a. Sex.   Intuitively, one expects that pheromone receptors in Lepidoptera or binding proteins should be restricted to male moth antennal chemosensory sensilla. Indeed, this specificity of tissue location is a key to identifying pheromone-binding proteins involved in olfaction as opposed to general lipid binding. However, this intuition is biased by the paucity of data on female responses to female-produced lepidopteran pheromones. It is likely that females can also smell both female-produced and male-produced pheromones for at least four possible reasons: (1) the need to monitor their own release rates; (2) the need to monitor conspecific release of pheromone to enable spacing in space or in time; (3) the need to monitor heterospecific presences; (4) the need for evaluation of the male. It is important to correlate the appearance of putative binding proteins in antennae of either sex with behaviors known to be pheromone mediated.

b. Time. There is now evidence that pheromone biosynthesis by females and pheromone responsiveness by males varies with photoperiod, with age of the moth, and with the occurrence of mating (see Morse and Meighen, Chapter 4, this volume; Raina and Menn, Chapter 5). Clearly, one must control for these variables when collecting antennal tissues with the null hypothesis that proteins involved in reception can undergo similar variations in abundance or affinity. While this may be incorrect, it remains an untested but intriguing hypothesis.

c. Whole Antenna versus Sensory Hair. Since the pheromone impinges on the whole antenna (indeed, the whole moth), one school of thought, espoused by the Seewiesen group, is that the most realistic system to examine is the whole antenna, with all its connections, hemolymph, and nonreceptive cuticle (see, for example, Kanaujia and Kaissling, 1985). Vogt (1984) has shown that homogenates of antennae produce extremely complex protein patterns on electrophoretic gels due to contamination by hemolymph proteins. Sensory hair homogenates give simpler gel patterns and allow clear visualization of sensory hair–specific binding and catabolic proteins. When working on the molecular processing of pheromones, we feel it is wiser to keep the biochemical complexity to a minimum, as defined by only those tissues intimately involved with processing and perception.

d. Soluble versus Membrane-Bound Proteins. The evidence of Vogt and Riddiford (1980, 1986b) strongly suggests that sensory hairs of many moths will contain male-specific, low molecular weight soluble binding proteins in the receptor lymph. The function of these may be buffering, phase partitioning, sequestration–inactivation (*sensu* Kaissling, 1986) of pheromone, or pheromone transport in the sensory hair lumen. At the other extreme are the elusive receptor proteins, presumed to exist in the dendritic membrane in association with transmembrane ion channels. If one is concerned with inactivation of pheromone, it is common that the enzymatic processing is in the soluble fraction. (This is true for *Choristoneura, Antheraea, Heliothis,* and others but not for the gyspy moth, *Lymantria.*) On the other hand, if one wishes to study the details of chemoreception, the dendritic membrane is the most crucial tissue for finding receptor and ion channel proteins (see Steinbrecht, Chapter 11, this volume; De Kramer and Hemberger, Chapter 13; Kaissling and Thorson, 1980; Boeckh, 1984).

2.   Substrates, Competitors, and Affinity Labels

a. Natural Pheromone.   Two fundamental assumptions in biochemical studies on pheromone binding are that the tritium-labeled pheromone is essentially indistiguishable from its protium isotopomer and that the natural pheromone should be either the most tightly bound or the most efficacious in opening an ion channel when it binds specifically. The first assumption overlooks the increased hydrophobicity of the tritium–carbon linkage relative to the carbon–hydrogen bond. There is little one can do to make the situation better, except to convince oneself that the marginal difference in hydrophobicity is small relative to the much larger effect of the long hydrocarbon chain. The second assumption will yield to experimentation. There may well be pheromonelike molecules which can be chemically more tightly bound or which will be more effective at producing an electrical signal.

b. Unnatural Pheromone Analogs.   As soon as a pheromone structure has become known, organic chemists have enthusiastically generated new synthetic routes and a plethora of pheromone analogs for evaluation by their often distant biological collaborators. The literature is replete with structure–activity studies for lepidopteran, hymenopteran, orthopteran, isopteran, dipteran, and coleopteran pheromones. The analogs fall into five classes: (1) chain length (homologs) or chain-branched analogs; (2) functional group analogs, including π system mimics and heteroatom replacements; (3) regiochemical analogs, with relocated double bonds or carbonyls; (4) diastereoisomers, including alkene geometrical isomers; and (5) enantiomers of the active structure. With such readily prepared compounds, which ones are most advantageous for biochemical studies?

For determination of binding specificity, a reliable and rapid binding assay is required. To date, none exists for accurate determination of the affinity of a pheromone for its putative receptor macromolecule or for the abundant sensillum lymph proteins. In principle, a competitive binding assay allows the most versatility, since a number of unlabeled analogs can be evaluated in competition with a single radiolabeled ligand, in our case the radioactive pheromone. The relative binding affinities tell only part of the story, and a true dissociation constant for the pheromone–protein binding equilibrium is best obtained by measurement of association and dissociation rates. Methodology for these measurements in the pheromone area has yet to be developed.

c. Chemical Affinity Labels.   In analyzing ligand–receptor interactions it is frequently possible to design a reactive mimic of a ligand which can covalently label the binding site. In contrast to suicide substrates, one cannot rely on a catalytic transformation to unmask the reactive group. Thus, chemical affinity labeling involves a partitioning of the label between decomposition in the solvent, nonspecific labeling of proteins, and the desired covalent attachment at the binding site of the receptor. In addition, modification of a pheromone to introduce a chemically reactive functional group may substantially alter its ability to cause an electrophysiological or behavioral response. The pheromonal efficacy of a reactive mimic should be determined, particularly in terms of cross-adaptation to the response to the authentic pheromone.

Most chemical affinity labels are alkylating or acylating agents which covalently modify nucleophilic sites on proteins. Thus, pheromone haloacetates, α-haloketones, α-haloaldehydes, acyl halides, and similar reactive mimics of pheromonal components would be most suitable for examination.

d. Photoaffinity Labels. A solution to the intrinsic reactivity of chemical affinity labels can be found in the use of photoaffinity labels. Analogs which retain biological activity and which also contain a diazocarbonyl, arylazide, or diazirine function are capable of light-induced loss of N_2 with production of a reactive cabene. The carbene can undergo direct insertion into X—H bonds, for $X = C$, N, O, and S, or it can rearrange to a less reactive form subject to attachment to a nucleophilic residue at the binding site. The uses of photoaffinity labels in insect systems have been described by Prestwich *et al.* (1984b, 1985a), while a more complete analysis of the process is provided by Bayley (1983). Photoaffinity labeling has been applied to the *Antheraea* pheromone-binding proteins as described in Section III,D.

3. Binding Assays

a. Methods of Analysis. Equilibrium dissociation constants are typically calculated from the ratio of the dissociation rate to the association rate, or from measurement of binding of the labeled ligand in the presence of increasing amounts of the unlabeled ligand. In all assays for binding, there must be a rapid and efficient separation of bound and free ligand, such that one or both can be quantified prior to reestablishment of an equilibrium. The lipophilicity of pheromones and the suspected membrane-bound nature of the receptors is problematical (Venter and Harrison, 1984a,b). However, a wealth of information is available to aid in the design of receptor binding assays (Jacobs and Cuatrecasas, 1981). We are pursuing several approaches for determining pheromone–protein binding, including (1) rapid filtration through G-15 Sephadex to bind macromolecules and elute unbound ligand and (2) rapid filtration through nitrocellulose or pretreated glass fiber filters to immobilize bound ligand and elute free ligand. The determination of binding constants and numbers of binding sites from the radiochemical data for bound and free ligand is a source of some controversy (Klotz, 1982), but Scatchard plots are commonly used.

  b. Competition by Analogs. The competitive binding assay is preferred for rapid screening of potential tight-binding analogs. Indeed, as outlined below, the search for high affinity pheromone analogs will be crucial in further characterization of the receptor proteins.

  c. Affinity Labeling. Covalent modification is achieved by (1) use of chemical affinity labels, (2) photoaffinity labeling, or (3) two-step modification in which a reversible binding is made irreversible by a reduction or oxidation. Specific examples of each of these will be given below. In each case, the covalently modified protein can be further analyzed under denaturing conditions. For impure preparations, the modified receptor can be followed during purification if a radiolabeled ligand was employed as the affinity label.

III. SPECIFIC EXAMPLES

  Detailed chemical and biochemical studies of pheromone catabolism and binding have been performed for very few insects (Blomquist and Dillwith, 1983), and most examples are from the Lepidoptera. Earlier examples are discussed first to show how increasing chemical input and biochemical sophistication have led to a clearer molecular picture of pheromone processing.

A. *Trichoplusia ni*

  The first demonstration of pheromone catabolism in an insect was the apparent conversion of Z7-12 : Ac (**I**) to the alcohol by esterases in tissues of the noctuid moth *Trichoplusia ni* (Ferkovich *et al.*, 1973) (Fig. 1). The cabbage looper was selected on the basis of known behavioral and electrophysiological responses and availability of synthetic pheromone. In these first experiments, binding of pheromone as a 1 mM (!) suspension to soluble antennal proteins (in a 0.5 M sucrose buffer) was observed by difference ultraviolet (UV) spectroscopy. The time-dependent diminution in binding was correlated with the appearance of Z7-12 : OH (**II**), an inhibitor of mating, as detected by GC.

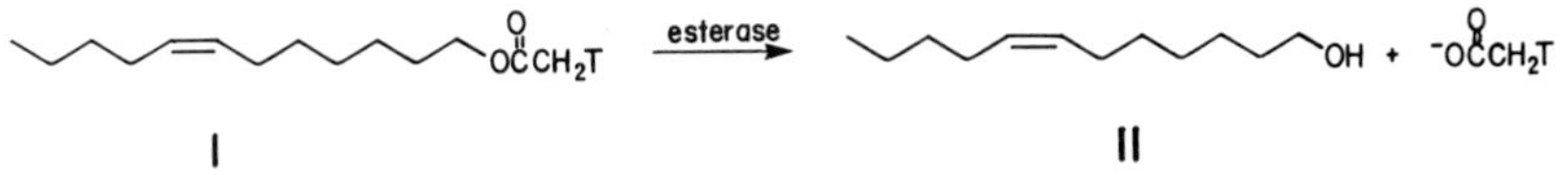

Fig. 1. Hydrolysis of *Trichoplusia ni* pheromone (T = H, ^{3}H).

Mayer (1975) then demonstrated substrate specificity for the antennal enzymes at short exposure times (4 sec) for isomers and analogs of Z7-12 : Ac; for longer exposures, no specific degradation was observed. Again, legs or antennae were dipped into suspensions of pheromone at >1 mM, with detection by GC. These experiments were then repeated *in vitro* (Mayer *et al.*, 1976) with a fluid obtained by sonic fracture of the hairs and elution of the receptor lymph and membrane fragments. Enzymatic degradation was found both in the membrane fraction and soluble fraction; after gel filtration, partially purified fractions were obtained which hydrolyzed three alkene regioisomers and the saturated 12 : Ac faster than the natural pheromone. At these high pheromone levels necessary for GC detection of products, it is difficult to interpret these results in a true biological context.

Later, Ferkovich and co-workers switched to a radiochemical assay using Z7-12 : Ac, tritium-labeled in the acetate group at 0.2–0.8 Ci/mmol. Metabolism was detected by a partition assay, since labeled acetic acid was released upon hydrolysis. Unfortunately, the unlabeled alcohol product could not be verified, and the levels of pheromone required for these assays were still 10 μM, well above the solubility of the pheromone in aqueous solution and well above the expected concentration *in vivo*. Nonetheless, Taylor *et al.* (1981) demonstrated an increase in pheromone hydrolysis by antennal esterases 1–3 days after eclosion in both males and females, corresponding to an increase in responsiveness of the *T. ni* males. They reported three esterase bands in polyacrylamide gel electrophoresis (PAGE) of antennal extracts and noticed that a paraoxon-resistant esterase in antennae which is absent from legs appears to be responsible for hydrolysis of the pheromone.

The antennal specificity and lower activity of the female enzymes were confirmed by Ferkovich *et al.* (1982a,b), with further attention to cuticular hydrolytic activity. Thus, in 1-min assays with acetate-labeled Z7-12 : Ac at 2–15 μM and detection of disappearance of acetate by TLC, homogenates degraded pheromone in the order antennae > legs > wings. In contrast, elution of activity with Ringer's solution gave esterase activity in the order wings > legs > antennae. They interpreted this to imply that the antennal esterases in the sensillum lymph and/or dendritic membrane must play an important role in the olfactory process as a pheromone-inactivation process. The cuticular esterase could function in preventing surface accumulation of pheromone, a role later documented for a non-elutable wing scale esterase of *Antheraea polyphemus* (Vogt and Riddiford, 1986a). The work of the Gainesville group has been nicely summarized by Ferkovich (1982).

In an unpublished study, B. D. Hammock, A. Sylwester, and L. K. Gaston (personal communication) examined the effects of series of general esterase inhibitors and trifluoromethyl ketone transition state analog-type inhibitors on degradation of two tritium-labeled pheromone components of *T. ni*. The minor component, dodecyl acetate (12 : Ac), was labeled at 5 Ci/mmol in the carbon chain, while the major component, Z7-12 : Ac (**I**), was labeled at 0.5 Ci/mmol in the acetate ester. They found that EPPAT was a potent irreversible inhibitor of this esterase in the low micromolar range and that the volatile 1,1,1-trifluoro-2-tetradecanone (**III**) was a potent nanomolar inhibitor of the antennal esterase activity (Fig. 2). Trifluoroketones with pheromonelike hydrocarbon chains were better inhibitors and showed electroantennogram responses similar to the natural acetate pheromone component. However, wind tunnel experiments and field trapping experiments with trifluoromethyl ketone analogs of pheromones did not produce overt behavioral responses. Thus, in the field, neither the potent esterase inhibitor–pheromone analog (Z)-1,1,1-trifluoropentadec-10-en-2-one (**IV**) nor the aromatic analog 3-phenyl-1,1,1-trifluoropropan-2-one (**IVa**) attracted male moths when used alone in a trap. These two trifluoromethyl ketones also failed to inhibit trap catch when used in conjunction with Z7-12 : Ac.

Nonetheless, this was the first example of the use of an inhibitor of pheromone catabolism to attempt to modify insect olfaction, a line of research which is actively pursued in my laboratories at Stony Brook at this time. As discussed above, this approach is different in principle from the mating disruption techniques using behavioral inhibitors (which stimulate other neurons) or pheromonal confusion methods (which prevent mate location by odor saturation). The pros and cons of these methods are discussed in earlier literature (Mitchell, 1981; Beevor and Campion, 1979; Wall, 1984).

B. *Bombyx mori*

The first pheromone deduced for an insect was E10,Z12-16 : OH (bombykol, **VI**); this is also one of the first insects in which pheromone metabolism and

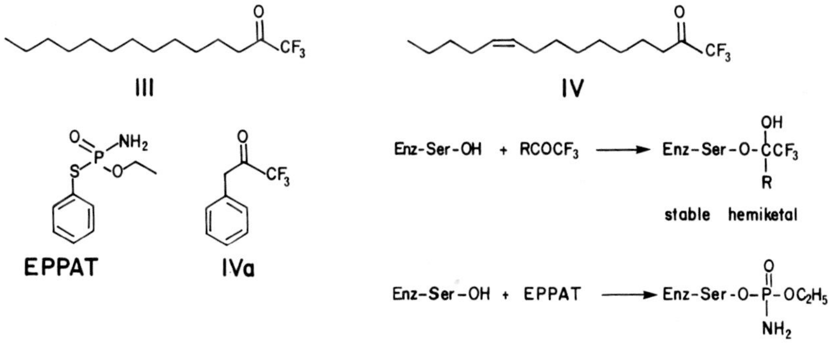

Fig. 2.   Inhibitors of *Trichoplusia ni* antennal esterases by a transition state analog and by a phosphoramidothiolate.

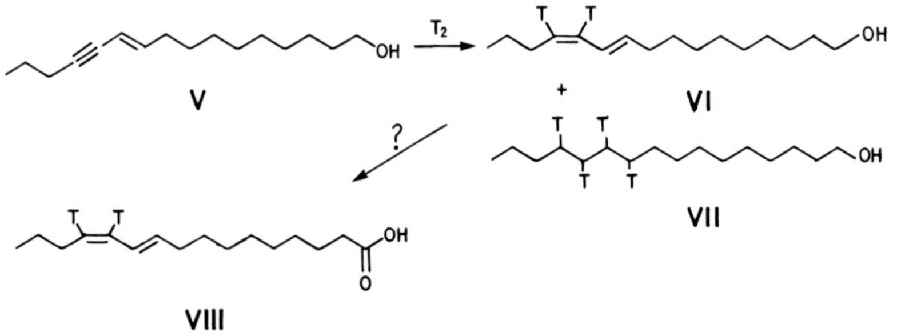

Fig. 3. Synthesis and metabolism of tritium-labeled bombykol.

perception were examined (for excellent retrospectives, see Schneider, 1984; Hecker and Butenandt, 1984). Labeled bombykol (*VI*) was prepared by Kasang (1968) by semitritiation of the 12-alkynyl compound (**V**) over a Lindlar catalyst; the tetrahydro analog (**VII**) was also obtained as a by-product and used to demonstrate specificity in later experiments (Fig. 3). Indeed, this first preparation of high specific activity pheromone was a landmark in understanding the molecular level of perception and catabolism of pheromones. Thus, it was calculated that single molecules impinge on the antenna at a rate of 100 hits/sec, and that several hundred hits would be required to reach a behavioral threshold (Kaissling and Priesner, 1970).

Whole antennae of the male silkworm moth, *Bombyx mori*, degrade labeled bombykol to "ester" and "acid" metabolites (**VIII**) (Kasang, 1974; Kasang and Weiss, 1974). At exposures of $10^{11}-10^{12}$ molecules per antenna, both male and female antennae showed a half-life for pheromone uptake of the order of 1 min. Much slower uptake was found in legs, heads, and wing scales, which lack the pore tubules by which pheromone enters the cuticular sensory hairs. "Uptake" was determined by the quantity of pentane-elutable labeled pheromone recovered; the remaining radioactivity was extracted with chloroform–methanol or was found in an insoluble residue. The metabolic half-life was also longer (3.8 min) for the conversion of the alcohol to labeled bombyk acid (**VIII,** R = H) and an unidentified ester (Kasang and Weiss, 1974). It is unfortunate that more confirmatory chemical studies were not performed. No attempts to manipulate or describe the binding or catabolic proteins were undertaken in this historically important species. As will become apparent below, the alcohol could either undergo oxidase and dehydrogenase reactions to the acid (as seen in *Heliothis,* Section III,E, and *Choristoneura,* Section III,F), or it could be susceptible to an ω-oxidation as seen in *Reticulitermes* antennae (Section III,G).

C. *Lymantria dispar*

1. Epoxidation

The correct structure of disparlure was deduced by epoxidation of glandular alkenes (Bierl *et al.,* 1970). Prelininary work on the biosynthesis of disparlure from the high specific activity (40 Ci/mmol) (Z)-2-methyl-7-octadecene (**X**) from the alkyne (**IX**) (Sheads and Beroza, 1973) and on the uptake and turnover of racemic disparlure by gypsy moth antennae was first performed by the Seewiesen group (Fig. 4). Thus, aqueous ethanolic suspensions of the labeled alkene (**X**) were injected into female pupae 2 days preemergence, and 30% of the label was recovered as disparlure (**XI**) by TLC of extracted female glands after eclosion (Kasang and Schneider, 1974). The controls using male pupae were not performed, and it is possible that in this 72-hr period many mixed-function oxidases could act on the alkene as a substrate. In addition, there was no direct evidence of pheromone gland involvement in this conversion; in view of the known diel periodicity and life cycle variation of disparlure release and production (Charlton and Cardé, 1982), this needs careful reinvestigation. The detailed information on the ultrastructure of the gland (Hollander *et al.,* 1982) and on neural control of calling (Hollander and Yin, 1982) makes this an attractive system to study a specific monooxygenase which could be temporally regulated. A preliminary experiment with clipped female glands and glandular homogenates indicates to us that conversion of the alkene precursor to labeled disparlure is very slow. Indeed, the regulation may occur at the level of alkene synthesis from an appropriate fatty acid. Further studies with our supply of 58 Ci/mmol alkene are planned, particularly with regard to the rate and enantioselectivity of the enzymatic monooxygenation.

2. Catabolism: Early Work

The early studies on catabolism of disparlure are also very sketchy (Kasang *et al.,* 1974), and we have recently begun detailed reinvestigation (Prestwich *et al.,* 1986b) as described below. In the Seewiesen study, whole antennae were ex-

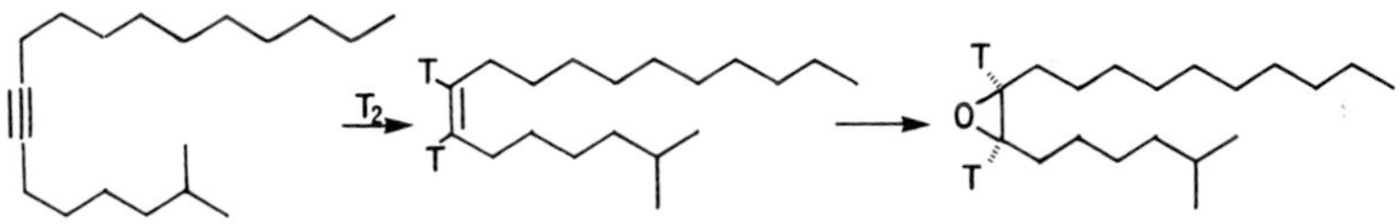

Fig. 4. Synthesis of labeled racemic disparlure.

posed to 5×10^{11} molecules / antenna of racemic [7,8-^{3}H]disparlure (**XI**) (40 Ci/mmol) and the pentane-elutable pheromone measured with time. About 2.5 min was required for disappearance with one-half the labeled epoxide, appearance of two uncharacterized polar metabolites, and appearance of about one-third of the label in polar material which did not move on TLC. Comparisons were made for differential uptake of disparlure (**XI**). and bombykol (**VI**), and "tetrahydrobombykol" (**VII**, hexadecanol); however, the claims for specificity of uptake and turnover are based on small differences in exponentially decaying curves in an experimental design lacking in key controls. For disparlure, the (+) isomer (stimulatory) and (−) isomer (inhibitory) were present in equal amounts. No attempts were made to examine specific sensory hair–associated biochemical events.

3. Catabolism and Binding: Recent Results

It has been clearly demonstrated that *Lymantria dispar* males possess separate receptor cells for the (+) and (−) enantiomers of disparlure (Hansen, 1984; Miller *et al.*, 1977). In addition, several groups have demonstrated the attractancy of the (+) enantiomer and inhibition of attraction by the (−) enantiomer in field, wind tunnel, and tethered flight situations (see, for example, Cardé *et al.*, 1977; Cardé and Hagaman, 1979; Miller and Roelofs, 1978; Preiss and Kramer, 1983; Yamada *et al.*, 1976). We felt that it was crucial to distinguish biochemical events in sensory hairs and in other nonreceptive tissues on the basis of the binding and catabolism of the high specific activity, tritium-labeled enantiomers of disparlure, as well as to reexamine the binding and catabolism of racemic disparlure.

a. Synthesis of Labeled Pheromone. We first repeated the semitritiation and epoxidation seqeunce of Sheads and Beroza (1973) using tetrahydrofuran as solvent for the tritium gas reduction to give racemic [7,8-^{3}H]disparlure (**XI**) at >55 Ci/mmol (Fig. 4). The material showed high radiochemical purity by autoradiography of the TLC-separated compound. For the preparation of the >95% e.e. (enantiomeric excess) disparlure enantiomers bearing high specific activity tritium labels, we selected the Sharpless asymmetric epoxidation over the Mori procedure (Mori *et al.*, 1976) to provide the desired chirality. Thus, alkynol **XII** was semihydrogenated to Z2-13 : OH (**XIII**) which was then epoxidized in the presence of (+) or (−)-diethyl tartrate to give the epoxy alcohols (−)-**XIV** and (+)-**XIV**, respectively (Fig. 5) (Rossiter *et al.*, 1981). Oxidation to the epoxy aldehydes followed by Wittig olefination provided the 5,6-dehydro analogs (+)-**XV** and (−)-**XV**. These alkenyl oxiranes were then reductively tritiated using a stoichiometric amount of tritium-presaturated tris(triphenylphosphine) chlororhodium (Wilkinson's catalyst), following a method optimized for the preparation of optically pure juvenile hormones from their 12,13-dehydro ana-

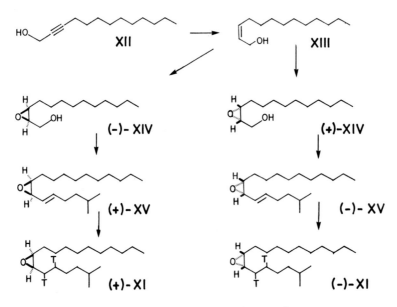

Fig. 5.   Synthesis of tritiated disparlure enantiomers.

logs (Prestwich and Wawrzeńczyk, 1985). Thus, both (+)-**XI** and (−)-**XI**, the enantiomers of disparlure, were obtained in high enantiomeric purity, radiochemical purity, and specific activity (52–58 Ci/mmol) (Prestwich *et al.*, 1987). The labeled 8-keto compound, resulting from a rearrangement and then reduction, comigrates with the epoxides and must be removed by sodium borohydride reduction to the 8-hydroxy compound followed by chromatography on silica gel (S. Graham, unpublished results).

b. Catabolic Enzymes.   Pheromone degradation occurs exclusively in sensory hair homogenates (R. G. Vogt and G. D. Prestwich, unpublished results). Thus, incubations of 100 n*M* solutions of labeled disparlure in Tris or phosphate buffers containing homogenates of leg tissue, hemolymph, whole antennae, and isolated sensory hairs (males only) were followed by extraction with hexane–ethyl acetate, separation by TLC, and autoradiography or β counting of the TLC plate. Our initial studies have demonstrated antennal-specific epoxide hydrolase (EH) activity in both male and female moths. Furthermore, the antennal branches themselves are devoid of EH activity, indicating that the sensory hairs contain the degradatory enzyme. Ultracentrifugation of the antennal homogenates at 100,000 *g* for 90 min affords an essentially inactive supernatant, while the resuspended membrane pellet is high in EH activity.

The product of disparlure catabolism is expected to be the *threo*-diols (**XVI**)

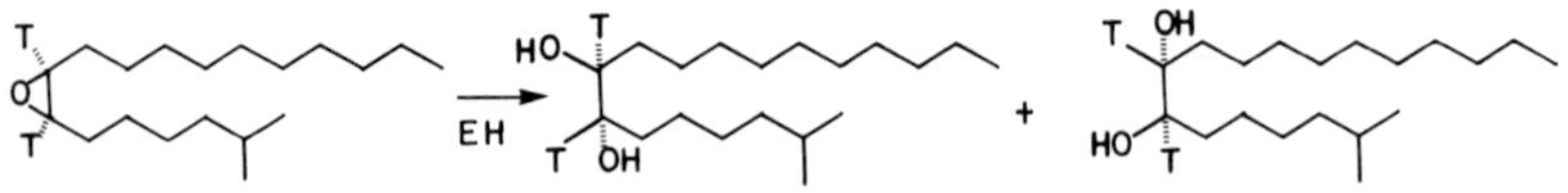

Fig. 6. Enzymatic hydrolysis of labeled disparlure.

arising from an anti opening of the *cis*-epoxide by water (Fig. 6). The synthetic diol mixture (S. Graham, unpublished results; Ujvary *et al.,* 1987; Lin *et al.,* 1984) comigrates with the labeled disparlure metabolite. We have not yet found an analytical method to distinguish the two possible enantiomeric diols **XVIa** and **XVIb.** The location of the tritium label and the chemical identity of the labeled diol have been confirmed by oxidative loss of tritium and by conversion to the diacetate, respectively (S. Graham, unpublished results; Prestwich *et al.,* 1987).

Curiously, the racemic, (+)-, and (−)-disparlure isomers all appear to be degraded at similar rates by the total antennal EH preparation (S. Graham, R. G. Vogt and G. D. Prestwich, unpublished results). Current work in this area is moving in three directions: (1) design, synthesis, and evaluation of specific inhibitors of the antennal EH; (2) demonstration of tissue and substrate specificity of the antennal EH; and (3) purification and characterization of the antennal EH. We hope these efforts will enable design of a new generation of gypsy moth control with chemically reactive sex attractant analogs (cf. Beroza and Knipling, 1972).

c. *Binding Proteins.*   The sensory hairs of the male gypsy moth can be readily isolated in high yield, free from hemolymph and epidermal contamination, following the procedure of Klein and Keil (1984) as modified by Vogt (1984). Native PAGE of isolated sensory hairs has shown two predominant low molecular weight proteins (R. G. Vogt, unpublished results). Interaction of the enantiomers of high specific activity disparlure with these antennal-specific proteins is currently being investigated, and binding assays are being developed to locate high-affinity membrane-associated receptor proteins and to determine their abundance and dissociation constants. Affinity labels for these proteins are being prepared in our laboratories.

D.   *Antheraea polyphemus*

Sensory hair lymph from antennae of males of the wild silkmoth, *Antheraea polyphemus,* contains several male-specific soluble proteins involved in pheromone processing, including a 2 μ*M* concentration of a specific pheromone esterase, 55,000 daltons, and 20 mM of a 15,000-dalton binding protein (Vogt and Riddiford, 1980, 1981, 1986a,b; Vogt, 1984). Models for the interaction of these two soluble proteins in the transport, perception, and degradation of the pheromone, E6,Z11-16 : Ac (Kochansky et al., 1975), have been developed by Vogt (1984) and Vogt and Riddiford (1986a,b). Comparisons of alternative models for the biochemistry of pheromone perception in this moth are presented elsewhere in this volume (Vogt, Chapter 12, this volume).

In the presence of the sensillar esterase under physiological conditions, the pheromone has an estimated half-life of 15–30 msec in the hair lumen. This suggests a molecular model for reception in which the binding protein acts as a carrier (or as a sequestration medium) and the enzyme acts as a rapid inactivator to maintain a low stimulus noise level in the sensillum. This two-component system damps the concentration differences outside the hair and delivers a relatively constant concentration of pheromone to the postulated receptor protein located in the dendritic membrane.

In this section, I shall first describe the synthesis of labeled pheromone and then discuss our efforts to unravel the biological chemistry of the esterase, the binding protein, and the receptor protein.

1. Synthesis of Labeled Substrates

A new synthetic pathway was needed to allow the preparation of high specific activity tritiated E6,Z11-16 : Ac, in particular one which allowed catalytic semi-tritiation of the 11-alkyne in the last step. A route to the acetate E6,Z11-16 : OAc (**XVIII**) via ester **XVII** was developed by Dr. Simon Golec in 1978 (see Vogt and Riddiford, 1981) and later repeated by us (Prestwich et al., 1984a) to provide several curies of [11,12-^{3}H$_2$]-labeled pheromone (**XIX**) and its di-azoacetate analog (**XX**) (Fig. 7). This material was hydrogenated over a Pt

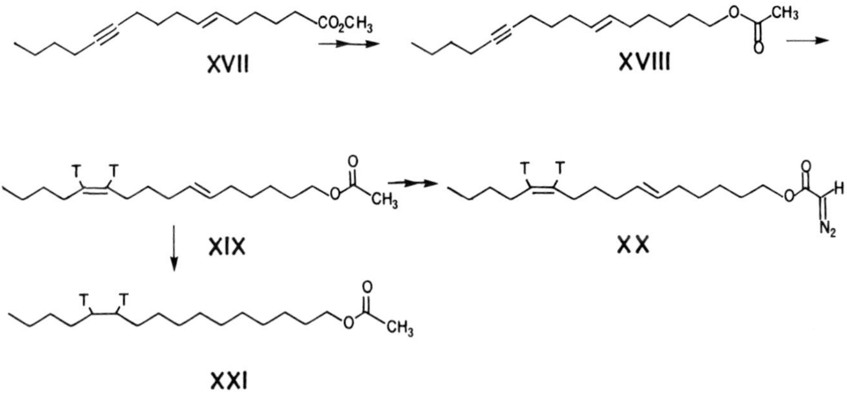

Fig. 7.   Synthesis of the tritiated acetates and a diazoacetate for *Antheraea polyphemus*.

catalyst to provide the labeled saturated hexadecyl acetate (**XXI**). These samples had specific activities in the 25–35 Ci/mmol range as a result of using methanol as the solvent during the tritium gas reduction.

2. Esterases

a. Sensillar Esterase. The hydrolytic activity and substrate specificity of the sensillar esterase (Fig. 8) have been studied in depth (Vogt and Riddiford, 1981, 1986b; Vogt *et al.*, 1985; Prestwich *et al.*, 1986a,b) both in the absence and presence of the sensillar binding protein. For purified enzyme, the K_m is 1.5 μM for 2-naphthyl acetate (**XXII**) and 2.2 μM for the natural pheromone (**XIX**); the maximal velocities per antennal equivalent are 3.3×10^{11} and 0.54×10^{11} mol liter^{-1} sec^{-1}, respectively. Degradation of tritium-labeled E6,Z11-16:Ac (≈ 100 nM) by the purified enzyme was subject to competitive inhibition by the corresponding diazoacetate, E6,Z11-16:Dza ($I_{50} \approx 20$ μM) but not by its Z-6 stereoisomer or by the 11-alkynyl analog ($I_{50} > 100$ μM). The same relative competitive abilities were found for the hydrolysis of 2-naphthyl acetate at a 10-fold lower inhibitor concentration. The more sterically crowded 1-naphthyl acetate (**XXIII**) was not a good substrate for the sensillar esterase. The serine esterase transition state analog inhibitor 1,1,1-trifluorotetradecan-2-one (**IV**) (Hammock *et al.*, 1982) was a potent but reversible inhibitor ($I_{50} = 5$ nM); EPPAT (**III**) ($I_{50} = 3$ μM) was an irreversible inhibitor. Other typical serine

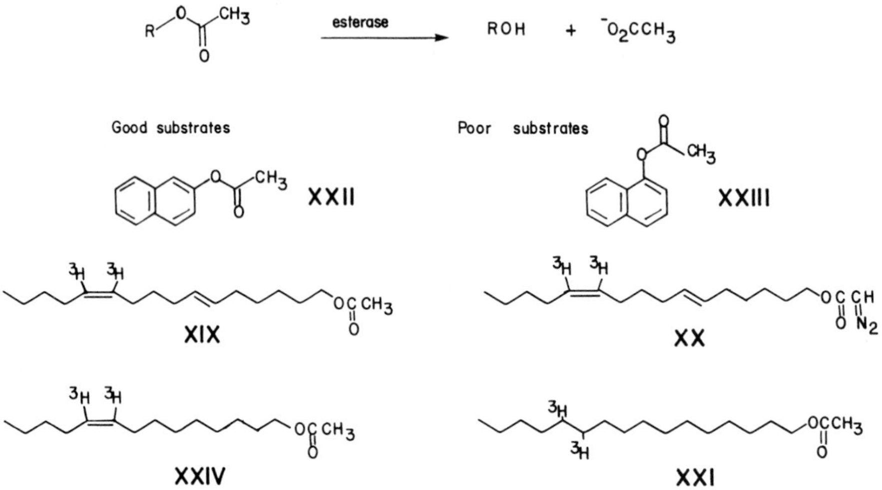

Fig. 8. Substrate selectivity of the sensillar esterase.

esterase inhibitors did not affect the sensillar enzymes (Vogt *et al.*, 1985). Chemically, it appeared that the enzyme preferentially bound fatty alcohol esters, particularly those possessing the correct side-chain geometry.

Enzymatic hydrolysis of the labeled acetate or diazoacetate moiety was also examined for three pheromone analogs (Fig. 8) each labeled with tritium: (a) E6,Z11-16:Dza (**XX**), the diazoacetate analog of the acetate pheromone; (b) 16:Ac (**XXI**), the saturated analog of the pheromone; and (c) Z9-14:Ac (**XXIV**), a shorter chain acetate with a Z olefinic linkage (Prestwich *et al.*, 1986c). The first two are poor substrates over four decades of concentration. The Z9-14:Ac, however, is the best alternative substrate for this *in vitro* pheromone catabolism system, which included the "buffering" effect of the pheromone binding protein (Vogt, Chapter 12, this volume). This finding acquires new significance in view of the recent report that E4,Z9-14:Ac is a new minor component of the *A. polyphemus* pheromone and that a third receptor neuron responds to it (Kaissling, 1986). (The second neuron identified responds optimally to the aldehyde, E6,Z11-16:Al; Kaissling and Thorson, 1980.)

b. Other Esterases. Based on the findings of Ferkovich (1982), Morse and Meighen (Chapter 4, this volume), and Ding and Prestwich (1986) with other insects, one anticipates esterase activities to be distributed throughout the insect. In particular, the insect integument is rich in esterases which can degrade pheromonal acetate esters. Vogt and Riddiford (1986a) recently described the presence of two esterases in *Antheraea polyphemus* which degrade pheromone: a soluble integumental esterase in antennal branches, legs, and wing scales, and a nonelutable (covalently bound?) wing scale esterase. The soluble enzymes were detected by 2-naphthyl acetate esterase staining in an electrophoretic gel, while the cuticle-bound scale esterase activity was detected only in detergent-suspended scale preparations. In the latter, the scales degraded greater than 30% of 10 nM pheromone to the alcohol in 5 min, while degradation of 2-naphthyl acetate was only seen above 50 μM. Scales of related saturniids did not hydrolyze tritium-labeled E6,Z11-16:Ac, further indicating species specificity of the scale esterase. As proposed earlier for *Trichoplusia ni* (Ferkovich *et al.*, 1982a,b), these external esterases probably serve an important cleaning function, removing adsorbed pheromone (both conspecific and heterospecific acetates) to reduce the level of olfactory noise reaching the male sensilla.

c. Whole Antennae. Isolated antennae of *A. polyphemus* adsorbed 32% of ^{3}H-labeled E6,Z11-16:Ac (**XIX**) from an airstream, with 80% of this on the sensory hairs (Kanaujia and Kaissling, 1985). The amount of pentane-elutable pheromone decreased with time, and a half-life of 3–8 min was calculated. This is much slower than one would predict from the esterase kinetics reported by Vogt *et* *al.* (1985). It is unresolved as to where the pheromone is "hiding" during this experiment, but a key role for the 15,000-dalton binding protein cannot be ruled out.

3. Binding Protein

The identification of a male antenna–specific soluble protein which could bind the pheromone (Vogt and Riddiford, 1980, 1981) was a major step forward in unraveling the biochemistry of insect olfaction. Models of how this protein is involved in the overall process of reception and transduction are discussed in depth by Vogt (Chapter 12, this volume). This discovery stimulated our interest in the chemistry of pheromone perception, since it followed soon after an equally intriguing observation that the diazoacetate analog of the *A. polyphemus* pheromone had 10% of the electrophysiological activity of the natural acetate pheromone (Ganjian *et al.*, 1978). Indeed, K.-E. Kaissling (personal communication) has indicated that the activity may equal that of the pheromone, since the release of the more polar diazoacetate from a filter paper source is 10% of that of the natural acetate pheromone. The existence of an olfactory-active photoactivatable analog of a pheromone suggested that binding proteins and membrane-associated receptor proteins could be selectively and efficiently photoaffinity-labeled, leading to a chemical understanding of pheromone perception.

Thus, we prepared the photoactivatable diazoacetate (**XX**) labeled with tritium at 25–35 Ci/mmol (Prestwich *et al.*, 1984a) in order to covalently modify the binding protein located in the receptor lymph and the putative receptor protein located in the dendritic membrane (Fig. 9). Indeed, irradiation of sensory hair homogenates containing 1–100 nM of tritium-labeled E6,Z11-16 : Dza for 10–60 sec with four 254-nm mercury vapor lamps resulted in selective photoattachment to male antennal proteins in both the soluble and membrane-associated sensillar fractions (Prestwich *et al.*, 1986b). Photoaffinity labeling of these proteins can be competed with unlabeled acetate pheromone and diazo analog, and no labeling

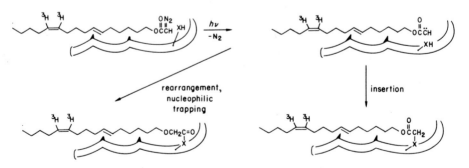

Fig. 9. Schematic photoaffinity labeling of binding proteins for E6,Z11-16 : Dza.

occurs when photolysis is omitted (Fig. 10). No soluble proteins labeled competitively in brain, muscle, or leg tissue. However, in female antennae a new soluble protein, M_r 70,000 on sodium dodecyl sulfate (SDS)–PAGE, showed competitive labeling (R. G. Vogt, G. D. Prestwich, and Y.-S. Ding, unpublished).

The nature of the binding protein is currently under investigation. Purified protein can be sequenced, and photoaffinity-labeled binding protein will be subjected to proteolysis and sequencing of the label-bearing polypeptide fragment(s). Given the presence of the male-specific binding proteins in moths like *Manduca sexta, Antheraea pernyi,* and *Hyalophora cecropia,* it will be intriguing to examine homologies in this class of proteins.

4. Receptor Protein

In sensory hairs collected by the mechanical breakage method (Klein and Keil, 1984) or by ultrasonic breakage (Ferkovich, 1982), the dendritic membranes become dislodged. For *A. polyphemus,* when lyophilized sensory hairs are homogenized, the cuticular debris removed at 12,000 g, and the supernatant further ultracentrifuged at 100,000 g, then a membrane pellet can be obtained (R. Vogt

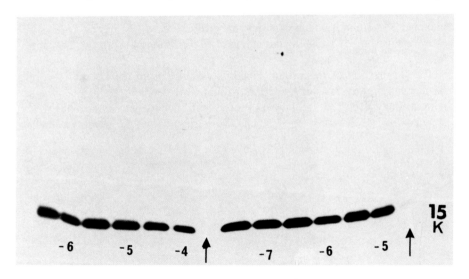

Fig. 10. SDS–PAGE separation of photoaffinity-labeled proteins from male *Antheraea polyphemus* antenna (200 nM tritiated E6,Z11-16:Dza) with increasing half-log concentrations (10^{-6}–10^{-4} M) of unlabeled diazoacetate (left) and of 10^{-7}–10^{-5} M of the pheromone E6,Z11-16:Ac (right). Arrows indicate that competitive displacement is seen at the highest concentration of each ligand.

has observed the vesicles microscopically; see Chapter 12, this volume). When the photoaffinity labeling experiment is repeated on washed or unwashed membrane vesicles, we find rapid and selective attachment of ^{3}H-labeled E6,Z11-16 : Dza (**XX**) to a 70,000-dalton membrane protein. Again, this protein is absent from all female tissues and absent from all other male tissues.

E. *Heliothis virescens*

1. Synthesis of Labeled Substrates

The two major pheromonal aldehydes, Z9-14 : Al and Z11-16 : Al, were synthesized with high specific activity tritium labels in the vinylic positions (Ding and Prestwich, 1986). As explained above (Section II,A,2,a), these compounds are most easily prepared by semitritiation of the corresponding C_{14} and C_{16} alkynyl acetates **XXV** and **XXVI** with tritium gas using a palladium on barium sulfate catalyst poisoned with quinoline (Fig. 11). The tritiations were carried out at 740 torr on a 0.1 mmol scale at the National Tritium Labeling Facility to give several curies of the labeled pheromone precursors **XXIV** and **XXVII**. When methanol was used as a solvent, we obtained specific activities in the range of 25–35 Ci/mmol; with anhydrous tetrahydrofuran as solvent, the specific activity was the maximal 58 Ci/mmol within experimental error. (Indeed, the largest error is in safely and accurately weighing out less than 10 mg of several curies of a volatile liquid!)

The localization of the tritium labels is assumed from the known reaction mechanism; however, as of late 1986, tritium NMR has now become available both at Stony Brook and at the NTLF. The high specific activity acetates were stored below $-20°C$ in heptane–toluene. Most importantly, the acetates were the

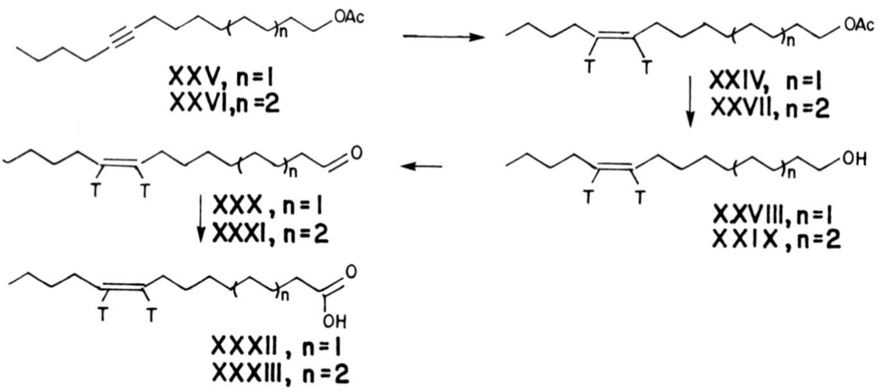

Fig. 11. Synthesis and interconversions of *Heliothis virescens* pheromones and congeners.

most useful form for both synthesis and storage of these stoichiometrically tritiated compounds. The labeled alcohols **XXVIII** and **XXIX** showed slow oxidation over the course of months, and the aldehydes **XXX** and **XXXI** decomposed with half-times of a few weeks; the acetates suffered less than 10% decomposition per year and were readily repurified from polar impurities by flash chromatography.

The preparation of the high specific activity aldehydes required a judicious choice of reagent. Of the techniques available for the partial oxidation of a primary alcohol to an aldehyde, pyridinium dichromate gave good radiochemical yields ($>70\%$) even when using less than 0.5 ml of dichloromethane containing a 100- to 1000-fold excess of oxidant and 10 mCi ($\sim$200 nmol) of labeled alcohol. The use of pyridinium chlorochromate, Jones reagent, chromium trioxide–pyridine complex, or polymeric chromium(VI) reagents led to either overoxidation or difficulty in product isolation.

2. Tissues Employed

Since the discovery by Raina and Klun (1984) of a brain factor in *Heliothis* species which triggers the release of pheromone during scotophase, we chose to collect all tissues from virgin male and female moths 1–2 days after eclosion and 2 hr after lights-off (long day photoperiod). It now appears likely that the enzymology *in vitro* is unaffected by the precise timing of tissue collection (Raina and Menn, Chapter 5, this volume), although one anticipates age dependence of the enzyme activities during the 1-week lifetime of the moths. We initially used whole antennae (clipped and stored at $-80°C$ or used fresh), legs, and the clipped, extruded female pheromone gland or male hairpencil–genitalia organ complex (Ding and Prestwich, 1986). This selection thus includes pheromone degrading/receiving tissues, control cuticle/hemolymph tissue, and pheromone-producing tissues. For each tissue, we assayed three extracts for enzymatic activity: soluble, solubilized with 0.1% Triton X-100, and residual. Enzyme assays were also conducted using the ultrasonic hair-fracture technique described by Ferkovich (1982), in which 50 pairs of antennae were sonicated for 60 min in an ultrasonic cleaning bath at 0°C in a pH 7.4 phosphate buffer with 0.5 M sucrose. Finally, an adaptation by M. Blackburn and J. Nelson (personal communication) of the cryogenic technique of Klein and Keil (1984) for sensory hair collection afforded relatively uncontaminated sensillar proteins from these filiform antennae with short sensilla.

3. Enzyme Assays

Following the procedures described by Morse and Meighen (1984a,b, 1986, Chapter 4, this volume) for the measurement of biosynthetic enzymes in *Choristoneura fumiferana*, we developed radiochemical assays for three key enzymes in the target tissues. Our results using Z9-14:Ac (**XXIV**) have been reported, and studies with Z11-16:Ac (**XXVII**) gave similar values (Table II). The most

TABLE II

Comparison of Maximal Rates of Conversion for Three Crude Antennal Enzymes from *Heliothis virescens* Moths for the (Z)-11-Hexadecenyl and (Z)-9-Tetradecenyl Substrates[a]

Enzyme (substrate)	Source (antennae)	Conversion to product[b]	
		Z9-14 series	Z11-16 series
Esterase (Ac)	Female	18%	24%
	Male	19%	11%
Alcohol oxidase (OH)	Female	27%	9%
	Male	28%	11%
Aldehyde dehydrogen-	Female	70%	56%
ase (Al)	Male	69%	58%

[a]Y.-S. Ding, unpublished results. For each assay, 2 antennal pair equivalents per assay were used, and soluble enzymes were obtained by homogenization and centrifugation at 12,000 g. The substrate employed determined which enzyme activity was being measured: Ac denotes the acetate esters of the Z11-16 or Z9-14 series; OH, the alcohols; Al, the aldehydes.

[b]Expressed as means of triplicate determinations, using 30 min incubations at 20°C with 100 nM radiolabeled substrate. Results corrected for nonenzymatic conversions. Recovery of radiolabel was >80% for the acetate and alcohol substrates but in the 40–50% range for the more labile aldehydes; these values are calculated from the quantity of radiolabel added to the assay tube and the fraction actually counted from the TLC plates. See text and Table I for precautions on surface adsorption problems.

striking difference is the threefold lower oxidase activity for the longer chain alcohol in both sexes. All our assays were performed at 20–50 nM with high specific activity pheromones freshly prepared in phosphate buffer solutions. Thus, esterase activity was measured using tritium-labeled Z9-14:Ac or Z11-16:Ac as substrates, alcohol oxidase activity was measured using labeled Z9-14:OH (**XXVIII**) or Z11-16:OH (**XXIX**) as substrates, and aldehyde dehydrogenase activity was determined with NAD$^+$ or NADP$^+$ cofactors and the labeled Z9-14:Al (**XXX**) or Z11-16:Al (**XXXI**) as substrates. In each case, the reaction was quenched by vortex mixing with ethyl acetate, and the labeled organics were separated by TLC for LSC analysis of product and substrate radioactivity.

The distribution of enzyme activities is displayed in Fig. 12. The key features include the following: (1) Aldehyde dehydrogenase is the primary enzyme activity found in both leg and antennal tissues of male and female moths. This is important in its implications for pheromone clearance from cuticular surfaces as

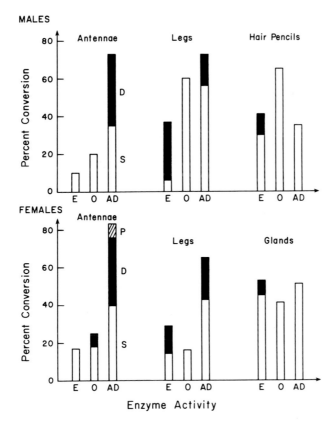

Fig. 12. Processing of pheromone by tissues of *Heliothis virescens* moths. E, Esterase; O, alcohol oxidase; AD, aldehyde dehydrogenase. Reproduced from Ding and Prestwich (1986), with permission of Plenum Publishing Corp.

well as from receptor lymph. We have not yet examined the specificity of this process nor do we know the number of enzymes involved. (2) Alcohol oxidase activity [O_2 required, no NAD(P) required] is low in antennae but relatively higher in male legs and glandular tissues of both sexes. The existence of a cuticular alcohol oxidase in the female gland (Teal *et al.*, 1983) is now thoroughly documented in three *Heliothis* species by Teal and Tumlinson (1986; Tumlinson and Teal, Chapter 1, this volume). They find that aldehyde production (detected by capillary GC) occurs on the surface of the gland and that the conversion is greatest for C_{12} to C_{16} primary alcohols but is relatively unaffected by degree of unsaturation. (3) Esterase activity is low in antennae, higher in leg tissues, and highest in the glandular tissues.

The high activity of the antennal aldehyde dehydrogenase is shown relative to

TABLE III

Dilution Series for Two Soluble Antennal Enzymes of *Heliothis virescens*[a]

Antennal equivalent per ml solution	Esterase (%)[b]				Aldehyde dehydrogenase (%)[b]			
	Male		Female		Male		Female	
	Z9-14 : Ac[c]	Z11-16 : Ac[c]	Z9-14 : Ac[c]	Z11-16 : Ac[c]	Z9-14 : Al[c,d]	Z11-16 : Al	Z9-14 : Al[c,d]	Z11-16 : Al
360	27	14	30	19	—	—	—	—
120	10	10	5	19	—	—	—	—
80	0	—	0	—	62	51	53	54
36	—	3	—	12	—	—	—	—
26.67	—	—	—	—	50	45	33	49
12	—	0	—	5	—	—	—	—
8.0	—	—	—	0	50	40	33	45
2.67	—	—	—	—	31	29	15	27
0.8	—	—	—	—	10	17	15	22
0.267	—	—	—	—	0	0	0	8
0.08	—	—	—	—	—	—	—	0

[a] Y.-S. Ding, unpublished results; Ding and Prestwich, 1986.

[b] All values are percent conversion to product, measured in duplicate or triplicate TLC assays and corrected for nonenzymatic hydrolysis or oxidation. Concentration of radiolabeled substrate, 100 nM.

[c] Data from Ding and Prestwich, 1986.

[d] Incubation time 50 min; all others 60 min.

the esterase in Table III. The hydrolysis of labeled Z9-14 : Ac (**XXIV**) cannot be observed in 1 hr incubations below 5 antennal equivalents (AE) per assay tube, while the aldehyde dehydrogenase activity of Z9-14 : Al (**XXX**) was still detectable at 0.04 AE per assay. (Note that each assay uses 50 μl of the enzyme solution indicated in the table.) Relative to the 14-carbon substrates, the esterase activity for labeled Z11-16 : Ac (**XXVII**) was detectable at a 10-fold lower enzyme concentration in females, and the aldehyde dehydrogenase activity on Z11-16 : Al was detectable at a threefold lower level in females. These differences were not as pronounced for male-derived enzymes. Further purification of this antennal aldehyde dehydrogenase and studies of its kinetics and substrate specificity are in progress.

4. Reactive Pheromone Mimics for Sensory Disruption

Alteration of the aldehyde function to produce a chemically reactive analog capable of sensory disruption is a primary goal of our research. This strategy was mentioned by Ritter and Persoons (1976) and by Prestwich (1987). One such methylcarbamate-containing antipheromone was reported by Baker and co-workers (Albans *et al.*, 1984) and was patented for reduction of oviposition on cotton by *Heliothis virescens* (Baker *et al.*, 1981). They prepared Z9-14 : Nmc (*N*-methylcarbamate) (**XXXIV**), Z9-14 : Tfa (trifluoroacetate) (**XXXV**), Z9-14 : Tca (trichloroacetate) (**XXXVI**), and (Z)-12-heptadecen-2-one (**XXXVII**) to act as competitive antipheromones for *H. virescens* and found reversible inhibition of electrophysiological and behavioral responses (Fig. 13). Exposure to 100 mg of these four analogs led to inhibition of male responsiveness to the natural seven-component pheromone blend. In contrast, exposure to a variety of saturated

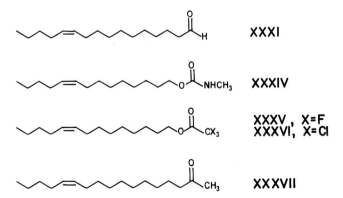

Fig. 13. Antipheromones which block responses of *Heliothis virescens* males to the natural pheromone blend.

analogs, alkenyl regioisomers, monohaloacetates, alcohols, alkenes, acrylates, dimethylcarbamates, and methyl carbonates showed no inhibition of response.

Figure 14 shows a model invoked to explain the antipheromonal effect, in which stabilization of a tetrahedral hemiketal adduct can lead to slow dissociation of a blocker when the side-chain geometry is correct. This is essentially the same mechanism proposed for the esterase inhibition by the trifluoromethyl ketones (see Section III,A and Hammock *et al.*, 1982). Recently, I. Ujvary and M. Toth (personal communication) have found no disruption of the perception of Z11-16:Ac in *Mamestra brassicae* by the "carbamone" Z11-16:Nmc. While Z11-16:Nmc elicited an EAG response only slightly less than Z11-16:Ac, the saturated 12:Nmc and 16:Nmc produced neither EAG signal nor disruption. Although the esterase activity was not examined by either group, we expect that inhibition of an antennal esterase or aldehyde dehydrogenase by the carbamone could explain in part the efficacy of these materials. This is currently under investigation in our laboratories at Stony Brook.

In 1984, we had reasoned that replacement of the aldehydic hydrogen by fluorine to give an acyl fluoride would produce a reactive mimic capable of sensory disruption in *Heliothis virescens* or other aldehyde pheromone-using insects (Prestwich, 1985, 1986). By analogy with the visual transduction mechanism involving a protonated Schiff base of retinal and opsin, we postulated that aldehyde perception might involve a transient iminium intermediate important in ion channel opening (Fig. 15). Thus, retinoyl fluoride reacts with opsin to give retinoyl rhodopsin, which is a nonfunctional pigment (Wong and Rando, 1982). An acyl fluoride could jam this channel in either an open or closed state, leading to either hyperactivation or anosmia, respectively. Indeed, we found the Z9-14:Acf (**XXXVIII**) and Z11-16:Acf (**XXXIX**) to be potent hyperagonists, causing aphrodisia in male *H. virescens* at high doses and disorientation at lower doses (Prestwich *et al.*, 1986a,b). This effect was similar to the interspecific couplings

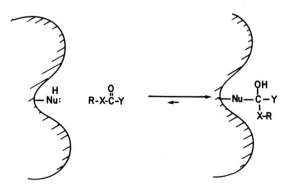

Fig. 14. Tight binding to receptor site nucleophile.

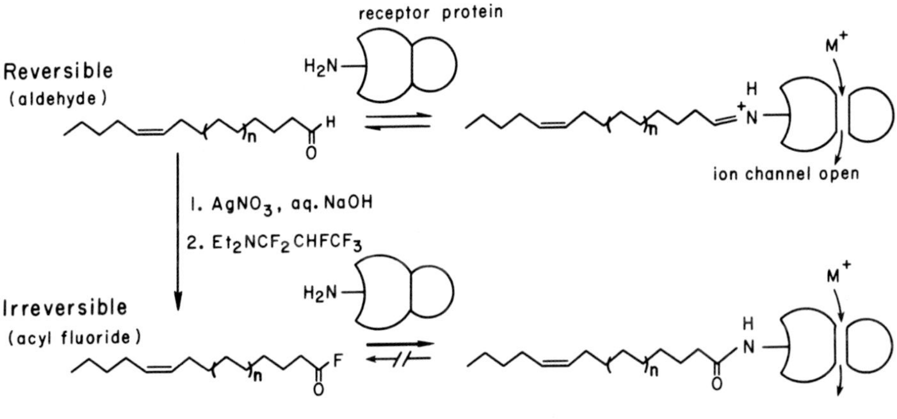

Fig. 15. Hypothetical model for the interaction of acyl fluoride pheromone analogs with receptor molecule. Adapted from Prestwich *et al.* (1986a), with permission of Birkhäuser Verlag.

caused by Z9-14 : Al as observed by Stadelbacher *et al.* (1983) and by Hendricks *et al.* (1982). The maximal effect, which included irreversible extrusion of the genitalia and hairpencils as well as *in copulo* locking, was observed with a 9 : 1 blend of the 16- and 14-carbon acyl fluorides.

How does one test for compounds capable of sensory disruption by either competitive or irreversible binding to a receptor site or by inactivation of pheromone-catabolizing enzyme? For the synthetic materials we prepare, four levels of biological evaluation are desirable. First, biochemical assays on antennal proteins allow observation of effects on catabolism or on receptor binding. We are actively developing rapid and quantitative competitive ligand-binding assays for evaluation of synthetic materials for receptor affinity. Second, we need to know how a single sensory cell responds to a volatile stimulus. Single hair recordings from the small sensilla of *Heliothis* antennae are difficult but possible (Blackburn and Nelson, 1987). The response of the whole antenna in an electroantennogram will also provide overall information with respect to electrical stimulation or suppression by reactive pheromone mimics. Third, a behavioral assay is needed to show how a compound affects the sequence of behaviors from initiation of flight to mate location and copulation. Finally, field assessment of the most behaviorally active compounds provides the crucial evidence of the ultimate utility of the compound under natural circumstances.

We have prepared a variety of aldehyde mimics (Fig. 16) which are currently undergoing screening for biochemical, electrophysiological, and in some cases behavioral activity. The acyl fluorides **XXXVIII** and **XXXIX** are readily hydrolyzed, with half-lives of 2–6 hr in air and in water, respectively. On the other hand, the so-called diolefin analogs (e.g., **XL**) (Carlson and McLaughlin,

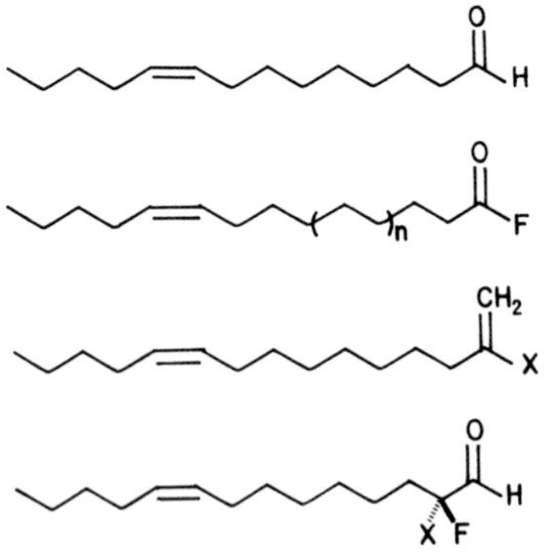

XXX

XXXVIII, n= I
XXXIX, n= 2

XL, X=H
XLI, X= F

XLII, X=H
XLIII, X=F

Fig. 16. Fluorinated pheromone analogs for *Heliothis virescens.*

1982,a,b), in which an alkene π system is substituted for a carbonyl, are very unreactive and stable disruptants. Similarly, the formate analogs, in which a methylene is replaced by an oxygen, are also stable olfactory-active analogs (Mitchell *et al.,* 1975). We prepared the 2-fluorovinyl analog **XLI** in an attempt to moderate the reactivity (Y.-S. Ding, unpublished results). This compound is surprisingly sensitive to acid and hydrolyzes on acidic silica gel. The 2-fluoroaldehydes **XLII** (cf. Rozen and Filler, 1985) and the 2,2-difluoroaldehydes **XLIII** (cf. Gelb *et al.,* 1985) have also been prepared, in the expectation that the tendency of the carbonyl to become tetrahedral by addition of a nucleophile would result in either inhibition of the antennal aldehyde dehydrogenase or tight binding to a receptor protein analogous to the model in Fig. 14. Other functional groups are also being prepared and examined *in vitro* and *in vivo.* For further information on the use of fluorine substitution in studying insect hormones and pheromones, see Prestwich (1986) and Camps *et al.* (1984a,b).

5. Affinity Labeling of Receptors

We have embarked on two approaches to the labeling of putative aldehyde receptors in *Heliothis virescens* sensillar dendrites. The first is a chemical affinity labeling technique based on the two-step covalent modification of olfactory cells reported to produce selective anosmia in tiger salamanders (Mason and Morton, 1984a,b; Mason *et al.,* 1985). Thus, male antennae were sonicated to fracture sensory hairs and elute soluble and membrane-associated proteins. After removal of debris, centrifugation at 100,000 *g* was used to separate these subcellular fractions. The supernatant and pellet fractions were incubated with labeled Z9-14:Al in three separate treatments: (a) no fixer, (b) $NaBH_4$ as fixer, and (c) $NaBH_3CN$ as fixer. Only the last treatment selectively reduces protonated Schiff bases in the presence of aldehydes. Electrophoretic separation of soluble and membrane proteins showed two major bands of protein, one enriched in the membrane fraction, which can be visualized by fluorescence autoradiography (Y.-S. Ding and G. D. Prestwich, unpublished results). While this does not yet provide convincing evidence for a membrane receptor, it gives us the technique to examine competitive displacement by pheromone analogs and selective attachment of other labeled aldehydes available in our laboratories (e.g., 16 : Al, Z11-16 : Al, and Z11-14 : Al). The major drawback is that 30–50 antennae per gel lane are required for adequate sensitivity, making this a very insect-intensive experimental protocol.

As an alternative to the two-step procedure, we can use radiolabeled reactive pheromone mimics to locate receptor proteins. In this regard, we have prepared the tritium-labeled Z9-14 : Acid (**XXXII**) (by tritiation of the alkynyl ester and hydrolysis) for conversion to the labeled acyl fluoride as a chemical affinity label. The 2-fluoro or 2-bromo aldehydes (e.g., **XLIV**) (Fig. 17) can also be prepared in labeled form, and these α-halocarbonyls would be reactive toward nucleophilic residues. For example, Fried and Tu (1984) have used [1-^{14}C]2-bromodecanal (**XLV**) as a chemical affinity label for the fatty aldehyde–using bacterial luciferase.

Photoaffinity labeling is also possible if the diazoketone analog shows binding to the active site. This was shown to be a viable aldehyde analog for the bacterial luciferase system by Tu and Henkin (1983), who photoattached 1-diazo-2-undecanone (**XLVI**) to the enzyme isolated from *Vibrio harveyi*. Our experience with photoaffinity labeling of proteins which bind insect hormones and pheromones suggests that **XLVII** may well be a viable ligand for labeling antennal aldehyde receptors.

F. *Choristoneura fumiferana*

In contrast to the extensive work on pheromone biosynthetic enzymes of the eastern spruce budworm moth by Morse and Meighen (1984a,b, 1986, Chapter 4, this volume), much less is known concerning the specific enzymes involved in

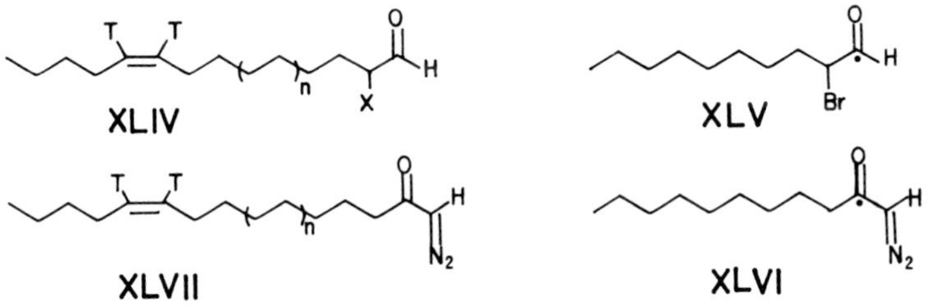

Fig. 17. Receptor site affinity labels for aldehyde-binding macromolecules.

the degradation of pheromone in the antennal tissues. This moth uses a 96 : 4 mixture of E and Z11-14 : Al (**XLVIII**) for pheromonal attraction, and the evidence is that the acetate is the storage form in the gland. Recently, Lonergan (1986) provided unambiguous chemical and spectral confirmation that the major component, E11-14 : Al, is converted *in vivo* and *in vitro* to the E11-14 : Acid (**XLIX**) as the sole metabolite (Fig. 18). When exposed to a saturated atmosphere of the aldehyde pheromone, male and female antennae, wings, and legs all accumulated the acid metabolite with an exponential increase over an 8-hr period. On a wet weight basis, the relative activities were quite similar. *In vitro,* homogenized tissues gave more effective conversion than incubation of unhomogenized tissues with the same 60 μM pheromone concentration, particularly from the male antenna (from 28% conversion to 75% for a 1 hr incubation).

The substrate selectivity of this enzymatic transformation, presumed to be mediated by an aldehyde dehydrogenase based on the findings of Morse and Meighen (1984a), was probed with various 12- to 16-carbon analogs. The saturated 12-, 13-, and 14-carbon analogs were equally good substrates when compared to E11-, Z11-, and 13-14 : Al. Pentadecanal was a modest substrate, while hexadecanal and the unsaturated Z13-16 : Al and Z11-16 : Al were not metabolized. This contrasts with the equally rapid degradation of Z11-16 : Al and

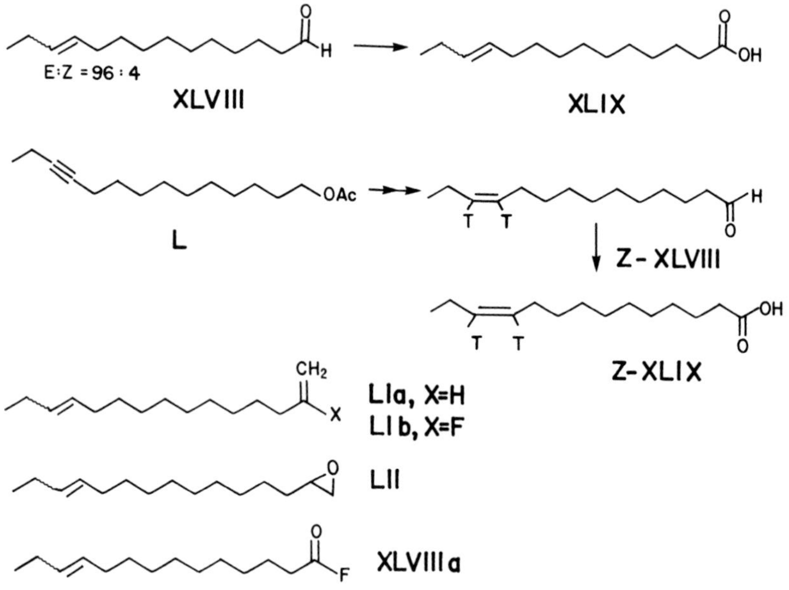

Fig. 18. Aldehyde dehydrogenase activity of *Choristoneura fumiferana* and aldehyde analogs tested as stereoelectronic pheromone mimics.

Z9-14 : Al in *Heliothis*. Finally, preliminary studies were conducted at Stony Brook with tritium-labeled Z11-14 : Al [(Z)-**XLVIII**] prepared from the corresponding 11-alkynyl acetate (**L**) by methods detailed above. Aldehyde dehydrogenase activity was indeed observed in male and female antennae and legs, with rapid conversion to labeled Z11-14 : Acid [(Z)-**XLIX**] (G. D. Prestwich, G. Lonergan, C. Sack, and Y.-S. Ding, unpublished results; see Fig. 18).

As in the *Heliothis* system, the diolefin anlog **LIa** (Z1,12-17 : Hy) will disrupt mating and maintain upwind flight by pheromone-activated *C. fumiferana* males (Silk and Kuenen, 1986; Silk *et al.*, 1985). We (Y.-S. Ding, and G. Lonergan, unpublished results) prepared the 96 : 4 *E* : *Z* mixture of acyl fluorides (E and Z11-14 : Acf) (**XLVIIIa**), the 2-fluorovinyl analog of the diolefin (**LIb**), and the oxirane analog **LII**. In preliminary wind tunnel trials, the acyl fluoride **XLVIIIa** (0.3 µg) did not significantly affect response (flight distance or number of source contacts) to the pheromone **XLVIII**. At 100-fold higher doses, shorter flights were observed. The fluorodiene **LIb** and the epoxide **LII** were essentially inactive as agonists or antagonists in these assays (P. Silk and L. P. S. Kuenen, personal communication).

G. *Reticulitermes flavipes*

1. Synthesis of Labeled Substrates

The trail-following pheromone obtained from the subterranean termite *Reticulitermes virginicus* (Isoptera: Rhinotermitidae) and from an associated brown-rot fungus was identified as (Z,Z,E)-3,6,8-dodecatrien-1-ol (**LIII**) (Tai *et al.*, 1969). In order to examine the metabolic deactivation of the trail pheromone in the closely related termite *Reticulitermes flavipes*, we prepared a series of ω-fluorinated (**LIV**) and ω-tritiated (**LV**) analogs of this dodecatrienol (Carvalho and Prestwich, 1984) (Fig. 19). Specifically, we made the (Z,Z)-3,6-dodecadien-1-ol analogs which had been demonstrated to possess essentially the same level of trail activity for this termite species (Ritter *et al.*, 1977; Tai *et al.*, 1971). The synthesis of the 12-^{3}H-labeled Z3,Z6-12 : OH (**LV**) and its 12-fluorinated

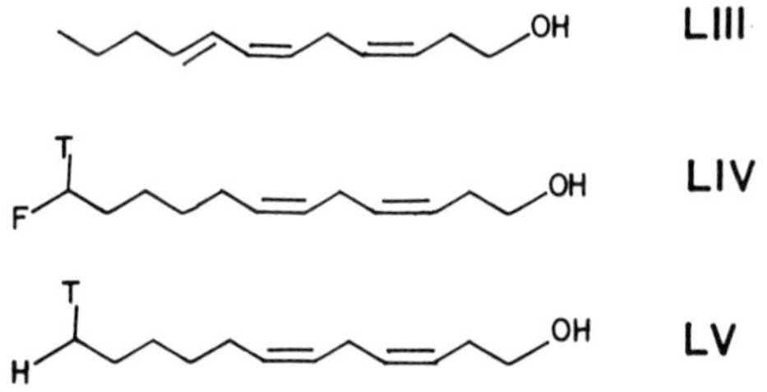

Fig. 19. Termite trail pheromone and analogs.

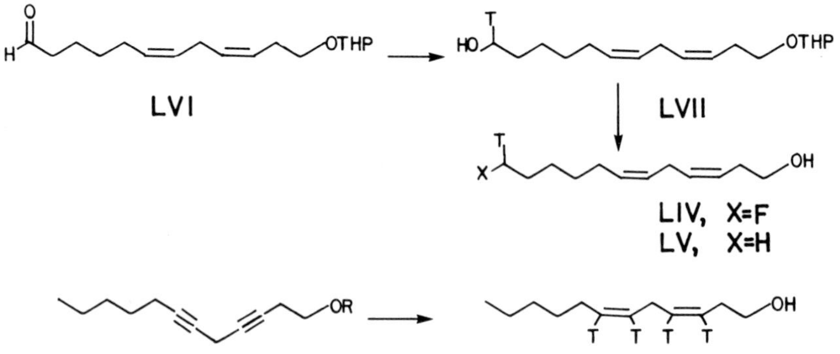

Fig. 20. Synthesis of labeled trail pheromone analogs.

analog (**LIV**) are shown in Fig. 20. The diene aldehyde **LVI** was reduced with sodium borotritide, and the labeled alcohol **LVII** was either fluorinated and deprotected to **LIV** or converted via its mesylate to diol **LV**. We had chosen to tritium-label the terminal methyl (fluoromethyl) group for two reasons: (1) we expected catabolism to occur via oxidation to the carboxylic acid, and (2) we planned to isolate the 2-^{3}H-labeled 2-fluorocitrate known to be produced by β-oxidation of the 16-tritio-16-fluorohexadecenoic acid (and its alcohol precursor). Moreover, the NTLF was not operational for atmospheric carrier-free tritium gas reductions at the time of these experiments. Future experiments would use the catalytic bis-semitritiation **LVIII** to **LIX** shown in Fig. 20; this method has been used to prepare the unlabeled dienol (Carvalho and Prestwich, 1984).

2. Metabolism of the Unfluorinated Dienol

Preliminary experiments on the catabolism of 12-^{3}H-labeled Z3,Z6-12 : OH (**LV**) by freshly excised antennae of *R. flavipes* workers were carried out at Stony Brook by Prof. John J. Brown (Washington State University). The labeled pheromone showed poor stability in aqueous buffers, particularly if oxygen was incompletely removed. Nonetheless, the most important unpublished results are summarized below. At the time of these experiments, we had not identified the product of the enzymatic pheromone degradation, although experiments with the 12-fluorinated analog discussed below strongly suggest that the 1,12-diol is the product; it is clearly not the carboxylic acid which might be expected from an oxidation/dehydrogenation sequence analogous to that in *Heliothis*.

Freshly excised antennae of worker *R. flavipes* (0.5 μg/pair) were homogenized in an insect Ringers solution containing 10% glycerol (pH 7.0) or a 50 m*M* Tris · HCl, 500 m*M* sucrose buffer (pH 7.5) and incubated with 100 n*M* of

12-³H-labeled Z3,Z6-12 : OH. The reactions were quenched with ethyl acetate, and the product distribution was determined by TLC–LSC. The alcohol is cleanly converted to a nonhydrolyzable polar compound (which comigrated with a simple monoglyceride) with a half-life of 6 min (Fig. 21a). The alcohol dehydrogenase inhibitors pyrazole, metronidazole, isobutyramide, propranolol, and butynediol, all at approximately 1 mM, showed no effect on the turnover, but boiling the homogenate prior to addition of labeled dienol abolished enzymatic activity. Saturation analysis with unlabeled dienol showed a sigmoidal curve with half-maximal velocity at approximately 35 nM (Fig. 21b).

Finally, the tissue, caste, and species specificity of the dienol turnover were examined (Fig. 22). The hemolymph and legs of workers also catalyzed the dienol degradation, but they were ≥10-fold less active than worker antennae per

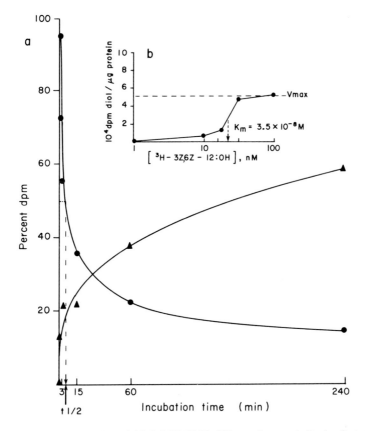

Fig. 21. Rapid conversion of labeled Z3,Z6-12 : OH to polar metabolite by *Reticulitermes flavipes* antennal homogenate. (a) Time course. (b) Saturation experiment, 4 hr incubation.

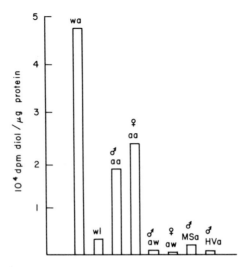

Fig. 22. Tissue and species specificity of Z3,Z6-12 : OH catabolism. wa, Worker antennae; wl, worker legs; aa, alate antennae; aw, alate wings; MSa, *Manduca sexta* male antennae; HVa, *Heliothis virescens* male antennae. Values are shown for 4 hr incubations.

microgram protein. Both male and female alate antennae showed half the activity of worker antennae. Alate wings showed essentially no conversion. Similarly, antennae and hemolymph of *Manduca sexta* and *Heliothis virescens* male moths showed very low rates of conversion of this dodecadienol.

3. Metabolism of the 12-Fluorododecadienol

The topical application of 16-^{3}H-labeled (*E*)-16-fluorohexadec-9-enoic acid and the corresponding alcohol (**LX**) resulted in the metabolic production of the toxic *erythro*-[2-^{3}H]-2-fluorocitrate (**LXI**) in approximately 0.02% overall conversion (Prestwich *et al.*, 1985b) (Fig. 23). The lipid metabolites consisted largely of acylglycerol derivatives and some free fatty acids. Curiously, termites treated with 12-^{3}H-labeled (*Z,Z*)-12-fluorododeca-3,6-dien-1-ol (**LIV**) showed less than 0.0004% conversion to labeled fluorocitrate, although considerable labeled citrate was produced. Moreover, the lipid products of this conversion were not the dodecadienoic acid and acyl glycerol derivatives as expected. The single polar product was chemically identified as the [12-^{3}H](*Z,Z*)-3,6-dodeca-dien-1,12-diol (**LXII**) (Fig. 23). This surprising identification by Dr. R. Yamaoka (Prestwich *et al.*, 1985b) is based on GC–mass spectral (MS) evidence for the dienediol and its diacetate derivative, and on the identity of the hydrogenated tetrahydro compound with authentic 1,12-diacetoxydodecane.

We have postulated that a unique antennal ω-oxidase catalyzes this transformation in both the 12-fluorinated and unfluorinated substrates. The existence of

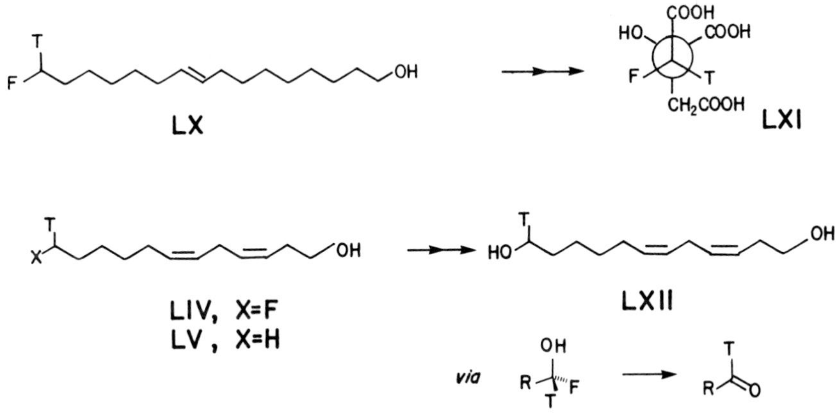

Fig. 23. Degradation of labeled fatty alcohols in *Reticulitermes flavipes*.

such ω-oxidases is also likely in pheromone biosynthesis in certain stored-product beetles (Vanderwel and Oehlschlager, Chapter 6, this volume). As shown in Fig. 23, the 12-fluorine substituent would be expected to be lost during such an oxidation. We further propose that this process constitutes a substrate-selective pheromone deactivation pathway for this termite species, whereby a volatile, hydrophobic, and behaviorally active lipid is rendered less volatile, more water soluble, and behaviorally inactive.

H. Other Examples

Five further studies have been reported which constitute chemical investigations into insect pheromone perception, but which have not been followed up to the extent of the earlier examples. These include (1) traditional structure–activity relationships such as those for gypsy moth pheromone (Schneider *et al.*, 1974; Schneider *et al.*, 1977) and tortricid and noctuid moths (Priesner, 1979), (2) metabolism of a fly-produced mating stimulus, (3) preparation of some chemical analogs of acetates, (4) exploration of the chiral conformations of achiral molecules interacting with receptor sites, and (5) metabolism of a primer pheromone, the honeybee queen substance.

1. *Dacus cucurbitae* and *D. dorsalis*

Metcalf *et al.* (1983) attempted to map the binding requirements for the olfactory receptor of two major tephritid flies in the Dacini tribe. While the melon fly *D. cucurbitae* responded optimally to raspberry ketone and other *p*-hydroxyphenylpropanoids, the oriental fruit fly *D. dorsalis* responded to the 3,4-dimethoxyphenylpropanoids. The responses to 40 related molecules were examined, and the antennal receptor site geometries were compared in terms of the coevolution of the flies with their host plants.

2. Drosophila melanogaster

Esterase 6, a polymorphic enzyme from the ejaculatory duct of male flies, is transferred to the female during mating along with Z11-18 : Ac (cis-vaccenyl acetate), a potential substrate for the enzyme. Indeed, Mane et al. (1983) proposed that Z11-18 : Ac is rapidly hydrolyzed to the corresponding alcohol and that both Z11-18 : Ac and Z11-18 : OH (or derivatives thereof) produced an anti-aphrodisiac effect by decreasing male courtship of inseminated females (Zawistowski and Richmond, 1986). Although no substrate specificities or kinetics were reported, this was alleged to be an example of the transfer of a substrate and enzyme by a male in a fashion which increases his genetic transfer. Unfortunately, this work was called into question (Vander Meer et al., 1987) when sensitive capillary GC methods failed to detect Z11-18 : OH in either sex and when esterase 6 was shown not to hydrolyze Z11-18 : Ac.

3. Agrotis segetum

The responses of sensory cells from male antennae of the turnip moth, A. segetum (Noctuidae), were measured upon stimulation with analogs of Z7-12 : Ac (**I**, the pheromone) in which the structure of the acetate was varied (Liljefors et al., 1984) (Fig. 24). Replacement of the alcohol oxygen with a methylene to obtain the methyl ketone (**LXIII**) afforded a weakly active stimulus. In contrast, the formate (**LXIV**), the propionate (**LXV**), the trifluoroacetate (**LXVI**), and the ethyl ether

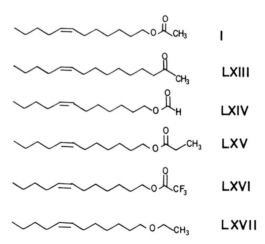

Fig. 24. Stereoelectronic analogs of Z7-12 : Ac tested with *Agrotis segetum*.

(**LXVII**) analogs were all essentially inactive. All portions of the acetate group, electronic and steric, are important to pheromonal activity for this moth. In addition, chain-elongated analogs of the Z5-10 : Ac component were studied by EAG and molecular mechanics calculations (Liljefors *et al.*, 1985); conformational energies and biological activity are strongly correlated.

It is noteworthy that the monohaloacetates and diazoacetate, which we have proposed as the best candidates for chemical or photoaffinity labels for pheromone receptors of acetates, were not examined in this study. To correct this deficiency, we have recently prepared a complete series of mono-, di-, and trihaloacetate analogs of Z11-16 : Ac for evaluation using whole antennae and homogenates of *Plutella xylostella* (L. Streinz and G. Prestwich, unpublished).

4. Ostrinia nubilalis and Argyrotaenia velutinana

Ostrinia nubilalis and *Argyrotaenia velutinana* are among the insects using Z11-14 : Ac (**LXVIII**) as a pheromone component. Chapman *et al.* (1978) prepared optically active cyclic analogs (*S*)-(−)-**LXIX** and (*R*)-(+)-**LXIX** of two possible chiral conformations of the acyclic pheromone and examined their attractiveness to the European corn borer and the redbanded leaf roller. Their bioassays provided evidence demonstrating the presence of two stereospecific chemoreceptors for the achiral pheromone, each with a different sense of chiral coiling of the Z11-14 : Ac (Fig. 25). This chemically novel approach to receptor mapping has not been further explored, and further evidence in support of the existence of two chiral chemoreceptive sites remains elusive.

5. Apis mellifera

Two studies on the metabolic fate of the queen honeybee primer pheromone, (*E*)-9-oxo-2-decenoic acid (**LXIX**), have been reported (Fig. 26). Butler *et al.* (1974) reported the exchange of the α-protons with tritiated water to give a low specific activity labeled compound (**LXIX**) which was used to study translocation on the surface and internally. The lability of the α-tritons precluded mean-

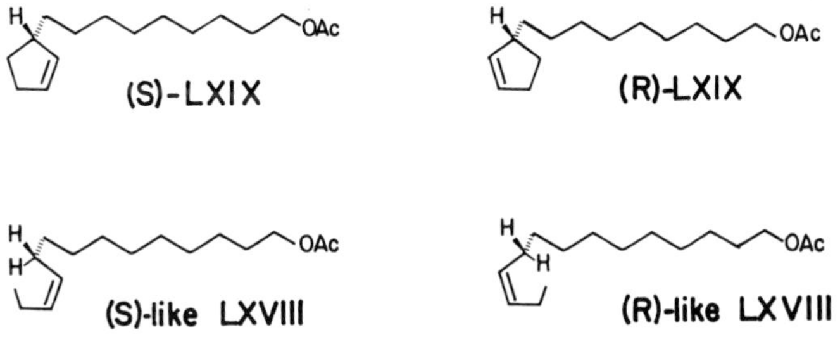

Fig. 25. Enantiomeric cyclic analogs of chiral conformations of an achiral pheromone.

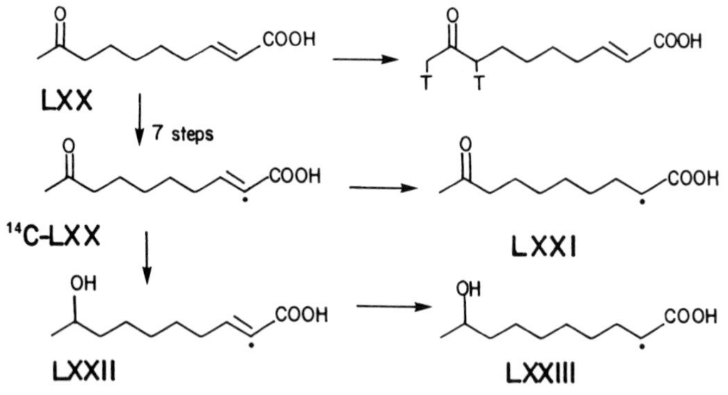

Fig. 26. Synthesis and metabolism of labeled queen bee pheromone.

ingful interpretation of the data. Better information was obtained earlier by Johnston *et al.* (1965), using 2-^{14}C-labeled **LXX,** obtained in seven synthetic steps by protection of the carbonyl, ozonolytic removal of two carbons, and reconstruction of the α,β-unsaturated acid from [^{14}C]malonic acid. They found as the major product the saturated 9-oxodecanoic acid (**LXXI**), with minor amounts of the unsaturated alcohol **LXXII** and the saturated alcohol **LXXIII.** We have recently prepared [4,5-[3]H$_2$]-labeled pheromone **LXX** for studies of pheromone processing in drones and worker bees (G. Prestwich and F. X. Webster, unpublished).

IV. CONCLUSION

Chemical studies of pheromone metabolism and pheromone binding to macromolecules in several moths and a termite have been facilitated by the availability of high specific activity tritium-labeled pheromones and pheromone analogs. The catabolism of pheromones is important in clearing external surfaces as well as in maintaining a low stimulus noise level in the lumen of the sensory hair. Inhibition of this pheromone breakdown can be achieved with chemically reactive pheromone analogs, and may lead to novel control strategies based on sensory disruption. In addition, the molecules which bind pheromones are targets for both chemically reactive and photoactivatable affinity labels. Such receptor protein–targeted reagents open the door to intensive study of pheromone perception on a molecular level, and they may lead to mating disruption by chemically induced selective anosmia to the pheromone.

ACKNOWLEDGMENTS

I thank the National Science Foundation (DMB-8316931 and PCM-8112755), the U.S. Department of Agriculture (85-CRCR-11736), and the Velsicol Chemical Corporation for grants in support of this research. Special thanks are due to Stuart Pharmaceuticals and to Rohm and Haas Co. for unrestricted awards. Research fellowship from the Alfred P. Sloan Foundation and the Camille and Henry Dreyfus Foundation are acknowledged with gratitude. This chapter would not have been possible without the contributions of my research group members and collaborators, and I wish to express my appreciation for their efforts and their permission to cite unpublished results.

REFERENCES

Albans, K. R., Baker, R., Jones, O. T., Justum A. R., and Turnbull, M. D. (1984). Inhibition of response of *Heliothis virescens* to its natural pheromone by antipheromones. *Crop Prot.* **3,** 501–506.

Aune, R. G., Gordon, B. E., Erwin, W. R., Peng, C. T., and Lemmon, R. M. (1982). A high-level tritium facility at the Lawrence Berkeley Laboratory. *In* "Synthesis and Application of Isotopically Labeled Compounds" (W. P. Duncan and A. B. Susan, eds.), pp. 437–438. Elsevier, Amsterdam.

Baker, R., Green, A., Justum, A. R., and Turnbull, M. D. (1981). Protecting plants from insect pests. Eur. Patent Appl. EP 42,448 [*Chem. Abstr.* **96,** 138030 (1982)].

Bayley, H. (1983). "Photogenerated Reagents in Biochemistry and Molecular Biology." Elsevier, Amsterdam.

Beevor, P. S., and Campion, D. G. (1979). The field use of "inhibitory" components of lepidopterous sex pheromones and pheromone mimics. *In* "Chemical Ecology: Odour Communication in Animals" (F. J. Ritter, ed.), pp. 313–325. Elsevier/North-Holland, Amsterdam.

Beroza, M., and Knipling, E. F. (1972). Gypsy moth control with the sex attractant pheromone. *Science* **177,** 19–27.

Bierl, B. A., Beroza, M., and Collier, C. W. (1970). Potent sex attractant of the gypsy moth: Its isolation, identification, and synthesis. *Science* **170,** 87–89.

Bjostad, L. B., and Roelofs, W. L. (1986). Sex pheromone biosynthesis in the redbanded leafroller moth studied by mass-labeling with stable isotopes and chemical ionization mass spectrometry. *J. Chem. Ecol.* **12,** 431–450.

Blackburn, M. B., and Nelson, J. O. (1987). Characterization of sex pheromone receptors of male *Heliothis virescens* using electroantennogram techniques. *J. Insect Physiol.* (in press).

Blomquist, G. J., and Dillwith, J. W. (1983). Pheromones: Biochemistry and physiology. *In* "Endocrinology of Insects" (R. G. H. Downer and H. Laufer, eds.), pp. 527–542. Alan R. Liss, New York.

Boeckh, J. (1984). Neurophysiological aspects of insect olfaction. *In* "Insect Communication" (T. Lewis, ed.), pp. 83–104. Royal Entomol. Society of London, London.

Butler, C. G., Callow, R. K., Greenway, A. R., and Simpson, J. (1974). Movement of the pheromone, 9-oxodec-2-enoic acid, applied to the body surfaces of honeybees (*Apis mellifera*). *Ext. Exp. Appl.* **17,** 112–116.

Cagan, R. H., and Kare, M. R. (1981). "Biochemistry of Taste and Olfaction." Academic Press, New York.

Camps, F., Coll, J., Fabrias, G., and Guerrero, A. (1984a). Synthesis of dienic fluorinated analogs of insect sex pheromones. *Tetrahedron* **40,** 2871–2878.

Camps, F., Coll, J., Fabrias, G., Guerrero, A., and Riba, M. (1984b). Fluorinated analogs of insect sex pheromones. *Experientia* **40,** 933–934.

Cardé, R. T., and Hagaman, T. E. (1979). Behavioral responses of the gypsy moth in a wind tunnel to air-borne enantiomers of disparlure. *Environ. Entomol.* **8,** 475–484.

Cardé, R. T., Doane, C. C., Baker, T. C., Iwaki, S., and Marumo, S. (1977). Attractancy of optically active pheromone for male gypsy moths. *Environ. Entomol.* **6,** 768–772.

Carlson, D. A., and McLaughlin, J. R. (1982a). Diolefin analog of a sex pheromone component of *Heliothis zea* active in disrupting mating communication. *Experientia* **38,** 309–310.

Carlson, D. A., and McLaughlin, J. R. (1982b). Disruption of mating communication in *Heliothis zea:* Synthesis and tests of olefinic analogs of a sex pheromone component. *Prot. Ecol.* **4,** 361–369.

Carvalho, J. F., and Prestwich, G. D. (1984). Synthesis of ω-tritiated and ω-fluorinated analogues of the trail pheromone of subterranean termites. *J. Org. Chem.* **49,** 1251–1258.

Chapman, O. L., Mattes, K. C., Sheridan, R. S., and Klun, J. A. (1978). Stereochemical evidence of dual chemoreceptors for an achiral sex pheromone in Lepidoptera. *J. Am. Chem. Soc.* **100,** 4878–4881.

Charlton, R. E., and Cardé, R. T. (1982). Rate and diel periodicity of pheromone emission from female gypsy moths (*Lymantria dispar*) determined with a glass-adsorption collection system. *J. Insect Physiol.* **28,** 423–430.

Coates, R. M., Hegde, S., and Pearce, C. J. (1982). The preparation and use of lithium triethylborotritide as a labeling reagent. *In* "Synthesis and Applications of Isotopically Labeled Compounds" (W. P. Duncan and A. B. Susan, eds.), pp. 429–430. Elsevier, Amsterdam.

Ding, Y.-S., and Prestwich, G. D. (1986). Metabolic transformation of tritium-labeled pheromone by tissues of *Heliothis virescens* moths. *J. Chem. Ecol.* **12,** 411–429.

Dodd, G., and Persaud, K. (1981). Biochemical mechanisms in verbrate primary olfactory neurons. *In* "Biochemistry of Taste and Olfaction" (R. H. Cagan and M. R. Kare, eds.), pp. 333–357. Academic Press, New York.

Evans, E. A. (1974). "Tritium and Its Compounds." Butterworths, London.

Evans, E. A. (1975). "Self-Decomposition of Radiochemicals: Principles, Control, Observations and Effects." Amersham Corporation, Arlington Heights, Illinois.

Evans, E. A., Warrell, D. C., Elvidge, J. A., and Jones, J. R. (1985). "Handbook of Tritium NMR Spectroscopy and Applications." Wiley, New York.

Ferkovich, S. M. (1982). Enzymatic alteration of insect pheromones. *In* "Perception of Behavioral Chemicals" (D. M. Norris, ed.), pp. 165–185. Elsevier/North-Holland, Amsterdam.

Ferkovich, S. M., Mayer, M. S., and Rutter, R. R. (1973). Conversion of the sex pheromone of the cabbage looper. *Nature (London)* **242,** 53–55.

Ferkovich, S. M., Oliver, J. E., and Dillard, C. (1982a). Comparison of pheromone hydrolysis by the antennae with other tissues after adult eclosion in the cabbage looper moth, *Trichoplusia ni. Entomol. Exp. Appl.* **31,** 327–328.

Ferkovich, S. M., Oliver, J. E., and Dillard, C. (1982b). Pheromone hydrolysis by cuticular and interior esterases of the antennae, legs, and wings of the cabbage looper moth. *Trichoplusia ni* (Hübner). *J. Chem. Ecol.* **8,** 859–866.

Filthuth, H. (1982). State of the art in scanning TLC. *In* "Synthesis and Applications of Isotopically Labeled Compounds" (W. P. Duncan and A. B. Susan, eds.), pp. 447–452. Elsevier, Amsterdam.

Fried, A., and Tu, S.-C. (1984). Affinity labeling of the aldehyde site of bacterial luciferase. *J. Biol. Chem.* **259,** 10754–10759.

Ganjian, I., Pettei, M. J., Nakanishi, K., and Kaissling, K.-E. (1978). A photoaffinity-labelled insect sex pheromone for the moth *Antheraea polyphemus*. *Nature (London)* **271**, 157–158.

Gelb, M. H., Svaren, J. P., and Abeles, R. H. (1985). Fluoro ketone inhibitors of hydrolytic enzymes. *Biochemistry* **24**, 1813–1821.

Guilford, G. L., Evans, E. A., Warrell, D. C., Jones, J. R., Elvidge, J. A., Lenk, R. M., and Tang, Y. S. (1982). Studies of catalysis. *In* "Synthesis and Applications of Isotopically Labeled Compounds" (W. P. Duncan and A. B. Susan, eds.), pp. 327–330. Elsevier, Amsterdam.

Hammock, B. D., Wing, K. D., McLaughlin, J., Lovell, V., and Sparks, T. C. (1982). Trifluoromethyl ketones as possible transition state analog inhibitors of juvenile hormone esterase. *Pest. Biochem. Physiol.* **17**, 76–88.

Hansen, K. (1984). Discrimination and production of disparlure enantiomers by the gypsy moth and the nun moth. *Physiol. Entomol.* **9**, 9–18.

Hecker, E., and Butenandt, A. (1984). Bombykol revisited—Reflections on a pioneering period and on some of its consequences. *In* "Techniques in Pheromone Research" (H. E. Hummel and T. A. Miller, eds.), pp. 1–44. Springer-Verlag, New York.

Hendricks, D. E., Perez, C. T., and Guerra, R. J. (1982). Disruption of *Heliothis* spp. mating behavior with chemical sex attractant components. *Environ. Entomol.* **11**, 859–866.

Hollander, A. L., and Yin, C.-M. (1982). Neurological influences on pheromone release and calling behaviour in the gypsy moth, *Lymantria dispar*. *Physiol. Entomol.* **7**, 163–166.

Hollander, A. L., Yin, C.-M., and Schwalbe, C. P. (1982). Location, morphology and histology of sex pheromone glands of the female gypsy moth, *Lymantria dispar* (L.). *J. Insect Physiol.* **28**, 513–518.

Jacobs, S., and Cuatrecasas, P. (1981). "Membrane Receptors. Methods for Purification and Characterization." Chapman and Hall, London and New York.

Johnston, N. C., Law, J. H., and Weaver, N. (1965). Metabolism of 9-keto-dec-2-enoic acid by worker honeybees (*Apis mellifera*). *Biochemistry* **4**, 1615–1621.

Kaissling, K.-E. (1986). Chemo-electrical transduction in insect olfactory cells. *In* "Molecular Entomology" (J. Law, ed.), Alan R. Liss, New York.

Kaissling, K.-E., and Priesner, E. (1970). Die Riechswelle des Seidenspinners. *Naturwissenschaften* **57**, 23–28.

Kaissling, K.E., and Thorson, J. (1980). Insect olfactory sensilla: Structural, chemical and electrical aspects of the functional organization. *In* "Receptors for Neurotransmitters, Hormones and Pheromones in Insects" (D. B. Satelle and T. Narahashi, eds.), pp. 261–282. Elsevier/North-Holland, Amsterdam.

Kaissling, K.-E., Klein, U., De Kramer, J. J., Keil, T. A., Kanaujia, S., and Hemberger, J. (1985). Insect olfactory cells: Electrophysiological and biochemical studies. *In* "Molecular Basis of Nerve Activity" (J. P. Changeux, F. Hucho, A. Maelicke, and E. Neumann, eds.), pp. 173–183. de Gruyter, Berlin and New York.

Kanaujia, S., and Kaissling, K.-E. (1985). Interactions of pheromone with moth antennae: Adsorption, desorption and transport. *J. Insect Physiol.* **31**, 71–81.

Kasang, G. (1968). Tritium—Markierung des sexuallockstoffes Bombykol. *Z. Naturforsch B* **23**, 1331–1335.

Kasang, G. (1974). Uptake of the sex pheromone ^{3}H-Bombykol and related compounds by male and female *Bombyx* antennae. *J. Insect Physiol.* **20**, 2407–2422.

Kasang, G., and Schneider, D. (1974). Biosynthesis of the sex pheromone disparlure by olefin–epoxide conversion. *Naturwissenschaften* **61**, 130–131.

Kasang, G., and Weiss, N. (1974). Thin-layer chromatographic analysis of radioactively labelled insect pheromones. Metabolites of [^{3}H]bombykol. *J. Chromatog.* **92**, 401–417.

Kasang, G., Knauer, B., and Beroza, M. (1974). Uptake of the sex attractant ^{3}H-disparlure by gypsy male moth antennae *(Lymantria dispar) [=Porthetria dispar]*. *Experientia* **30**, 147–148.

Klein, U., and Keil, T. A. (1984). Dendritic membrane from insect olfactory hairs: Isolation method and electron microscopic observations. *Cell. Mol. Neurobiol.* **4**, 385–396.

Klotz, I. M. (1982). Numbers of receptor sites from Scatchard graphs: Facts and fantasies. *Science* **217**, 1247–1249.

Kochansky, J., Tette, J., Taschenberg, E. F., Cardé, R. T., Kaissling, K.-E., and Roelofs, W. L. (1975). Sex pheromone of the moth *Antheraea polyphemus. J. Insect Physiol.* **21**, 1977–1983.

Liljefors, T., Thelin, B., and van der Pers, J. N. C. (1984). Structure–activity relationships between stimulus molecule and response of a pheromone receptor cell in turnip moth, *Agrotis segetum:* Modifications of the acetate group. *J. Chem. Ecol.* **10**, 1661–1675.

Liljefors, T., Thelin, G., van der Pers, J. N. C., and Lofstedt, C. (1985). Chain-elongated analogues of a pheromone component of the turnip moth, *Agrotis segetum:* A structure-activity study using molecular mechanics. *J. Chem. Soc.* (Perkin Trans.) **II**, 1957–1962.

Lin, G.-Q., Wu, B.-C., Liu, L.-Y., Wang, X.-Q., and Zhou, W.-S. (1984). Studies on the identification and synthesis of insect pheromone. *Acta Chim. Sinica* **42**, 74–81.

Liu, X., Macaulay, E. D. M., and Pickett, J. A. (1984). Propheromones that release pheromonal carbonyl compounds in light. *J. Chem. Ecol.* **10**, 809–822.

Lonergan, G. (1986). Metabolism of pheromone components and analogs by cuticular enzymes of *Choristoneura fumiferana. J. Chem. Ecol.* **12**, 483–496.

Mane, S. D., Tompkins, L., and Richmond, R. C. (1983). Male esterase 6 catalyzes the synthesis of a sex pheromone in *Drosophila melanogaster* females. *Science* **222**, 419–421.

Mason, J. R., and Morton, T. H. (1984a). Selective deficits in the sense of smell caused by chemical modification of the olfactory epithelium. *Science* **226**, 1092–1094.

Mason, J. R., and Morton, T. H. (1984b). Fast and loose covalent binding of ketones as a molecular mechanism in vertebrate olfactory receptors. *Tetrahedron* **40**, 483–492.

Mason, J. R., Leong, F. C., Plaxco, K. W., and Morton, T. H. (1985). Two-step covalent modification of proteins. Selective labelling of Schiff base-forming sites and selective blockade of the sense of smell *in vivo. J. Am. Chem. Soc.* **107**, 6075–6084.

Mayer, M. S. (1975). Hydrolysis of sex pheromone by the antennae of *Trichoplusia ni. Experientia* **31**, 452–454.

Mayer, M. S., Ferkovich, S. M., and Rutter, R. R. (1976). Localization and reactions of a pheromone degradative enzyme isolated from an insect antenna. *Chem. Senses Flavor* **2**, 51–61.

Meighen, E. A., and Grant, G. G. (1985). Bioluminescence analysis of long chain aldehydes: Detection of insect pheromones. *In* "Bioluminescence and Chemiluminescence: Instruments and Applications" (K. Van Dyke, ed.), pp. 253–268. CRC Press, Boca Raton, Florida.

Meighen, E. A., Slessor, K. N., and Grant, G. G. (1981). Bacterial bioluminescence: Applications to entomology. *In* "Bioluminescence an Chemoluminescence" (J. Knox, ed.), pp. 409–416. Academic Press, New York.

Metcalf, R. L., Mitchell, W. C., and Metcalf, E. R. (1983). Olfactory receptors in the melon fly *Dacus cucurbitae* and the oriental fruit fly *Dacus dorsalis. Proc. Natl. Acad. Sci. U.S.A.* **80**, 3143–3147.

Miller, J. R., and Roelofs, W. L. (1978). Gypsy moth responses to pheromone enantiomers as evaluated in a sustained-flight tunnel. *Environ. Entomol.* **7**, 42–44.

Miller, J. R., Mori, K., and Roelofs, W. L. (1977). Gypsy moth field trapping and electroantennogram studies with pheromone enantiomers. *J. Insect Physiol.* **23**, 1447–1453.

Mitchell, E. R. (1981). "Management of Insect Pests with Semiochemicals." Plenum, New York.

Mitchell, E. R., Jacobson, M., and Baumhover, A. H. (1975). *Heliothis* spp.: Disruption of pheromonal communication with (Z)-9-tetradecen-1-ol formate. *Environ. Entomol.* **4**, 577–579.

Mori, K., Takigawa, T., and Matsui, M. (1976). Stereoselective synthesis of optically active disparlure, the pheromone of the gypsy moth (*Porthetria dispar* L.). *Tetrahedron Lett.* **44**, 3953–3956.

Morse, D., and Meighen, E. (1984a). Detection of pheromone biosynthetic and degradative enzymes *in vitro. J. Biol. Chem.* **259**, 475–480.

Morse, D., and Meighen, E. (1984b). Aldehyde pheromones in Lepidoptera: Evidence for an acetate ester precursor in *Choristoneura fumiferana. Science* **226**, 1434–1436.

Morse, D., and Meighen, E. (1986). Pheromone biosynthesis and the role of functional groups in pheromone specificity. *J. Chem. Ecol.* **12**, 335–351.

Muccino, R. R. (1983). "Organic Syntheses with Carbon-14." Wiley, New York.

Oldham, K. G. (1977). Radiotracer techniques for enzyme assays and enzymatic assays. *In* "Radiotracer Techniques and Applications" (E. A. Evans and M. Muramatsu, eds.), pp. 823–890. Dekker, New York.

Pevsner, J., Sklar, P. B., and Snyder, S. H. (1986). Odorant-binding protein: Localization to nasal glands and secretions. *Proc. Natl. Acad. Sci. U.S.A.* **83**, 4942–4946.

Priesner, E. (1979). Specificity studies on pheromone receptors of noctuid and tortricid Lepidoptera. *In* "Chemical Ecology: Odour Communication in Animals" (F. J. Ritter, ed.), pp. 57–71. Elsevier/North-Holland, Amsterdam.

Preiss, R., and Kramer, E. (1983). Stabilization of altitude and speed in tethered flying gypsy moth males: Influence of (+)- and (−)-disparlure. *Physiol. Entomol.* **8**, 55–68.

Prestwich, G. D. (1985). Reactive pheromone mimics for insect mating disruption. U.S. Patent, 4,544,504.

Prestwich, G. D. (1986). Fluorinated sterols, hormones, and pheromones: Enzyme-targeted disruptants in insects. *Pestic. Sci.* **37**, 430–440.

Prestwich, G. D. (1987). Proinsecticides: Metabolically activated toxicants. *In* "Safer Insecticides: Development and Use" (E. Hodgson and R. Kuhr, eds.). Dekker, New York.

Prestwich, G. D., and Wawrzeńczyk, C. (1985). High specific activity enantiomerically enriched juvenile hormones: Synthesis and binding assay. *Proc. Natl. Acad. Sci. U.S.A.* **82**, 5290–5294.

Prestwich, G. D., Golec, F. A., and Andersen, N. H. (1984a). Synthesis of a highly tritiated photoaffinity labeled pheromone analog for the moth *Antheraea polyphemus. J. Labelled Compd. Radiopharm.* **21**, 593–601.

Prestwich, G. D., Singh, A. K., Carvalho, J. F., Koeppe, J. K., Kovalick, G. E., and Chang, E. (1984b). Photoaffinity labels for insect juvenile hormone binding proteins. *Tetrahedron* **40**, 529–537.

Prestwich, G. D., Koeppe, J. K., Kovalick, G. E., Brown, J. J., Chang, E. S., and Singh, A. K. (1985a). Experimental techniques for photoaffinity labeling of juvenile hormone binding proteins of insects with epoxyfarnesyl diazoacetate. *In* "Methods in Enzymology" (J. H. Law and H. C. Rilling, eds.), Vol. 111, pp. 509–530. Academic Press, New York.

Prestwich, G. D., Yamaoka, R., and Carvalho, J. F. (1985b). Metabolism of tritiated ω-fluorofatty acids and alcohols in the termite *Reticulitermes flavipes* Kollar (Isoptera: Rhinotermitidae). *Insect Biochem.* **15**, 205–209.

Prestwich, G. D., Carvalho, J. F., Ding, Y.-S., and Hendricks, D. E. (1986a). Acyl fluorides as reactive mimics of aldehyde pheromones: Hyperactivation and aphrodisia in *Heliothis virescens. Experientia* **42**, 964–966.

Prestwich, G. D., Vogt, R. G., and Ding, Y.-S. (1986b). Chemical studies of pheromone catabolism and reception. *In* "Molecular Entomology" (UCLA Symposia on Molecular and Cellular Biology, New Series) (J. Law, ed.), Alan R. Liss, New York.

Prestwich, G. D., Vogt, R. G., and Riddiford, L. M. (1986c). Binding and hydrolysis of radiolabeled pheromone and several analogs by male-specific antennal proteins of the moth *Antheraea polyphemus. J. Chem. Ecol.* **12**, 323–333.

Prestwich, G. D., Graham, S., Kuo, J. W., and Vogt, R. G. (1987). Tritium-labeled enantiomers of disparlure: Synthesis and *in vitro* metabolism (submitted).

Price, S. (1981). Receptor proteins in vertebrate olfaction. *In* "Biochemistry of Taste and Olfaction" (R. H. Cagan and M. R. Kare, eds.), pp. 69–84. Academic Press, New York.

Raina, A. K., and Klun, J. A. (1984). Brain factor control of sex pheromone production in the female corn earworm moth. *Science* **225**, 531–532.

Ritter, F. J., and Persoons, C. J. (1976). Insect pheromones as a basis for the development of more effective selective pest control agents. *In* "Drug Design" (A. Ariens, ed.), pp. 59–114. Academic Press, New York.

Ritter, F. J., Bruggeman, I. E. M., Persoons, C. J., Talman, E., vanOosten, A., and Verviewl, P. E. J. (1977). Evaluation of social insect pheromones in pest control, with special reference to subterranean termites and pharaoh's ants. *In* "Crop Protection Agents: Their Biological Evaluation" (N. R. McFarlane, ed.), pp. 195–216. Academic Press, New York.

Roberts, T. R. (1978). "Radiochromatography." Elsevier, Amsterdam.

Rossiter, B. E., Katsuki, T., and Sharpless, K. B. (1981). Asymmetric epoxidation provides shortest routes to four chiral epoxy alcohols which are key intermediates in syntheses of methymycin, erythromycin, leukotriene C-1, and disparlure. *J. Am. Chem. Soc.* **103**, 464–465.

Rozen, S., and Filler, R. (1985). α-Fluorocarbonyl compounds and related chemistry. *Tetrahedron* **41**, 1111–1153.

Schneider, D. (1984). Insect olfaction—Our research. *In* "Foundations of Sensory Science" (W. W. Dawson and J. M. Enoch, eds.), pp. 381–418. Springer-Verlag, Heidelberg.

Schneider, D., Lange, R., Schwarz, F., Beroza, M., and Bierl, B. A. (1974). Attraction of male gypsy and nun moths to disparlure and some of its chemical analogues. *Oecologia* **14**, 19–36.

Schneider, D., Kafka, W. A., Beroza, M., and Bierl, B. A. (1977). Odor receptor responses of male gypsy and nun moths (Lepidoptera, Lymantriidae) to disparlure and its analogues. *J. Comp. Physiol. A* **113**, 1–15.

Sheads, R. E., and Beroza, M. (1973). Preparation of tritium-labeled disparlure, the sex attractant of the gypsy moth. *J. Agric. Food Chem.* **21**, 751–753.

Sheppard, G. (1975). "The Radiochromatography of Labelled Compounds." Amersham Corporation, Arlington Heights, Illinois.

Shulman, S. D., and Kobayashi, Y. (1986). Imaging scanners for the analysis of radiolabeled TLC and other biological samples. *In* "Synthesis and Applications of Isotopically Labeled Compounds 1985" (R. R. Muccino, ed.), pp. 459–46. Elsevier, Amsterdam.

Silk, P. J., and Kuenen, L. P. S. (1986). Spruce budworm (*Choristoneura fumiferana*) pheromone chemistry and behavioral responses to pheromone components and analogs. *J. Chem. Ecol.* **12**, 367–383.

Silk, P. J., Kuenen, L. P. S., and Lonergan, G. C. (1985). A biologically active analogue of the primary sex pheromone components of spruce budworm, *Choristoneura fumiferana* (Lepidoptera: Tortricidae). *Can. Entomol.* **117**, 257–260.

Sklar, P. B., Anholt, R. R. H., and Snyder, S. H. (1986). The odorant-sensitive adenylate cyclase of olfactory receptor cells: Differential stimulation by distinct classes of odorants. *J. Biol. Chem.* **261**, 15538–15543.

Stadelbacher, E. A., Barry, M. W., Raina, A. K., and Plimmer, J. R. (1983). Fatal interspecific mating of two *Heliothis* species induced by synthetic sex pheromone. *Experientia* **39**, 1174–1176.

Still, W. C., Kahn, M., and Mitra, A. (1978). Rapid chromatographic technique for preparative separations with moderate resolution. *J. Org. Chem.* **43**, 2923–2925.

Tai, A., Matsumura, F., and Coppel, H. C. (1969). Chemical identification of the trail-following pheromone for a southern subterranean termite. *J. Org. Chem.* **34**, 2180–2182.

Tai, A., Matsumura, F., and Coppel, H. C. (1971). Synthetic analogues of the termite trail-following pheromone: Structure and biological activity. *J. Insect Physiol.* **17**, 181–188.

Taylor, T. R., Ferkovich, S. M., and van Essen, F. (1981). Increased pheromone catabolism by antennal esterases after adult eclosion of the cabbage looper moth. *Experientia* **37**, 729–731.

Teal, P. E. A., and Tumlinson, J. H. (1986). Induced *in vivo* biosynthesis of bombykal by sex pheromone glands of *Heliothis virescens* and *H. zea*. *J. Chem. Ecol.* **12**, 353–366.

Teal, P. E. A., Carlysle, T. C., and Tumlinson, J. H. (1983). Epidermal glands in terminal abdominal segments of female *Heliothis virescens* (F.) (Lepidoptera: Noctuidae). *Ann. Entomol. Soc. Am.* **76**, 242–247.

Tu, S.-C., and Henkin, J. (1983). Characterization of the aldehyde binding site of bacterial luciferase by photoaffinity labeling. *Biochemistry* **22**, 519–523.

Ujvary, I., Voight, E., and Lesko, K. (1986). Synthesis of a possible degradation product of (+)-disparlure, the sex pheromone of the gypsy moth, *Lymantria dispar*. *Acta Chim. Hungarica*, in press.

Vander Meer, R. K., Obin, M. S., Zawistowski, S., Sheehan, K. B., and Richmond, R. C. (1987). A reevaluation of the role of *cis*-vaccenyl acetate, *cis*-vaccenol and esterase 6 in the regulation of mated female sexual attractiveness in *Drosophila melanogaster*. *J. Insect Physiol.* **32**, 681–686.

Venter, J. C., and Harrison, L. C. (1984a). "Membranes, Detergents and Receptor Solubilization." Alan R. Liss, New York.

Venter, J. C., and Harrison, L. C. (1984b). "Molecular and Chemical Characterization of Membrane Receptors." Alan R. Liss, New York.

Vogt, R. G. (1984). The biochemical design of sex pheromone reception in the wild silk moth *Antheraea polyphemus*. Ph.D. thesis, University of Washington.

Vogt, R. G., and Riddiford, L. M. (1980). Pheromone deactivation by antennal proteins of Lepidoptera. *In* "Scientific Papers of the Institute of Organic and Physical Chemistry of Wroclaw Technical University" (F. Sehnal, A. Zabza, J. J. Menn, and B. Cymborowski, eds.), pp. 955–967. Technical Univ. Press, Wroclaw.

Vogt, R. G., and Riddiford, L. M. (1981). Pheromone binding and inactivation by moth antennae. *Nature (London)* **293**, 161–163.

Vogt, R. G., and Riddiford, L. M. (1986a). Scale esterase: A pheromone-degrading enzyme from the scales of the silk moth *Antheraea polyphemus*. *J. Chem. Ecol.* **12**, 469–482.

Vogt, R. G., and Riddiford, L. M. (1986b). Pheromone reception: A kinetic equilibrium. *In* "Mechanisms of Perception and Orientation to Insect Olfactory Signals" (T. Payne, R. Cardé, and J. Boeckh, eds.), pp. 201–205. Oxford Univ. Press, Oxford.

Vogt. R. G., Riddiford, L. M., and Prestwich, G. D. (1985). Kinetic properties of a pheromone degrading enzyme: The sensillar esterase of *Antheraea polyphemus*. *Proc. Natl. Acad. Sci. U.S.A.* **82**, 8827–8831.

Wall, C. (1984). The exploitation of insect communication by man—fact or fantasy? *In* "Insect Communication" (T. Lewis, ed.), pp. 379–400. Royal Entomol. Society of London, London.

Wieland, D. M., Tobes, M. C., and Mangner, T. J. (1985). "Analytical and Chromatographic Techniques in Radiopharmaceutical Chemistry." Springer-Verlag, New York.

Wong, C. G., and Rando, R. R. (1982). Inactivation of bovine opsin by all-*trans*-retinoyl fluoride. *J. Am. Chem. Soc.* **104**, 7374–7375.

Yamada, M., Saito, T., Katagiri, K., Iwaki, S., and Marumo, S. (1976). Electroantennogram and behavioural responses of the gypsy moth to enantiomers of disparlure and its *trans* analogues. *J. Insect Physiol.* **22**, 755–761.

Zawistowski, S., and Richmond, R. C. (1986). Inhibition of courtship and mating of *Drosophila melanogaster* by the male-produced lipid, *cis*-vaccenyl acetate. *J. Insect Physiol.* **32**, 189–192.

15

Molecular Mechanisms of Vertebrate Olfaction: Implications for Pheromone Biochemistry

U. PACE
D. LANCET

Department of Membrane Research
The Weizmann Institute of Science
Rehovot 76 100, Israel

I. INTRODUCTION

Although the sense of smell is a key for survival and adaptation in the animal world and has been the subject of intense interest and research, the molecular mechanisms underlying its function are still largely unknown. In recent years there has been consistent progress in our understanding of the biochemistry of vertebrate odor recognition, as well as a refinement of the corresponding electrophysiological and neuroanatomical techniques. The aim of this chapter is to describe the most recent results in the biochemistry of vertebrate olfaction and to indicate the possible directions of future research. The accent will be on research principles and on their possible application to the study of insect olfaction and pheromone reception. Complementary information can be found in other chapters in this volume (in particular, De Kramer and Hemberger, Chapter 13, and Vogt, Chapter 12).

Pheromone Biochemistry

II. OLFACTORY MEMBRANE PREPARATIONS

The sense of smell in both vertebrates and invertebrates has been studied mainly using electrophysioloigcal techniques. These techniques include the electroolfactogram (EOG) and the electroantennogram (EAG), summated generator potential recordings, as well as intracellular and extracellular single unit recordings. The sense of smell appears to be similar to other neuronal reception systems, with the odorant or pheromone playing a role analogous to that of neurotransmitters, reacting with specialized receptors to activate conductance changes at the dendritic membrane; these changes give rise in turn to action potentials.

In contrast to the detailed knowledge obtained by electrophysiological and neuroanatomical studies (Moulton and Beidler, 1967; Gesteland, 1976; Getchell et al., 1984; Getchell, 1986), the biochemical aspects of the olfactory processes have only recently begun to be elucidated (Price, 1981; Dodd and Persaud, 1981; Lancet, 1984, 1986a,b; Synder et al., 1986). One of the reasons for this relative ignorance is the fact that a reproducible membrane preparation suitable for biochemical studies has not been available until recently. Two major obstacles hindered the development of membrane preparations from olfactory epithelium. First, there is no reliable and specific marker for monitoring olfactory activity in vitro. Second, the transductory machinery is concentrated in a specific area of the epithelium (the cilia) and is therefore largely diluted in preparations from whole epithelia. Thus, Kurihara and co-workers (Kurihara and Koyama, 1972) and Dodd and co-workers (Menevse et al., 1977) measured adenylate cyclase activity in homogenates from whole epithelia or in partially purified epithelial membrane preparations, but they were not able to show odorant activation of this enzyme.

Once the importance of olfactory cilia (the dendritic extensions of chemosensory neurons) in the mechanism of olfactory transduction was recognized (Fig. 1), Cagan and co-workers (Rhein and Cagan, 1980) developed a preparation of purified cilia from the olfactory organ of fish and measured its binding of radiolabeled amino acid odorants. These experiments marked the establishment of a useful olfactory membrane preparation amenable to biochemical analysis. More recently a cilia preparation from the olfactory epithelium of frogs was developed (Chen and Lancet, 1984; Chen et al., 1986c; Anholt et al., 1986a) and used both for the characterization of proteins which could be involved in olfactory reception, and for the study of transductory elements such as GTP-binding proteins (G-proteins) and adenylate cyclase (Pace et al., 1985; Pace and Lancet, 1986; Sklar et al., 1986; Shirley et al., 1986; Lancet and Pace, 1987).

The technique used for isolating olfactory cilia is known as the calcium shock procedure, in which olfactory epithelium is abruptly exposed to a rise in Ca^{2+} concentration. These and similar procedures give a preparation which accounts for a few percent of the total membrane material of the epithelium but which is

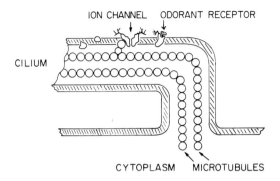

Fig. 1.   Schematic representation of an olfactory cilium. Olfactory cilia are extension of the dendritic membrane of the chemosensory neurons. They contain the microtubular axoneme (tubulin monomers schematically represented by circles) and are ensheathed with lipid bilayer that contains the transduction molecular machinery. Shown here are the odorant receptor and an ion channel, both depicted as transmembrane glycoproteins. It is possible that some of these components are specifically anchored to the microtubular cytoskeleton.

highly enriched in some specific proteins and enzymatic activities (tubulin, GTP-binding proteins, some glycoproteins, adenylate cyclase) (Pace *et al.*, 1985; Chen *et al.*, 1986b,c; Chen and Lancet, 1984). Cilia preparations of this kind have now been developed in our laboratory and elsewhere also for the mammalian olfactory epithelium (Pace and Lancet, 1986; Sklar *et al.*, 1986; Shirley *et al.*, 1986). As previously pointed out (Lancet, 1986a,b), the cilia preparation resembles isolated rod outer segment preparations from retina, and it is similarly useful in elucidating the biochemical processes underlying sensory transduction (see Stryer, 1986).

As for the development of membrane preparations from insect chemosensory organs, there have been recent reports about preparations of dendritic membranes from antennae of *Anteraea polyphemus,* and preliminary biochemical studies have been described (Klein and Keil, 1984). One of the problems in obtaining membrane preparations from insect antennae is in the interaction of the cell membranes with the cuticular structures, which hinders efficient homogenization and prevents the release of membrane vesicles. Thus, it was necessary to add to the homogenization buffers detergents such as Triton X-100 or sodium dodecyl sulfate, with consequent loss of activity (Klein, 1980). Only recently have these problems been overcome, and this could be the starting point of the biochemical study of insect pheromone reception, using similar tools and contents to those established for studies of vertebrate olfaction. Recent biochemical and chemical results with soluble and membrane-associated olfactory proteins are described by De Kramer and Hemberger (Chapter 13), Vogt (Chapter 12), and Prestwich (Chapter 14, this volume).

III. TRANSDUCTORY ENZYMES
AND SECOND MESSENGERS

The transduction of stimuli across the membrane is a key step in every sensory mechanism, including chemoreception. Chemosensory transduction constitutes a chain of events which take place following the binding of odorous molecules to specific cell surface receptor proteins. The transductory events may underlie many of the characteristics of the chemoreceptive response, including time course, amplification, and adaptation. Transduction mechanisms can be broadly divided into two groups: (1) direct gating of ion channels by the extracellular ligand, and (2) gating of channels through a chain of biochemical reactions which involves cytoplasmic second messenger(s). A transduction mechanism of the first kind has been thoroughly studied in the case of the nicotinic acetylcholine receptor (AchR). In this case the receptor and the ion channel are one and the same polypeptide complex, and binding of the agonist modulates ion channel opening (Changeaux *et al.*, 1984). This transduction system enables a fast response but, on the other hand, affords little amplification.

The second class of transduction mechanisms involves the production of second messengers and has been the subject of intense studies in recent years, leading to a unified picture of its components, namely, the receptor (R), the GTP-binding protein (G), and the catalytic subunit (C). Two such systems have been studied in detail: (1) the hormone- and neurotransmitter-dependent adenylate cyclase, and (2) the light-dependent cGMP phosophdiesterase of the vertebrate visual rod outer segment (ROS). In the first case, various receptors, such as the β-adrenergic receptor, act via the the stimulatory GTP-binding protein (G_s), and the catalytic component is the enzyme adenylate cyclase (Gilman, 1984; Schramm and Selinger, 1984). In the ROS, the receptor is the photoactivated protein rhodopsin, and the G-protein is called transducin (Stryer, 1986; Kaupp and Koch, 1986).

The mechanism proposed for these transduction systems is as follows. The primary event is binding of the hormone or neurotransmitter to the receptor or the absorption of a photon by rhodopsin. The activated receptors catalyzes the binding of GTP to the G-protein which is in turn activated. The activated G-protein turns on the catalytic component, and this activation ceases upon hydrolysis of GTP to GDP, leaving the G-protein inactive and ready for a new cycle of activation (Figs. 2 and 3).

This chain of events involves two amplification steps: the first is at the level of the R–G interaction, since an activated receptor may activate a large number of G-proteins (500 in the case of rhodopsin–transducin interaction; Stryer, 1986). The second phase is at the catalytic unit level: an activated cyclase or phosphodiesterase molecule may synthesize or hydrolyze a large number of cAMP or

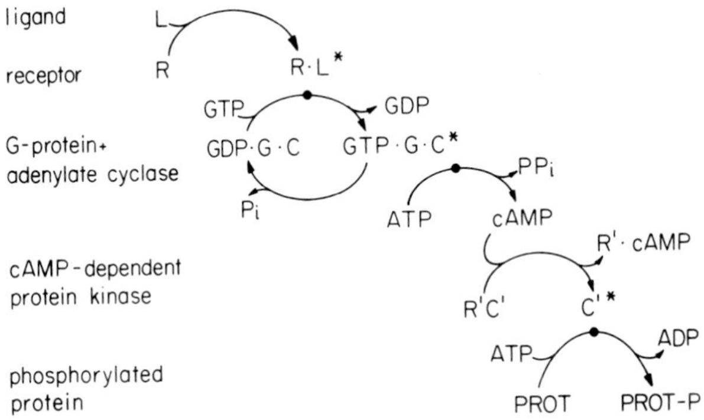

Fig. 2. The cyclic nucleotide–enzyme cascade. The ligand (L) binds to a receptor (R), thereby activating it (* indicates an activated component). The active RL complex catalyzes the exchange of GDP to GTP at the GTP-binding protein (G-protein, G) (● indicates a catalytic step). Amplification is effected by the ability of one molecule of activated receptor to catalyze such exchange at up to several hundred G-proteins. Activated G associates with (or may exist in a preformed complex with) the catalytic unit of adenylate cyclase (C). The complex containing GTP-G and C is active, capable of catalyzing the conversion of ATP to cyclic AMP (cAMP) and pyrophosphate (PP_i). Adenylate cyclase activity is spontaneously turned off through the hydrolysis of GTP to GDP and phosphate (P_i) at the GTP binding site of G. cAMP binds to the regulatory subunit (R′) of cAMP-dependent protein kinase, thereby releasing the kinase catalytic subunit (C′) in its active form. C′ catalyzes the phosphorylation of proteins (PROT): covalent linking of phosphate (P) transferred from ATP to the hydroxyl groups of serine and threonine residues.

cGMP molecules (500 in the case of ROS). Thus the overall amplification in ROS is $>10^5$ and for the adenylate cyclase is probably similarly high.

Another enzyme which has been suggested to be under the control of a G-protein is phospholipase C, which is specific for phosphatidyl inositol (PI) (Cockcroft and Gomperts, 1985). Breakdown of PI is thought to give rise to two different second messengers (inositol triphosphate and diacylglycerol), which act synergistically in activating a protein kinase (protein kinase C) (Joseph, 1985; Berridge and Irvine, 1984; Fig. 6).

As for transduction systems in olfaction, considerable evidence has accumulated indicating that they involve adenylate cyclase. This is not surprising, since responses to extraneous ligands (neurotransmitters) at dendritic membranes of many neuron types has been suggested to involve cAMP (Fig. 4). The role of adenylate cyclase (which generates cAMP) in olfaction was first recognized by Minor and Sakina (1973), who used an electrophysiological method, modified electroolfactogram recordings, for probing the effect of cAMP and of its membrane-penetrable analog dibutyryl cAMP. They found that these agents, but not other similar nucleotides such as AMP, GMP, or cGMP, mimic the effect of the odorant, as it would be expected if odorants act by raising the intracellular cAMP

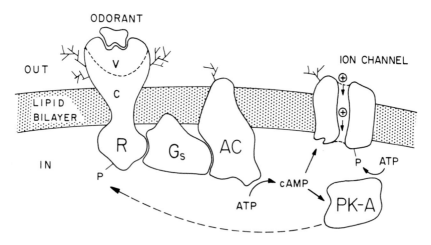

Fig. 3. Model showing the proposed involvement of the cyclic nucleotide cascade in olfaction. Some features have already been supported by experimental data as described in the text. It is hypothesized that there exists a family of receptor proteins (R) which share common structural regions (c) but differ at a variable region (v) containing different odorant binding sites in different receptor types (see also Fig. 7). The receptor is presumed to be a transmembrane glycoprotein, its carbohydrate moieties shown as attached branching structures which form part of the common region. Odorants bind extracellularly, and transduction events occur in the cytoplasm. The receptor interacts with the intracellular, membrane-associated G-protein of the stimulatory type (G_S). This, in turn, activates adenylate cyclase (AC, now believed to be a transmembrane glycoprotein) to generate cAMP. This second messenger may activate cAMP-dependent protein kinase (PK-A) leading to phosphorylation of polypeptides that may be related to ion channel conductance. Alternatively, cAMP could interact directly with an ion channel structure, a mechanism homologous to that found in retinal photoreceptor cells. Protein phosphorylation could also affect the receptor in a feedback-type mechanism.

concentration. Moreover, caffeine or theophylline, which are known inhibitors of cyclic nucleotide phosphodiesterase (the enzyme that degrades cAMP), potentiate the effect of odorants. Later Menevse *et al.* (1977) confirmed and extended some of the latter findings.

The development of cilia preparations led to further clarification of this point. We succeeded in demonstrating odorant activation of the adenylate cyclase of olfactory cilia (Pace *et al.*, 1985). The olfactory adenylate cyclase appears to be regulated by a stimulatory G-protein analogous to hormone-coupled G_s (Gilman, 1984), since odorant activation is seen only in the presence of GTP (Pace *et al.*, 1985; Pace and Lancet, 1986). The α subunit of the G-protein of olfactory cilia (Fig. 5) could also be identified by a covalent label (ADP-ribosylation) catalyzed by cholera toxin, or by specific antisera. ADP ribosylation is also found to increase adenylate cyclase activity, as expected, again indicating that the G-m-Cholinergic β_2- Adrenergic D_2- Dopaminergic   Opiate   Olfactory

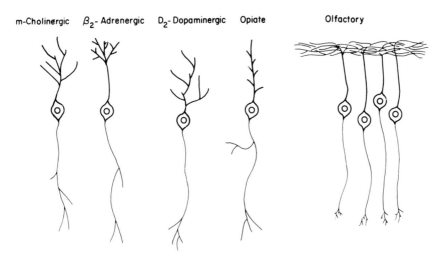

Fig. 4. Types of neurons that respond to chemical stimulation at their dendritic membrane by changes in intracellular cAMP levels.

protein involved is of the G_s kind (Pace *et al.*, 1985; Pace and Lancet, 1986; Anholt *et al.*, 1986b; see Gilman, 1984; Schramm and Selinger, 1984, for general reviews).

Sklar *et al.* (1986) screened a variety of odorants for their effect on olfactory adenylate cyclase and found GTP-dependent activation by certain odorant classes. Many other odorants (e.g., aliphatic acids, amines, and some organic solvents), however, do not activate adenylate cyclase beyond the GTP-stimulated level. The authors suggest that additional odorant-activated transduction mechanisms may exist in olfactory cilia, e.g., the activation of phospholipase-C, which acts on a membrane lipid (phosphatidylinositol bisphosphate) to produce two second messengers (Fig. 6). Huque and Bruch (1986) reported the activation of phosphoinositide turnover in olfactory cilia by odorants and found that GTP was also involved in this process. One of the second messengers produced by this pathway, diacylglycerol, is known to activate protein kinase C, a calcium/phospholipid–activated enzyme. The existence of protein kinase C in olfactory cilia was inferred from phorbol ester binding measurements (Anholt *et al.*, 1986b), but this point requires further clarification in view of the lack of directly measured protein kinase C activity in olfactory cilia (Heldman and Lancet, 1986).

There is no direct biochemical evidence regarding the mechanism of transduction in insect olfactory systems. However, there are indications that cyclic nucleotides are involved in the process. Villet (1978) showed that cyclic nucleotide analogs and phosphodiesterase inhibitors enhance the response of prefused an-

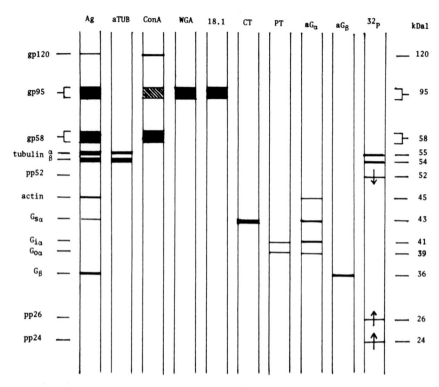

Fig. 5. Identified polypeptides of olfactory cilia from frogs. Polypeptides are marked on the left, molecular masses on the right. At the top are the different methods used for polypeptide detection. The tubulin dimer (α, β) is a prominent component seen by silver staining (Ag) and by immunoblotting with anti-tubulin antibodies (aTUB) (Chen and Lancet, 1984). The lectins concanavalin A (Con A) and wheat germ agglutinin (WGA) detect three important glycoproteins: gp120, gp95, and gp58 (Chen and Lancet, 1984; Chen et al., 1986b). The first is a minor while the last two are major components in silver staining. gp95 is also labeled by a specific monoclonal antibody 18.1 (Chen et al., 1986a). Bacterially derived cholera toxin (CT) and pertussis toxin (PT) label, respectively, the α subunits of the stimulatory G-protein ($G_{s\alpha}$) and of the inhibitory ($G_{i\alpha}$) and brain-specific ($G_{o\alpha}$) G-proteins. Monoclonal antibody 569 (aGα) labels all these G-protein α subunits as well as a band near actin, possibly a G_s subtype (Anholt et al., 1986b; U. Pace and D. Lancet, unpublished). The common β subunit of these G-proteins is labeled by specific antisera (Anholt et al., 1986a,b; U. Pace and D. Lancet, unpublished) and is also prominently seen in silver staining, together with $G_{s\alpha}$ which is a weaker band (Chen et al., 1986c; Pace and Lancet, 1986). ^{32}P-Labeled phosphoproteins detected in olfactory cilia are α and β tubulin, pp52 (possibly the regulatory subunit of the cAMP-dependent protein kinase), and pp26 and pp24 (Heldman and Lancet, 1986). Arrows mark decreased or increased phosphorylation induced by cAMP.

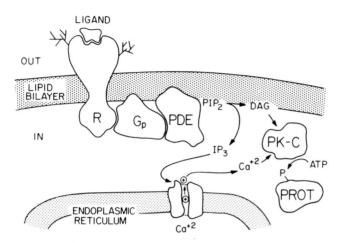

Fig. 6. The phosphatidylinositol cycle. A ligand-activated receptor (R) activates a G-protein (G_p, not yet fully identified) that in turn activates the enzyme phosphatidylinositol biphosphate (PIP_2) phosphodiesterase (PDE). The membrane lipid PIP_2 is broken down into two second messengers: membrane-associated diacylglycerol (DAG) and soluble inositol trisphosphate (IP_3). The first product activates protein kinase C (PK-C) which phosphorylates various protein substrates. The second product enhances the release of calcium ions (Ca^{2+}) from the internal stores in the lumen of the endoplasmic reticulum, increasing cytoplasmic calcium. Calcium synergizes with DAG in activating PK-C.

tennae to pheromones (as measured by EAG). Data from single unit recordings from olfactory cells of *A. polyphemus* indicate that there is a large delay between stimulus presentation and channel opening (Kaissling, 1986). This finding is consistent with the activation of a cyclic nucleotide cascade by the odorant or the pheromone. Also the extreme sensitivity of pheromone-sensitive cells may be due to the presence of an amplification mechanism of the kind afforded by the cyclic nucleotide cascade. Clearly further biochemical studies are required in order to understand the mechanism by which the pheromone signals are transduced. An interesting possibility is that vertebrate and invertebrate olfaction utilizes different second messengers, as in the case for visual transduction, where cyclic GMP and phosphatidylinositol are respectively operative (Stryer, 1986; Kaupp and Koch, 1986; Vandenberg and Montal, 1984; Selinger *et al.*, 1986).

The elucidation of the olfactory second messenger system can also be used as a tool for the identification of the receptor for odorants, since components of the adenylate cyclase system may be separated and reconstituted in both homologous and heterologous systems (May *et al.*, 1985; Levitzki, 1985). It may thus be possible to use the G-protein and adenylate cyclase as detection devices for the receptor (Lancet 1986a,b; see Section V).

IV. ION CHANNELS AND THEIR MODULATION

All the electrical properties of excitable cells are due to their ion channels and stimulation by neurotransmitters is thought to finally modulate the ion conductance of such channels. There are a number of ways by which ion channels are modulated. One way (mentioned above) is gating of the channels by the external ligand, as it is the case of the acetylcholine receptor–linked Na^+/K^+ channel (Changeaux *et al.*, 1984). In this case the receptor is the channel itself, or is in close association with it, and the conformational change induced by the ligand causes the opening or closure of the channel.

A second way by which a channel can be modulated is by means of a phosphorylation–dephosphorylation cycle. This mechanism may be controlled by second messengers, such as Ca^{2+} or cAMP, which are known to activate protein kinases. In particular, phosphorylation of membrane proteins by the cAMP-dependent protein kinase has been claimed to be involved in many cases in which an electrophysiological response follows stimulation by a ligand that activates adenylate cyclase. This mechanism has been tested, for example, in the case of the modulation of the response of *Aplysia* motor neurons (Castellucci *et al.*, 1982; Byrne, 1985). In this case a neurotransmitter elicits a response mediated by K^+ channels. A second neurotransmitter, which is linked to adenylate cyclase, modulates the response of the first one. It has been found that injection of cAMP or of the catalytic subunit of the cAMP-dependent protein kinase may mimic the effect of the second transmitter.

The third and most newly discovered mechanism of modulation of the ion channels is direct gating by the second messenger. This has so far been demonstrated only in the case of ROS, where cGMP was shown to open Na^+ channels in the plasma membrane (Fesenko *et al.*, 1985; Yau and Nakatani, 1985; Stryer, 1986; Kaupp and Koch, 1986). Since, as mentioned before, the primary effect of light in ROS is reduction of the cGMP concentration, the final result of light activation is the blocking of Na^+ influx, leading to a hyperpolarization of the rod cell (Miller, 1983; Stryer, 1986; Kaupp and Koch, 1986).

The studies of ion channels in olfaction have increased recently owing to the development of new techniques, such as patch clamp recordings. This is done either by directly recording from the olfactory receptor neuron (at the soma and dendritic knob) or by using reconstituted systems, in which proteins from the membranes of the olfactory organ are incorporated into artificial lipid bilayers. Preliminary studies of the ionic channels in isolated olfactory sensory neurons have been reported by Maue and Dionne (1984) and by Firestein and Werblin (1985). Both report the characterization of several K^+-selective channels. Potassium selective channels has also been detected by Vodyanoy and Murphy (1983) by reconstitution of the membrane proteins of olfactory epithelia into artificial lipid bilayer. They could also show that the mean opening time of these channels is increased by some odorants. Early studies (Takagi *et al.,* 1969) done by classical electrophysiological methods have shown that K^+ or Na^+ conductance was involved in the response of odorants.

One of the most interesting points to be clarified is whether the olfactory ion channels are directly gated by the cyclic nucleotide second messenger. A recent patch clamp study of toad olfactory cilia (Nakamura and Gold, 1987) strongly supports this mechanism (Fig. 5). In parallel, protein phosphorylation could be involved in ion channel modulation. We find that cAMP-dependent protein kinase, as well as two specific polypeptide substates for it [of 24 and 26 kDa (kilodaltons)], are present in frog olfactory cilia (Heldman and Lancet, 1986, and Fig. 5). The role of such components in olfactory transducation/adaptation is yet to be elucidated.

The ionic currents which generate receptor potentials in pheromone-sensitive cells have been studied in *A. polyphemus* (Kaissling, 1986). The data indicate that application of pheromone causes opening of single channels in the dendritic membrane. The biochemical nature and ion specificities of these channels are not known. However, since the sensillum lymph has a very high K^+ concentration (>200 mM), it is possible that these depolarizing currents are mediated by K^+ influx as a consequence of a pheromone-mediated channel opening.

V. OLFACTORY RECEPTOR PROTEINS:
PROBLEMS AND PROSPECTS

The search for olfactory receptor proteins has been a major goal of research in chemoreception. As described before, our concept of the olfactory transduction process postulates the existence of a protein receptor, probably a transmembrane protein, which interacts with a second messenger system, in all likelihood adenylate cyclase. The binding of the odorants to this receptor initiates the chain of events which eventually produces the firing of action potentials by the olfactory sensory neuron (see Getchell *et al.,* 1984; Lancet, 1986a,b; Fig. 3).

Some authors have suggested that olfactory receptor proteins may not exist, and that the interaction of odorants with the sensory cell are mediated by the lipid bilayer, since most odorants are lipophilic and readily enter the bilayer (Kashiwayanagi and Kurihara, 1984). This view is contradicted by a number of basic findings, however, which support the role of a protein receptor in olfactory transduction.

1. Olfactory reception is affected by compounds which modify proteins, such as alkylating reagents (Getchell and Gesteland, 1972; Shirley *et al.,* 1983a; Delaleu and Holley, 1980), or by molecules which bind surface proteins, such as lectins (Shirley *et al.,* 1983b; Chen *et al.,* 1986d).

2. The response to some odorants is stereospecific (Beets, 1971), and this fact cannot be accounted for by simple physical (nonspecific) interactions with the membrane.

3. The fact that there are genetically determined specific anosmias (odor blindnesses) in man (Amoore, 1982), in other vertebrates (Wysocki *et al.*, 1977), and in insects (Rodrigues and Siddiqi, 1978; Venard and Pichon, 1984), implies the involvement of gene products, i.e., specific proteins, in the recognition process.

4. Finally, the involvement of adenylate cyclase in the transduction process (Pace *et al.*, 1985; Sklar *et al.*, 1986) also implies the mediation of a protein receptor, as in many similar receptor systems.

It has been proposed (Boyse *et al.*, 1982; Lancet, 1984) that such a receptor would constitute a membrane protein, possibly a glycoprotein, which has a constant region, providing the interaction with the common transductory system, and a variable region, which interacts with different odorants (Figs. 3 and 7). The variability could be provided by mechanisms similar to those that generate different antibody amino acid sequences through DNA recombination and somatic mutations (Hood *et al.*, 1985). If this is true, the genetic organization of the olfactory receptor protein(s) may resemble that of immunoglobulin genes in B lymphocytes. This may imply that individual sensory neurons would express a single kind of receptor, in analogy to the principle of "one cell, one antibody" which is valid for the B lymphocytes. Indeed, the electrophysiological recordings of single cells which show that each olfactory neuron has a unique pattern of activation by odorants (Sicard and Holley, 1984) are consistent with this possibility, although not disproving the notion that one cell has several receptor types (see Gesteland, 1976).

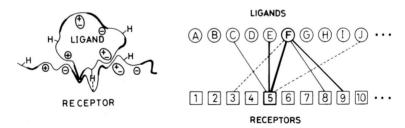

Fig. 7. Scheme showing the types of possible interactions between a typical receptor and its ligand. + or −, Ionic or dipolar interactions; H, hydrogen atoms potentially forming hydrogen bonds; bold lines, hydrophobic interactions. Different receptors may vary in the binding surface they present, hence have different ligand binding specificity. In a group of receptors, such as immunoglobulins and possibly olfactory receptors, any receptor can bind more than one ligand, and each ligand may bind to more than one receptor. Such relations may partly explain the broad odorant specificity spectra of the sensory neurons (see Lancet 1986a,b).

In recent years the field of neuronal receptors has greatly advanced, owing to the refinement of the various techniques of radioactive ligand binding (see Snyder, 1984). The application of such methods led to the discovery of odorant binding proteins in olfactory tissue (reviewed in Getchell *et al.*, 1984; Getchell, 1986; Lancet, 1986a,b; Snyder *et al.*, 1986). However, it is important to bear in mind that theoretical and practical considerations indicate that the study of olfactory receptor proteins poses some unique difficulties to the application of ligand binding techniques (see Price, 1981; Lancet, 1986a).

1. Olfactory receptors most probably have low equilibrium binding constants and high dissociation rate constants, conditions which hinder the application of most receptor binding techniques (Mason and Morton, 1984; Lancet, 1986a).

2. Odorants are lipophilic and they easily bind to nonreceptor proteins and to the lipids of the membrane. This may result in a high degree of nonspecific binding.

3. Olfactory receptors are, as pointed out above, likely to be heterogeneous: a biochemical preparation from entire epithelia will contain many receptor types. Odorants may bind to more than one receptor type, leading to complex saturation curves.

Fruitful binding studies with radiolabeled odorants have been performed in fish, where many of the above-mentioned problems are alleviated: odorants are few and nonlipophilic (mainly amino acids) and receptor heterogeneity is less pronounced. Binding of radiolabeled amino acids to olfactory cilia of fishes has been demonstrated by several researchers (Cagan and Zeiger, 1978; Rhein and Cagan, 1980; Fesenko *et al.*, 1983), and a correlation has been found between binding and electrophysiological potency (Cagan and Zeiger, 1978).

In terrestrial vertebrates binding sites for some odorants such as pyrazine (Bignetti *et al.*, 1985; Pevsner *et al.*, 1985) and camphor (Fesenko *et al.*, 1979) have been described, and proteins which bind these odorants have been isolated from nasal tissue. The pyrazine-binding protein is water soluble, and immunohistological studies have shown that it is not found in the sensory neurons but in the secretory cells near the basal lamina of respiratory and olfactory epithelia (Pevsner *et al.*, 1985, 1986). It may constitute an odorant carrier, similar to the pheromone-binding protein of *A. polyphemus* (see below). Salamanders have been studied *in vivo* using a two-step chemical modification to correlate behavior with a molecular understanding of odorant binding (Mason and Morton, 1984; Mason *et al.*, 1984).

Insect pheromone receptors may be useful for the application of ligand binding techniques because of their high specificity and presumed homogeneity and high affinity. Yet specific binding of pheromones to dendritic membranes from olfactory sensilla has not been completely described. A pheromone-binding protein with relatively low affinity and low specificity has been isolated from antennae of *A. polyphemus* (Vogt and Riddiford, 1981; Vogt, Chapter 12, this volume). This is a soluble protein present in the sensillum lymph at a very high concentration, suggesting that it may have a role as a pheromone carrier. However, an intriguing possibility is that the pheromone-binding protein *is* the receptor, i.e., it serves as a soluble receptor which, when occupied, may bind to a membrane protein to initiate transduction events. In this way, it may be similar to periplasmic chemoattractant receptors of bacteria (Koshland, 1980).

An alternative approach to the identification of olfactory receptor proteins has been proposed (Lancet, 1986a; Chen and Lancet, 1984), based on the accumulating knowledge of the molecular components of the olfactory transduction system (Fig. 5). We and other groups started with the characterization, by functional, immunochemical, and biochemical criteria, of major proteins, which are good candidates to be olfactory receptor proteins. In particular, a glycoprotein (gp95) with transmembrane receptor properties has recently been isolated and purified, and its biochemical characteristics have been studied in depth (Chen *et al.*, 1986b) (Fig. 5). This glycoprotein is a major component of the ciliary membrane, and it has been shown by specific monoclonal antibodies (Fig. 5) to be localized in the surface layer of olfactory epithelia (Chen *et al.*, 1986a). It is an integral membrane protein and it binds strongly the lectin wheat germ agglutinin (WGA). We have shown that WGA inhibits the EOG response to various odorants as well as the *in vitro* activation of adenylate cyclase by odorants (Chen *et al.*, 1986d). These findings point to the possible involvement of gp95 in the process of transduction of the odorant signal. The purification of gp95 is now underway, with the intention to obtain partial sequence analysis and finally clone the gene(s) coding for it (Lancet and Pace, 1987).

The discovery of odorant-dependent adenylate cyclase allows another research route to the study of olfactory receptor protein(s), based on the fact that the adenylate cyclase system is universal and its components may be exchanged among different kinds of cells and across species. Thus, receptors of various sources may react with different G-proteins and activate different cyclases in reconstituted systems (May *et al.*, 1985; Schramm and Selinger, 1984; Levitzki, 1985). In one kind of reconstitution study, receptors for β-adrenergic agonists or glucagon were inserted into cells which do not have them and were shown to activate adenylate cyclase there (Schramm *et al.*, 1977). Other reconstitution studies showed the interaction between purified β-adrenergic receptors and G_s reconstituted in liposomes (Asano *et al.*, 1984). In a much similar way it has been shown that purified muscarinic acetylcholine receptor interacts with the purified G-proteins from brain, Gi and Go when reconstituted in phospholipid vesicles (Florio and Sternweis, 1985; Kurose *et al.*, 1986). We intend to use this approach as an assay for olfactory receptor activity, and to try to identify olfactory receptor proteins after fractionation and purification of the ciliary proteins that serve as receptor candidates.

REFERENCES

Amoore, J. E. (1982). Odor theory and odor classification. *In* "Fragrance Chemistry: The Science of the Sense of Smell" (E. T. Theimar, ed.), pp. 27–76. Academic Press, New York.

Anholt, R. H., Aebi, U., and Snyder, S. H. (1986a). A partially purified preparation of isolated chemosensory cilia from the olfactory epithelium of the bull frog, *Rana catesbeiana*. *J. Neurosci.* **6**, 1962–1969.

Anholt, R. H., Mumby, S. M., Stoffers, D. A., Girard, P. R., Kuo, J. F., and Snyder, S. H. (1986b). Transductory proteins of olfactory receptor cells: Identification of guanosine nucleotide binding proteins and protein kinase C. *Biochemistry* **26**, 788–795.

Asano, T., Pedersen, S. E., Scott, C. W., and Ross, E. M. (1984). Reconstitution of catecholamine-stimulated binding of guanosine 5'-O-(3-thiotriphosphate) to the stimulatory GTP-binding protein of adenylate cyclase. *Biochemistry* **23**, 5460–5467.

Beets, J. T. (1971). Olfactory response and molecular structure. *In* "Handbook of Sensory Physiology" (L. M. Beidler, ed.), Vol. 4(1), pp. 257–321. Springer-Verlag, Berlin and New York.

Berridge, M. J., and Irvine, R. F. (1984). Inositol triphosphate, a novel second messenger in cellular signal transduction. *Nature (London)* **312**, 315–321.

Bignetti, E., Cavaggioni, A., Pelosi, P., Persaud, K. C., Sorbi, R. T., and Trindelli, R. (1985). Purification and characterization of an odorant-binding protein from cow nasal tissue. *Eur. J. Biochem.* **149**, 227–231.

Boyse, E. A., Beauchamp, G. K., Yamazaki, K., Bard, J., and Thomas, L. (1982). Chemosensory communication: A new aspect of the major histocompatibility complex and other genes in the mouse. *Oncodev. Biol. Med.* **4**, 101–16.

Byrne, J. H. (1985). Neural and molecular mechanisms underlying information storage in *Aplysia:* Implications for learning and memory. *Trends Neurosci.* **8**, 478–482.

Cagan, R. H., and Zeiger, W. N. (1978). Biochemical studies of olfaction: Binding specificity of radioactively labeled stimuli to an isolated olfactory preparation from rainbow trout (*Salmo giardinieri*). *Proc. Natl. Acad. Sci. U.S.A.* **75**, 4679–4683.

Castellucci, V. F., Nairn, A., Greengard, P., Schwartz, J. H., and Kandel, E. R. (1982). Inhibitor of adenosine 3':5'-monophosphate-dependent protein kinase blocks presynaptic facilitation in *Aplysia*. *J. Neurosci,* **2**, 1673–1681.

Changeaux, J. P., Davillers-Thiery, A., and Chemouilli, P. (1984). Acetylcholine receptor: An allosteric protein. *Science* **225**, 1335–1345.

Chen, Z., and Lancet, D. (1984). Membrane proteins unique to olfactory cilia: Candidates for sensory receptor molecules. *Proc. Natl. Acad. Sci. U.S.A.* **81**, 1859–1863.

Chen, Z., Ophir, D., and Lancet, D. (1986a). Monoclonal antibodies to ciliary glycoproteins of frog olfactory neurons. *Brain Res.* **368**, 329–338.

Chen, Z., Pace, U., Ronen, D., and Lancet, D. (1986b). Polypeptide gp95: A unique glycoprotein of olfactory cilia with transmembrane receptor properties. *J. Biol. Chem.* **261**, 1299–1305.

Chen, Z., Pace, U., Heldman, J., Shapira, A., and Lancet, D. (1986c). Isolated frog olfactory cilia: A preparation of dendritic membranes from chemosensory neurons. *J. Neurosci.* **6**, 2146–2154.

Chen, Z., Pace, U., Lev, M., and Lancet, D. (1986d). Functional studies of a candidate chemoreceptor protein: An *in-vitro* adenylate cyclase assay for olfactory response. *Mol. Pharmacol.* (submitted).

Cockcroft, S., and Gomperts, B. D. (1985). Role of guanine nucleotide binding protein in the activation of polyphosphoinositide phosphodiesterase. *Nature (London)* **314**, 534–536.

Delaleu, J. C., and Holley, A. (1980). Modification of transduction mechanism in the frog's olfactory mucosa using a thiol reagent as olfactory stimulus. *Chem. Senses Flavour* **3**, 205–218.

Dodd, G., and Persaud, K. (1981). Biochemical mechanisms in vertebrate primary olfactory neurons. *In* "Biochemistry of Taste and Olfaction" (R. H. Cagan and M. R. Kare, eds.), pp. 333–358. Academic Press, New York.

Fesenko, E. E., Novoselov, V. I., Krapivinskaya, L. D. (1979). Molecular mechanism of olfactory reception IV. Some biochemical characteristic of the camphor receptor from rat olfactory epithelium. *Biochim. Biophys. Acta* **587**, 424–433.

Fesenko, E. E., Novoselov, V. I., Krapivinskaya, L. D., Mjasvedov, N. F., and Zolotarev, J. A. (1983). Molecular mechanism of odor sensing. VI. Some biochemical characteristics of a possible receptor for amino acids from the olfactory epithelium of the skate *Dasyetis pastinaca* and carp *Cyprinus carpio*. *Biochim. Biophys. Acta* **759**, 250–256.

Fesenko, E. E., Kolesnikov, S. S., and Lynbersky, A. L. (1985). Induction by cyclic GMP of cationic conductance in plasma membrane of retinol rod outer segment. *Nature (London)* **313**, 310–313.

Firestein, S., and Werblin, F. (1985). Electrical properties of olfactory cells isolated from the epithelium of the tiger salamander. *Neurosci. Abstr.* **11**, 970–970.

Florio. V. A., and Sternweis, P. C. (1985). Reconstitution of resolved muscarinic cholinergic receptors with purified GTP-binding proteins. *J. Biol. Chem.* **261**, 3477–3483.

Gesteland, R. C. (1976). Physiology of olfactory reception. *In* "Frog Neurobiology" (R. Llinas and W. Precht, eds.), pp. 234–249. Springer-Verlag, Berlin and Heidelberg.

Getchell, M. L., and Gesteland, R. C. (1972). The chemistry of olfactory reception: Stimulus specific protection from sulfhydryl reagent inhibition. *Proc. Natl. Acad. Sci. U.S.A.* **96**, 1494–1498.

Getchell, T. V. (1986). Functional properties of vertebrate olfactory receptor neurons. *Physiol. Rev.* **66**, 772–817.

Getchell, T. V., Margolis, F. L., and Getchell, M. L. (1984). Perireceptor and receptor events in vertebrate olfaction. *Prog. Neurobiol.* **23**, 317–345.

Gilman, A. G. (1984). G-proteins and dual control of adenylate cyclase. *Cell* **36**, 577–579.

Heldman, J., and Lancet, D. (1986). Cyclic AMP dependent phosphorylation in olfactory cilia. *J. Neurochem.* **47**, 1527–1533.

Hood, L., Kronenberg, M., and Hunkapiller, T. (1985). T-Cell antigen receptor and the immunoglobulin supergene family. *Cell* **40**, 225–229.

Huque, T., and Bruch, R. C. (1986). Odorant- and guanine nucleotide-stimulated phosphinositide turnover in olfactory cilia. *Biochem. Biophys. Res. Commun.* **137**, 37–42.

Joseph, S. K. (1985). Receptor stimulated phosphoinositide metabolism: A role for GTP-binding proteins? *Trends Biochem. Sci.* **10**, 297–298.

Kaissling, K. E. (1986). Chemo-electrical transduction in insect olfactory receptors. *Annu. Rev. Neurosci.* **9**, 121–145.

Kashiwayanagi, M., and Kurihara, K. (1984). Neuroblastoma cells as model for olfactory cells: Mechanism of depolarization in response to various odorants. *Brain Res.* **293**, 251–258.

Kaupp, U. B., and Koch, K. W. (1986). Mechanism of photoreception in vertebrate vision. *Trends Biochem. Sci.* **11**, 43–47.

Klein, U. (1980). Investigation of proteins from isolated insect olfactory hairs. *In* "Olfaction and Taste VII" (H. van der Starre, ed.), p. 89. IRL Press, London.

Klein, U., and Keil, T. A. (1984). Dendritic membranes from insect olfactory hairs: Isoelectric method and electron microscopic observations. *Cell. Mol. Neurobiol.* **4**, 385–396.

Koshland, D. E. (1980). Bacterial chemotaxis in relation to neurobiology. *Annu. Rev. Neurosci.* **3**, 43–75.

Kurihara, K., and Koyama, N. (1972). High activity of adenyl cyclase in olfactory and gustatory organ. *Biochem. Biophys. Res. Commun.* **48**, 30–34.

Kurose, H., Katada, T., Haga, T., Haga, K., Ichiyama, A., and Ui, M. (1986). Functional interaction of purified muscarinic receptor with purified inhibitory guanine nucleotide regulatory protein reconstituted in phospholipid vesicles. *J. Biol. Chem.* **261**, 6423–6428.

Lancet, D. (1984). Molecular view of olfactory reception. *Trends Neurosci.* **7**, 35–36.

Lancet, D. (1986a). Vertebrate olfactory reception. *Annu. Rev. Neurosci.* **9**, 329–355.

Lancet, D. (1986b). Molecular components of olfactory reception and transduction. *In* "Molecular Neurobiology of the Olfactory System" (F. L. Margolis and T. V. Getchell, eds.), Plenum, New York. (in press).

Lancet, D., and Pace, U. (1987). The molecular basis of odor recognition. *Trends Biochem. Sci.* **12**, 63–66.

Levitzki, A. (1985). Reconstitution of membrane–receptor systems. *Biochim. Biophys. Acta* **822**, 127–153.

Mason, J. R., and Morton, T. H. (1984). Fast and loose covalent binding of ketones as a molecular mechanism in vertebrate olfactory receptors. *Tetrahedron* **40**, 483–492.

Mason, J. R., Clark, L., and Morton, T. H. (1984). Selective deficits in the sense of smell caused by chemical modification of the olfactory epithelium. *Science* **226**, 1092–1094.

Maue, R. A., and Dionne, V. E. (1984). Ion channel activity in isolated murine olfactory receptor neurons. *Soc. Neurosci. Abstr.* **10**, 655–655.

May, D. C., Ross, E. M., Gilman, A. G., and Smigel, M. D. (1985). Reconstitution of catecholamine-stimulated adenylate cyclase activity using three purified proteins. *J. Biol. Chem.* **260**, 15829–15833.

Menevse, A., Dodd, G., and Poynder, T. M. (1977). Evidence for the specific involvement of cAMP in the olfactory transduction. *Biochem. Biophys. Res. Commun.* **77**, 671–677.

Miller, W. H. (1983). Does cyclic GMP hydrolysis control visual transduction in rods? *Trends Pharm. Sci.* **4**, 509–511.

Minor, A. V., and Sakina, N. L. (1973). Role of cyclic adenosine-3′-5′-monophosphate in olfactory reception. *Neurofysiologya* **5**, 415–422.

Moulton, D. G., and Beidler, L. M. (1967). Structure and function in the peripheral olfactory system. *Physiol. Rev.* **47**, 1–52.

Nakamura, T., and Gold, G. H. (1987). A cyclic nucleotide-gated conductance in olfactory receptor cilia. *Nature (London)* **325**, 442–444.

Pace, U., and Lancet, D. (1986). Olfactory GTP-binding protein: Signal transducing polypeptide of vertebrate chemosensory neurons. *Proc. Natl. Acad. Sci. U.S.A.* **83**, 4947–4951.

Pace, U., Hansky, E., Salomon, Y., and Lancet, D. (1985). Odorant sensitive adenylate cyclase may mediate olfactory reception. *Nature (London)* **316**, 255–258.

Pevsner, J., Trifiletti, R. R., Stritmatter, S. M., and Snyder, S. H. (1985). Isolation and characterization of an olfactory receptor protein for odorant pyrazines. *Proc. Natl. Acad. Sci. U.S.A.* **82**, 3050–3054.

Pevsner, J., Sklar, P. B., and Snyder, S. H. (1986). Odorant binding protein: Localization to nasal glands and secretion. *Proc. Natl. Acad. Sci. U.S.A.* **83**, 4942–4946.

Price, S. (1981). Receptor proteins in vertebrate olfaction. *In* "Biochemistry of Taste and Olfaction" (R. H. Cagan and M. R. Kare, eds.), pp. 69–84. Academic Press, New York and London.

Rhein, L. D., and Cagan, R. H. (1980). Biochemical studies of olfaction: Isolation, characterization and odorant binding activity of cilia from rainbow trout olfactory rosettes. *Proc. Natl. Acad. Sci. U.S.A.* **77**, 4412–4416.

Rodrigues, V., and Siddiqi, O. (1978). Genetic analysis of chemosensory pathways. *Proc. Ind. Acad. Sci. B* **87**, 147–160.

Schramm, M., and Selinger, Z. (1984). Message transmission: Receptor controlled adenylate cyclase system. *Science* **225**, 1350–1356.

Schramm, M., Orly, J., Eimerl, S., and Korner, M. (1977). Coupling of hormone receptors to adenylate cyclase of different cells by cell fusion. *Nature (London)* **268**, 310–313.

Selinger, Z., Devary, O., Blumenfeld, A., Heichal, O., and Minke, B. (1986). Light activated GTP hydrolysis and breakdown of phosphoinositides in *Musca* eye membranes. "Abstracts of the Cold Spring Harbor Meeting on G-Proteins and Signal Transduction," p. 50. Cold Spring Harbor Laboratories, Cold Spring Harbor, New York.

Shirley, S., Polak, E., and Dodd, G. (1983a). Chemical modification studies on rat olfactory mucosa using a thiol-specific reagent and enzymatic iodination. *Eur. J. Biochem.* **132**, 485–494.

Shirley, S., Polak, E., and Dodd, G. (1983b). Selective inhibition of rat olfactory receptors by Concanavalin A. *Biochem. Soc. Trans.* **11**, 780–781.

Shirley, S. G., Robinson, C. J., Dickinson, K., Aujla, R., and Dodd, G. H. (1986). Olfactory adenylate cyclase of the rat. *Biochem. J.* **240**, 605–607.

Sicard, G., and Holley, A. (1984). Receptor cell responses to odorants: Similarities and differences among odorants. *Brain Res.* **292**, 283–296.

Sklar, P. B., Anholt, R. H., and Snyder, S. H. (1986). The odorant sensitive adenylate cyclase of olfactory receptor cells: Differential stimulation by distinct classes of odorants. *J. Biol. Chem.* **261**, 15538–15543.

Snyder, S. (1984). Drug and neurotransmitter receptors in the brain. *Science* **224**, 22–31.

Snyder, S. H., Sklar, P. B., and Pevsner, J. (1986). Olfactory receptor mechanisms: Odorant binding protein and adenylate cyclase. *In* "Molecular Neurobiology of the Olfactory System" (F. L. Margolis and T. V. Getchell, eds.). Plenum, New York.

Stryer, L. (1986). Cyclic GMP cascade of vision. *Annu. Rev. Neurosci.* **9**, 87–119.

Takagi, S. F., Kitamura, H., Imai, K., and Takeuchi, H. (1969). Further studies on the roles of sodium and potassium in the generation of the electroolfactogram, effects of mono-, di-, and trivalent cations. *J. Gen. Physiol.* **59**, 115–130.

Vandenberg, C. A., and Montal, M. (1984). Light-regulated biochemical events in invertebrate photoreceptors: Light regulated phosphorylation of rohodopsin and phosphoinositides in squid photoreceptor membranes. *Biochemistry* **23**, 2347–2352.

Venard, R., and Pichon, Y. (1984). Electrophysiological analysis of the peripheral response to odors in wild type and smell deficient olf C mutant of *Drosophila melanogaster*. *J. Insect. Physiol.* **30**, 1–5.

Villet, R. H. (1978). Mechanism of insect sex pheromone sensory transduction: Role of adenyl cyclase. *Comp. Biochem. Physiol.* **61**, 389–394.

Vodyanoy, V., and Murphy, R. B. (1983). Single channel fluctuations in biomolecular lipid membranes induced by rat olfactory epithelial homogenates. *Science* **220**, 710–719.

Vogt, R. G., and Riddiford, L. M. (1981). Pheromone binding and inactivation by moth antennae. *Nature (London)* **293**, 161–163.

Wysocki, C. J., Whitney, G., and Tucker, D. (1977). Specific anosmias in the laboratory mouse. *Behav. Genet.* **7**, 171–188.

Yau, K. W., and Nakatani, K. (1985). Light suppressible, cyclic GMP-sensitive conductance in the plasma membrane of a truncated rod outer segment. *Nature (London)* **317**, 252–255.

Index